NEWLY REVISED AND EXPANDED

THE COMPLETE & UP-TO-DATE

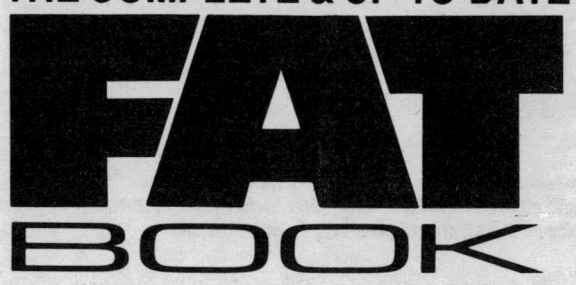

FAT
BOOK

A GUIDE TO THE FAT, CALORIES, AND FAT PERCENTAGES IN YOUR FOOD

KAREN J. BELLERSON

AVERY PUBLISHING GROUP

Garden City Park, New York

SOURCES

Food manufacturers and processors direct, as well as their product labels.

United States Department of Agriculture Handbook No. 8, revised, "Composition of Foods, Raw, Processed, Prepared," sections 8-1 through 8-22; Agriculture Handbook No. 456, "Nutritive Value of American Foods In Common Units"; Home and Garden Bulletin No. 232, "Nutrition and Your Health: Dietary Guidelines for Americans."

Individual fast food chains.

Cover designers: Rudy Shur, Evan Schwartz, and Ann Vestal
In-house editors: Bonnie Freid, Joanne Abrams, Elaine Will Sparber, and Marie Caratozzolo
Typesetters: Evan Schwartz, Bonnie Freid, and Kerri Matheson

Library of Congress Cataloging-in-Publication Data

Bellerson, Karen J.
   The complete & up-to-date fat book : a guide to the fat,
calories, and fat percentages in your food / Karen J. Bellerson.
     p. cm.
     Chiefly tables.
     ISBN 0-89529-561-X
   1. Food—Fat content—Tables. 2. Food—Caloric content—Tables.
I. Title. II. Title: Complete and up to date fat book.

TX551.B39 1993   641.1'4
                                                QBI92-20337

Printed in the United States of America

10 9 8 7 6 5 4

Contents

To David,
Thank you for all of your loving contributions.

Acknowledgments

In finalizing a complex book such as *The Complete and Up-to-Date Fat Book,* it takes a team effort, and I want to thank all those of Avery Publishing Group for being on my team. You are a great group with whom it is a privilege to work!

I also wish to say thank you to those of you who have written to ask questions and/or to offer comments, suggestions, and even criticisms. They have all been valuable to me.

Preface

"A wise man should consider that health is the greatest of all human blessings. . ."
—Hippocrates

Since *The Complete and Up-to-Date Fat Book* first came out, many things have changed. All we have to do is look at our grocery shelves to see the evidence that we, as consumers, are listening and learning about better nutrition and making it known to the food manufacturers that we want healthier choices when we shop for food. And the food manufacturers are getting the message, offering us more and more low-fat and fat-free products to choose from!

Other changes show up in the amount of poultry, fruits, vegetables, and different grains being consumed today compared to yesteryear, as well as the appearance of the new Food Guide Pyramid, put out by the United States Department of Agriculture, which has taken the place of the Four Food Groups (see page 2).

We see fast-food restaurants making changes, offering healthier choices such as leaner hamburgers, salad selections with low- or no-fat salad dressings, grilled chicken entrees, and fat-free muffins. Why, Burger King even carries Weight Watchers low-fat entrees!

Schools are educating our young people to recognize where the fat is in their diets and to understand the importance of making wiser, healthier selections when they eat. After all, there is strong evidence that fat begins to clog our arteries in childhood, and forming healthy eating habits while young helps to establish good lifelong habits. *Please note* that children under two years of age should not have their diets restricted, as these years are an important period of rapid growth and development.

The one thing that remains constant, however, is the relationship of a high-fat diet (a diet in which more than 30 percent of daily calories comes from fat) and higher risks of developing a life-threatening disease such as cancer, heart disease, diabetes, or high blood pressure (hypertension). The importance of watching the amount of fat we consume in our diets is reflected by the statistics released this past summer by the National Center for Health Statistics for the ten leading causes of death in the United States. These figures are for 1989, the latest year for which up-to-date figures have been compiled.

Top Ten Killers	Deaths Per Year
1. Heart Disease	737,867
2. Cancer	496,152
3. Stroke	145,551
4. Accidents (automobile, airplane, etc.)	95,028
5. Chronic Lung Diseases (bronchitis, emphysema, etc.)	84,344
6. Pneumonia and Influenza	76,550
7. Diabetes	46,833*
8. Suicide	30,232
9. Liver Disease and Cirrhosis	26,694
10. Homicides and "Legal Interventions"	22,909

*This figure does not include all diabetes-complicated deaths, which would make this figure closer to 150,000 according to the American Diabetes Association.

Physicians, nutrition experts, and other health-care professionals and organizations continue to promote the very real health benefits of a low-fat nutritional lifestyle, while studies continue to show the correlation of a high-fat diet and these life-threatening diseases.

My goal for this book is to keep you as up to date as possible on what products are available. I completed this revision of The Complete and Up-to-Date Fat Book as soon as possible because of the flood of new foods now being offered by the food manufacturers. I shall continue to refine and update future editions of The Complete and Up-to-Date Fat Book for you, the consumer, to provide you with the information you need to reduce the fat in your diet.

Karen J. Bellerson
St. Charles, Missouri

Introduction

"The single most influential dietary change one can make to lower the risk of these diseases is to reduce intake of foods high in fats and to increase the intake of foods high in complex carbohydrates and fiber."
–The Surgeon General's Report on Nutrition and Health (1988)

"It is calculated that, if intake of dietary fat were reduced from the present 40 percent of total calorie intake to 25 percent, about 9,000 lives would be saved annually."
–National Cancer Institute, *Annual Review of Public Health*

"Eating less fat can reduce the risk of colon, prostate, and breast cancer."
–National Research Council, "Diet And Health" (1989)

For decades, studies have shown the influence of diet on the development of disorders such as high blood pressure, diabetes, osteoarthritis, heart disease, and some forms of cancer. Much of what we know today about the diet-disease relationship dates back to World War II, when the incidence of death from heart attacks among the people of Western Europe declined in great numbers while the war was going on. The cause of this dramatic decline was found to be the rationing of foods such as meat, dairy products, and eggs during the war. Once the war was over and these foods were once again available, the incidence of heart disease again rose. In-depth studies were begun in earnest to find out about the negative effects of these foods.

Countless studies continue to prove that there is a very real relationship between our diet and the risk of developing a life-threatening disease. In response to these findings, the United States Department of Agriculture has replaced the Four Basic Food Groups of milk, meat, vegetables and fruits, and breads and cereals with the new Food Guide Pyramid (see Figure 1).

Notice that fats, oils, and sweets are the smallest part of the new Food Guide Pyramid. This new pyramid reflects advice from all the major health organizations recommending a diet consisting of 55 to 60 percent carbohydrates, 15 percent protein, and *no more than 30 percent fat*. There are some who feel that only 25 percent or less of our calories should come from fat, in order to lower our risk of heart disease and some kinds of cancer.

Okay, you're convinced that you need to get the fat out of your diet, but where do you begin? Before we go into some simple guidelines, let's look at a few basic facts about fat.

1

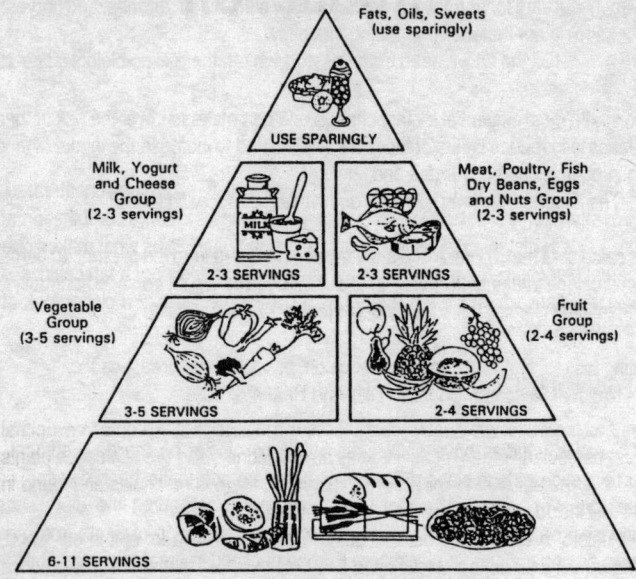

Figure 1 shows the Food Guide Pyramid with the following labels:

Fats, Oils, Sweets (use sparingly) — USE SPARINGLY

Milk, Yogurt and Cheese Group (2-3 servings) — 2-3 SERVINGS

Meat, Poultry, Fish Dry Beans, Eggs and Nuts Group (2-3 servings) — 2-3 SERVINGS

Vegetable Group (3-5 servings) — 3-5 SERVINGS

Fruit Group (2-4 servings) — 2-4 SERVINGS

6-11 SERVINGS

Bread, Cereal, Rice, and Pasta Group (6–11 servings)

Figure 1.   The Food Guide Pyramid.

FAT IS REQUIRED BY THE BODY

The fact is that we need some fat in our diets. Adults need a minimum daily intake of 15 to 25 grams of dietary fat to meet the body's needs. (Children under the age of two years should not have their dietary fat restricted, however, because of the possible interference with their development.)

Our bodies use fat in numerous ways—ways in which most of us are unaware. We use fat in manufacturing antibodies to fight disease. Fats act as carriers for the fat-soluble vitamins A, D, E, and K. Fat deposits cushion, protect, and hold in place vital organs such as the kidneys, heart, and liver. Fat is the body's insulation against environmental temperature changes and is what gives the body its shape. While fat is one of the three nutrient energy sources, it also aids in digestion by slowing down the stomach's secretions of hydrochloric acid, which is what produces that satisfying feeling of fullness after a meal. So, as you can see, fat should not be totally eliminated from our diets!

There are two types of fat in the body. They are the nonessential fatty acids, which our body is able to manufacture, and the essential fatty acids, which we cannot make and have to get through our diets. These essential (unsaturated) fatty acids are necessary for normal growth; for healthy skin, blood, arteries, and nerves; and for keeping our metabolism running smoothly.

We can get all the fat we need from unsaturated fat; there is no biological need for saturated fat!

CHOLESTEROL AND DIETARY FAT

There are three main types of fats in the foods we eat. They are polyunsaturated, monounsaturated, and saturated. Most processed foods contain a combination of all three kinds of dietary fat. The percentage of each type of fat is what makes one food a healthier choice than another food. While cholesterol is not a fatty acid, it is a fat-like substance and is often referred to as a "fat." Let's take a closer look at each of these substances.

Cholesterol (HDL and LDL)

Cholesterol is a white, waxy, fatty substance found in all foods that come from animal sources, particularly organ meats such as brains, kidney, and liver. Because plants do not have the ability to manufacture cholesterol, there is no cholesterol found in plants; this includes oils that come from vegetable sources.

Cholesterol is essential to our well-being. We don't need a lot of it in our blood, clogging up our arteries, but we do need it to help build cell membranes, to produce hormones (estrogen, progesterone, and testosterone), and to manufacture bile acids that are needed to eliminate excess cholesterol from the body. About 75 percent of the cholesterol found in our body (all our body needs) is manufactured in our liver, even if we don't eat animal products; the other 25 percent comes from our diet.

The cholesterol manufactured by our liver is carried through our bloodstream by LDLs (low-density lipoproteins). High levels of LDLs in the bloodstream can result in clogged arteries, causing high blood pressure, stroke, or heart disease. This is why LDL is referred to as the "bad" cholesterol or, as I refer to it, the "lethal" cholesterol. LDL levels can be reduced through proper diet.

Now we come to the HDLs (high-density lipoproteins), the "good" cholesterol (I refer to it as the "healthy" cholesterol). HDLs carry excess cholesterol from different body tissues to the liver, where it is metabolized by the liver and then processed through the intestines and eliminated from the body. High levels of these HDLs are correlated with a decreased risk of coronary heart disease. HDL levels can be raised through regular exercise.

Polyunsaturated Fats

Polyunsaturated fats are found in most foods, including certain fish (Omega-3), but mainly in nuts, oils from plants, seeds, and soybeans (Omega-6). These fats are liquid at room temperature. Polyunsaturated fats reduce blood cholesterol, but an excess may lower the protective "good" cholesterol, HDL. (Some studies speculate that there is a link between polyunsaturates and breast cancer.)

Foods with high contents of polyunsaturated fats include the following:

- Bagels
- Barbecue Sauce
- Bread (French, Italian, Raisin, Oatmeal, Pumpernickel, and Rye)
- Chickpeas (Garbanzo Beans)
- Corn Chips
- Corn Meal
- Fish (Bluefish, Cod, Haddock, Herring, Mackerel, Salmon, Sardines, Mussels, Oysters, Rainbow Trout, Scallops, and Whitefish)
- Lentils
- Nuts (Pine, Walnuts, and Brazil)
- Popcorn (air popped)
- Potato ChipsPotato Salad (made with mayonnaise)
- Refried Beans
- Salad Dressings (most types—check your labels)
- Seeds (Pumpkin, Sesame, Squash, and Sunflower)
- Soybeans
- Squash
- Sweet Potatoes
- Tuna Salad (made with mayonnaise)
- Tofu
- Vegetable and Nut Oils (see chart on page 325)

Monounsaturated Fats

Monounsaturated fats are found in most foods, but mainly in vegetable and nut oils such as olive, peanut, and canola (rapeseed). These fats are also liquid at room temperature. Monounsaturated fats reduce total blood cholesterol while not having the side effect of lowering the protective "good" cholesterol, HDL.

Be aware that both polyunsaturated and monounsaturated fats can be hydrogenated. Hydrogenation is a process of adding hydrogen to an oil in order to make it more solid at room temperature so that it can be used in processing foods such as baked goods, non-dairy creamers, and whipped toppings. Hydrogenation of unsaturated fats makes them saturated. When reading product labels, watch for the words "hydrogenated" or "partially hydrogenated."

The following foods have high contents of monounsaturated fats. Those foods marked with an asterisk (*) are also high in saturated fats.

- Almonds
- Animal Fats* (most types)
- Avocados
- Beef* (leaner cuts)
- Biscuits
- Bread* (most types— read your labels)
- Brownies
- Cake* (most types)
- Chicken

- Cookies* (most types)
- Croissants*
- Donuts* (most types)
- Eggs*
- Fruitcake
- Gingerbread
- Lard*
- Margarine (stick)
- Muffins*
- Nuts (Hazelnuts, Cashews, Chestnuts, Macadamia, Peanuts, Pecans, and Pistachio)
- Oatmeal
- Ocean Perch
- Pastry* (includes pie crust)
- Peanut Butter
- Pies* (most types)
- Popcorn (popped in vegetable oil)
- Pork*
- Sausage* (most types)
- Shortening (vegetable)
- Spaghetti (with tomato sauce)
- Taco*
- Veal* (leaner cuts)
- Vegetable and Nut Oils (see chart on page 325)

Saturated Fats

Foods containing saturated fats include all meat and dairy products. The tropical oils, coconut, palm, and palm kernel, although from plant origin, are also high in saturated fat. Cocoa butter, the oil used in making chocolate, is also a highly saturated fat source. Use powdered cocoa instead in all your recipes calling for chocolate. Saturated fats are generally solid at room temperature. Remember that saturated fats—more than dietary cholesterol—raise total blood cholesterol.

The following foods have high contents of saturated fats. For other foods high in these fats, see the list of high-monounsaturated-fat foods, as those foods marked with asterisks (*) are also high in saturated fats.

- Beef (fattier cuts)
- Beef Tallow
- Boston Brown Bread (canned)
- Butter
- Cake (snack, most types, and those with chocolate frosting)
- Cheese (most types)
- Cheesecake
- Chili (with beef)
- Chocolate
- Cocoa butter
- Cocoa mixes
- Coconut (and all coconut products)
- Cottage cheese (4 percent fat)
- Cream
- Custard (baked)
- Duck
- Eggnog
- Fried Foods (using saturated oils)
- Garlic Spread
- Granola
- Gravy (brown—packaged)
- Hot Dogs
- Ice Cream
- Ice Milk
- Lamb
- Luncheon Meats (Corned beef, Bologna, etc.)
- Malts
- Milk (whole, 2%, & 1%)
- Non-Dairy Creamers (especially powdered)
- Non-Dairy Whipped Cream
- Pies (Cream)

- Pizza
- Pompano
- Popcorn (most microwave brands)
- Pork (fattier cuts)
- Puddings
- Pumpkin (canned)
- Quiche
- Sauces (Bearnaise, Hollandaise, White, Cheese, etc.)
- Seaweed
- Shakes
- Soups (most cream types)
- Sour Cream
- Turkey (dark meat)
- Turkey (self-basting)
- Veal (fattier cuts)
- Vegetable and Nut Oils (Particularly Coconut, Palm, and Palm Kernel; see chart on page 325)
- Yogurt (made from whole milk solids)

THE NEW FOOD LABEL

More than two years after the need for labeling reforms was acknowledged by the Food and Drug Administration (FDA), the long-awaited food label was finally chosen in December 1992. Since there had been disagreements between the Department of Health and Human Services and the United States Department of Agriculture (USDA) on the final format of the label, the White House was brought in to help resolve the conflict. A compromise recommended by President George Bush and his administration was accepted by both agencies.

The new labels could appear on some foods by the middle of 1993, and will be required on all processed foods regulated by the FDA and on all processed meat products regulated by the USDA by May of 1994. Some industry groups are unhappy with the final choice, saying that the label will be cluttered and confusing for the consumer. See Figure 2 on page 7 for a model of the new food label.

According to Louis W. Sullivan, M.D., Secretary of Health and Human Services, the FDA will be working with a broad coalition of industry, consumer, and public health groups to familiarize consumers nationwide with the new food label, and to help consumers use the label to make nutritionally sound choices.

Let's take a look at some of the food label reforms. One of the most controversial changes was the elimination of the well-known USRDAs (the United States Recommended Daily Allowances) for different nutrients. Instead, the label will list the grams of fat, sodium, and other nutrients found in each serving, and will place the listed amount in the context of a recommended daily diet of 2,000 calories. For instance, in the label shown in Figure 2, the total fat is listed as 5 percent of the "Daily Value"—in other words, one serving will provide you with 5 percent of the recommended maximum daily intake of that nutrient. Suggested nutrient levels have been based on current scientific recommendations.

The new food label will also include the following:

- Defined, standardized serving sizes to make food comparisons more exact.

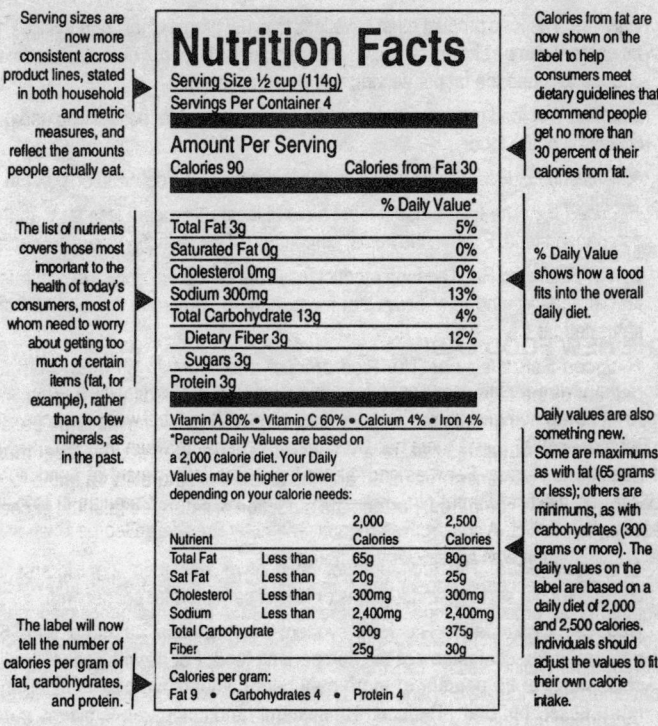

Serving sizes are now more consistent across product lines, stated in both household and metric measures, and reflect the amounts people actually eat.

The list of nutrients covers those most important to the health of today's consumers, most of whom need to worry about getting too much of certain items (fat, for example), rather than too few minerals, as in the past.

The label will now tell the number of calories per gram of fat, carbohydrates, and protein.

Calories from fat are now shown on the label to help consumers meet dietary guidelines that recommend people get no more than 30 percent of their calories from fat.

% Daily Value shows how a food fits into the overall daily diet.

Daily values are also something new. Some are maximums, as with fat (65 grams or less); others are minimums, as with carbohydrates (300 grams or more). The daily values on the label are based on a daily diet of 2,000 and 2,500 calories. Individuals should adjust the values to fit their own calorie intake.

Nutrition Facts

Serving Size ½ cup (114g)
Servings Per Container 4

Amount Per Serving

Calories 90   Calories from Fat 30

         % Daily Value*

Total Fat 3g	5%
Saturated Fat 0g	0%
Cholesterol 0mg	0%
Sodium 300mg	13%
Total Carbohydrate 13g	4%
Dietary Fiber 3g	12%
Sugars 3g	
Protein 3g	

Vitamin A 80% • Vitamin C 60% • Calcium 4% • Iron 4%

*Percent Daily Values are based on a 2,000 calorie diet. Your Daily Values may be higher or lower depending on your calorie needs:

Nutrient		2,000 Calories	2,500 Calories
Total Fat	Less than	65g	80g
Sat Fat	Less than	20g	25g
Cholesterol	Less than	300mg	300mg
Sodium	Less than	2,400mg	2,400mg
Total Carbohydrate		300g	375g
Fiber		25g	30g

Calories per gram:
Fat 9 • Carbohydrates 4 • Protein 4

Figure 2. The New Food Label.

- Definitions of food descriptions and claims such as "Low Fat" and "Reduced Cholesterol."

- Only certain "approved" health claims.

- The listing of all sweeteners together in the ingredients list, under the collective term "Sweeteners," when more than one sweetener is used in a product.

- The identification of "fake fats," such as Simplesse and caseinate, as milk derivatives, when used in foods that claim to be non-dairy, such as coffee whiteners and frozen desserts.

As stated above, the new label will include specific definitions of food descriptions and claims. Those definitions related to fat and cholesterol are as follows:

- *Fat Free.* The food product must have less than 0.5 grams of fat per serving. The fat content can be shown as "less than one gram (< 1)" or the manufacturer may choose to round the fat per serving to the nearest gram.

- *Low Fat.* The food product must have 3 grams or less of fat per serving and per 50 grams of the food.

- *% (Percent) Fat Free.* The food product must meet the FDA's definition of "Low Fat."

- *Reduced Fat.* The food product must have at least 25 percent less fat than the comparison food. Further, the actual percentage of the reduction must be stated.

- *Low in Saturated Fat.* The food product may contain 1 gram or less of saturated fat per serving, and may derive not more than 15 percent of its calories from saturated fat.

- *Reduced Saturated Fat.* The food product must contain no more than 50 percent of the saturated fat of the comparison food. Foods with a reduction of 25 percent or greater may have a comparative claim using the term "Less." If "Reduced Saturated Fat" or a comparative claim is used, the label must indicate the percent or reduction and the amount of saturated fat in the food with which it is compared. Further, the reduction of saturated fat must exceed 1 gram.

- *Cholesterol Free.* The food product must have less than 2 milligrams of cholesterol per serving, and 2 grams or less of saturated fat per serving.

- *Reduced Cholesterol.* The food product must contain no more than 50 percent of the cholesterol of the comparison food. Foods with reductions in cholesterol of 25 percent or more may bear comparative claims using the term "Less," but both "Reduced Cholesterol" and comparative claims must be fully explained, and the reduction in cholesterol must exceed 20 milligrams per serving.

GUIDELINES FOR REDUCING THE FAT IN YOUR DIET

As I mentioned earlier, fat is needed for healthy body functions and should not be totally eliminated from our diets. The Surgeon General's Report on Nutrition and Health (1988) conveyed, "Adults need a minimum daily intake of 15 to 25 grams of fat to meet these necessities."

The American Heart Association; the American-Health Foundation; the American Cancer Society; the National Heart, Lung, and Blood Institute; the National Center for Nutrition and Dietetics; the American Diabetes Association; and the Surgeon General all recommend that no more than 30 percent of our daily calories should come from fat, and no more than one-third of those fats (or 10 percent of our daily calories) should be saturated fats! Below, I will show you how to calculate this 30 percent and even 20 percent (in case you want to lower your fat intake even more).

FAT CALORIES *ARE* DIFFERENT!

Fat calories are indeed different from carbohydrate and protein calories. That difference is very important for us to understand, because we can actually replace fat with more carbohydrates and protein and still be eating fewer calories! Yes, it's true!

Why? Not only does fat have 9 calories per gram, while carbohydrates and protein have only 4 calories each per gram, but the way our body metabolizes dietary fat is different from the way it processes carbohydrates or protein. Dietary fat is very similar in chemical composition to our body fat, so it takes less energy to convert it to body fat. It takes only 3 percent of the calories in the fat we eat to turn that food into body fat, while it takes at least 25 percent of the carbohydrate and protein calories we eat to convert them into body fat. What does this mean? It means that reducing the fat in our diets is not only the most healthy way to eat, it is also an excellent way to control our weight! Maybe there really is something to that old saying about fat, "You eat it, you wear it!" Remember, though, that if you eat more calories than your body needs, regardless of the nutrient providing these calories, the excess will be stored as body fat.

THE FAT GRAM BUDGET FORMULA

Fortunately, if you have decided to reduce your dietary fat, there is a simple formula that will let you know exactly how many fat grams you should allow yourself on a daily basis. To find out your maximum daily allowance, multiply your daily calorie intake by .30, and divide that total by 9 (there are 9 calories in each gram of fat). For a daily intake of 1,500 calories, your equation would look like this:

$$1500 \times .30 \div 9 = 50 \quad OR \quad 1500 \times .30 = 450.00 \div 9 = 50$$

Of course, to calculate your daily fat gram budget, you need to know your daily calorie intake. To find this out, if you don't already know, just use *The Complete and Up-to-Date Fat Book* to keep a diary for three or four days. This will help you determine more precisely your actual daily calorie intake. Write down everything you eat and drink for these days, add up the totals, then divide by the number of days you kept track. Remember that just because you have budgeted X amount of fat grams for the day, you *don't have to eat that amount of fat.* Just make sure not to go over budget!

So you will have a means of comparison, I have taken the guesswork out of it for you by listing the fat gram budgets for the following daily calorie intakes. The following table shows both 30-percent and 20-percent maximum daily fat gram budgets.

Maximum Daily Fat Gram Budget

Daily Calorie Intake	Fat Grams Allowed		Daily Calorie Intake	Fat Grams Allowed	
	20%	30%		20%	30%
1,200	27	40	2,200	49	73
1,300	29	43	2,300	51	76
1,400	31	46	2,400	53	80
1,500	33	50	2,500	56	83
1,600	36	53	2,600	58	86
1,700	38	56	2,700	60	90
1,800	40	60	2,800	62	93
1,900	42	63	2,900	64	96
2,000	44	66	3,000	67	100
2,100	47	70			

Note that this data has been rounded off by dropping all decimal places. This chart begins at 1,200 calories, as it is not recommended for anyone to eat fewer than 1,200 calories (for women) or 1,500 calories (for men) in order to meet her or his daily nutritional needs.

MAKING SMARTER, HEALTHIER CHOICES

The following are some tips to keep in mind as you take stock of your eating habits and begin your quest for better nutrition by reducing your intake of dietary fat.

- Eat more chicken, turkey, and fish in place of red meat. Be sure to remove the skin on your chicken and turkey before or after cooking (it doesn't matter), and to avoid frying. If beef is on the menu, make your choice from the leaner cuts and trim all fat away before cooking. Select cuts with between 4 and 9 grams of fat for a 3-ounce serving, broiled, roasted, or braised. If you prefer pork, be sure to check out the new "Leaner Pork" on page 389. When making meatballs out of extra-lean ground beef, you can add moisture by mixing it with raw grated potatoes or carrots.

  Nutritionists recommend that you keep red meat consumption down to only once or twice a week. Since red meat is high in saturated fat, this will help you to control your saturated fat intake.

- Don't forget the "fat-free" or reduced-fat mayonnaise on the market today when throwing together a macaroni, potato, tuna, or turkey salad.

- Use a reduced-fat margarine or spread instead of butter or regular margarine. Try Krafts's Touch of Butter or Land O' Lakes spread with sweet cream for that "real butter" flavor. Try using smaller amounts and you will find yourself enjoying the taste of the food itself more. The reduced-fat margarines can be used in your cooking, as well.

- There is a great selection of low-fat and fat-free salad dressings on the market today. They come in many flavors and styles; try them until you find one or more to your taste. Remember that you can save as many as 6 to 10 grams of fat *per tablespoon* by not using regular salad dressings!

- Instead of rich desserts like ice cream, try the wide range of frozen yogurt desserts now available in your grocery store's freezer section. Again, because of the wide range of tastes, you may have to try more than one or two to find the ones for you. There are also "lighter" ice creams now available in a wide range of such gourmet flavors as caramel nut fudge sundae and mocha almond fudge. The low-fat and fat-free bakery goods now on the market give us almost unlimited choices for our sweet tooth.

- Substitute low-fat, reduced-fat, or fat-free cheese for those cheeses higher in fat. The fat saved here is between 6 and 10 grams per ounce!

- Most breads are low in fat (1 gram per slice), but be careful when you reach for a croissant to make that sandwich. Croissants can have as many as 14 grams of fat in them.

- Try dry cereals for a great tasting snack. Most of them have 0–3 grams of fat per serving. Do read the labels on the granola-type cereals, which are higher in fat.

- Canadian bacon is a tasty low-fat substitute for bacon. Bacon bits also have less fat and can be used as pizza toppings, too.

- While ten French fries have 8 grams of fat, a 1.5-ounce package of potato chips has a whopping 15 grams of fat!

- You can thicken sauces without using fat by substituting puréed vegetables for cream or whole milk.

- Make your own bread coatings with plain bread crumbs and your choice of spices. Dip food into skim milk or egg whites before coating and baking in a hot oven.

- Instead of non-dairy creamer, try powdered low-fat or skim milk.

- Reduce the amount of fat in your recipes by a third to a half, replacing the amount reduced with water or fruit juice. Try to buy only those commercial mixes to which you add the fat or oil, so you can control the amount.

- Instead of pan frying or deep frying, try basting your meat, fish, or poultry with wine, lemon juice or other fruit juices, broth, tomato juice, or low-fat or fat-free salad dressing to keep it from drying out.

- Instead of using whole eggs, replace each yolk with two egg whites or a low-fat egg substitute. Omelettes can be made with one whole egg and an additional egg white or two.

- Whenever using oil, make sure it's the least saturated oil available to you and remember that although it may be low in saturated fat, *all oils have 14 grams of fat for each tablespoon.* (See Oils, pages 324–325.)

- Cocoa powder is an excellent low-fat substitute for baking chocolate, which is high in fat. Three tablespoons of cocoa equal one square of baking chocolate.

- Use a nonstick skillet sprayed with a small amount of nonstick cooking spray. Or use a paper towel to spread a small amount of oil over the surface of the frying pan.

These simple changes can easily be made. Learn the low-fat substitutes to use in your cooking at home, and stay away from too many "bought" high-fat bakery products. Read your labels! Once you have learned to recognize the fat content of the foods available to you by using *The Complete and Up-to-Date Fat Book,* making healthier eating choices will become a way of life!

LET'S GET STARTED!

By following the suggestions in this book *a little at a time* and educating yourself about the sources of dietary fat, you will be on your way to a healthy, low-fat lifestyle. Using *The Complete and Up-to-Date Fat Book,* check the fat content of the foods you usually eat against your daily fat gram budget and see what may need to be changed or replaced by a lower-fat food. Then, find appropriate low-fat substitutes for these higher-fat foods to bring you in line with your budget. Sound easy? With the wide range of choices of lower-fat foods on the market today, it's easier than ever!

You will be startled by exactly how much dietary fat you have been eating. You may even find that if a favorite food takes a big enough bite (no pun intended) out of your daily fat gram budget, you will want that favorite food less often and will automatically begin to make more nutritionally-sound food selections!

LET'S WRITE IT DOWN

In the beginning, as you acquaint yourself with *The Complete and Up-to-Date Fat Book,* you will find that keeping a daily account of your food intake is invaluable. Keep track of everything you eat as you begin to count up the fat grams and calories for each day. This way, you will be able to get a better idea of exactly what you are eating and where you need to make adjustments. Keeping close track of your eating habits, as you begin to form new ones, will also enable you to:

- Recognize your eating patterns.
- Gain control over what you eat.
- Budget your fat grams and calories more realistically.
- Think twice about deviating from a healthy low-fat lifestyle.
- Take pride in seeing your progress in writing.

LET'S GET ACQUAINTED WITH
THE COMPLETE AND UP-TO-DATE FAT BOOK

Although extreme care has been taken in recording all data in *The Complete and Up-to-Date Fat Book*, you may come across an occasional discrepancy between it and the nutritional data on product labels or other sources of nutritional information. There are a number of reasons why this might occur.

Manufacturers are given a slightly flexible range in which they are able to "round off" their data and still be in accordance with governmental regulations on product labeling. For example, if the fat gram data for a certain product is 2.3 grams, the manufacturer is able to list the fat content in this particular product as being 2 grams, dropping the .3. The same is done with data on calories. If a product serving has 134 calories, the manufacturer is able to list the calorie content of this product as being 130 or 135. Wherever possible, I have kept the nutritional data intact without "rounding off" for either fat or calorie content.

When I gathered data from product labels and compared this with data I received directly from the manufacturer, there would occasionally be a difference between them. This difference was caused by the product label listing the nutritional data of the old formula, while the manufacturer was providing the most up-to-date data after the product formula had been changed. In these cases, the data directly from the manufacturer was always used.

Product serving sizes would also change and cause a change in nutritional data. So, be sure, when comparing products, that you are comparing the same serving size, i.e., ¼ cup against ¼ cup.

Other differences can be caused by analytical methods and sampling techniques used by the different nutritional sources.

As you can see, data is listed in four columns. "Amount" means the serving size of food served or used in a recipe. Remember that any deviation of serving size will cause a change in the rest of the data given in all of the other columns. Fat content of each food is listed in fat grams (the measurement used for dietary fat); and the calorie column needs no explanation.

Further, I have listed the percentage of calories from fat under "% Fat Calories" for all listings. If you need to figure the percentage of fat in a food not listed, the formula is:

Fat Grams X 9 = Total Fat Calories (TFC);
Divide TFC by the total calorie content of your chosen food.

> *EXAMPLE:*   1 oz Cheddar Cheese = 9 fat grams and 110 calories.
>
>   9 X 9 = 81 TFC   81 divided by 110 = 73%

Since a high-fat food is any food in which 30 percent or more of the calories come from fat, this cheddar cheese would be considered a high-fat food.

Remember that some of the data has been rounded off, as mentioned, and the percentage might be off slightly, but not to the point that it matters. For example, all oils and fats have 100 percent of their calories in fat. However, if you look at a fat such as BUTTER, you will see that the "% Fat Calories" (100%) deviates slightly from the calculated amount—i.e., 11 fat grams X 9 = 99%. Because we know that all oils and fats contain 100 percent fat calories, I did not want to mislead you by using the rounded-off data and listing 99% instead of the absolute 100%.

You will find both generic and brand name products in these tables. The listing of a product by brand name is not necessarily meant as an endorsement. Brand name products not listed had no nutritional data available at the time, and their omission is for that reason only.

HOW TO USE THIS BOOK

The Complete and Up-to-Date Fat Book is an in-depth and comprehensive reference book. As you shop for and prepare low-fat foods, this book will be an invaluable source of information.

Serving amount, fat grams, total calories, and percentage of fat calories are provided for every product listed. In most cases, the foods are listed alphabetically for ready-reference. Some foods, where appropriate, are listed in groups, i.e., Frozen Entree/Dinner, Mexican Food, Oriental Food, etc. Following this A-to-Z food list, you will also find a separate section of fast food franchises.

Since cereals and soups are frequently prepared with milk, quick-reference charts for adding milk can be found in these sections. Also, because when we use oil in our food preparation it's important that we choose the least saturated oil available to us, I have prepared a chart on page 325, showing the breakdown by percentage of saturated, polyunsaturated, and monounsaturated fat contents of the most commonly used fats and oils.

As far as style, the book is organized with main headings for food capitalized and bold, and subheadings smaller (also capitalized and bold) with solid boxes before them. Descriptions of foods are upper/lower case, with brand names in parentheses.

If you are unable to find a particular food, look for the listing of a similar food. The nutritional data should be close, if not exact, for any product not listed. When doing this, make sure you are comparing the same serving size. Also, be sure you are comparing weight measure against weight measure and volume measure against volume measure. The Table of Equivalent Measures (see page 16) should help you, not only in comparing serving sizes, but in making your exchanges easier as well. Note that all cooked vegetable amounts are drained of liquid, unless otherwise noted.

You will find *The Complete and Up-to-Date Fat Book* a valuable companion as you begin to take control of your eating habits. And you will discover that adopting a low-fat lifestyle reaps many rewards—rewards such as more energy, better sleep, lower grocery bills, more control over your weight, and, perhaps most important, radiant health!

EXPLANATION OF ABBREVIATIONS AND SYMBOLS USED

~	=	Approximately		Pkt	=	Packet
Choc	=	Chocolate		Lb	=	Pound
Dia	=	Diameter		Sand	=	Sandwich
"	=	Inch		Tbs	=	Tablespoon
<	=	Less Than		Tsp	=	Teaspoon
Oz	=	Ounce		w/	=	With
Pkg	=	Package		w/o	=	Without

Regarding dishes noted as "Standard Home Recipe," "Homemade," and "Home Recipe," the data listed refer to standard ingredients being used in preparation; no low-fat substitutes were used in these recipes. The data listed is to be used as a guideline for the same dish you might make in your home. You should also keep this in mind for the data on box mix dishes, as they are prepared according to package directions and, unless noted otherwise, low-fat ingredients were not used.

TABLE OF EQUIVALENT MEASURES

VOLUME

1 tablespoon	=	3 teaspoons
		½ fluid ounce
2 tablespoons	=	1 fluid ounce
4 tablespoons	=	¼ cup
		2 fluid ounces
16 tablespoons	=	1 cup
		½ pint
⅓ cup	=	5⅓ tablespoons
½ cup	=	8 tablespoons
		4 fluid ounces
⅔ cup	=	10⅔ tablespoons
¾ cup	=	12 tablespoons
1 cup	=	8 fluid ounces
2 cups	=	1 pint
2 pints	=	1 quart
4 quarts	=	1 gallon

WEIGHT

1 ounce	=	28.35 grams
3.5 ounces	=	100 grams
4 ounces	=	¼ pound
8 ounces	=	½ pound
12 ounces	=	¾ pound
16 ounces	=	1 pound
		454 grams

A

Food and Description	Amount	Fat Grams	Total Calories	% Fat Calories
ABALONE				
fried	3 oz	5.77	161	32%
raw	3 oz	1	90	10%
ACEROLA/raw	1	–	2	–
	1 cup	–	31	–
ACEROLA JUICE	8 oz	.7	51	12%
ACORN				
dried	1 oz	8.9	145	55%
raw	1 oz	6.8	105	58%
ACORN FLOUR				
full fat	1 oz	9	142	57%
ADZUKI BEANS				
boiled	½ cup	<1	147	3%
canned-sweetened	½ cup	<1	351	1%
raw	½ cup	<1	325	1%
ALBACORE (*See* TUNA)				
ALE (*See* BEER, ALE, AND MALT LIQUOR)				
ALEWIFE(herring)/raw	4 oz	5.6	144	35%
ALFALFA SPROUTS/raw	1 cup	–	10	–
ALLIGATOR/raw	3 oz	3	200	14%
ALLSPICE	1 tsp	–	6	–
ALMOND				
blanched-slivered				
(Azar)	1 oz	15	170	79%
(Dole)	1 oz	14	170	74%
dried				
blanched	1 oz	14.9	166	81%
unblanched	1 oz	14.8	167	80%
dry roasted	1 oz	14.65	167	79%
(Blue Diamond)	1 oz	14	179	70%
hickory smoked	1 oz	15	166	81%
honey roasted				
(Eagle)	1 oz	12	150	72%
oil roasted				
blanched	1 oz	16	174	83%

Food and Description	Amount	Fat Grams	Total Calories	% Fat Calories
(Planters)				
blanched				
sliced	1 oz	15	170	79%
slivered	1 oz	15	170	79%
whole	1 oz	15	170	79%
dry roasted	1 oz	15	170	79%
honey roasted	1 oz	13	170	69%
roasted-salted (Blue Diamond)	1 oz	15	150	90%
slices (Azar)	1 oz	15	170	79%
Smokehouse (Blue Diamond)	1 oz	14	150	84%
sour cream & onion (Blue Diamond)	1 oz	14	150	84%
toasted	1 oz	14	167	75%
ALMOND BUTTER				
honey & cinnamon	1 Tbs	8	96	75%
plain	1 Tbs	9.5	101	85%
raw (Hain) natural	2 Tbs	18	190	85%
toasted blanched (Hain)	2 Tbs	19	220	78%
ALMOND MEAL/partially defatted	1 oz	5	116	39%
ALMOND PASTE	1 Tbs	7.7	127	55%
	1 cup	62	1010	55%
ALMOND POWDER				
full fat	1 oz	15	168	80%
	1 cup	34	385	80%
partially defatted	1 oz	5	112	40%
	1 cup	10	255	35%
ALOE VERA JUICE	2 oz	–	5	–
AMARANTH				
box (Health Valley)				
fat-free fast menu				
w/garden vegetables	7.5 oz	2.7	140	17%
cooked	½ cup	–	14	–
raw	1 cup	–	7	–
ANCHOVY, EUROPEAN				
canned in oil	5 fish	1.9	42	41%
fresh-raw	3 oz	4	62	58%
pate	1 tsp	.8	14	51%
ANISE	1 tsp	–	7	–
APPLE				
(Del Monte) sliced	2 oz	–	140	–
Generic				
canned-slices-sweetened	½ cup	.5	68	7%
cooked w/o skin	1 cup	.6	91	6%
dried				
cooked	1 cup	–	144	–

Food and Description	Amount	Fat Grams	Total Calories	% Fat Calories
cooked w/sugar	1 cup	–	232	–
uncooked	1 cup	–	209	–
uncooked	10 rings	–	155	–
raw w/skin	1	.5	81	6%
slices	1 cup	–	64	–
raw w/o skin	1	–	72	–
slices	1 cup	–	62	–
(Luck's) fried-canned	8 oz	–	190	–
(Mariani)	¼ cup	–	150	–
(Nature's Favorite) Apple Chips				
cinnamon	1 oz	5	120	38%
golden delicious	1 oz	5	120	38%
original	1 oz	5	120	38%
(Sun Maid) chunks	2 oz	–	150	–
(Tree Top) Apple Chips				
cinnamon	½ oz	< 1	55	8%
regular	½ oz	< 1	55	8%
(Weight Watcher's) Chips	¾ oz	–	70	–
APPLE BUTTER	1 Tbs	–	33	–
	1 cup	2	525	3%
(Smucker's) Autumn Harvest Natural & Cider Apple Butter	1 tsp	–	12	–
(Smucker's) Spiced	2 tsp	–	25	–
APPLE CIDER				
Bottled				
Generic - Sweet	8 oz	–	124	–
(Indian Summer)				
Apple-Cherry	6 oz	–	100	–
Apple-Cranberry	6 oz	–	100	–
Plain	6 oz	–	80	–
(Mussleman's) Lucky Leaf	6 oz	–	90	–
(Tree Top)	6 oz	–	90	–
Mix				
(Alpine)				
low-cal	8 oz	–	16	–
regular	8 oz	–	80	–
APPLE DRINK				
(Alpine)				
Spiced Cider Mix	8 oz	–	80	–
sugar-free	8 oz	–	16	–
(Juice Works) Apple	6 oz	–	97	–
APPLE DUMPLINGS				
(Pepperidge Farm) frozen	3 oz	13	260	45%
Standard Home Recipe (USDA)	1 average	16	275	52%

Food and Description	Amount	Fat Grams	Total Calories	% Fat Calories
APPLE JUICE				
Bottled, boxed, or canned				
(Campbell's) Juice Bowl-Apple	6 oz	–	110	–
(IGA) unsweetened	6 oz	–	74	–
(Indian Summer)	6 oz	–	90	–
(Kraft) Pure 100%	6 oz	–	80	–
(Martinelli's) Sparkling	6 oz	–	100	–
(Minute Maid)				
Juices to Go	9.6 oz	–	145	–
On the Go	10 oz	–	152	–
(Mott's)	8.45 oz	–	124	–
natural style	6 oz	–	88	–
(Ocean Spray) unsweetened	6 oz	–	90	–
(President's Choice)				
Cox's Orange Pippin	6 oz	–	90	–
(Red Cheek)				
Natural Style	6 oz	–	97	–
100% Pure	6 oz	–	97	–
(S&W)	6 oz	–	85	–
(Seneca)	6 oz	–	90	–
Sparkling	6 oz	–	80	–
(Sippin' Pak) from concentrate	8.45 oz	–	110	–
(Sunglo)	8.45 oz	–	130	–
(Sunkist)				
from frozen concentrate	8 oz	–	79	–
(Tree Top)	6 oz	–	90	–
(TreeSweet)	6 oz	–	90	–
(Tropicana)	8 oz	–	116	–
(Welch's) Sparkling	6 oz	–	100	–
(White House)	6 oz	–	87	–
Frozen				
(Birds Eye)	6 oz	–	80	–
(Minute Maid)	6 oz	–	90	–
(Seneca)	6 oz	–	90	–
(Sunkist)	8 oz	–	79	–
(Tree Top)	6 oz	–	90	–
APPLE JUICE COCKTAIL				
(Welch's Orchard)				
Apple-Grape-Cherry	6 oz	–	110	–
Cocktails-In-A-Box	8.45 oz	–	150	–
Apple-Grape-Raspberry	6 oz	–	100	–
Cocktails-In-A-Box	8.45 oz	–	140	–
Apple-Orange-Pineapple	6 oz	–	100	–
Cocktails-In-A-Box	8.45 oz	–	140	–

Food and Description	Amount	Fat Grams	Total Calories	% Fat Calories
APPLE NECTAR				
cinnamon	6 oz	–	110	–
plain (Kern's)	6 oz	–	110	–
APPLE-BERRY DRINK				
(Juice Works) Appleberry	6 oz	–	96	
APPLE-BOYSENBERRY JUICE				
(Knudsen)	8 oz	–	110	–
APPLE-CHERRY DRINK	8 oz	–	116	–
APPLE-CHERRY JUICE				
(Red Cheek)	6 oz	–	113	–
APPLE-CRANBERRY DRINK				
(Mott's)	10 oz	–	176	–
	9.5 oz	–	167	–
(Tropicana) single serve	10 oz	–	175	–
APPLE-CRANBERRY JUICE				
(Mott's)	6 oz	–	80	–
	8.45 oz	–	136	–
(Tree Top)	6 oz	–	100	–
APPLE-GRAPE JUICE				
(Libby's) Juicy Juice	6 oz	–	90	–
(Mott's)	6 oz	–	86	–
	8.45 oz	–	128	–
(Red Cheek)	6 oz	–	109	–
(Tree Top)	6 oz	–	100	–
APPLE-PEAR JUICE				
(Tree Top)	6 oz	–	90	–
APPLE-RASPBERRY DRINK				
(Mott's)	10 oz	–	158	–
	9.5 oz	–	150	–
APPLE-RASPBERRY JUICE				
(Mott's)	9.45 oz	–	134	–
(Red Cheek)	6 oz	–	113	–
(Tree Top)	6 oz	–	100	–
APPLESAUCE				
canned				
sweetened	1 cup	–	194	–
unsweetened	1 cup	–	106	–
(Del Monte)				
sweetened	½ cup	–	90	–
Lite	½ cup	–	50	–
(Hunt's) Snack Pack				
natural	4.25oz	–	50	–
regular	4.25 oz	–	80	–
raspberry	4.25 oz	–	80	–

Food and Description	Amount	Fat Grams	Total Calories	% Fat Calories
strawberry	4.25 oz	–	80	–
(Mott's)				
chunky	4 oz	–	57	–
cinnamon	4 oz	–	72	–
natural	4 oz	–	44	–
regular	4 oz	–	88	–
(Nutradiet) unsweetened	½ cup	–	55	–
(S&W)				
sweetened	½ cup	–	90	–
unsweetened	½ cup	–	55	–
(Seneca)				
cinnamon	½ cup	–	90	–
100% natural	½ cup	–	50	–
McIntosh	½ cup	–	90	–
regular	½ cup	–	90	–
sweetened	½ cup	–	90	–
(Tree Top)				
cinnamon	½ cup	–	80	–
natural	½ cup	–	60	–
original	½ cup	–	80	–
(Wilderness)				
raspberry	½ cup	–	82	–
strawberry	½ cup	–	90	–
APRICOT				
candied	1 oz	–	96	–
canned				
(Del Monte)				
halves unpeeled	½ cup	–	100	–
whole unpeeled	½ cup	–	100	–
(Del Monte) Lite halves				
unpeeled	½ cup	–	60	–
(Nutradiet)				
halves	½ cup	–	35	–
whole peeled	½ cup	–	28	–
(S&W)				
halves unpeeled in heavy syrup	½ cup	–	110	–
whole peeled in heavy syrup	½ cup	–	100	–
canned in water w/o skin	1 cup	–	51	–
canned in water w/skin	1 cup	–	65	–
in juice	1 cup	–	119	–
in light syrup	1 cup	–	160	–
in heavy syrup	1 cup	–	214	–
dried				
cooked	½ cup	–	106	–

Food and Description	Amount	Fat Grams	Total Calories	% Fat Calories
uncooked	½ cup	.6	155	4%
(Del Monte)	2 oz	–	140	–
(Mariani)	¼ cup	–	140	–
(Sun Maid)	2 oz	–	140	–
fresh	3 fruit	.5	51	9%
	1 cup	–	74	–
frozen, sweetened	½ cup	–	119	
APRICOT JUICE				
unsweetened	8 oz	–	123	–
APRICOT NECTAR	1 cup	–	141	–
(Del Monte)	6 oz	–	100	–
(Libby's)	8 oz	–	140	–
(S&W)	6 oz	–	100	–
APRICOT-ORANGE NECTAR				
(Kern's)	6 oz	–	112	–
APRICOT-PINEAPPLE NECTAR				
(Kern's)	6 oz	–	110	–
(Nutradiet)	½ cup	–	35	–
(S&W)	6 oz	–	120	–
ARMADILLO/raw	3 oz	4	150	24%
ARROWHEAD/plant				
cooked	Medium Corm	.5	9	50%
raw	Medium Corm	.5	12	38%
ARTICHOKE				
canned-marinated crowns				
(Cara Mia)	1 oz	–	12	–
fresh-cooked	Medium	–	53	–
frozen-cooked	½ cup	–	36	–
Jerusalem Artichoke raw/slices	½ cup	–	57	–
raw	Medium	–	65	–
ARTICHOKE HEARTS				
canned-marinated				
(Cara Mia)	1 oz	2	27	67%
(S & W)	3.5 oz	25	225	100%
fresh-cooked	½ cup	–	37	–
frozen (Birds Eye)	3 oz	–	30	–
ASPARAGUS				
canned	½ cup	.78	24	29%
All Green (Nutradiet)	½ cup	–	17	–
All Green Fancy (S & W)	½ cup	–	18	–
All Green cut spears (Del Monte)	½ cup	–	20	–
spears & tips (Del Monte)	½ cup	–	20	–

Food and Description	Amount	Fat Grams	Total Calories	% Fat Calories
Colossal Spears (S&W)	½ cup	–	20	–
Green Tipped (Del Monte)	½ cup	–	20	–
50% Less Salt (Green Giant)	½ cup	–	20	–
spears (Green Giant)	½ cup	–	20	–
whole spears (Thank You)	½ cup	–	25	–
fresh-cooked/cuts & tips	½ cup	–	22	–
	4 spears	–	15	–
frozen cuts (Birds Eye)	½ cup	–	25	–
frozen spears				
(Birds Eye)	3.3 oz	–	25	–
(Pictsweet)	3.3 oz	–	25	–
raw	½ cup	–	15	–
	4 spears	–	13	–
ASPARAGUS SOUP, CREAM OF (*See* SOUP)				
AVOCADO				
California				
mashed	1 cup	36	407	80%
raw	1	30.79	324	86%
Florida	1	27	340	72%

B

Food and Description	Amount	Fat Grams	Total Calories	% Fat Calories
BABY FOOD				

(NOTE: A low-fat nutrition program is not recommended for any child under two years of age.)

■ **BAKED GOODS**

(Gerber)				
Animal Crackers	.4 oz	2	50	36%
Animal Shaped Cookies	.4 oz	2	60	30%
Arrowroot Cookies	.4 oz	2	50	36%
Pretzels	.4 oz	–	50	–
Toddler Biter Biscuits	.4 oz	1	50	18%
Zwieback Toast	.5 oz	2	70	26%
(Nabisco)				
Zwieback Teething Toast	2 pieces	1	60	15%

Food and Description	Amount	Fat Grams	Total Calories	% Fat Calories
■ **CEREALS**				
(Beech-Nut Stages)				
Dry-Ready-To-Serve				
Barley-dry	½ oz	–	50	–
w/whole milk	2.4 oz	3	100	27%
High Protein-dry	½ oz	1	50	18%
w/whole milk	2.4 oz	4	100	36%
Mixed-dry	½ oz	1	50	18%
w/whole milk	2.4 oz	4	100	36%
Oatmeal-dry	½ oz	1	50	18%
w/whole milk	2.4 oz	4	100	36%
Oatmeal w/Bananas-dry	½ oz	1	60	15%
w/whole milk	2.4 oz	4	100	36%
Rice-dry	½ oz	1	60	15%
w/whole milk	2.4 oz	4	100	36%
Rice w/Bananas-dry	½ oz	1	60	15%
w/whole milk	2.4 oz	4	100	36%
Stage 2				
Mixed w/Applesauce & Bananas	4.5 oz	–	80	–
Oatmeal w/Applesauce & Bananas	4.5 oz	1	90	10%
Rice w/Applesauce & Bananas	4.5 oz	–	100	–
(Gerber)				
Dry-Ready-To-Serve (½ oz = 4 Tablespoons)				
Barley-dry	½ oz	1	60	15%
w/whole milk	2.4 oz	4	100	36%
High Protein-dry	½ oz	1	50	18%
w/whole milk	2.4 oz	4	100	36%
High Protein w/Apple & Orange				
dry	½ oz	1	60	15%
w/whole milk	2.4 oz	4	100	36%
Mixed-dry	½ oz	1	60	15%
w/whole milk	2.4 oz	4	100	36%
Oatmeal-dry	½ oz	1	60	15%
w/whole milk	2.4 oz	1	100	36%
Oatmeal w/Banana-dry	½ oz	1	60	15%
w/whole milk	2.4 oz	4	100	36%
Rice-dry	½ oz	1	60	15%
w/whole milk	2.4 oz	4	100	36%
Rice w/Banana				
dry	½ oz	1	60	15%
w/whole milk	2.4 oz	4	100	36%
Junior With Fruit				
Mixed w/Applesauce & Bananas	6 oz	2	140	13%
Oatmeal w/Applesauce & Bananas	6 oz	2	130	14%
Rice w/Mixed Fruit	6 oz	1	140	6%

Food and Description	Amount	Fat Grams	Total Calories	% Fat Calories
Strained With Fruit				
Mixed w/Applesauce & Bananas	1 jar/4.5 oz	1	100	9%
Oatmeal w/Applesauce & Bananas	1 jar/4.5 oz	1	100	9%
Rice w/Applesauce & Bananas	1 jar/4.5 oz	1	100	9%
(Heinz)				
Instant				
Barley-dry	½ oz	1	60	15%
w/whole milk	2.4 oz	4	100	36%
Mixed-dry	⅓ oz	1	50	18%
w/whole milk	2.4 oz	4	90	40%
Oatmeal-dry	½ oz	2	60	30%
w/whole milk	2.4 oz	5	100	45%
Rice-dry	½ oz	1	60	15%
w/whole milk	2.4 oz	4	100	36%
Instant With Fruit				
Mixed w/Bananas & Apple Juice	½ oz	1	50	18%
Rice w/Bananas & Apple Juice	½ oz	1	60	15%
Oatmeal w/Bananas & Apple Juice	½ oz	1	60	15%
Rice w/Bananas & Apple Juice	½ oz	1	60	15%
Rice w/Pears & Apple Juice	½ oz	1	50	18%
■ DESSERTS				
Apple Betty				
junior	~ 7.8 oz	–	153	–
strained	~ 4.8 oz	–	97	–
(Beech-Nut Stages)				
Caramel Pudding				
junior	~ 7.5 oz	1.9	167	10%
strained	~ 4.8 oz	.9	104	8%
Cherry Vanilla Pudding				
junior	~ 7.8 oz	< 1	152	3%
strained	~ 4.8 oz	< 1	91	5%
Chocolate Custard				
junior	~ 7.8 oz	3.5	195	16%
strained	~ 4.5 oz	2	107	17%
Stage 2				
Banana Custard Pudding	4.5 oz	1	120	8%
Banana Pineapple	4.5 oz	–	100	–
Dutch Apple	4.5 oz	–	80	–
Guava Tropical Fruit	4.5 oz	–	100	–
Mango Tropical Fruit	4.5 oz	–	90	–
Mixed Fruit & Yogurt	6 oz	1	140	6%
	4.5 oz	1	110	8%
Papaya Tropical Fruit	4.5 oz	–	80	–
Peaches & Yogurt	4.5 oz	1	110	8%
Vanilla Custard Pudding	4.5 oz	3	130	21%

Food and Description	Amount	Fat Grams	Total Calories	% Fat Calories
Stage 3				
Banana Custard	7.5 oz	2	200	9%
Mixed Fruit & Yogurt	7.5 oz	1	170	5%
Peaches & Yogurt	7.5 oz	2	190	10%
Vanilla Custard	7.5 oz	5	210	21%
(Heinz)				
Instant (Dry Serving Size)				
Banana Pudding	4 Tbs	1	60	15%
Dutch Apple Pie	4 Tbs	–	50	–
Peach Cobbler	4 Tbs	1	60	15%
Vanilla Custard	4 Tbs	2	60	30%
(Gerber)				
Junior				
Dutch Apple	6 oz	2	130	14%
Fruit	6 oz	1	130	7%
Hawaiian Delight	6 oz	1	150	6%
Peach Cobbler	6 oz	1	130	7%
Vanilla Custard Pudding	6 oz	2	150	7%
Strained				
Banana Apple	4.5 oz	1	90	10%
Cherry Vanilla Pudding	4.5 oz	1	90	10%
Chocolate Custard Pudding	4.5 oz	2	110	16%
Dutch Apple	4.5 oz	2	100	18%
Fruit	4.5 oz	1	100	9%
Hawaiian Delight	4.5 oz	1	120	8%
Orange Pudding	4.5 oz	1	110	8%
Peach Cobbler	4.5 oz	1	100	9%
Vanilla Custard Pudding	4.5 oz	1	100	9%
Peach Melba				
junior	~ 7.8 oz	–	132	–
strained	~ 4.8 oz	–	81	–
Pineapple Pudding				
junior	~ 7.8 oz	.9	192	4%
strained	~ 4.5 oz	< 1	104	4%
■ DINNERS				
(Beech-Nut Stages)				
Stage 2				
Beef & Egg Noodles w/Vegetables	4.5 oz	4	90	40%
Beef Dinner Supreme	4.5 oz	7	120	53%
Chicken & Rice w/Vegetables	4.5 oz	3	80	34%
Chicken Noodle w/Vegetables	4.5 oz	3	90	30%
Macaroni, Tomato & Beef	4.5 oz	3	90	30%
Turkey Dinner Supreme	4.5 oz	5	110	41%
Turkey Rice w/Vegetables	4.5 oz	2	70	26%
Vegetable Beef	4.5 oz	3	90	30%

Food and Description	Amount	Fat Grams	Total Calories	% Fat Calories
Vegetable Chicken	4.5 oz	3	90	30%
Vegetable Ham	4.5 oz	3	90	30%
Vegetable Lamb	4.5 oz	3	90	30%
Stage 3				
Beef & Egg Noodles w/Vegetables	6 oz	8	150	48%
	7.5 oz	5	150	30%
Beef Dinner Supreme	7.5 oz	9	180	45%
Chicken Noodles w/Vegetables	6 oz	2	100	18%
	7.5 oz	4	140	26%
Macaroni, Tomato & Beef	6 oz	8	160	45%
	7.5 oz	5	150	30%
Spaghetti, Tomato & Beef	7.5 oz	5	170	27%
Turkey Dinner Supreme	7.5 oz	8	190	38%
Turkey Rice w/Vegetables	7.5 oz	4	130	28%
Vegetable Bacon	7.5 oz	9	180	45%
Vegetable Beef	6 oz	7	160	39%
	7.5 oz	5	150	30%
Vegetable Chicken	6 oz	2	90	20%
	7.5 oz	5	140	32%
Vegetable Lamb	7.5 oz	5	140	32%
Table Time				
Beef Stew	6 oz	4	140	26%
Pasta Squares in Meat Sauce	6 oz	4	140	26%
Soups				
Hearty Chicken w/stars	6 oz	9	180	45%
Hearty Vegetable	6 oz	–	70	–
Spaghetti Rings in Meat Sauce	6 oz	4	160	23%
Vegetable Stew w/Chicken	6 oz	8	190	38%
(Gerber)				
Chunky Products				
Homestyle Noodles & Beef	6 oz	6	150	36%
Macaroni Alphabets w/beef & tomato sauce	6.25 oz	4	140	26%
Noodles & Chicken w/Carrots & Peas	6 oz	3	110	25%
Rice w/Beef & Tomato Sauce	6.25 oz	4	140	26%
Saucy Rice w/Chicken	6 oz	3	120	23%
Spaghetti-Tomato Sauce & Beef	6.25 oz	5	160	28%
Vegetables & Beef	6.25 oz	5	130	35%
Vegetables & Chicken	6.25 oz	5	140	32%
Vegetables & Ham	6.25 oz	5	130	35%
Vegetables & Turkey	6.25 oz	4	120	30%
Junior				
Beef Egg Noodle	6 oz	4	120	30%

Food and Description	Amount	Fat Grams	Total Calories	% Fat Calories
Chicken Noodle	6 oz	3	100	27%
Macaroni Tomato Beef	6 oz	2	110	16%
Spaghetti Tomato Sauce Beef	6 oz	3	120	23%
Split Peas Ham	6 oz	3	130	21%
Turkey Rice	6 oz	4	110	33%
Vegetable Bacon	6 oz	6	140	39%
Vegetable Beef	6 oz	3	110	25%
Vegetable Chicken	6 oz	3	100	27%
Vegetable Ham	6 oz	4	120	30%
Vegetable Lamb	6 oz	5	120	38%
Vegetable Turkey	6 oz	3	100	27%
Junior Lean Meat Dinners				
Beef w/Vegetables	4.5 oz	3	100	27%
Chicken w/Vegetables	4.5 oz	3	90	30%
Ham w/Vegetables	4.5 oz	4	110	33%
Turkey w/Vegetables	4.5 oz	4	100	36%
Strained				
Beef Egg Noodle	4.5 oz	3	90	30%
Chicken Noodle	4.5 oz	3	90	30%
Macaroni Cheese	4.5 oz	3	90	30%
Macaroni Tomato Beef	4.5 oz	2	80	23%
Turkey Rice	4.5 oz	3	80	34%
Vegetable Bacon	4.5 oz	5	100	45%
Vegetable Beef	4.5 oz	4	90	40%
Vegetable Chicken	4.5 oz	2	80	23%
Vegetable Ham	4.5 oz	3	80	34%
Vegetable Lamb	4.5 oz	4	90	40%
Vegetable Liver	4.5 oz	1	60	15%
Vegetable Turkey	4.5 oz	2	70	26%
Strained Lean Meat Dinners				
Beef w/Vegetables	4.5 oz	3	90	30%
Chicken w/Vegetables	4.5 oz	3	90	30%
Ham w/Vegetables	4.5 oz	4	100	36%
Turkey w/Vegetables	4.5 oz	4	100	36%
(Heinz)				
Instant (Dry Serving Size)				
Beef Noodle	5 Tbs	3	70	39%
Chicken Noodle	5 Tbs	2	70	26%
Chicken Rice	6 Tbs	2	60	30%
Tuna Noodle	6 Tbs	1	60	15%
Turkey Rice	5 Tbs	2	70	26%
Vegetables & Beef	5 Tbs	3	70	39%
Vegetables & Chicken	5 Tbs	2	70	26%
Vegetables & Ham	5 Tbs	2	70	26%

Food and Description	Amount	Fat Grams	Total Calories	% Fat Calories
Vegetables & Turkey	5 Tbs	2	60	30%
■ FINGER FOODS				
(Gerber) Toddler				
Chicken Sticks	2.5 oz	8	120	60%
Meat Sticks	2.5 oz	7	110	57%
Turkey Sticks	2.5 oz	9	120	68%
■ FROZEN FOODS				
(Growing Healthy)				
Chunky Products				
Pasta, Chicken & Vegetables	6 oz.	2	140	13%
Vegetables & Beef	6 oz.	1	120	8%
Vegetables & Chicken	6 oz.	1	110	8%
Junior				
Pasta, Chicken & Vegetables	6 oz.	2	120	15%
Vegetables & Beef	6 oz.	1	110	8%
Vegetables & Chicken	6 oz.	1	100	9%
Strained				
Bananas	4 oz.	–	9	–
Carrots	4 oz.	–	43	–
Garden Vegetables	4 oz.	–	46	–
Pasta, Chicken, & Vegetables	4 oz.	1	80	11%
Peaches	4 oz.	–	64	–
Peas	4 oz.	–	23	–
Sweet Potatoes	4 oz.	–	106	–
Vegetables & Beef	4 oz.	1	70	13%
Vegetables & Chicken	4 oz.	1	60	15%
■ FRUIT JUICES				
(Beech-Nut Stages)				
Stage 1				
Apple	4.2 oz	–	60	–
Pear	4.2 oz	–	60	–
White Grape	4.2 oz	–	60	–
Stage 2				
Juice Plus	4 oz	–	80	–
Unstaged				
Apple	4 oz	–	60	–
Apple Banana	4.2 oz	–	60	–
Apple Cherry	4.2 oz	–	50	–
Apple Cranberry	4.2 oz	–	60	–
Apple Grape	4.2 oz	–	60	–
Apple Pear	4.2 oz	–	60	–
Mixed Fruit	4.2 oz	–	60	–
Orange	4.2 oz	–	60	–
Pear	4 oz	–	60	–
Tropical Blend	4 oz	–	70	–

Food and Description	Amount	Fat Grams	Total Calories	% Fat Calories
(Gerber)				
Strained				
Apple	4.2 oz	–	60	–
Apple-Apricot	4.2 oz	–	60	–
Apple-Banana	4.2 oz	–	70	–
Apple-Cherry	4.2 oz	–	60	–
Apple-Grape	4.2 oz	–	60	–
Apple-Peach	4.2 oz	–	60	–
Apple-Pineapple	4.2 oz	–	60	–
Apple-Plum	4.2 oz	–	60	–
Apple-Prune	4.2 oz	–	70	–
Mixed Fruit	4.2 oz	–	70	–
Orange	4.2 oz	–	70	–
Pear	4.2 oz	–	60	–
Toddler				
Apple	4 oz	–	60	–
Apple-Cherry	4 oz	–	60	–
Apple-Grape	4 oz	–	60	–
Apple'N Berry	4 oz	–	60	–
Fruits-A-Plenty	4 oz	–	60	–
Fruits Of The Sun	4 oz	1	60	15%
Mixed Fruit	4 oz	1	60	15%
Pear	4 oz	–	60	–
■ FRUITS				
(Beech-Nut Stages)				
Stage 1				
Barlett Pears	2.8 oz	–	50	–
	4.5 oz	–	60	–
Chiquita Bananas	2.8 oz	–	70	–
	4.5 oz	–	100	–
Golden Delicious Applesauce	2.8 oz	–	45	–
	4.5 oz	–	60	–
Yellow Cling Peaches	2.8 oz	–	40	–
	4.5 oz	–	60	–
Stage 2				
Apples & Grapes	4.5 oz	–	90	–
Apples & Strawberries	4.5 oz	–	90	–
Applesauce & Apricots	4.5 oz	–	60	–
Applesauce & Bananas	4.5 oz	–	60	–
Applesauce & Cherries	4.5 oz	–	70	–
Apples, Mandarin Oranges & Bananas	4.5 oz	–	90	–
Apples, Peaches & Strawberries	4.5 oz	–	100	–
Apples, Pears & Bananas	4.5 oz	–	90	–
Apricots, w/Pears & Applesauce	4.5 oz	–	70	–

Food and Description	Amount	Fat Grams	Total Calories	% Fat Calories
Bananas w/Pears & Applesauce	4.5 oz	–	90	–
Bartlett Pears & Pineapple	4.5 oz	–	70	–
Cottage Cheese w/Pineapple	4.5 oz	1	110	8%
Fruit Dessert	4.5 oz	–	80	–
Island Fruits	4.5 oz	–	90	–
Pears & Applesauce	4.5 oz	–	70	–
Plums w/rice	4.5 oz	–	110	–
Prunes w/Pears	4.5 oz	–	120	–
Stage 3				
Apples & Grapes	7.5 oz	–	190	–
Apples & Strawberries	7.5 oz	–	160	–
Applesauce	6 oz	–	80	–
	7.5 oz	–	100	–
Applesauce & Bananas	7.5 oz	–	110	–
Applesauce & Cherries	7.5 oz	–	110	–
Apples, Mandarin Oranges & Bananas	7.5 oz	–	150	–
Apples, Peaches & Strawberries	7.5 oz	–	160	–
Apples, Pears & Bananas	7.5 oz	–	160	–
Apricots w/Pears & Apples	6 oz	–	110	–
	7.5 oz	–	120	–
Bananas w/Pears & Apples	6 oz	–	120	–
	7.5 oz	–	160	–
Bartlett Pears	6 oz	–	90	–
	7.5 oz	–	110	–
Bartlett Pears & Pineapple	7.5 oz	–	120	–
Cottage Cheese w/Pineapple	6 oz	2	160	11%
	7.5 oz	2	190	10%
Fruit Dessert	7.5 oz	–	130	–
Island Fruits	7.5 oz	–	150	–
Peaches	6 oz	–	100	–
	7.5 oz	–	150	–
(Gerber)				
First Foods				
Applesauce	2.5 oz	–	40	–
Bananas	2.5 oz	–	60	–
Peaches	2.5 oz	–	30	–
Pears	2.5 oz	–	40	–
Prunes	2.5 oz	–	70	–
Junior				
Apple Blueberry	6 oz	1	80	11%
Applesauce	6 oz	1	90	10%
Apricots w/Tapioca	6 oz	1	130	7%
Bananas w/Tapioca	6 oz	1	140	6%

Food and Description	Amount	Fat Grams	Total Calories	% Fat Calories
Bananas w/Pineapple & Tapioca	6 oz	1	90	10%
Peaches	6 oz	1	110	8%
Pear Pineapple	6 oz	1	100	9%
Pears	6 oz	1	100	9%
Plums w/Tapioca	6 oz	1	130	7%
Strained				
Apple Blueberry	4.5 oz	1	60	15%
Applesauce	4.5 oz	1	60	15%
Applesauce & Apricot	4.5 oz	1	70	13%
Apricots w/Tapioca	4.5 oz	1	90	10%
Bananas w/Tapioca	4.5 oz	1	110	8%
Bananas w/Pineapple & Tapioca	4.5 oz	–	60	–
Peaches	4.5 oz	1	90	10%
Pear Pineapple	4.5 oz	1	80	11%
Pears	4.5 oz	1	80	11%
Plums w/Tapioca	4.5 oz	–	90	–
Prunes w/Tapioca	4.5 oz	1	100	9%
Strained Tropical Fruits				
Guava w/Tapioca	4.5 oz	1	90	10%
Mango Bananas & Passion Fruit w/Tapioca	4.5 oz	–	100	–
Mango w/Tapioca	4.5 oz	1	90	10%
Papaya w/Tapioca	4.5 oz	1	80	11%
Peaches Mango w/Tapioca	4.5 oz	1	100	9%
Tropical Fruits w/Tapioca	4.5 oz	1	80	11%
(Heinz)				
Instant				
Apples	1 serving	–	50	–
Bananas	1 serving	–	50	–
Peaches	1 serving	–	50	–
Pears	1 serving	–	50	–
Instant Fruit Combinations				
Apples & Apricots	1 serving	–	50	–
Apples & Bananas	1 serving	–	50	–
Apples & Peaches	1 serving	–	50	–
Apples & Pears	1 serving	–	50	–
Apricots w/Pears & Bananas	1 serving	–	50	–
Mixed Fruit	1 serving	–	50	–
Peaches & Pears	1 serving	–	50	–
Pears & Pineapple	1 serving	–	50	–
■ MEATS				
(Beech-Nut Stages)				
Stage 1				
Beef	2.8 oz	7	100	63%
	3.5 oz	8	120	60%

Food and Description	Amount	Fat Grams	Total Calories	% Fat Calories
Chicken	2.8 oz	6	90	60%
	3.5 oz	6	110	49%
Lamb	2.8 oz	6	90	60%
	3.5 oz	8	130	55%
Turkey	2.8 oz	6	100	54%
	3.5 oz	7	120	53%
Veal	2.8 oz	7	100	63%
	3.5 oz	7	120	53%
(Gerber)				
Junior Meats				
Beef	2.5 oz	4	80	45%
Chicken	2.5 oz	7	110	57%
Ham	2.5 oz	5	90	50%
Turkey	2.5 oz	6	100	54%
Veal	2.5 oz	4	80	45%
Strained Meats & Egg Yolks				
Beef	2.5 oz	4	80	45%
Chicken	2.5 oz	7	110	57%
Egg Yolks	2.25 oz	11	130	76%
Ham	2.5 oz	5	90	50%
Lamb	2.5 oz	3	70	39%
Pork	2.5 oz	5	90	50%
Turkey	2.5 oz	6	100	54%
Veal	2.5 oz	4	80	45%
Ham				
junior	~ 3.5 oz	6.6	123	48%
strained	~ 3.5 oz	5.7	110	48%
Liver-strained	~ 3.5 oz	3.7	100	33%
■ VEGETABLES				
(Beech-Nut Stages)				
Stage 1				
Butternut Squash	2.8 oz	–	20	–
	4.5 oz	–	40	–
Green Beans	4.5 oz	–	40	–
Regal Imperial Carrots	4.5 oz	–	40	–
Sweet Potatoes	2.8 oz	–	40	–
	4.5 oz	–	70	–
Tender Sweet Peas	4.5 oz	–	70	–
Stage 2				
Creamed Corn	4.5 oz	–	90	–
Garden Vegetables	4.5 oz	–	60	–
Mixed Vegetables	4.5 oz	–	50	–
Peas & Carrots	4.5 oz	–	60	–
Stage 3				
Carrots	7.5 oz	–	60	–

Food and Description	Amount	Fat Grams	Total Calories	% Fat Calories
Green Beans	7.5 oz	–	60	–
Mixed Vegetables	7.5 oz	–	90	–
Sweet Potatoes	7.5 oz	–	120	–
(Gerber)				
First Foods				
Carrots	2.5 oz	1	40	23%
Green Beans	2.5 oz	–	20	–
Peas	2.5 oz	1	40	23%
Squash	2.5 oz	–	20	–
Sweet Potatoes	2.5 oz	–	50	–
Junior				
Carrots	6 oz	1	50	18%
Creamed Green Beans	6 oz	1	80	11%
Mixed Vegetables	6 oz	1	70	13%
Peas	6 oz	1	90	10%
Squash	6 oz	1	60	15%
Sweet Potatoes	6 oz	1	110	8%
Strained				
Beets	4.5 oz	1	60	15%
Carrots	4.5 oz	1	40	23%
Creamed Corn	4.5 oz	1	80	11%
Creamed Spinach	4.5 oz	1	60	15%
Garden Vegetables	4.5 oz	1	50	18%
Green Beans	4.5 oz	1	50	18%
Mixed Vegetables	4.5 oz	1	60	15%
Peas	4.5 oz	1	60	15%
Squash	4.5 oz	1	40	23%
Sweet Potatoes	4.5 oz	1	80	11%
(Heinz)				
Instant (Dry Serving Size)				
Beets	3 Tbs	–	50	–
Carrots	5 Tbs	2	70	26%
Creamed Corn	6 Tbs	1	60	15%
Creamed Peas	5 Tbs	1	00	15%
Creamed Spinach	6 Tbs	2	60	30%
Garden Vegetables	5 Tbs	1	60	15%
Green Beans	4 Tbs	1	60	15%
Mixed Vegetables	5 Tbs	2	70	26%
Peas & Carrots	5 Tbs	1	60	15%
Squash	5 Tbs	1	50	18%
Sweet Potatoes	4 Tbs	1	60	15%
Spinach				
junior	~ 7.5 oz	3	90	30%
strained	~ 4.5 oz	1.7	48	32%

Food and Description	Amount	Fat Grams	Total Calories	% Fat Calories
BABY/INFANT FORMULA				
(Carnation) Canned				
Good Start	5 oz	5.1	100	46%
Follow Up	5 oz	4.1	100	37%
(SMA) Canned				
Lo Iron	5 oz	5.3	100	48%
With Iron				
Liquid	5 oz	5.3	100	48%
Powder				
prepared	5 oz	5.3	100	48%
BACON (*See also* LUNCHEON MEAT)				
Breakfast Strips				
cooked	3 slices	12.5	156	72%
(Eckrich) Sizzlean				
cooked	2 slices	8	90	80%
(Oscar Meyer) Lean & Tasty				
heated	1 slice	4	50	72%
(Swift) Premium-brown				
sugar cured	2 slices	9	110	74%
Canadian Bacon				
cold	2 slices/ 2 oz	3.95	89	40%
grilled	2 slices/ 2 oz	3.9	86	41%
(Hormel)	1 oz	2	35	51%
(Oscar Meyer) 93% fat-free	1 oz	1	35	26%
Cured Breakfast Strips				
Black Label (Hormel) cooked	2 slices	5	60	75%
pan-fried or roasted	3 slices	9	109	74%
Range Brand (Hormel) cooked	2 slices	9	110	74%
Red Label (Hormel) cooked	3 slices	10	110	82%
Thick-sliced	1 slice	19	190	90%
BACON BITS				
(Hormel)	1 Tbs	2	30	60%
(Oscar Meyer)	¼ oz	1	21	43%
BACON-LIKE BITS	1 serving	.5	10	45%
BACON SUBSTITUTES				
Bacon Bits (Betty Crocker)	2 tsp	1	25	36%
Bacon Flavor Sprinkles				
(Molly McButter)	½ tsp	–	4	–
BacOs (Betty Crocker)	2 tsp	1	25	36%
(Durkee)				
Bacon Chips	1 Tbs	2	44	41%
Imitation Bacon Bits	1 Tbs	2	50	36%

Food and Description	Amount	Fat Grams	Total Calories	% Fat Calories
(McCormick/Schilling)				
Bac'n Bits	1 Tbs	1	25	36%
Bac'n Chips	1 Tbs	1	26	36%
BAGEL				
Generic				
Plain - 3" dia	1	.8	64	11%
Pumpernickel - 3" dia	1	.5	152	3%
Whole Wheat - 3" dia	1	.6	152	4%
(International-Bailys)				
Garlic	1-1.5 oz	< 1	110	4%
Onion	1-1.5 oz	< 1	110	4%
Plain	1-1.5 oz	< 1	110	4%
(Lenders) Frozen Bagelettes	1	.5	70	6%
Big 'N Crusty	1	1	230	3%
Blueberry	1	1	190	4%
Cinnamon Raisin	1	1	200	4%
Egg	1	1	150	6%
Garlic, Onion	1	1	160	5%
Oat Bran	1	2	170	10%
Plain	1	1	150	6%
Poppy	1	1	160	5%
Pumpernickel	1	1	160	5%
Raisin & Honey	1	1	190	4%
Rye	1	1	150	6%
Sesame	1	1	160	5%
Soft	1	3	210	13%
Wheat & Honey	1	1	190	4%
(Sara Lee) Frozen				
Cinnamon & Raisin	1	2	240	7%
Egg	1	2	250	7%
Oat Bran	1	1	220	4%
Onion	1	1	230	4%
Plain	1	1	230	4%
Poppy Seed	1	1	230	4%
Sesame Seed	1	3	260	10%
BAGEL CHIPS				
(Burns & Ricker) Bagel Crisps				
Cinnamon	6 pieces	5	130	35%
Garlic	6 pieces	8	130	55%
Oat Bran	6 pieces	8	150	48%
Onion	6 pieces	9	130	62%
Plain	6 pieces	6	130	42%
Sea Salt	6 pieces	8	130	55%
Sesame	6 pieces	9	130	62%

Food and Description	Amount	Fat Grams	Total Calories	% Fat Calories
(New York Style)				
Garlic	¾ oz	3	90	30%
Garlic-Bite Size	½ oz	2	60	30%
Hot'N Spicy	¾ oz	2	90	20%
Plain	¾ oz	3	90	30%
Sea Salt	¾ oz	3	90	30%
BAKE & FRY MIX (*See also* SEASONINGS)				
(Arrowhead) Biscuit Mix	2 oz	1	100	9%
(Bisquick)	2 oz	8	240	30%
Reduced Fat	½ cup	4	210	17%
(Feam)				
Brown Rice	½ cup	3	215	13%
Rice	½ cup	1	260	4%
Whole Wheat	½ cup	2	210	9%
(Golden Dipt)				
Batter Mix	1 oz	–	90	–
Beer Batter	1 oz	–	100	–
Breading Frying Mix	1 oz	–	90	–
Cajun Style Fish Fry	⅔ oz	–	60	–
Chicken Frying Mix	1 oz	–	90	–
Corny Dog Batter	1 oz	–	100	–
Fish & Chips Batter	1¼ oz	–	120	–
Fish Fry	⅔ oz	–	60	–
Funnel Cake	7/10 oz	1	100	9%
Hush Puppy Deluxe	1¼ oz	–	120	–
Hush Puppy w/Onion	1¼ oz	–	120	–
Jalapeno Hush Puppy	1¼ oz	–	120	–
Onion Ring Mix	1 oz	–	100	–
Seafood Frying	⅔ oz	–	60	–
Tempura Batter	1 oz	–	100	–
(Hain)				
Whole Wheat	1.5 oz	1	150	6%
(Jiffy)	1 oz	3	115	24%
(Krusteaz)	2 Tbs	–	48	–
(Martha White)				
Recip-Ease	½ cup	8	240	30%
BAKING POWDER	1 tsp	–	5	–
(Calumet)	1 tsp	–	4	–
(Davis)	1 Tbs	–	15	–
BAKING SODA	1 tsp	–	5	–
BALSAM PEAR/raw	1 cup	–	15	–
leaf tips				
cooked	½ cup	–	10	–
raw	½ cup	–	7	–

Food and Description	Amount	Fat Grams	Total Calories	% Fat Calories
pods				
cooked	½ cup	–	12	–
raw	½ cup	–	8	–
BAMBOO SHOOT				
canned	1 cup	< 1	25	18%
canned (La Choy)	¾ cup	–	6	–
cooked	1 cup	–	14	–
raw	½ cup	–	21	–
BANANA				
(Del Monte)				
chips-freeze dried	¼ cup	4	124	29%
flakes	⅓ cup	1	22	41%
fresh	1 medium	< 1	101	5%
mashed	1 cup	1	207	4%
powder	2 oz	–	194	–
sliced	1 cup	–	130	–
Plantain Banana	1	1	220	4%
cooked-sliced	1 cup	< 1	180	3%
BANANA NECTAR				
(Libby's)	6 oz	–	110	–
BANANA-ORANGE DRINK	8 oz	–	126	–
BANANA-PINEAPPLE NECTAR				
(Kern's)	6 oz	–	120	–
BARBECUE LOAF (See LUNCHEON MEAT)				
BARBECUE SAUCE (See SAUCE)				
BARLEY				
Generic				
Pearled				
Cooked	4 oz	.5	139	3%
	1 cup	.7	193	3%
Dry	1 oz	< 1	100	4%
	1 cup	2	704	3%
Raw	1 oz	.7	100	6%
	1 cup	4	651	6%
Pearled				
(Arrowhead Mills)	2 oz	1	200	5%
(Quaker/Scotch)				
Medium pearled	¼ cup	1	170	5%
Quick	⅓ cup	.5	172	3%
BARRACUDA				
baked or broiled	3 oz	5	135	33%
breaded & fried	3 oz	7.5	169	40%
BASIL				
ground	1 tsp	–	3	–

Food and Description	Amount	Fat Grams	Total Calories	% Fat Calories
leaves	1 tsp	–	3	–
BASS				
Black				
cooked-dry heat	3 oz	14.5	215	61%
raw	3 oz	1	80	11%
Freshwater				
raw	3 oz	3	97	28%
Mixed				
raw	3 oz	3	97	28%
Striped				
cooked-dry heat	3 oz	1.98	82	22%
BAY LEAF/crumbled	1 tsp	–	5	–
BEAN (*See* individual names)				
BEAN, BAKED & VARIETY				
canned				
baked				
(B&M)				
BBQ	~ 1 cup	6	310	17%
Honey	~ 1 cup	2	280	6%
Red Kidney	~ 1 cup	7	290	22%
Small Pea	~ 1 cup	8	330	22%
Tomato	~ 1 cup	3	230	12%
Vegetarian	~ 1 cup	2	280	6%
Yellow Eye	~ 1 cup	7	362	17%
(Green Giant)				
baked w/bacon & brown sugar	½ cup	1	130	7%
(S&W) Brick Oven	½ cup	2	160	11%
(Stagg)	½ cup	2.5	145	16%
(Van Camp's)	1 cup	2	260	7%
Deluxe	1 cup	4	320	11%
Garden Style Special Recipe	½ cup	.8	110	7%
baked w/beef	½ cup	4.59	161	26%
baked w/brown sugar	½ cup	2.5	142	16%
baked w/crumbled bacon	½ cup	4	160	23%
baked w/franks	½ cup	8	182	40%
baked w/molasses & brown sugar	½ cup	1.5	133	10%
baked w/pork	½ cup	1.96	133	13%
baked w/pork & sweet sauce	½ cup	1.85	140	12%
baked w/pork & tomato sauce	½ cup	1	123	7%
barbecue (Campbell's)	7⅛ oz	4	210	17%
Boston Baked	½ cup	6.7	193	31%
(Health Valley)	½ cup	1	110	8%
Boston Baked-No Salt				
(Health Valley)	½ cup	1	110	8%

Food and Description	Amount	Fat Grams	Total Calories	% Fat Calories
Cajun Beans & Sauce (Lipton)	½ cup	.6	130	4%
Homestyle (Campbell's)	½ cup	2	115	16%
	8 oz	4	230	16%
Maple Sugar (S&W)	½ cup	1	150	6%
New England Style				
(Special Recipe)	½ cup	2.5	148	15%
Old Fashioned (Campbell's)	½ cup	1.5	115	12%
Old Fashioned (Campbell's)	8 oz	3	230	12%
Pork & Beans				
(Campbell's)	8 oz	3	190	14%
(Heinz)	8 oz	4	250	14%
(Hormel) Micro Cup	7.5 oz	5	250	18%
(Hunt's)	4 oz	1	140	6%
(Van Camp's)	1 cup	2	220	8%
Pork & Molasses (Libby)	½ cup	2	140	13%
Pork & Tomato Sauce (Libby)	½ cup	2	140	13%
Pork'N Beans (S&W)	½ cup	2	130	14%
Ranchero (Campbell's)	7¾ oz	4	190	19%
Smokey Ranch (S&W)	½ cup	2	130	14%
Texas Style Barbecue (S&W)	½ cup	1	135	7%
Vegetarian				
(Heinz)	8 oz	1	230	4%
(Libby)	½ cup	1	130	7%
Vegetarian Seasoned in Tomato Sauce				
(Campbell's)	½ cup	1	210	4%
Vegetarian Style Beans				
(Van Camp's)	1 cup	1	210	4%
Vegetarian w/miso				
(Health Valley)	½ cup	1	90	10%
homemade (includes white beans, molasses, brown				
sugar, salt pork & spices)	½ cup	6.5	190	31%
BEAN MEALS, BAKED				
Beanee Weenee /canned				
(Van Camp's)	1 cup	15	330	41%
Beans'N Franks (Heinz)	7¾ oz	15	330	41%
BEAN SALAD, MIXED				
Four Bean Salad				
canned				
(Hanover)	½ cup	–	80	–
(Joan of Arc)	½ cup	–	100	–
Garden Salad-marinated				
jar (S&W)	½ cup	1	90	10%
Mixed Bean Salad-marinated				
canned (S&W)	½ cup	1	90	10%

Food and Description	Amount	Fat Grams	Total Calories	% Fat Calories
Mixed Beans (Pinto & Great Northern) seasoned w/pork				
canned				
(Luck's)	7.25 oz	5	200	23%
	7.5 oz	7	220	29%
Three Bean Salad				
canned				
(Green Giant)	½ cup	–	70	–
(Joan Of Arc)	½ cup	–	80	–
homemade	1 cup	15	300	45%
BEAN SOUP (*See* SOUP)				
BEAN SPROUT				
Kidney/boiled	4 oz	< 1	37	12%
raw	1 cup	< 1	53	8%
Mung/boiled	1/2 cup	–	13	–
raw	4 oz	–	40	–
stir fried	1/2 cup	–	31	–
Navy/boiled	1 cup	< 1	88	5%
raw	4 oz	< 1	70	6%
Pinto/boiled	4 oz	–	25	–
raw	4 oz	1	70	13%
Soy/boiled	1/2 cup	2	38	47%
raw	10 sprouts	.6	12	45%
stir fried	4 oz	8	143	50%
BEAVER/roasted	3 oz	11.6	211	50%
BEECHNUT/dried	1 oz	14	164	77%
BEEF				

(Note: Serving sizes are for cooked beef, unless otherwise stated. "Lean only" means beef trimmed of all separable fat before cooking. "Lean and fat" means untrimmed and cooked or eaten as purchased. Prime cuts have the most fat, Choice cuts less, and Select/Good cuts the least amount of all cuts.)

■ **BEEF CUTS**				
Brisket				
Whole/lean & fat-braised	3 oz	27.6	332	75%
Whole/lean only-braised	3 oz	10.9	205	48%
Chuck				
Arm pot roast/lean & fat				
Choice	3 oz	22.5	301	67%
Good	3 oz	20.8	287	65%
Arm pot roast/lean only				
Choice-braised	3 oz	8.8	199	40%
Good-braised	3 oz	7.6	189	36%
Blade/lean & fat				
All grades-braised	3 oz	25.9	325	72%
Blade/lean only				
All grades-braised	3 oz	13	230	51%

Food and Description	Amount	Fat Grams	Total Calories	% Fat Calories
Ground (Chef's Grind) 20% Fat				
Uncooked	3 oz	15	200	68%
Rib roast or steaks/lean & fat				
Choice-braised	3 oz	31	364	77%
Good-braised	3 oz	25.8	321	72%
Rib roast or steaks/lean only				
Choice-braised	3 oz	15.6	218	64%
Good-braised	3 oz	8.7	187	42%
Stew meat-boneless				
Lean & fat				
Braised or stewed	3 oz	20	279	65%
Lean only				
Braised or stewed	3 oz	8	183	39%
Club Steak/lean & fat				
Choice-broiled	3 oz	34.5	386	30%
Corned Beef				
Boneless				
Roasted	3 oz	25.8	316	74%
Flank				
Lean and fat/Choice				
Braised	3 oz	13	218	54%
Broiled	3 oz	13.9	216	58%
Lean only				
Choice-braised	3 oz	11.8	208	51%
Choice-broiled	3 oz	12.7	207	55%
Ground (Note: 4 oz raw ground meat is equal to 3 oz cooked ground meat.)				
Extra lean 15% fat				
Broiled medium	3 oz	13.9	215	58%
Broiled well-done	3 oz	13	225	52%
Fried medium	3 oz	14	216	58%
Fried well-done	3 oz	13.6	224	55%
Raw	4 oz	19	265	65%
Extra Lean 10% Fat				
Raw	4 oz	11	202	49%
Broiled well done	3 oz	9.6	186	46%
(Healthy Choice)	4 oz	4	130	28%
Lean 21% Fat				
Raw	4 oz	24	303	71%
Broiled medium	3 oz	15.7	231	61%
Broiled well-done	3 oz	15	238	57%
Fried medium	3 oz	16	234	62%
Fried well-done	3 oz	15	235	57%
Regular				
Raw	4 oz	30	351	77%

Food and Description	Amount	Fat Grams	Total Calories	% Fat Calories
Broiled medium	3 oz	17.6	246	64%
Broiled well-done	3 oz	16.5	248	60%
Fried medium	3 oz	19	260	66%
Fried well-done	3 oz	16	243	59%
London Broil, 100% lean				
Choice-braised	3 oz	6	167	32%
Rib				
Whole/lean & fat				
Choice-broiled	3 oz	26	313	75%
Choice-roasted	3 oz	27.6	328	76%
Good-broiled	3 oz	26	313	75%
Good-roasted	3 oz	24.9	306	73%
Whole/lean only				
Choice-broiled	3 oz	11.5	198	52%
Choice-roasted	3 oz	12.6	209	54%
Rib Eye				
Lean & fat				
Choice-broiled	3 oz	17.5	250	63%
Lean only				
Choice-broiled	3 oz	9.9	191	47%
Ribs, Short				
Lean & fat				
Choice-braised	3 oz	35.7	400	80%
Lean only				
Choice-braised	3 oz	15	251	54%
Round				
Bottom/lean & fat				
Choice-braised	3 oz	13	224	52%
Good-braised	3 oz	12	215	50%
Prime-braised	3 oz	16	253	57%
Bottom/lean only				
Choice-braised	3 oz	8	191	38%
Good-braised	3 oz	7	182	35%
Prime-braised	3 oz	11	212	47%
Eye of/lean & fat				
Choice-roasted	3 oz	12	207	52%
Good-roasted	3 oz	12	201	54%
Prime-roasted	3 oz	13	213	55%
Eye of/lean only				
Choice-roasted	3 oz	6	156	35%
Good-roasted	3 oz	5	150	30%
Prime-roasted	3 oz	7	168	38%
Full Cut/lean & fat				
Choice-broiled	3 oz	15.5	233	60%

Food and Description	Amount	Fat Grams	Total Calories	% Fat Calories
Good-broiled	3 oz	14	222	57%
Full Cut/lean				
Choice-broiled	3 oz	6.8	165	37%
Good-broiled	3 oz	5.9	157	34%
Ground (Chef's Grind) 15% Fat				
Uncooked	3 oz	12	170	64%
Tip/lean & fat				
Choice-roasted	3 oz	13	216	54%
Good-roasted	3 oz	12	205	53%
Prime-roasted	3 oz	16	242	60%
Tip/lean only				
Choice-roasted	3 oz	7	164	38%
Good-roasted	3 oz	6	156	35%
Prime-roasted	3 oz	9	181	45%
Top/lean & fat				
Choice-broiled	3 oz	8	181	40%
Good-broiled	3 oz	7	156	40%
Prime-broiled	3 oz	10	201	45%
Top/lean only				
Choice-broiled	3 oz	5	165	27%
Good-broiled	3 oz	5	156	29%
Prime-broiled	3 oz	8	201	45%
Rump Roast				
Lean & fat				
Choice-roasted	3 oz	23	295	70%
Good-roasted	3 oz	19.9	269	67%
Lean only				
Choice-roasted	3 oz	7.9	177	40%
Good-roasted	3 oz	6	162	33%
Shank Crosscuts				
Lean & fat				
Choice-simmered	3 oz	10	208	43%
Lean only				
Choice-simmered	3 oz	5	171	26%
Sirloin				
Ground (Chef's Grind) 10% Fat				
Uncooked	3 oz	8	140	51%
Lean & fat				
All grades-broiled	3 oz	15	238	57%
Lean only				
All grades-broiled	3 oz	7	177	36%
Steak				
Porterhouse/lean & fat				
Choice-broiled	3 oz	18	254	64%

Food and Description	Amount	Fat Grams	Total Calories	% Fat Calories
Porterhouse/lean only				
Choice-broiled	3 oz	9	185	44%
T-bone/lean & fat				
Choice-broiled	3 oz	20.9	276	68%
T-bone/lean only				
Choice-broiled	3 oz	8.8	182	44%
Tenderloin				
Lean & fat				
Choice-broiled	3 oz	15	230	59%
Choice-roasted	3 oz	19	262	65%
Good-broiled	3 oz	13	216	54%
Good-roasted	3 oz	17	245	62%
Prime-broiled	3 oz	19.9	270	66%
Lean only				
Choice-broiled	3 oz	8	176	41%
Choice-roasted	3 oz	9.9	189	47%
Good-broiled	3 oz	7	167	38%
Good-roasted	3 oz	8.6	177	44%
Prime-broiled	3 oz	10.5	197	48%
Top Loin				
Lean & fat				
Choice-broiled	3 oz	16.6	243	62%
Good-broiled	3 oz	14	223	57%
Prime-broiled	3 oz	22	288	69%
Lean only				
Choice-broiled	3 oz	8	176	41%
Good-broiled	3 oz	6	162	33%
Prime-broiled	3 oz	11.6	208	50%
Wedge-Bone Sirloin				
Lean & fat				
Choice-broiled	3 oz	16	240	56%
Good-broiled	3 oz	15	232	58%
Prime-broiled	3 oz	19	271	63%
Lean only				
Choice-broiled	3 oz	6	178	30%
Good-broiled	3 oz	7	170	37%
Prime-broiled	3 oz	10	201	45%
■ BEEF CUTS, ORGAN, OTHER				
Brains				
Fried	3 oz	13.5	167	73%
Simmered	3 oz	10.6	136	70%
Heart/braised	3 oz	4.8	148	29%
Kidneys/simmered	3 oz	2.9	122	21%
Liver				
Braised	3 oz	4	137	26%

Food and Description	Amount	Fat Grams	Total Calories	% Fat Calories
Fried	3 oz	6.8	184	33%
Lungs/braised	3 oz	3	102	27%
Pancreas/braised	3 oz	14.7	232	57%
Spleen/braised	3 oz	4	123	29%
Sweetbreads/braised	3 oz	19.7	272	65%
Thymus/braised	3 oz	21	273	69%
Tongue				
Braised-medium fat	3 oz	22	208	95%
Simmered	3 oz	17.6	241	66%
Tripe/raw	4 oz	4	111	32%
BEEF BROTH (See SOUP)				
BEEF DISHES (See also FROZEN ENTREE/DINNER; individual listings)				
Beef Bourguignoine				
Standard Home Recipe (USDA)	¾ cup	8	194	37%
Beef Pot Pie				
Frozen				
(Banquet)	7 oz	33	510	58%
(Morton)	7 oz	31	430	65%
(Swanson)	7 oz	20	380	47%
	16 oz	36	700	46%
Standard Home Recipe (USDA)				
(⅓ of 9" dia pie)	~7 oz	30	515	52%
Beef Stew				
Canned				
(Bounty) vegetable	7.6 oz	3	144	19%
(Chef Boyardee) Meat Ball	8 oz	24	350	62%
(Dinty Moore) 24 oz can	8 oz	12	220	49%
(Dinty Moore) 40 oz can	8 oz	11	210	47%
(Estee) vegetable	7.5 oz	11	210	47%
(Healthy Choice)	7.5 oz	2	140	13%
(Heinz) vegetable	7.5 oz	9	210	34%
(Libby's) vegetable	7.5 oz	5	160	28%
	8 oz	6	170	32%
Frozen				
(Banquet)	7 oz	5	140	32%
Microwaveable				
(Lunch Bucket)	8.5 oz	6	170	32%
Standard Home Recipe (USDA)	1 cup	11	220	45%
Beef Stroganoff				
Frozen (Weight Watchers)	9 oz	13	320	37%
Standard Home Recipe (USDA)				
w/noodles	1 cup	20	342	53%
Beef Wellington				
Standard Home Recipe (USDA)	4 oz	18	325	50%

Food and Description	Amount	Fat Grams	Total Calories	% Fat Calories
Beefaroni				
Canned (Chef Boyardee)	7 oz	6	200	27%
Beef-o-getti				
Canned (Chef Boyardee)	7 oz	9	210	39%
Breaded Beef Steaks				
Frozen (Hormel)	4 oz	30	370	73%
Corned Beef (See CORNED BEEF, CORNED BEEF HASH)				
Creamed Dried Beef				
Standard Home Recipe (USDA)	¾ cup	18	275	59%
Goulash				
Canned				
(Heinz)	7.5 oz	11	240	41%
(Hormel) Short Order	7.5 oz	12	230	47%
Great Beginnings (Hormel) Box prepared				
w/Chunky Beef	5 oz	7	136	46%
Hamburger (See also FAST FOOD, FROZEN ENTREE/DINNER, HAMBURGER HELPER)				
Mini Beef Cheeseburger (Jimmy Dean)				
Refrigerated-microwaveable	1 burger	5	120	38%
(International Lites) Microwaveable Box				
Beef Peking	10 oz	3	230	61%
Beef Stroganoff	10 oz	8	260	28%
Enchilada Acapulco	10 oz	8	250	29%
Milano Lasagna	10 oz	7	280	23%
Kid's Kitchen (Hormel) Microwaveable Box				
Beef Ravioli	7.5 oz	2	160	11%
Chunky Vegetables & Beef	7.5 oz	1	120	8%
Spaghetti w/meatballs	7.5 oz	8	200	36%
(Light Balance) Microwaveable lunch buckets				
Beef Americana	8.25 oz	3	170	16%
Beef & Pasta Bordeaux	8.25 oz	1	180	5%
Stuffed Green Peppers (homemade)				
With beef & bread crumbs	1 med pepper	10.5	325	29%
With beef & rice	½ pepper	13	219	53%
BEEF, FROZEN ENTREE (See BEEF DISHES, FROZEN ENTREE/DINNER)				
BEEF PRODUCTS (See also LUNCHEON MEAT)				
Beef Spread				
(Underwood)				
Roast beef	2⅛ oz	11	140	71%
Beef Tallow	1 cup	205	1849	100%
	1 Tbs	12.8	115	100%
Breakfast Strips				
(Oscar Meyer) Lean'N Tasty	1 slice	4	45	80%

Food and Description	Amount	Fat Grams	Total Calories	% Fat Calories
(Sizzlean) cooked	2 strips	5	70	64%
Dried or Chipped Beef	2.5 oz	4	145	25%
Dried/Sliced				
(Armour Star)	8 slices	2	60	30%
(Hormel)	1 oz	1	45	20%
Smoked Chopped Beef	1 oz	1	38	24%
Smoked Sliced Beef (Hormel)	1 oz	3	50	54%
Steak-Umm (Gagliardi)				
Frozen-sandwich steaks	2 oz	16	180	80%
BEEF SAUSAGE (See LUNCHEON MEAT; SAUSAGE)				
BEEF SEASONING (See SEASONINGS)				
BEEF SOUP (See SOUP)				
BEER, ALE, AND MALT LIQUOR				
Ale-generic	12 fl oz	–	155	–
(Amstel) Light	12 fl oz	–	95	–
(Anheuser-Busch)	12 fl oz	–	153	–
(Anheuser-Busch) Natural Light	12 fl oz	–	110	–
(Augsberger)	12 fl oz	–	175	–
(Beck's)	12 fl oz	–	143	–
Dark	12 fl oz	–	156	–
Light	12 fl oz	–	132	–
Beer-generic				
Light	12 fl oz	–	100	–
Regular	12 fl oz	–	146	–
(Black Horse)	12 fl oz	–	158	–
(Blatz)	12 fl oz	–	136	–
(Blatz) Light	12 fl oz	–	96	–
(Bud) Dry	12 fl oz	–	127	–
(Bud) Light	12 fl oz	–	108	–
(Budweiser)	12 fl oz	–	144	–
(Busch)	12 fl oz	–	144	–
(Busch) Light	12 fl oz	–	110	–
(Carling's) Black Label	12 fl oz	–	136	–
(Carlsburg)	12 fl oz	–	149	–
(Carlsburg) Light	12 fl oz	–	110	–
Champale-Extra dry	12 fl oz	–	169	–
(Cheers) non-alcoholic	12 fl oz	–	55	–
(Classic)	12 fl oz	–	144	–
(Colt 45)	12 fl oz	–	156	–
(Coors)				
Dry	12 fl oz	–	119	–
Extra Gold	12 fl oz	–	151	–
Light	12 fl oz	–	103	–
Original	12 fl oz	–	137	–

Food and Description	Amount	Fat Grams	Total Calories	% Fat Calories
(Coqui) Malt Liquor	12 fl oz	–	208	–
(Corona Light	12 fl oz	–	105	–
(Cutter)	12 fl oz	–	76	–
(Elephant) Malt Liquor	12 fl oz	–	211	–
(Foster's) Lager	12 fl oz	–	120	–
(Gablinger's)	12 fl oz	–	96	–
(Goebel)	12 fl oz	–	131	–
(Guinness) Extra Stout	12 fl oz	–	192	–
(Hamm's)				
Light	12 fl oz	–	96	–
Regular	12 fl oz	–	136	–
(Heidelberg) Light	12 fl oz	–	115	–
(Heileman's)				
Old Style	12 fl oz	–	147	–
Light	12 fl oz	–	110	–
Special Export	12 fl oz	–	151	–
Light	12 fl oz	–	115	–
Special Export Dark	12 fl oz	–	155	–
(Heineken)	12 fl oz	–	152	–
Special Dark	12 fl oz	–	192	–
(Herman Joseph's)	12 fl oz	–	157	–
(Hofbrau) Dark Reserve	12 fl oz	–	204	–
(Keystone)				
Dry	12 fl oz	–	121	–
Light	12 fl oz	–	100	–
Original	12 fl oz	–	121	–
(Killian's)	12 fl oz	–	127	–
(King Cobra)	12 fl oz	–	182	–
(Kingsbury) non-alcoholic malt	12 fl oz	–	60	–
(Knickerbocker)	12 fl oz	–	140	–
(Kronenbourg)	12 fl oz	–	170	–
(LA)	12 fl oz	–	112	–
Lite Genuine Draft	12 fl oz	–	98	–
Lite Ultra	12 fl oz	–	77	–
(Lowenbrau)	12 fl oz	–	157	–
Dark Special	12 fl oz	–	158	–
Special	12 fl oz	–	158	–
(Michelob)	12 fl oz	–	160	–
Classic Dark	12 fl oz	–	164	–
Dry	12 fl oz	–	130	–
Light	12 fl oz	–	134	–
(Mickeys) Malt Liquor	12 fl oz	–	156	–
(Miller)				
Genuine Draft	12 fl oz	–	147	–

Food and Description	Amount	Fat Grams	Total Calories	% Fat Calories
High Life	12 fl oz	–	147	–
Lite	12 fl oz	–	96	–
Magnum	12 fl oz	–	162	–
(Milwaukee's) Best Light	12 fl oz	–	98	–
(Molson) Light	12 fl oz	–	109	–
(Moussy) non-alcoholic	11.1 fl oz	–	50	–
Natural Light (Anheuser-Busch)	12 fl oz	–	110	–
Near Beer	12 fl oz	–	32	–
(Nordik Wolf) Light	12 fl oz	–	110	–
(O'Doul's)	12 fl oz	–	70	–
(Old Milwaukee)	12 fl oz	–	145	–
Light	12 fl oz	–	120	–
(Old Style) Light	12 fl oz	–	115	–
(Olympia) Gold Light	12 fl oz	–	70	–
(Ortieb's)	12 fl oz	–	140	–
(Pabst Blue Ribbon)	12 fl oz	–	144	–
(Pabst Blue Ribbon) Extra Light	12 fl oz	–	70	–
(Pabst) NA (non-alcoholic)	12 fl oz	–	55	–
(Piels)	12 fl oz	–	134	–
(Pilsner)	12 fl oz	–	145	–
(Prior) Double Dark	12 fl oz	–	171	–
(Rainier)	12 fl oz	–	142	–
(Red Bull) Malt Liquor	12 fl oz	–	192	–
(Red White & Blue) Light	12 fl oz	–	115	–
(Rheingold)	12 fl oz	–	148	–
Light	12 fl oz	–	96	–
(Schaefer)	12 fl oz	–	138	–
Light	12 fl oz	–	111	–
(Schlitz)	12 fl oz	–	145	–
Light	12 fl oz	–	121	–
Malt Liquor	12 fl oz	–	177	–
(Schmidt)	12 fl oz	–	142	–
Light	12 fl oz	–	96	–
Select (non alcoholic malt)	12 fl oz	–	00	–
Sharp's (Miller) non-alcoholic	12 fl oz	–	68	–
(St. Pauli Girl)				
Dark	12 fl oz	–	156	–
Light	12 fl oz	–	144	–
(Stroh's)				
American Lager	12 fl oz	–	145	–
Bock	12 fl oz	–	157	–
Bohemian	12 fl oz	–	148	–
Light	12 fl oz	–	115	–
Signature	12 fl oz	–	150	–

Food and Description	Amount	Fat Grams	Total Calories	% Fat Calories
(Tiger Head) Ale	12 fl oz	–	166	–
BEERWURST (*See* LUNCHEON MEAT)				
BEET				
canned	½ cup		36	–
crinkle cut pickled				
(Del Monte) Salad Bar Vegetables	½ cup	–	80	–
Harvard-slices	½ cup	–	89	–
Julienne French Style (S&W)	½ cup	–	40	–
party sliced pickled w/red				
wine vinegar (S&W)	½ cup	–	70	–
pickled	½ cup	–	75	–
(Libby & Seneca)	½ cup	–	35	–
pickled-sliced (Libby)	½ cup	–	80	–
pickled-sliced				
w/red wine vinegar (S&W)	½ cup	–	70	–
pickled-Whole-Extra Small (S&W)	½ cup	–	70	–
sliced				
(Del Monte)	½ cup	–	35	–
(Libby)	½ cup	–	35	–
(Nutradiet)	½ cup	–	35	–
small sliced (Freshlike)	½ cup	–	40	–
small Tender sliced (S&W)	½ cup	–	40	–
small whole				
(Freshlike)	½ cup	–	40	–
(S&W)	½ cup	–	40	–
tender diced (S&W)	½ cup	–	40	–
whole or tiny whole				
(Del Monte)	½ cup	–	35	–
fresh /cooked	½ cup	–	26	–
BEET DISHES				
Beets in Orange Sauce/frozen				
(Birds Eye) Specialty Classics	5 oz	3	110	25%
BEET GREENS				
fresh				
cooked	½ cup	–	20	–
raw	½ cup	–	4	–
BERRY DRINK				
Berries & Berries (Tropicana)				
single serve	10 oz	–	156	–
Berry Blend (Crystal Light)				
mix-diet	8 oz	–	3	–
(Hi-C) Wild	6 oz	–	92	–
	8.45 oz	–	129	–
Very Berry (Hawaiian Punch)	6 oz	–	90	–

Food and Description	Amount	Fat Grams	Total Calories	% Fat Calories
BERRY JUICE				
Juicy Juice (Libby's)	6 oz	–	90	–
BISCUITS (*See also* BAKE & FRY MIX)				
Frozen (Bridgeford)				
heat & serve-microwave	1	6	190	28%
Homemade 2" dia	1	5	100	45%
Mix				
Baking mix (Krusteaz) 2" dia	1	4	110	33%
BixMix (Martha White)	1	3	100	27%
Generic	1	3	95	28%
Ruskets biscuits (La Loma)	2	–	110	–
Refrigerated				
Baking Powder 1869 Brand (Pillsbury)	1	5	100	45%
Big Country Butter Tastin' (Pillsbury)	1	4	100	36%
Big Country Buttermilk (Pillsbury)	1	4	100	36%
Big Country Southern Style (Pillsbury)	1	4	100	36%
Big Premium Heat'n Eat (Pillsbury)	2	15	280	48%
Butter (Pillsbury)	1	< 1	50	9%
Butter Tastin' 1869 Brand (Pillsbury)	1	5	100	45%
Butter Tastin' Flaky (Hungry Jack)	1	4	100	36%
Buttermilk 1869 Brand (Pillsbury)	1	5	100	45%
Buttermilk (Pillsbury)	1	1	50	18%
Buttermilk, Extra Rich (Hungry Jack)	1	1	50	18%
Buttermilk, Flaky (Hungry Jack)	1	4	90	40%
Buttermilk, Fluffy (Hungry Jack)	1	4	80	45%
Buttermilk, Big Country (Hungry Jack)	2	8	200	36%
Buttermilk, Deluxe Heat 'n Eat (Pillsbury)	2	15	280	48%
Buttermilk, Heat'nEat (Pillsbury)	2	5	170	26%
Buttermilk, Flaky Extra Lights (Pillsbury)	2	4	110	33%
Buttermilk, Tenderflake (Pillsbury)	2	5	110	41%
Country (Pillsbury)	1	1	50	18%
Good'N Buttery	2	10	180	50%
Grands! (Pillsbury)				
Butter Tastin'	1	9	190	43%
Cinnamon Raisin	1	7	190	33%
Flaky	1	8	190	38%
Honey Tastin' Flaky (Hungry Jack)	1	4	90	40%
OvenReady (Ballard)	1	< 1	50	9%
OvenReady, Buttermilk (Ballard)	1	< 1	50	9%
Plain - Generic	1	2	65	29%
Southern Style Flaky (Hungry Jack)	1	4	80	45%

Food and Description	Amount	Fat Grams	Total Calories	% Fat Calories
Tender Layer Buttermilk (Pillsbury)	1	2	60	30%
Tenderflake Baking Powder (Pillsbury)	2	5	110	41%
BLACK BEAN / boiled	½ cup	< 1	113	4%
BLACK BEAN SOUP (*See* SOUP)				
BLACK CHERRY DRINK				
Bottled	8 oz	–	117	–
Mix (Kool Aid)	8 oz	–	100	–
BLACK CHERRY JUICE				
(Smucker's)	8 oz	–	130	–
BLACK CHERRY JUICE CONCENTRATE				
(Hain)	1 oz	–	70	–
BLACK TURTLE BEANS				
(Hain) canned	4 oz	1	70	13%
BLACK TURTLE SOUP				
boiled	½ cup	< 1	121	4%
canned	½ cup	–	109	–
(Progresso)	8 oz	1	205	4%
BLACKBERRY				
canned in water	1 cup	1.5	60	23%
canned in juice	½ cup	< 1	41	11%
canned in heavy syrup	½ cup	< 1	94	5%
fresh	1 cup	1	75	12%
frozen/no sugar	½ cup	< 1	97	5%
BLACKBERRY JUICE				
canned	½ cup	1	46	20%
(Smucker's)	8 oz	1.5	91	15%
BLACK-EYED PEA				
canned				
(Progresso)	8 oz	1	165	6%
Seasoned w/Pork				
(Luck's)	7.5 oz	6	200	27%
dried-boiled	½ cup	.6	100	5%
dried-raw	½ cup	1	131	7%
dry (Joan of Arc/Green Giant)	½ cup	1	90	10%
frozen-cooked	½ cup	1	115	8%
frozen (Freshlike)	3.3 oz	1	95	10%
young pods w/seeds				
boiled	1 cup	–	32	–
raw	1 cup	–	42	–
BLACK-EYED PEA DISHES				
Black-eyed Peas & Corn seasoned w/pork				
canned (Luck's)	7.5 oz	7	220	29%

Food and Description	Amount	Fat Grams	Total Calories	% Fat Calories
BLUEBERRY				
canned				
in heavy syrup	1 cup	< 1	225	2%
(S&W)	½ cup	< 1	111	4%
in water	1 cup	< 1	94	5%
fresh	1 cup	< 1	82	6%
frozen				
no sugar	1 cup	< 1	88	5%
	3.5 oz	< 1	50	9%
sweetened	1 cup	< 1	190	2%
BLUEBERRY-CRANBERRY DRINK				
(Ocean Spray)	6 oz	–	120	–
BLUEFISH/raw	3 oz	3.6	105	31%
BOCKWURST (See LUNCHEON MEAT)				
BOLOGNA (See also LUNCHEON MEAT)				
4" dia	1 slice	8	89	81%
4½" dia	1 slice	6.5	72	81%
BORAGE				
cooked	½ cup	1	25	36%
raw	½ cup	< 1	9	50%
BORSCHT (See SOUP)				
BOYSENBERRY				
canned				
in water	1 cup	–	90	–
in heavy syrup	1 cup	–	226	–
fresh	½ lb	–	125	–
frozen				
no sugar	1 cup	–	66	–
sweetened	1 cup	–	144	–
BOYSENBERRY DRINK				
Plus-Nice & Natural	6 oz	–	60	–
BOYSENBERRY JUICE				
Delight	6 oz	–	80	–
(Omucker's) Naturally 100%	8 oz	–	120	–
BRAN				
Oat				
(Golden Harvest)	1 oz	2	90	20%
(Quaker)	½ cup	3.8	165	21%
(Roman Meal)	¼ cup	3	115	24%
Rice	3 oz	19	375	46%
(Golden Harvest)	½ cup	8	120	60%
Rite Bran				
(Uncle Ben's)	½ cup	9	100	81%
Toasted Wheat (Kretchmer)	⅓ cup	2	60	30%

Food and Description	Amount	Fat Grams	Total Calories	% Fat Calories
Unprocessed				
(Miller's)	1 oz/			
	6 Tbs	1	70	13%
(Quaker)	2 Tbs	–	8	–
BRANDY (*See* LIQUOR, DISTILLED)				
BRATWURST (*See* LUNCHEON MEAT)				
BRAZIL NUT/dried	1 oz	18.8	186	91%
BREAD (*See also* CRISPBREAD; CRUMPETS; MELBA TOAST; MUFFINS; ROLLS)				
Apple Walnut Cinnamon Swirl				
Bountiful Breads (Pepperidge Farm)	2 slices	6	160	34%
Banana Nut /homemade	1 slice	2	180	9%
Black	1 slice	–	64	–
Box mix-Quick (Pillsbury)				
Apple Cinnamon	1/12 loaf	6	190	28%
Banana	1/12 loaf	6	170	32%
Blueberry	1/12 loaf	6	180	30%
Cranberry	1/12 loaf	4	170	21%
Date	1/12 loaf	3	160	17%
Nut	1/12 loaf	6	170	32%
Bran	1 slice	2.9	110	24%
(Brownberry) Country Bakery Light	1 slice	< 1	40	11%
Bran & Honey (Roman Meal)	1 slice	1	66	14%
Bran'ola				
Country Oat (Brownberry)	1 slice	3	90	30%
Hearty Wheat (Brownberry)	1 slice	1.5	90	15%
Original (Brownberry)	1 slice	1	90	10%
Brown/canned				
(B&M) plain	1/2" slice	–	80	–
w/raisins	1/2" slice	–	80	–
(S&W) New England Recipe	2 slices	–	76	–
Boston/canned (3¼x½")	1 slice	1	95	10%
Cheese	1 slice	1	72	13%
Cinnamon Raisin	1 slice	1	80	11%
Cinnamon Swirl				
(Pepperidge Farm)	1 slice	3	90	30%
(Country Hearth)				
European Butter Sesame	1 slice	1	70	13%
Grainola	1 slice	1	75	12%
Honey Nugget	1 slice	1	70	13%
Indian	1 slice	1	100	9%
Old Fashioned Buttermilk	1 slice	1	70	13%
Old Fashioned Wheat	1 slice	1	70	13%
Old Fashioned Sandwich	1 slice	1	75	12%
7 Whole Grain	1 slice	1	80	11%

Food and Description	Amount	Fat Grams	Total Calories	% Fat Calories
Stone Ground Whole Wheat	1 slice	1	70	13%
Wheat Berry	1 slice	1	70	13%
Wheat Sandwich	1 slice	1	70	13%
Cracked Wheat	1 slice	1	75	12%
(Pepperidge Farm)	1 slice	1	65	14%
(Roman Meal)	1 slice	–	66	–
Date Nut/homemade	1 slice	3	100	27%
(Earth Grains)				
Barley Bran	1 slice	1	70	13%
Canadian Oat	1 slice	1	70	13%
Cracked Wheat	1 slice	1	70	13%
Deli Rye	1 slice	1	70	13%
French - San Francisco Style	1 slice	1	70	13%
Gold'N Bran	1 slice	1	70	13%
Honey N'Bran	1 slice	1	70	13%
Honey Multi-Grain	1 slice	1	70	13%
Honey Oat & Nut	1 slice	2	80	23%
Honey Oatberry	1 slice	1	70	13%
Oat & Nut	1 slice	2	80	23%
Oat Bran	1 slice	2	80	23%
Raisin Cinnamon Swirl	1 slice	2	80	23%
Wheat Berry	1 slice	1	70	13%
Yogurt Bran	1 slice	1	70	13%
Egg	1 slice	2.6	75	31%
French (5x2½x1")	1 slice	.8	100	7%
(Arnold) Francisco	1 slice	1	70	13%
(Continental Baking) Brown 'N Serve				
Bread du Jour	1 slice	1	70	13%
(International Hearth)	1 slice	1	70	13%
(Le Francais) Francisco Square	2 oz	1	150	6%
refrigerated Crusty (Pillsbury)	1 slice	.5	60	7%
Frozen bread doughs - baked				
French (Bridgeford)	2 slices	1	150	6%
Honey Wheat				
(Bridgeford)	1 slice	1	75	12%
(Rhodes)	1 slice	.5	75	6%
White				
(Bridgeford)	1 slice	1	75	12%
(Rhodes)	1 slice	.5	80	6%
(Rich's)	1 slice	.5	58	8%
Garlic	1 slice	3.8	100	34%
(Cole's) frozen-butter				
flavored mini loaf	1 oz	3	90	10%
(Oh Boy!) frozen w/cheese	2 oz	11	202	49%

Food and Description	Amount	Fat Grams	Total Calories	% Fat Calories
Gluten	1 slice	1	69	13%
Granola (Country Hearth)	1 slice	1	70	13%
(Pepperidge Farm)				
Oat & Honey	1 slice	2	65	28%
Wheat & Honey	1 slice	2	60	30%
(Grant's Farm)				
Buttermilk	1 slice	1	80	11%
Honey Cracked	1 slice	1	70	13%
Oat Bran	1 slice	1	70	13%
Oatmeal & Toasted Almonds	1 slice	2	80	23%
Stoneground Wheat & 7 Grain	1 slice	1	70	13%
Wheat Berry	1 slice	1	70	13%
Health Nut (Brownberry)	1 slice	2	70	26%
Hearth Breads (Pepperidge Farm)				
Baked				
Brown & Serve Italian	1 oz	1	80	11%
French Style Enriched	2 oz	2	150	12%
Twin French Style Enriched	1 oz	1	80	11%
Vienna Thick Sliced	1 slice	1	70	13%
Hi-Fibre (Monk's Bread)	1 slice	1	50	18%
Hillbilly (Holsum)	1 slice	1	70	13%
Homestyle Buttermilk	1 slice	1	75	12%
Honey Apple (Brownberry)	1 slice	1	60	15%
Honey Bran (Pepperidge Farm)				
1½-lb loaf	2 slices	2	180	10%
Honey Oat Bran (Roman Meal)	1 slice	1	71	13%
Honey, Nut & Oat (Roman Meal)	1 slice	1.5	72	19%
Honey Wheat Berry	1 slice	1	70	13%
(Roman Meal)	1 slice	1	66	14%
Honey-Buttered Split Top White				
(Family Recipe)	1 slice	1	80	11%
Wheat	1 slice	1	70	13%
Honeybran-Light (Roman Meal)	1 slice	–	40	–
Hush Puppies	1 slice	7	145	34%
Italian (4½x3¼x¾")	1 slice	–	85	–
(Brownberry) Bakery Light	1 slice	< 1	40	11%
(Kangaroo) Pocket				
Breakfast				
Cinnamon Raisin	1	–	65	–
Wheat Oat Bran	1	–	60	–
Sandwich	1	–	75	–
(King's Hawaiian)	½ oz	1	43	21%
Low Sodium	1 slice	.8	70	10%
Mixed Grain	1 slice	1	65	14%

Food and Description	Amount	Fat Grams	Total Calories	% Fat Calories
(Mrs. Wright's)				
Crushed Wheat	1 slice	1	80	11%
Crushed Wheat Sandwich	1 slice	1	70	13%
French Enriched	1 slice	1	70	13%
Homestyle Butter Top Wheat	1 slice	1	70	13%
Homestyle Butter Top White	1 slice	1	80	11%
Honey Bran	1 slice	1	90	10%
Honey Wheat Berry	1 slice	1	70	13%
Jewish Rye w/Seeds	1 slice	1	60	15%
Lite	1 slice	–	40	–
Multi Meal Sandwich	1 slice	1	70	13%
Old Fashioned Italian	1 slice	1	100	9%
Old World Style Black	1 slice	1	60	15%
Raisin	1 slice	1	70	13%
Roundtop Wheat	1 slice	1	80	11%
Sandwich Wheat	1 slice	1	80	11%
Supersoft Sandwich	1 slice	1	60	15%
Supersoft White	1 slice	1	80	11%
Unsalted Grain	1 slice	1	70	13%
Unsalted White	1 slice	1	80	11%
Multi-Bran (Roman Meal)	1 slice	1	64	14%
Oat (Roman Meal)	1 slice	1	70	13%
Oat Bran-Light				
(Rainbo/Colonial)	1 slice	.5	40	11%
Oat Bran & Honey				
(Roman Meal) Light	1 slice	.5	40	11%
Oatmeal				
(Brownberry)	1 slice	1	60	15%
Bakery Light	1 slice	< 1	40	11%
(Pepperidge Farm)				
Hearty Crunch Oat	2 slices	4	190	19%
Light Style	2 slices	–	90	–
Thin Sliced	1 slice	1	70	13%
Variety Breads	2 slices	2	140	13%
Very Thin	2 slices	2	80	23%
(Pepperidge Farm) 1½-lb loaf	2 slices	2	180	10%
Oatmeal & Oat Bran	1 slice	1	65	14%
(Oatmeal Goodness)				
Cinnamon Oatmeal	1 slice	1	80	11%
Oatmeal Bran	1 slice	1	80	11%
Oatmeal & Sunflower Seeds	1 slice	1	80	11%
Thinner Sliced White Oatmeal	1 slice	1	80	11%
Wheat Oatmeal	1 slice	1	80	11%
Oatnut Bread (Oroweat)	1 slice	2	100	28%

Food and Description	Amount	Fat Grams	Total Calories	% Fat Calories
(Oroweat) Light				
Country Oat	1 slice	–	40	–
Hearty Rye	1 slice	–	40	–
9 Grain	1 slice	–	40	–
100% Whole Wheat	1 slice	–	40	–
Sour Dough	1 slice	–	40	–
Pita-6 ½" dia	1 slice	.5	165	3%
8 ½" dia	1 slice	1	232	4%
Pita, Sesame-6 ½" dia	1 slice	1	140	6%
Pita, whole wheat-8 ½" dia	1 slice	2	200	9%
Potato	1 slice	.8	70	10%
Prepared Bread Dough				
(Pillsbury) Hearty Grains				
Cornbread Twists	1 piece	3	70	39%
Country Oatmeal Twists	1 piece	2	80	23%
Cracked Wheat & Honey	1 piece	2	80	23%
Multi-Grain	1 piece	2	80	23%
Oatmeal Raisin	1 piece	2	90	20%
Pumpernickel	1 slice	1	80	11%
(Pepperidge Farm)				
Family	1 slice	1	80	11%
party slices	4 slices	1	60	15%
Pumpernickel-Rye				
(Earth Grains)	1 slice	1	70	13%
(Brownberry)	1 slice	1	70	13%
Pumpkin-homemade	1 slice	5	130	35%
(Purity) Texas Toast	1 slice	2	150	12%
(Rainbo)				
IronKids	1 slice	1	60	15%
Light Sourdough	1 slice	< 1	40	11%
Raisin	1 slice	1	65	14%
homemade	1 slice	2	135	13%
(Monks' Bread)	1 slice	2	70	26%
Raisin Cinnamon				
(Brownberry)	1 slice	1	70	13%
(Pepperidge Farm)	2 slices	4	180	20%
Raisin Walnut				
(Brownberry)	1 slice	3	70	39%
Round Top (Roman Meal)	1 slice	1	68	13%
(Rubschlager)				
Cocktail Pumpernickel	2 slices	1	60	15%
Cocktail Rye	1 slice	1	50	18%
Danish Pumpernickel	1 slice	1	70	13%
European Style Whole Grain	1 slice	2	80	23%

Food and Description	Amount	Fat Grams	Total Calories	% Fat Calories
German Style Komissbrot	1 slice	1	70	13%
Jewish Deli Rye	1 slice	1	70	13%
Sandwich Malt	1 slice	2	90	20%
Sandwich Rye	1 slice	2	90	20%
Sandwich Wheat	1 slice	2	90	20%
Sweedish Limpa Rye	1 slice	1	60	15%
Westphalian Pumpernickel	1 slice	1	70	13%
Rye				
(Brownberry)				
Dill Rye	1 slice	< 1	70	6%
Natural UnSeeded	1 slice	1	70	13%
Natural UnSeeded Thin	1 slice	1	50	18%
Thin Sliced	1 slice	1	50	18%
(Pepperidge Farm)				
Family w/Seeds	1 slice	1	80	11%
Family Seedless	1 slice	1	80	11%
Party Slices	4 slices	1	60	18%
Rye, Caraway-Natural				
(Brownberry)	1 slice	1	70	13%
Rye, Dijon (Pepperidge Farm)	1 slice	1	50	18%
Hearty (Pepperidge Farm)	1 slice	1	70	13%
7-Grain (Pepperidge Farm)				
Hearty 7-Grain	2 slices	2	180	9%
Light Style	1 slice	–	40	–
Seven Grain (Roman Meal)	1 slice	1	68	13%
Light	1 slice	.5	40	11%
Sour Dough	1 slice	.8	72	10%
French				
brown n'serve				
(Colombo)	2 oz	–	150	–
(Earth Grains)	1 slice	1	70	13%
mini loaf (Earth Grains)	1 oz	1	80	11%
Spoonbread-homemade				
w/whole-ground cornmeal	2 oz	7	117	54%
Sprouted Wheat (Pepperidge Farm)	2 slices	2	140	13%
Sun Grain (Roman Meal)	1 slice	1	68	13%
Sunflower & Bran (Monks' Bread)	1 slice	1	70	13%
Triticale	1 slice	.5	61	7%
12-Grain				
(Aunt Hattie's)	1 slice	< 1	100	4%
(Brownberry) Natural	1 slice	1	60	15%
Vienna				
(4¾x4x½")	1 slice	1	70	13%
(Pepperidge Farm) Light Style	2 slices	–	90	–

Food and Description	Amount	Fat Grams	Total Calories	% Fat Calories
(Weight Watchers)				
Cinnamon Raisin	1 slice	1	60	15%
Light Cinnamon Raisin	1 slice	< 1	40	11%
Multi-grain	1 slice	< 1	40	11%
thin slice	2 slices	< 1	80	6%
Oat Bran	1 slice	< 1	40	11%
Rye	1 slice	< 1	40	11%
thin slice	2 slices	< 1	40	6%
Wheat	1 slice	< 1	40	11%
thin slice	2 slices	< 1	80	6%
White	1 slice	< 1	40	11%
thin slice	2 slices	< 1	80	6%
Wheat				
(Brownberry)				
Golden	1 slice	< 1	40	11%
Natural	1 slice	1	80	11%
Soft	1 slice	1	70	13%
(Pepperidge Farm)				
Cracked				
Thin Sliced	1 slice	1	60	15%
Variety Breads	2 slices	2	140	13%
Family-2 lb loaf	2 slices	2	140	13%
Hearty Sesame	2 slices	3	190	14%
Light Style	2 slices	–	90	–
1½-lb loaf	2 slices	4	180	26%
Wheat Berry-Light				
(Rainbo/Colonial)	1 slice	.5	40	11%
(Roman Meal)	1 slice	–	39	–
White	1 slice	1	65	14%
(Brownberry)				
Natural Country	1 slice	2	100	18%
Soft	1 slice	2	80	23%
(Fresh Horizons)	1 slice	1	50	18%
Light				
(Rainbo/Colonial)	1 slice	.5	40	11%
(Roman Meal)	1 slice	–	40	–
(Pepperidge Farm)	1 slice	1.5	75	18%
Hearty Country (1½ lb)	2 slices	2	190	9%
Large Family-2 lb loaf	2 slices	2	140	13%
Thin Sliced Enriched	2 slices	4	160	23%
8 oz size	2 slices	2	140	13%
Very Thin Sliced	2 slices	–	80	–
Refrigerated Pipin' Hot (Pillsbury)	1 slice	2	70	26%
Sandwich (Pepperidge Farm)	2 slices	2	130	14%

Food and Description	Amount	Fat Grams	Total Calories	% Fat Calories
Sandwich (Roman Meal)	1 slice	1	55	16%
Toasting (Pepperidge Farm)	1 slice	1	90	10%
Very Thin (Earth Grains)	1 oz	1	80	11%
Whole Bran-Natural (Brownberry)	1 slice	1	60	15%
Whole Grain (Roman Meal)	1 slice	1	66	14%
Whole Wheat	1 slice	1	65	14%
(Earth Grains)-Very Thin	1 oz	1	70	13%
(Fresh Horizons)	1 slice	1	50	18%
homemade	1 slice	1.6	67	22%
pound loaf	1 slice	1	70	13%
(Pepperidge Farm)	1 slice	1	60	15%
Thin Sliced (Pepperidge Farm)	2 slices	2	120	15%
8 oz size	2 slices	2	120	15%
Very Thin (Pepperidge Farm)	2 slices	–	70	–
(Pillsbury)-Refrigerated Pipin' Hot	1 slice	2	80	23%
(Rainbo/Colonial)-Light	1 slice	.5	40	11%
(Roman Meal)	1 slice	1	66	14%
(Roman Meal)-Light	1 slice	–	40	–
(Sunbeam)-Reduced Calorie	1 slice	.5	40	11%
(Wonder)				
Brown'N Serve				
du Jour Austrian	1 slice	1	70	13%
du Jour French	1 slice	1	70	13%
Light Fat-Free				
Beefsteak Soft Rye	1 slice	–	40	–
Italian	1 slice	–	40	–
Sour Dough	1 slice	–	40	–
Wheat	1 slice	–	40	–
White	1 slice	–	40	–
Rye Breads-Wonder Rye, Beefsteak Onion Rye, Beefsteak Soft Rye, Beefsteak Hearty Rye, Beefsteak Mild Rye, Beefsteak Wheatberry Rye & Braun's Old Allegheny	1 slice	1	70	13%
Wheat Breads				
Beefsteak Hearty Wheat	1 slice	1	70	13%
Beefsteak Multigrain	1 slice	1	70	13%
Beefsteak Soft	1 slice	1	70	13%
Country Grain	1 slice	1	70	13%
Cracked Wheat	1 slice	1	70	13%
Family Wheat	1 slice	1	70	13%
Fresh & Natural	1 slice	1	70	13%
High Fiber Wheat	1 slice	–	40	–
(Home Pride)	1 slice	1	70	13%
(Home Pride) Butter Top	1 slice	1	70	13%

Food and Description	Amount	Fat Grams	Total Calories	% Fat Calories
(Home Pride)				
7 Grain	1 slice	1	70	13%
Stoneground	1 slice	1	70	13%
100% Whole Wheat	1 slice	1	70	13%
100% Whole Wheat-soft	1 slice	1	70	13%
Wheat Light	1 slice	–	40	–
White Breads				
Beefsteak Robust	1 slice	1	70	13%
Home Pride Butter Top	1 slice	1	70	13%
Wonder High Fiber	1 slice	–	40	–
Wonder Thin Sliced	1 slice	1	50	18%
Wonder White	1 slice	1	70	13%
Wonder White Light	1 slice	–	40	–
Wonder White w/Buttermilk	1 slice	1	70	13%
(Wonder) Specialty Breads				
Cinnamon Raisin	1 slice	1	80	11%
DiCarlo Parisian French	1 slice	1	70	13%
DiCarlo Sour Dough	1 slice	1	70	13%
Hollywood Dark	1 slice	1	70	13%
Hollywood Light	1 slice	1	70	13%
Oatmeal Goodness	1 slice	2	90	20%
Wonder Family Italian	1 slice	1	70	13%
Wonder French	1 slice	1	70	13%
BREAD COATINGS (See BAKE & FRY MIX; SEASONINGS)				
BREAD CRUMBS (See also BAKE & FRY MIX; SEASONINGS)				
(Contadina)-seasoned	1 cup	3.6	426	6%
	1 Tbs	–	35	–
(Friday's) Seasoned	1 oz		56	
Generic - dry	1 cup	5	390	12%
(Kellogg's) corn flake crumbs	1 oz	–	111	–
(Old London)	1 oz	2	210	9%
soft-cubes	1 cup	1	81	9%
soft-crumbs	1 cup	1	122	7%
(Progresso)				
plain	2 Tbs	< 1	60	8%
Italian	2 Tbs	< 1	60	8%
BREAD CUBES (Brownberry)	1 oz	1	110	8%
BREAD PUDDING (See PUDDING & MOUSSE)				
BREAD STICKS				
Brown 'N Serve				
Garlic	1	< 1	70	6%
Italian Soft Breadstick	1	1	80	11%
Sour Dough (Continental Baking)				
Bread du Jour	1	1	130	7%

Food and Description	Amount	Fat Grams	Total Calories	% Fat Calories
(Fattorie & Pandea)				
traditional	3	1	60	15%
whole wheat	3	1	57	16%
(Gorton's) Crunchier	4	12	190	57%
(Lance)				
Cheese	1	1	10	90%
Garlic	1	1	15	60%
Plain	1	1	15	60%
Sesame	2	1	15	60%
(Oroweat)				
Cheese	1 oz	2	110	16%
Garlic	1 oz	2	113	16%
Plain	1 oz	2	110	16%
Sesame	1 oz	2	120	15%
(Pillsbury) Refrigerated soft	1	2	100	18%
(Stella D'Oro)				
Onion	1	1	40	23%
Pizza	1	1	43	21%
Plain	1	1	41	22%
Sesame	3	7	170	29%
	1	2	51	35%
Wheat	1	1	42	21%
BREAD STUFFING (See also STUFFING)				
dry	1 cup	31	500	56%
moist	1 cup	26	420	56%
BREADFRUIT/raw	¼ small	–	99	–
	1 cup	.5	227	2%
BREAKFAST BARS (See also GRANOLA/GRANOLA-TYPE BARS)				
(Carnation) Breakfast Bars				
Chocolate chip	1 bar	11	200	50%
Chocolate crunch	1 bar	10	190	47%
Peanut butter crunch	1 bar	10	190	47%
Peanut butter w/chocolate chips	1 bar	11	200	50%
(Carnation) Slender				
Chocolate, Chocolate chip	1 bar	7	135	47%
Chocolate peanut butter, Vanilla	1 bar	7.5	135	50%
(Fi-Bar) A.M.				
Apple Oatmeal & Spice	1 bar	3	150	18%
Banana Nut	1 bar	4	150	24%
Raisin Nut	1 bar	4	150	24%
Strawberry Oatmeal Almond	1 bar	4	150	24%
(Grist Mill) Oat Bran Bar				
Cinnamon	1 bar	4	110	33%
Honey	1 bar	4	110	33%

Food and Description	Amount	Fat Grams	Total Calories	% Fat Calories
Peanut	1 bar	5	115	39%
(Health Valley)				
Fat-Free Fruit	1 bar	< 1	95	5%
Fruit & Fitness Energy	2 bars	5	200	23%
Oat Bran Fruit				
Apples/dates	1 bar	4	150	24%
Fruit & nuts	1 bar	4	150	24%
Raisin/cinnamon	1 bar	4	140	26%
(Jack La Lane) High Energy Bar				
Original	1 bar	6	165	33%
(Kelloggs) Nutri-grain				
Apple	1 bar	5	150	30%
Blueberry	1 bar	5	150	30%
Raspberry	1 bar	5	150	30%
Strawberry	1 bar	5	150	30%
(Nature's Wafers)				
Oat Bran Bars				
Chocolate Creme	1 bar	2	80	23%
Peanut Butter	1 bar	2	80	23%
Vanilla	1 bar	3	80	34%
Yogurt Bars				
Chocolate Creme	1 bar	2	80	23%
Strawberry	1 bar	2	80	23%
Vanilla	1 Bar	2	80	23%
(Pillsbury) Figurines				
Chocolate	1 bar	5	100	45%
Chocolate caramel	1 bar	6	100	54%
Chocolate peanut butter	1 bar	6	100	54%
S'Mores	1 bar	5	100	45%
Vanilla	1 bar	5	100	45%
(Smart Start) Cereal Bars				
Corn Flakes	1 bar	7	180	35%
Nutri Grain-blueberry	1 bar	7	170	37%
Nutri Grain-strawberry	1 bar	7	170	37%
Oat bran	1 bar	6	170	32%
Raisin Bran	1 bar	6	170	32%
Rice Krispies	1 bar	6	130	42%
Strawberry	1 bar	7	180	35%
(Sunbelt)				
Baked apple bar	1.31 oz bar	2	130	14%
Muesli	1 oz bar	1	100	9%
Peanut butter naturals	1.56 oz bar	13	240	49%
(Tiger's Milk)				
Peanut butter	1 bar	7	160	39%

Food and Description	Amount	Fat Grams	Total Calories	% Fat Calories
Peanut butter & honey	1 bar	5	160	28%
Protein rich	1 bar	6	160	34%
Raisin nut crunch	1 bar	9	170	48%
(Worthington) Natural Touch				
Caroby Milk Bar	1 bar	9	150	54%

BREAKFAST DRINK (*See also* BREAKFAST BARS, NUTRITIONAL SUPPLE-MENTS)

NOTE:Drinks and mixes prepared according to package directions.

Food and Description	Amount	Fat Grams	Total Calories	% Fat Calories
(Alba)				
Chocolate, Marshmallow, Milk				
Chocolate, Rich chocolate	1	1	110	8%
(Alba) 77 Fit n Frosty				
Chococolate	1	1	70	13%
Chocolate marshmallow	1	1	70	13%
Double fudge	1	1	70	13%
Strawberry & vanilla	1	–	70	–
(Carnation) Instant Breakfast				
Diet-no sugar				
Chocolate	1 envelope	1	70	13%
w/8 oz 2% milk	8 oz	6	190	28%
Chocolate malt	1 envelope	2	70	26%
w/8 oz 2% milk	8 oz	6	190	28%
Strawberry	1 envelope	–	70	–
w/8 oz 2% milk	8 oz	5	190	24%
Vanilla	1 envelope	–	70	–
w/8 oz 2% milk	8 oz	5	190	24%
Original				
Chocolate	1 envelope	1	130	7%
w/8 oz whole milk	8 oz	9	280	29%
Chocolate Malt	1 envelope	2	130	8%
w/8 oz whole milk	8 oz	10	280	32%
Coffee	1 envelope	–	130	–
w/8 oz whole milk	8 oz	8	280	26%
Strawberry	1 envelope	–	130	
w/8 oz whole milk	8 oz	8	280	26%
Vanilla	1 envelope	–	130	–
w/8 oz whole milk	8 oz	8	280	26%
(Carnation) Slender				
Can				
Banana, Chocolate, Chocolate malt,				
Chocolate fudge, Milk chocolate,				
Strawberry, Peach, Vanilla	10 oz	4	220	16%
Dry				
Chocolate	1 envelope	1	110	8%

Food and Description	Amount	Fat Grams	Total Calories	% Fat Calories
Dutch chocolate	1 envelope	1	110	8%
French vanilla	1 envelope	.5	110	4%
(Lucerne) Instant Breakfast				
Chocolate	1 serving	1	130	7%
Coffee	1 serving	–	130	–
Vanilla	1 serving	–	130	–
(Pillsbury) Instant Breakfast				
Chocolate, Chocolate malt				
Dry	1 package	–	130	–
w/8 oz whole milk	1 serving	9	290	28%
Strawberry				
Dry	1 package	–	130	–
w/ 8 oz whole milk	1 serving	9	290	28%
Vanilla				
Dry	1 package	–	130	–
w/ 8 oz whole milk	1 serving	9	300	27%

BREAKFAST SANDWICH (*See also* EGG MEALS; individual FAST FOOD listings)

Food and Description	Amount	Fat Grams	Total Calories	% Fat Calories
Biscuits				
(Hormel) New Traditions-frozen				
Bacon & Egg	1	9	220	37%
Chicken	1	10	280	32%
Egg, Bacon, & Cheese	1	13	280	42%
Ham & Egg	1	8	230	31%
Sausage	1	22	350	57%
Sausage & Egg	1	21	350	54%
Sausage & Cheese	1	27	420	58%
Steak	1	15	330	41%
(Jimmy Dean) microwaveable				
Chicken	1	8	170	42%
Sausage	1	14	210	60%
Steak	1	11	190	52%
(Great Starts)				
Egg, Canadian Bacon & Cheese	1	22	420	47%
Egg, Sausage & Cheese	1	28	460	55%
Sausage	1	22	410	48%
(Haugin's Farm) Sausage	1	11	180	55%
(Hormel) New Traditions				
Canadian bacon/egg/cheese	1	16	350	41%
Sausage & Egg	1	19	350	49%
(Owens) microwaveable				
Ham 'N Cheese	1	6	150	36%
Sausage'N Biscuit	1	14	210	60%
Smoked Sausage	1	12	200	54%
(Schwan's) Country Steak	1	24	430	50%

Food and Description	Amount	Fat Grams	Total Calories	% Fat Calories
(Weight Watchers) Sausage	1	11	220	45%
Muffins				
(Healthy Choice)				
English Muffin Sandwich	1	3	200	14%
Turkey Sausage Omelet	1	4	210	17%
Western-Style Omelet	1	3	200	14%
(Hormel) New Traditions-frozen				
Canadian Bacon, Egg, & Cheese	1	8	250	29%
Sausage, Egg, & Cheese	1	22	380	52%
(Jimmy Dean) microwaveable				
Ham & cheese	1	4	130	28%
Sausage	1	11	190	52%
(Weight Watchers) English				
Muffin Sandwich	1	8	230	31%
Other				
(Weight Watchers)				
Garden Vegetable Omelet Sandwich	1	6	210	26%
Ham & Cheese Bagel Sandwich	1	6	210	26%
Tacos				
(Owens) Border Breakfasts				
Ham	1	6	90	60%
Sausage	1	12	190	57%
BREATH MINTS (*See* CANDY)				
BROADBEAN				
boiled	½ cup	< 1	93	5%
canned	½ cup	< 1	91	5%
raw				
immature	8 oz	1	238	4%
mature	8 oz	3.8	766	5%
BROCCOLI				
cooked/chopped	½ cup	–	23	–
frozen				
(Pictsweet)				
Express microwave	2.5 oz	–	20	–
frozen/baby spears (Birds Eye)	3.3 oz	–	30	–
frozen/chopped	3.3 oz	–	25	–
(Pictsweet)	3.3 oz	–	25	–
frozen/cut				
(Harvest Fresh)	½ cup	–	18	–
frozen/cuts				
(Green Giant)	½ cup	–	12	–
(Pictsweet)	3.3 oz	–	25	–
frozen/Florentine				
(Pictsweet)	3.2 oz	–	30	–

Food and Description	Amount	Fat Grams	Total Calories	% Fat Calories
frozen/florets (Birds Eye)	3.3 oz	–	25	–
frozen/spears				
(Birds Eye)	3.3 oz	–	25	–
(Harvest Fresh)	½ cup	–	20	–
(Pictsweet)	3.3 oz	–	25	–
frozen individually/spears (Green Giant)	½ cup	–	12	–
frozen w/butter sauce	½ cup	–	58	–
raw/chopped	½ cup	–	12	–
BROCCOLI DISHES				
Broccoli Crisp				
frozen (Ore Ida)	3 oz	11	190	52%
Broccoli Cuts in Cheese Sauce				
One serving vegetables				
frozen (Green Giant)	5 oz	3	70	39%
Broccoli in Butter Sauce				
One serving vegetables				
frozen (Green Giant)	4.5 oz	2	45	40%
Broccoli in Cheese Sauce				
frozen (Birds Eye)	5 oz	6	120	45%
Broccoli in Cheese Sauce, frozen				
Micro Quick (Freshlike)	4.5 oz	3	70	39%
Broccoli in Cheese Flavored Sauce				
frozen (Green Giant)	½ cup	2	60	30%
Broccoli in Creamy Italian Sauce				
frozen (Birds Eye)	4.5 oz	6	90	60%
Broccoli in White Cheddar Cheese Flavored Sauce				
frozen (Green Giant)	½ cup	3	50	54%
Broccoli Stuffed Shells				
frozen (Celentano)	6.75 oz	15	280	48%
BROCCOLI SOUP (See SOUP)				
BROTWURST (See LUNCHEON MEAT)				
BROWNIES (See also COOKIE)				
Box Mix				
(Betty Crocker)				
Chocolate Chip Supreme	1	6	140	39%
Frosted (Stir'n Frost)	1	9	250	22%
Frosted Supreme	1	6	160	34%
Fudge (regular size)	1	6	150	36%
Fudge (family size)	1	5	140	32%
German Chocolate Supreme	1	7	160	39%
Supreme Fudge	1	6	140	39%
Walnut	1	7	140	45%
(Betty Crocker) Bake Shop Brownie Mix				
Caramel Pecan	1	8	220	33%

Food and Description	Amount	Fat Grams	Total Calories	% Fat Calories
Chunky Chocolate Walnut	1	10	230	39%
(Betty Crocker) Microwave				
Frosted	1	7	180	35%
Fudge	1	6	150	36%
Walnut	1	7	160	39%
(Betty Crocker) Microrave Singles				
w/hot fudge topping	1	12	350	31%
(Duncan Hines)				
Chewy Recipe Fudge	1	5	130	35%
Gourmet Truffle	1	13	280	42%
Gourmet Turtle	1	9	200	41%
Gourmet Vienna White	1	12	240	45%
Milk Chocolate	1	7	160	39%
Original Double Fudge	1	6	150	36%
Peanut Butter Fudge	1	8	150	48%
(Estee) 2"x2"	1	2	45	40%
(Pillsbury)				
Deluxe Family-Sized Fudge	2" square	7	150	42%
Deluxe Fudge Brownie	2" square	6	150	36%
Deluxe Fudge Brownie w/walnuts	2" square	8	150	48%
Lovin' Lites-Fudge	1	2	100	18%
Microwave				
Fudge brownie	1	9	190	43%
Fudge brownie w/chocolate				
fudge frosting	1	11	240	41%
Walnut brownie	1	12	210	51%
Microwave ready fudge brownie				
w/choc-flavored chips	1	9	180	45%
Ultimate Caramel Fudge Chunk	2" square	7	170	37%
Ultimate Chunky Triple Fudge	2" square	7	170	37%
Ultimate Double Fudge	2" square	6	160	34%
Ultimate Rocky Road Fudge	2" square	8	170	42%
Commercial-w/Frosting	~ ¾oz	4	100	36%
Frozen				
(Weight Watchers)				
Ala Mode	1 piece	4	180	20%
Chocolate	1.25 oz	3	100	27%
Cheesecake	3.5 oz	5	200	23%
Mint Frosted	1.23 oz	2	100	18%
Peanut Butter Fudge	1.23 oz	3	100	27%
Swiss Mocha Fudge	1.23 oz	2	90	20%
Homemade				
Butterscotch (1-3/4x1-3/4x7/8")	1	5	115	39%
w/Frosting (1-3/4x1-3/4x7/8")	1	6	95	57%

Food and Description	Amount	Fat Grams	Total Calories	% Fat Calories
Pouch Mix (Robin Hood/Gold Medal) prepared				
Fudge Brownie	1	4	100	36%
Ready-To-Eat				
Brownie Nut Bar (Bakery Wagon)	1 cookie	4	97	37%
Fudge (Little Debbie)	2 oz	8	260	28%
	3 oz	12	340	32%
Fudge Brownie (Break Cake)	1 brownie	18	370	44%
BRUSSELS SPROUTS				
fresh-cooked	½ cup	–	30	–
frozen				
(Green Giant)	½ cup	–	25	–
(Freshlike)	3.3 oz	–	35	–
(Pictsweet)	3.3 oz	–	35	–
(Pictsweet)				
Express Microwave	2.5 oz	–	30	–
frozen-cooked	½ cup	–	33	–
BRUSSELS SPROUTS DISHES				
Baby Brussels Sprouts in cheese sauce, frozen				
(Birds Eye)	4.5 oz	6	110	49%
Brussels Sprouts in butter sauce, frozen				
(Green Giant)	½ cup	1	40	23%
Brussels Sprouts in cheese flavored sauce, frozen				
(Green Giant)	½ cup	2	70	26%
BUCKWHEAT KERNELS				
Kasha roasted, (Wolff's) cooked	4 oz	1	170	5%
BUFFALO (BISON)/raw	3 oz	1.8	93	17%
BULGUR/hard red winter				
dry-canned				
seasoned	1 cup	4.5	246	17%
unseasoned	1 serving	.9	227	4%
generic				
cooked	1 cup	< 1	152	3%
uncooked	1 cup	3	600	5%
BURBOT/raw	3 oz	.68	76	8%
BURDOCK-root				
cooked	1 cup	< 1	110	4%
raw	1 cup	< 1	85	5%
BURGER-LIKE MEAL ENHANCER	~ 4 oz	< 1	90	5%
BURGER MIX	1 oz	.7	90	7%
BUTTER (*See also* BUTTER BLENDS, BUTTER SUBSTITUTE, MARGARINE)				
sweet/salted and unsalted	1 pat	4	36	100%
	1 Tbs	11	100	100%
	1 stick/			
	4 oz	92	810	100%

Food and Description	Amount	Fat Grams	Total Calories	% Fat Calories
(Hotel Bar/Keller's)	1 tsp	4	35	100%
(Land O'Lakes)	1 Tbs	11	100	100%
	1 tsp	4	35	100%
whipped	1 pat	3	27	100%
	1 stick/			
	4 oz	61	542	100%
	1 Tbs	9	81	100%
(Land O'Lakes)	1 Tbs	7	60	100%
	1 tsp	3	25	100%
BUTTER BEAN				
canned				
(Joan of Arc/Green Giant)	½ cup	–	80	–
(Luck's) Speckled/Seasoned				
w/Pork	7.5 oz	8	230	31%
(S&W)				
tender cooked-dry	½ cup	–	100	–
(Van Camp's)	1 cup	1	160	6%
BUTTER BLENDS				
(Blue Bonnet)				
Stick and Tub	1 Tbs	11	90	100%
	4 oz	44	360	100%
(Buttery Blend) liquid	1 Tbs	14	120	100%
(Downey's) Honey Butter				
Cinnamon	1 Tbs	1	50	18%
Original	1 Tbs	1	50	18%
(Kraft) Touch of Butter Spread				
bowl	1 Tbs	5.5	50	100%
stick-50% fat	1 Tbs	7	60	100%
(Land O'Lakes) Country Morning Blend				
stick				
light	1 tsp	2	20	100%
salted	1 Tbs	11	100	100%
unsalted	1 Tbs	11	100	100%
	1 tsp	4	35	100%
tub				
light	1 tsp	2	20	100%
salted	1 Tbs	10	90	100%
unsalted	1 Tbs	10	90	100%
	1 tsp	3	30	100%
(Land O'Lakes) Spread				
w/sweet cream	1 tsp	3	25	100%
BUTTER SUBSTITUTE				
Best of Butter/plain	½ tsp	< 1	4	100%
cheddar cheese flavor	½ tsp	< 1	6	75%

Food and Description	Amount	Fat Grams	Total Calories	% Fat Calories
sour cream flavor	½ tsp	< 1	4	100%
Butter Buds Butter Flavored Mix	1 Tbs= ½ oz	–	6	–
Butter Buds Sprinkles	½ tsp	–	4	–
Butter Flavored Salt	no set amount	–	–	–
Butter Spray (Weight Watchers)	1 second spray	< 1	2	100%
Butter Sprinkles (Molly McButter)	½ tsp	–	4	–
Imitation Butter Flavor Salt	no set amount	–	–	–
BUTTERBUR				
cooked	½ cup	< 1	8	56%
raw	1 cup	< 1	13	35%
BUTTERFISH				
raw	3 oz	6.8	124	49%
BUTTERNUTS				
dried	1 oz	16	174	83%

C

Food and Description	Amount	Fat Grams	Total Calories	% Fat Calories
CABBAGE				
Chinese				
raw/shredded	½ cup	–	5	–
fresh-cooked	½ cup	–	10	–
Red, raw/shredded	½ cup	–	10	–
Savoy, raw	1 cup	–	12	–
Spoon, raw	1 cup	–	37	–
Swamp, fresh-cooked	1 cup	–	21	–
White				
raw/shredded	½ cup	–	12	–
fresh-cooked	½ cup	–	16	–
CABBAGE DISHES				
Stuffed, homemade	~ 5 oz	18	310	52%

Food and Description	Amount	Fat Grams	Total Calories	% Fat Calories
CAKE AND CAKE PASTRIES (*See also* DONUT; MUFFINS; PASTRY SHEET; PASTRY SHELL; PASTRY,TOASTER; SNACK CAKES)				
(NOTE: Homemade cakes were made with vegetable shortening. Homemade frostings were made with margarine.)				
Angelfood (Break Cake)	1 oz	–	70	–
Angelfood-box mix				
(Betty Crocker)				
Confetti	1/12 cake	–	150	–
Lemon Custard	1/12 cake	–	150	–
Traditional	1/12 cake	–	130	–
White	1/12 cake	–	150	–
(Duncan Hines)	1/12 cake	–	140	–
Apple Cinnamon Coffee cake-box mix				
(Pillsbury)	1/8 cake	7	240	20%
Apple Fruit Squares-frozen				
(Pepperidge Farm)	1	12	220	49%
Applesauce	3 oz	12	400	27%
Baklava/homemade	2 oz	18	250	65%
Banana-frozen				
(Sara Lee)	1 slice	6	170	32%
Black Forest-frozen				
(Sara Lee)	1 slice	8	190	38%
(Weight Watchers)	3 oz	5	180	25%
Boston Cream Pie (*See also* PIE)				
frozen				
(Pepperidge Farm)	2⅞ oz	14	290	43%
(Weight Watchers)	3 oz	4	190	19%
Box mixes				
(Betty Crocker) Classics Dessert Mixes				
Boston Cream Pie	1/8 pkg	6	270	20%
Golden Pound Cake	1/12 cake	9	200	41%
Lemon Chiffon Cake	1/12 cake	4	200	18%
(Betty Crocker) Microwave box mixes w/frosting				
Chocolate Fudge				
w/vanilla frosting	1/6 cake	16	310	47%
Lemon w/lemon frosting	1/6 cake	16	300	48%
German Chocolate				
w/coconut pecan frosting	1/6 cake	17	310	49%
Devil's Food				
w/chocolate frosting	1/6 cake	16	300	48%
Golden Vanilla				
w/rainbow chip frosting	1/6 cake	16	310	47%
Yellow w/chocolate frosting	1/6 cake	16	300	48%
Pineapple Upside-Down Cake	1/8 cake	10	250	36%

Food and Description	Amount	Fat Grams	Total Calories	% Fat Calories
(Betty Crocker) Microwave Singles				
Chocolate w/chocolate frosting	1 cake	18	440	37%
Yellow w/chocolate frosting	1 cake	19	440	39%
(Betty Crocker) Pudding Cake Mixes				
Chocolate & lemon	⅙ cake	5	230	20%
(Betty Crocker) Snackin' Cake				
Applesauce Raisin	⅑ cake	6	190	28%
Banana Walnut	⅑ cake	7	200	25%
Golden Chocolate Chip	⅑ cake	5	190	24%
(Betty Crocker) Stir 'N Frost w/frosting				
Chocolate Devil's Food				
w/chocolate frosting	⅙ cake	5	210	21%
Spice Cake w/vanilla frosting	⅟₁₆ cake	9	280	28%
Yellow Cake w/chocolate frosting	⅟₁₆ cake	8	220	33%
(Betty Crocker) Supermoist				
Apple Cinnamon	⅟₁₂ cake	10	250	36%
Butter Brickle	⅟₁₂ cake	10	250	36%
Butter Pecan	⅟₁₂ cake	11	250	40%
Butter Recipe/chocolate	⅟₁₂ cake	13	270	43%
Butter Recipe/yellow	⅟₁₂ cake	11	260	38%
Carrot	⅟₁₂ cake	11	250	40%
Cherry Chip	⅟₁₂ cake	3	190	14%
Chocolate Chip	⅟₁₂ cake	14	280	45%
Chocolate Chocolate Chip	⅟₁₂ cake	12	260	42%
Chocolate Fudge	⅟₁₂ cake	12	260	42%
Devil's Food	⅟₁₂ cake	12	260	42%
German Chocolate	⅟₁₂ cake	12	260	42%
Golden Vanilla	⅟₁₂ cake	14	280	45%
Lemon	⅟₁₂ cake	11	260	38%
Marble	⅟₁₂ cake	11	250	40%
Milk Chocolate	⅟₁₂ cake	12	260	42%
Rainbow Chip	⅟₁₂ cake	11	250	40%
Sour Cream Chocolate	⅟₁₂ cake	12	260	42%
Sour Cream White	⅟₁₂ cake	3	180	15%
Spice	⅟₁₂ cake	11	260	38%
White	⅟₁₂ cake	9	240	34%
Yellow	⅟₁₂ cake	11	260	38%
(Betty Crocker) Supermoist Light Mixes				
Devils Food				
No Cholesterol	⅟₁₂ cake	3	180	15%
Standard Recipe	⅟₁₂ cake	4	190	19%
White	⅟₁₂ cake	3	180	15%
Yellow				
No Cholesterol	⅟₁₂ cake	3	180	15%

Food and Description	Amount	Fat Grams	Total Calories	% Fat Calories
Standard Recipe	1/12 cake	4	190	19%
(Dromedary) Carrot Cake	1 piece	15	232	58%
(Duncan Hines) Delights				
Devil's Food	1/12 cake	5	180	25%
Fudge Marble	1/12 cake	4	180	20%
Lemon	1/12 cake	4	180	20%
Yellow	1/12 cake	4	180	20%
(Duncan Hines) Original Directions				
Angel Food	1/12 cake	–	140	–
Butter Recipe				
Fudge	1/12 cake	13	270	43%
Golden	1/12 cake	13	270	43%
Dark Dutch Fudge	1/12 cake	15	280	48%
Devil's Food	1/12 cake	15	280	48%
Fudge Marble	1/12 cake	11	260	38%
French Vanilla	1/12 cake	11	260	38%
Lemon Supreme	1/12 cake	11	260	38%
Pineapple Supreme	1/12 cake	11	260	38%
Spice	1/12 cake	11	260	38%
Strawberry Supreme	1/12 cake	11	260	38%
Swiss Chocolate	1/12 cake	15	280	48%
White	1/12 cake	10	250	36%
Yellow	1/12 cake	11	260	38%
(Duncan Hines) Tiarra Dessert Mixes				
Black Forest Mousse	1/12 cake	13	260	45%
Cherries & Cream	1/12 cake	11	250	40%
Chocolate Mousse	1/12 cake	16	270	53%
Chocolate Amaretto Mousse	1/12 cake	16	270	53%
(Estee) Chocolate-box mix	1/10 cake	2	100	18%
all other flavors	1/10 cake	2	100	18%
(Pillsbury)				
Bundt Brand Ring				
Black Forest Cherry	1/16 cake	12	270	40%
Boston Cream	1/16 cake	10	260	35%
Chocolate Caramel	1/16 cake	13	290	40%
Chocolate Eclair	1/16 cake	10	260	35%
Chocolate Macaroon	1/16 cake	14	280	45%
Pineapple	1/16 cake	11	280	35%
Pound	1/16 cake	9	230	35%
Tunnel of Fudge	1/16 cake	16	310	46%
Tunnel of Lemon	1/16 cake	9	270	30%
Lovin' Lites				
Devil's Food				
Egg Recipe	1/12 cake	3	170	16%

Food and Description	Amount	Fat Grams	Total Calories	% Fat Calories
Egg White Recipe	1/12 cake	2	160	11%
White				
Egg Recipe	1/12 cake	3	180	15%
Egg White Recipe	1/12 cake	2	170	11%
Yellow				
Egg White Recipe	1/12 cake	2	170	11%
Egg Recipe	1/12 cake	3	180	15%
Lovin' Loaf-Angel Food	1/8 cake	–	90	–
Streusel Swirl				
Blueberry	1/16 cake	11	280	35%
Cinnamon	1/16 cake	11	260	38%
Lemon	1/16 cake	11	260	38%
(Pillsbury) Microwave box mixes				
Chocolate Cake	1/8 cake	13	210	56%
Double Chocolate Supreme	1/8 cake	19	330	52%
Double Lemon Supreme	1/8 cake	15	300	45%
Lemon	1/8 cake	13	220	53%
Streusel Swirl-Cinnamon	1/8 cake	11	240	41%
Tunnel of Fudge Bundt	1/8 cake	17	290	53%
Yellow	1/8 cake	13	220	53%
(Pillsbury) Microwave box mixes w/frosting				
Chocolate cake				
w/chocolate frosting	1/8 cake	17	300	51%
Chocolate cake				
w/chocolate fudge frosting	1/8 cake	17	300	51%
Chocolate cake				
w/vanilla frosting	1/8 cake	17	300	51%
Lemon cake w/lemon frosting	1/8 cake	17	300	51%
Yellow cake				
w/chocolate frosting	1/8 cake	17	300	51%
(Pillsbury) Microwave snack cakes				
Banana Walnut	1/9 cake	12	210	51%
Carrot	1/9 cake	11	200	44%
(Pillsbury Plus)				
Applesauce	1/12 cake	11	250	40%
Applesauce Spice	1/12 cake	11	250	40%
Banana	1/12 cake	11	250	40%
Butter Recipe	1/12 cake	12	260	42%
Carrot & Spice	1/12 cake	11	260	38%
Chocolate Chip	1/12 cake	14	270	47%
Confetti	1/12 cake	9	240	34%
Dark Chocolate	1/12 cake	12	250	43%
Devil's Food	1/12 cake	14	270	47%
Fudge Marble	1/12 cake	12	270	40%

Food and Description	Amount	Fat Grams	Total Calories	% Fat Calories
German Chocolate	1/12 cake	11	250	40%
Lemon	1/12 cake	11	250	40%
Strawberry	1/12 cake	11	260	42%
White				
Basic Recipe	1/12 cake	10	230	39%
No Cholesterol Recipe	1/12 cake	4	190	19%
Yellow	1/12 cake	12	260	42%
Brownie Cheese Cake/frozen				
(Weight Watchers)	3.5 oz	5	200	23%
Butterscotch Pecan-frozen				
(Pepperidge Farm)	1 5/8 oz	7	160	40%
Caramel Cake-homemade				
no icing (8" dia)	1/12 cake	10	218	42%
w/caramel icing	1/12 cake	12	315	34%
Carrot w/cream cheese frosting				
frozen				
(Pepperidge Farm)	1 3/8 oz	8	140	51%
(Sara Lee)	1 slice	13	260	45%
(Weight Watchers)	3 oz	5	170	27%
homemade (10"dia)	1/10 cake	21	385	49%
Cheesecake (9" dia)	1/12 cake	18	280	58%
Frozen				
(Sara Lee) French	1 slice	13	200	59%
(Weight Watchers)				
Cherries & Cream	3 oz	2	130	14%
Strawberry	3.9 oz	4	180	20%
Home recipe (9"dia)	1/12 cake	18	280	58%
Mix				
(Jell-O)				
8" w/whole milk	1/8 cake	13	280	42%
Real Fruit Topping				
Cherry/dry	1/8 pkg	4	220	16%
prepared w/whole milk	1/8 pkg	13	330	35%
New York-no bake	1/8 cake	14	290	43%
Strawberry/dry	1/8 pkg	4	220	16%
prepared w/whole milk	1/8 pkg	13	330	35%
(Royal)-No Bake				
Lite	1/8 cake	3	130	21%
Real	1/8 cake	3	160	17%
Ready-To-Serve				
(Formagg) Le Creme				
Amaretto/almond	2 oz	6	130	42%
Pineapple	2 oz	6	130	42%
Plain	2 oz	6	130	42%

Food and Description	Amount	Fat Grams	Total Calories	% Fat Calories
Strawberry	2 oz	6	130	42%
Chocolate				
frozen				
(Pepperidge Farm)	2⅞ oz	17	310	49%
(Sara Lee) Free & Light	1 slice/1 oz	–	110	–
(Weight Watchers)	2.5 oz	5	180	25%
homemade				
no icing (9"dia)	½₂ cake	13	272	43%
w/chocolate icing	½₂ cake	16	365	40%
Chocolate Fudge-frozen				
(Pepperidge Farm)	1⅝ oz	10	180	50%
Chocolate Fudge Stripe-frozen				
(Pepperidge Farm)	1⅝ oz	9	170	48%
Chocolate Mint-frozen				
(Pepperidge Farm)	1⅝ oz	9	170	48%
Chocolate Mousse-frozen				
(Sara Lee)	1 slice	14	200	63%
Cinnamon bun				
frosted	1/~ 2 oz	5	185	24%
plain	1/~ 2 oz	5	174	26%
refrig w/icing (Hungry Jack)	2	14	290	43%
refrig w/icing (Pillsbury)	1	4.5	115	35%
Coconut-frozen-(Pepperidge Farm)	1⅝ oz	8	180	40%
Coffeecake				
box mix				
(Pillsbury) Apple Cinnamon	⅛ cake	7	240	26%
crumb	~ 2.5 oz	7	230	27%
(Hostess) 97% fat free				
Cinnamon Crumb Coffee Cake	1 cake	1	80	11%
(Pillsbury) refrigerated-Streusel Coffee Cake				
Cinnamon Swirl	1 slice	11	230	43%
Pecan Crumb	1 slice	12	230	47%
(Sara Lee) frozen				
Apple Cinnamon	1 cake	13	290	40%
Butter Streusel	1 cake	12	230	47%
Pecan	1 cake	16	280	51%
(Weight Watcher) frozen				
Streusel w/cinnamon	2.25 oz	7	190	33%
Cottage Pudding/homemade				
no sauce	3 oz	8	251	29%
w/chocolate sauce	3 oz	8.7	315	25%
Cream Puff w/custard filling				
(3⅓" dia 2" high)	1	18	303	54%
shell only	2 oz	10	136	66%

Food and Description	Amount	Fat Grams	Total Calories	% Fat Calories
frozen (Rich's)	1	8	146	49%
Cupcakes (See SNACK CAKES)				
Danish /Sweet Rolls				
(Aunt Fanny's)				
Individual				
Caramel Nut	2 oz	6	190	28%
Cinnamon	2 oz	5	190	24%
Cinnamon Duals (1 roll)	1.9 oz	5	180	25%
Dixie Fruit Roll	2 oz	4	180	20%
Old Fashioned Apple Cinnamon	2 oz	4	180	20%
Rectangular (11 oz.)				
Cinnamon	2 oz	4	181	20%
Cinnamon Raisin	2 oz	3	181	15%
Pecan	2 oz	4	183	20%
Strawberry	2 oz	4	190	19%
(Break Cake)				
Cinnamon Nut Rolls	2-3 oz	11	330	33%
(Earth Grains)				
Apple	2 oz	8	210	34%
Bear Claw	2.25 oz	11	260	38%
Cheese	1.92 oz	10	220	41%
Cherry	1.92 oz	8	210	34%
Cinnamon	1.67 oz	9	200	41%
Raisin Nut	1.67 oz	10	210	43%
Generic				
Plain (4½" dia)	1/~2 oz	12	220	49%
w/Fruit (4½" dia)	1/~2oz	13	235	50%
(Hostess)				
Apple	1 piece	20	360	50%
Butterhorn	1 piece	18	330	49%
Raspberry	1 piece	7	270	23%
(Pillsbury)-refrigerated				
Best Quick Cinnamon	1	5	110	41%
Caramel w/nuts	1	8	160	45%
Cinnamon Raisin w/icing	1	7	150	42%
Orange	1	7	150	42%
(Sara Lee)-frozen				
Apple	1	6	120	45%
Apple (Free & Light)	1	–	130	–
Cheese	1	8	130	31%
Cinnamon Raisin	1	8	150	27%
Cinnamon Roll				
All Butter	1	10	230	39%
w/icing	1	10	290	31%

Food and Description	Amount	Fat Grams	Total Calories	% Fat Calories
(Weight Watchers)-frozen				
Apple Sweet Roll	4.5 oz	4	160	23%
Cheese Sweet Roll	5 oz	5	180	25%
Devil's Food				
frozen (Pepperidge Farm)	1⅝ oz	9	180	45%
homemade w/choc icing (9" dia)	1/16 cake	8	235	31%
Double Fudge Cake				
(Weight Watchers) frozen	2.75 oz	4	180	20%
Eclair				
Frozen				
(Rich's) chocolate	1 piece	10	210	43%
(Weight Watchers) chocolate	2.1 oz	4	120	30%
Generic				
chocolate icing/custard filling	1 piece	13.6	239	51%
(Entenmann's) Fat Free				
Apple Buns	1 bun	–	50	–
Apple Cinnamon Twist	1.1 oz	–	90	–
Apple Spice Cake	1 oz	–	80	–
Apricot Twist	1.1 oz	–	90	–
Banana Loaf	1.3 oz	–	90	–
Bavarian Creme Pastry	1.3 oz	–	80	–
Blueberry Cheese Coffee Cake	1 oz	–	90	–
Blueberry Crunch Coffee Cake	1 oz	–	70	–
Cheese Filled Crumb Coffee Cake	1.2 oz	–	90	–
Cherry Cheese Coffee Cake	1.3 oz	–	90	–
Cinnamon Apple Twist	1.1 oz	–	90	–
Cinnamon Ring	1 oz	–	80	–
Chocolate Loaf	1 oz	–	70	–
Cranberry Orange Cake	1 oz	–	70	–
Fudge Iced Chocolate Cake	1.3 oz	–	90	–
Fudge Iced Gold Cake	1.3 oz	–	90	–
Golden Chocolatey Chip Loaf	1 oz	–	80	–
Golden French Crumb Cake	1 oz	–	70	–
Golden Loaf	1 oz	–	70	–
Holiday Ring	1 oz	–	80	–
Lemon Twist Coffee Cake	1.1 oz	–	80	–
Louisiana Crunch	1 oz	–	80	–
Marble Loaf	1 oz	–	70	–
Orange Cake	1 oz	–	70	–
Pineapple Crunch Cake	1.3 oz	–	90	–
Pineapple Crunch Loaf	1.3 oz	–	90	–
Raspberry Cheese Buns	1 bun	–	50	–
Raspberry Cheese Pastry	1.3 oz	–	100	–
Raspberry Twist	1.1 oz	–	90	–

Food and Description	Amount	Fat Grams	Total Calories	% Fat Calories
(Entenmann's) Regular Bakery Line				
All Butter French Crumb	1.6 oz	8	180	40%
All Butter Pound	1 oz	5	110	41%
Apple Puffs	1 puff	13	280	42%
Cheese Coffee Cake	1.6 oz	7	150	42%
Cheese Filled Crumb Coffee Cake	1.4 oz	6	130	42%
Cheese Topped Buns	1 bun	12	240	45%
Cinnamon Buns	1 bun	10	230	39%
Cinnamon Filbert Ring	1.5 oz	12	190	57%
Crumb Coffee Cake	1.3 oz	7	160	39%
Danish Ring	1.5 oz	10	180	50%
Fudge Iced Devil's Food Cake	1.2 oz	5	130	35%
Lemon Danish Twist	1.2 oz	7	140	45%
Louisiana Crunch Cake	1.7 oz	8	180	40%
Pecan Danish Ring	1.5 oz	11	180	55%
Old Fashioned Apple Strudel	1.5 oz	5	120	38%
Raspberry Danish Twist	1.2 oz	7	140	45%
Sour Cream Pound Loaf	1 oz	7	120	53%
Thick Fudge Golden Cake	1.2 oz	6	130	42%
Walnut Danish Ring	1.5 oz	10	180	50%
Fruit Squares-frozen				
(Pepperidge Farm)				
Apple	1	12	220	49%
Blueberry	1	11	220	45%
Cherry	1	12	230	47%
Fruitcake				
homemade-dark (7.5" dia)	⅟₃₂ cake	7	165	38%
(Manor)				
plain	2 oz	11	240	41%
Cherry Rapture	2 oz	15	260	52%
deluxe	2 oz	6	210	26%
French Apple Walnut	2 oz	16	260	55%
Macadamia Surprise	2 oz	14	240	53%
German Chocolate				
(Pepperidge Farm)	1⅝ oz	10	180	50%
frozen				
(Weight Watchers)	2.5 oz	7	200	32%
Gingerbread				
box mix				
(Betty Crocker)	⅑ pkg	7	220	29%
(Pillsbury)	⅑ pkg	5	180	25%
homemade (8"square)	⅑ cake	4	175	21%
Golden-frozen				
(Pepperidge Farm)	1⅝ oz	9	180	45%

Food and Description	Amount	Fat Grams	Total Calories	% Fat Calories
Honey Buns				
(Aunt Fanny's)				
Apple Bear	4 oz	26	460	51%
Birdie, Jelly-filled	4 oz	24	450	48%
Bogie, Creme-filled	4 oz	27	460	53%
Honey Bun-regular	3 oz	20	360	50%
Lemon Bear	4 oz	23	440	47%
Snow Bear	4 oz	24	480	45%
(Break Cake)	1-3 oz	28	410	62%
Hot Cross Bun	2 oz	8	190	38%
Lemon-frozen (Pepperidge Farm)				
Coconut	3 oz	13	280	42%
Cream	1⅝ oz	9	170	37%
Napoleon	1 medium	15	285	47%
Peach Melba-frozen				
(Pepperidge Farm)	3⅛ oz	7	270	23%
(Pepperidge Farm) Dessert Light-individual servings-frozen				
Apple'n Spice	1 pkg	2	170	11%
Cherry Cake Supreme	1 pkg	2	170	11%
Lemon Cake Supreme	1 pkg	5	170	27%
Peach Parfait	1 pkg	5	150	30%
Raspberry Vanilla Swirl	1 pkg	5	160	28%
Strawberry ShortCake	1 pkg	5	170	27%
Pineapple Cream-frozen				
(Pepperidge Farm)	2 oz	7	190	33%
Pound-(8½x3½x3¼")	1/17 cake	5	120	38%
frozen				
Butter (Sara Lee)	1 slice	7	130	49%
Cholesterol Free (Pepperidge Farm)	1	6	110	49%
Free & Light (Sarah Lee)	1 slice/1 oz	–	70	–
w/blueberry topping				
(Weight Watchers)	2.5 oz	6	180	30%
mix (Martha White)	1/10 cake	4	120	30%
Prune Whip (baked) homemade				
hot	1 cup	–	140	–
cold	1 cup	–	203	–
Raspberry Mocha-frozen				
(Pepperidge Farm)	3⅛ oz	14	310	41%
(Sara Lee) Lights-frozen				
Chocolate Mousse	1 pkg	9	180	45%
Double Chocolate	1 pkg	5	160	28%
French Cheese Cake	1 pkg	6	180	30%
Lemon Cream Cake	1 pkg	7	190	33%
Strawberry Cheese Cake	1 pkg	4	160	23%

Food and Description	Amount	Fat Grams	Total Calories	% Fat Calories
Sheet cake				
w/no-cook white frosting (9"sq)	⅛ cake	14	445	28%
w/o frosting	⅛ cake	12	315	34%
Spice-w/brown sugar frosting				
homemade (9"dia)	⅒ cake	16	411	35%
Sponge-tube-no icing				
homemade (9¾" dia)	1/12 cake	3.8	196	17%
Strawberry Cream-frozen				
(Pepperidge Farm)	2 oz	7	190	33%
Strawberry French C'Cake-frozen				
(Sara Lee)	1 slice	11	200	50%
Strawberry Short Cake-frozen				
(Sara Lee)	1 slice	8	190	38%
(Weight Watchers)	3 oz	4	160	23%
Strudel				
(Aunt Fanny's) Individual				
Apple	3 oz	18	330	49%
Cherry	3 oz	16	320	45%
Sweet Rolls (*See* Danish/Sweet Rolls in this listing)				
Torte - chocolate (8½" dia)-homemade	1/16 cake	22	317	63%
Turnovers				
frozen (Pepperidge Farm)				
Apple	1	17	300	51%
Blueberry	1	19	310	55%
Cherry	1	19	310	55%
Peach	1	18	310	52%
Raspberry	1	17	310	49%
refrigerated (Pillsbury) All flavors	1	8	170	42%
Vanilla-frozen (Pepperidge Farm)	1⅝ oz	8	190	38%
White cake-homemade-				
w/white frosting (9" dia)	1/16 cake	9	260	28%
w/coconut frosting (9" dia)	1/16 cake	10	289	31%
Yellow cake-homemade				
w/caramel frosting (9" dia)	1/16 cake	9.5	293	29%
w/choc frosting (9" dia)	1/16 cake	11	245	40%
CAKE ICING				
■ DECORATORS-CAKE & COOKIE (Pillsbury)				
Chocolate	1 Tbs	2	60	30%
Other flavors	1 Tbs	2	70	26%
■ FROSTING-BOX MIX				
(Betty Crocker)				
Chocolate fudge	1/12 cake	6	180	30%
Chocolate fudge creamy	1/12 cake	6	170	32%
Chocolate sour cream	1/12 cake	8	160	45%
Coconut pecan	1/12 cake	8	150	48%

Food and Description	Amount	Fat Grams	Total Calories	% Fat Calories
Creamy cherry	1/12 cake	6	180	30%
Creamy milk chocolate	1/12 cake	5	170	27%
Creamy vanilla	1/12 cake	5	170	27%
Fluffy	1/12 cake	–	70	–
Lemon	1/12 cake	6	100	54%
Rainbow chip	1/12 cake	6	180	30%
Sour cream chocolate fudge	1/12 cake	6	180	30%
Sour cream white	1/12 cake	5	170	27%
(Estee) All flavors	1½ Tbs	1-2	50-60	18%-30%
(Pillsbury)				
Chocolate/Frost It Hot	1/8 cake	–	50	–
Coconut almond	1/12 cake	10	160	56%
Coconut pecan	1/12 cake	7	150	42%
Fluffy white	1/12 cake	–	60	–
Fluffy white/Frost It Hot	1/8 cake	–	50	–
■ FROSTING-READY-TO-SPREAD				
(Betty Crocker)				
Butter pecan	1/12 cake	7	170	37%
Caramel nut	1/12 cake	8	160	45%
Cherry	1/12 cake	6	160	34%
Chocolate	1/12 cake	7	160	39%
Chocolate chip	1/12 cake	7	170	37%
Coconut pecan	1/12 cake	9	160	51%
Cream cheese	1/12 cake	7	170	37%
Dark dutch fudge	1/12 cake	7	160	39%
Lemon	1/12 cake	6	170	32%
Milk chocolate	1/12 cake	6	160	34%
Rainbow chip	1/12 cake	7	170	37%
w/mini morsels	1/12 cake	7	170	37%
Rocky road	1/12 cake	7	150	42%
w/mini morsels	1/12 cake	8	160	45%
Sour cream chocolate	1/12 cake	7	160	39%
Sour cream white	1/12 cake	6	160	34%
Vanilla	1/12 cake	6	160	34%
(Betty Crocker) Creamy Deluxe				
Light Chocolate	1/12 cake	2	130	14%
Light Vanilla	1/12 cake	2	140	13%
Party Frosting				
Chocolate w/Dinosaurs	1/12 cake	7	160	39%
Vanilla w/Teddy Bears	1/12 cake	6	160	34%
(Duncan Hines)				
Chocolate	1/12 cake	7	160	39%
Cream cheese	1/12 cake	8	160	45%
Dark Dutch fudge	1/12 cake	7	160	39%
Milk chocolate	1/12 cake	7	160	39%

Food and Description	Amount	Fat Grams	Total Calories	% Fat Calories
Polka dot pink & vanilla	1/12 cake	7	160	39%
Vanilla	1/12 cake	7	160	39%
(Pillsbury)				
Frosting supreme				
Butter fudge	1/12 cake	6	140	39%
Caramel pecan	1/12 cake	8	150	48%
Chocolate chip	1/12 cake	4	150	24%
Chocolate fudge	1/12 cake	6	150	36%
Coconut almond	1/12 cake	9	150	54%
Coconut pecan	1/12 cake	10	160	56%
Cream cheese	1/12 cake	6	160	34%
Double Dutch	1/12 cake	6	140	39%
Funfetti				
Chocolate	1/12 cake	6	140	39%
Pink	1/12 cake	6	150	36%
Sunshine vanilla	1/12 cake	6	150	36%
Vanilla	1/12 cake	6	150	36%
Lemon	1/12 cake	6	160	34%
Milk chocolate	1/12 cake	6	150	36%
Strawberry	1/12 cake	6	160	34%
Swirl				
Milk chocolate w/fudge	1/12 cake	6	150	36%
Vanilla w/fudge	1/12 cake	6	150	36%
Vanilla	1/12 cake	6	160	34%
(Lovin' Lites)				
Chocolate fudge	1/12 cake	2	130	14%
Milk chocolate	1/12 cake	2	130	14%
Vanilla	1/12 cake	2	130	14%
■ FROSTING-STANDARD HOME RECIPE (USDA)				
Boiled	1/4 cup	–	74	–
Caramel	1/4 cup	6	306	18%
Chocolate	1/4 cup	9.5	259	33%
Coconut	1/4 cup	3	151	18%
White	1/4 cup	5	300	15%
CALIFORNIA RED BEAN/boiled	1/2 cup	–	109	–
CANDY				
Almond Joy (Peter Paul)	1.76 oz	14	250	50%
(Andes) Creme De Menthe	1 oz	9	150	54%
Baby Ruth	1 oz	6	130	42%
Baby Ruth	2.2 oz	13	300	39%
nuggets	1 oz	6	130	42%
Bar None	1.5 oz	14	240	53%
Bit-O-Honey Bar (Nestle)	1.7 oz	4	200	18%
Black Cow-sucker	1 oz	3	127	21%
Bonkers!/all flavors	1	–	20	–

Food and Description	Amount	Fat Grams	Total Calories	% Fat Calories
(Bounty) dark chocolate & coconut bar	2.1 oz	8	150	48%
milk chocolate & coconut bar	2.1 oz	8	150	48%
(Brach's) candies				
Bridge Mix	1 oz	6	130	42%
Broxie-Big	1 oz	8	150	48%
Little	1 oz	8	150	48%
Butterscotch Disks	1 oz	–	110	–
Candy corn	1 oz	–	100	–
Chocolate Covered Buttercream Egg	1 oz	3	120	23%
Chocolate Covered Chelsea Chips	1 oz	6	140	39%
Chocolate Covered Cherries	1 oz	2	110	16%
Chocolate Covered Cherry Cream Egg	1 oz	2	110	16%
Chocolate Covered Coconut Cream Egg	1 oz	3	110	16%
Chocolate Covered Fruit & Nut Cream Egg	1 oz	2	110	16%
Chocolate Covered Maple Cream Eggs	1 oz	2	110	16%
Chocolate Covered Mint Patties	1 oz	2	110	16%
Chocolate Covered Vanilla Cream	1 oz	2	110	16%
Chocolate Covered Mint Cremes	1 oz	2	110	16%
Chocolate Covered Mints	1 oz	2	110	16%
Chocolate Covered Orange Sticks	1 oz	2	110	16%
Chocolate Covered Thin Mints	1 oz	2	110	16%
Chocolate Creme Cherries	1 oz	2	110	16%
Chocolate Jots	1 oz	5	130	35%
Chocolate Malted Milk Eggs	1 oz	5	130	35%
Christmas Jots	1 oz	5	130	35%
Christmas Mint Pearls	1 oz	1	110	8%
Christmas Nougats	1 oz	2	110	16%
Christmas Ornaments	1 oz	8	150	48%
Cinnamon Disks	1 oz	–	110	–
Cinnamon Imperials	1 oz	–	110	–
Coffee	1 oz	2	120	15%
Crazy Pumpkin Heads	1 oz	1	100	9%
Creme De Menthe Mint	1 oz	9	150	54%
Dark Chocolate Covered Cherries	1 oz	2	110	16%
Dark Chocolate Cov'd Hulachews	1 oz	8	140	51%
Dark Chocolate Nonpariels	1 oz	6	140	39%
Dark Chocolate X-Mas Nonpariels	1 oz	6	140	39%
Dessert Mints	1 oz	–	110	–
Easter Nougats	1 oz	1	100	9%
Filled Peanuts	1 oz	1	110	8%

Food and Description	Amount	Fat Grams	Total Calories	% Fat Calories
French Burnt Peanuts	1 oz	7	150	30%
Fruit Bunch	1 oz	–	100	–
Gumdinger Gum Balls	1 oz	2	110	16%
Gummy Worms	1 oz	–	100	–
Heart Box Candies	1 oz	2	110	16%
Holiday Mints	1 oz	1	110	8%
Jelly Beans	1 oz	–	100	–
Jelly Nougats	1 oz	1	100	9%
Jordan Apples	1 oz	2	120	15%
Jube Jels	1 oz	–	100	–
Lemon Drops	1 oz	–	110	–
Lollydrops	1 oz	–	110	–
Love	1 oz	8	150	48%
Kentucky Mints	1 oz	–	110	–
Licorice Twists	1 oz	1	100	9%
Marshmallow Eggs	1 oz	3	120	23%
Marshmallow Rabbits	1 oz	3	120	23%
Marshmallow Santas	1 oz	3	120	23%
Milk Chocolate Cashew Clusters	1 oz	5	130	35%
Milk Chocolate Covered Cherries	1 oz	2	110	16%
Milk Chocolate Covered Malt Balls	1 oz	5	130	35%
Milk Chocolate Covered Peanuts	1 oz	9	150	54%
Milk Chocolate Covered Putters	1 oz	9	150	54%
Milk Chocolate Peanut Clusters	1 oz	9	150	54%
Milk Chocolate Stars	1 oz	8	150	48%
Milk Maid Caramels	1 oz	2	110	16%
chocolate	1 oz	3	110	25%
Mint Filled Straws	1 oz	1	110	8%
Mint Jots	1 oz	2	120	15%
Mint Parfait	1 oz	9	150	54%
Mint Pearls	1 oz	2	120	15%
Neapolitan Coconuts	1 oz	2	120	15%
Nut Goodies	1 oz	4	130	28%
Orangettes	1 oz		100	
PBM Easter Eggs	1 oz	10	160	56%
PBM Heart	1 oz	9	150	54%
PBM Santas	1 oz	10	160	56%
PBM Squares	1 oz	9	150	54%
Panned Peanuts	1 oz	7	140	45%
Pastel Fiesta Eggs	1 oz	3	120	23%
Peanut Caramel Clusters	1 oz	8	150	48%
Peanut Clusters	1 oz	9	150	54%
Peanut Butter Kisses	1 oz	2	110	16%
Peanut Jots	1 oz	6	140	39%

Food and Description	Amount	Fat Grams	Total Calories	% Fat Calories
Peanut Parfait	1 oz	10	160	56%
Peanuts-chocolate covered	1 oz	10	160	56%
small	1 oz	7	140	45%
Peppermint Kisses	1 oz	1	100	9%
Petite	1 oz	9	150	54%
Raisins-chocolate covered	1 oz	5	130	35%
Red Laces	1 oz	–	100	–
Red Twists	1 oz	–	100	–
Robin's Eggs	1 oz	6	140	39%
Royals	1 oz	2	110	16%
Salt Water Taffy	1 oz	1	100	9%
Santa's Assortment	1 oz	2	110	16%
Santas-foiled-tray of 8	1 oz	7	140	45%
Snappy Tarts	1 oz	–	100	–
Solid Chocolate Eggs	1 oz	8	150	48%
Solid Chocolate Bells-foiled	1 oz	8	150	48%
Spearmint Leaves	1 oz	–	100	–
Spicettes	1 oz	–	100	–
Starlight Mints	1 oz	–	110	–
Targets	1 oz	3	120	23%
Ting-A-Ling	1 oz	8	150	48%
Toffee	1 oz	2	110	16%
Valentine Hearts	1 oz	2	110	16%
Valentine Nougat Kisses	1 oz	2	110	16%
Breath Savers Mints-sugar-free all flavors	1	–	8	–
Butterfinger	1 oz	5	134	34%
	2 oz	11	270	37%
Butternut	2 oz	13	270	43%
Butterscotch (Cadbury)	1 oz	1	113	8%
Dairy Milk	1 oz	8	150	48%
Roasted Almond	1 oz	9	150	48%
Candy Corn	¼ cup	1	180	5%
Carmello (Cadbury's)	1 oz	7	140	45%
Caramels (Kraft)	1	1	30	30%
Chocolate Fudgies	1	1	35	26%
(Storck) Chocolate Riesen	1 oz	4.7	130	33%
Caravelle	1 oz	5	127	35%
Charleston Chew/all flavors	2 oz	6	240	23%
Cherries-chocolate covered	1	3	90	30%
	1 oz	4	126	29%
Cherry Bites (Y&S)	1 oz	< 1	100	5%

Food and Description	Amount	Fat Grams	Total Calories	% Fat Calories
Chocolate				
dark sweet	1 oz	10	150	60%
milk-plain	1 oz	9	145	50%
milk w/almonds	1 oz	10	150	60%
milk w/peanuts	1 oz	11	155	64%
milk w/rice cereal	1 oz	7	140	45%
Roast Almonds (Cadbury)	1 oz	9	150	54%
Special Dark (Hershey)	1 bar	12	220	49%
Chocolate Covered Almonds	1 oz	12	161	67%
Peanuts (Nestle) Goobers	1⅜ oz	13	220	53%
Chocolate-Discs-sugar coated	1 oz	5.6	132	38%
Chocolate Mint Patty	1	1	50	18%
Chuckles-jellied candied				
fruit flavors	1 oz	–	100	–
jellied eggs	1 oz	–	110	–
Jujubes	1 oz	–	110	–
Juju Softees	1 oz	–	100	–
Licorice	1 oz	–	100	–
Chunky-milk chocolate	1 oz	4	120	30%
original	1 oz	7	143	44%
peanut	1 oz	9	151	54%
pecan	1 oz	8	148	49%
Clark Bar	1 oz	5	134	34%
Divinity (Home Recipe)	.5 oz	–	38	–
(Estee)				
Chocolate Covered Raisins	6 pieces	2	30	60%
Crunch Chocolate Bar	2 squares	3	45	60%
Estee-ets	5 pieces	2	35	51%
Gummy Bears	4 pieces	–	20	–
(Featherweight) Sweet Pretenders				
Chewy Caramels	1 piece	1	30	30%
Chocolate-flavored Almond Bar	¼ bar	7	90	70%
	2 oz	28	360	70%
Chocolate-flavored Crunch Bar	¼ bar	8	80	68%
	2 oz	24	320	68%
Milk Chocolate-flavored Bar	¼ bar	6	80	68%
	2 oz	24	320	68%
Peppermint Swirls	1 piece	–	20	–
5th Avenue	2 oz	12	280	39%
	1.16 oz/ 2 bars	7	160	39%
Fruit & Nut Bar (Cadbury)	1 oz	8	150	48%
Fudge-caramel & peanuts	1 oz	5	123	37%
chocolate	1 oz	4.5	122	33%

Food and Description	Amount	Fat Grams	Total Calories	% Fat Calories
chocolate w/nuts	1 oz	5.9	128	42%
vanilla	1 oz	3	113	24%
vanilla w/nuts	1 oz	5	120	38%
Golden Almond Chocolate Bar				
(Hershey)	1.5 oz	16	240	60%
Good & Plenty	1 oz	< 1	106	4%
Gum Drops/all flavors	1 oz	–	100	–
(Estee)	4 pieces	–	25	–
Hard candy	1 oz	–	110	–
(Estee)	2 pieces	–	25	–
Hot Tamales	1 oz	–	109	–
Jaw Breaker	1	–	20	–
Jelly Beans/all flavors	1 oz	–	100	–
	1 cup	1	807	1%
Junior Mints	1 oz	3	120	23%
Kisses (Hershey's) plain	1 kiss	1	25	36%
	9 pieces	13	220	53%
	1 oz/			
	~6 pieces	9	150	54%
w/almonds	1 oz	10	160	56%
Kit-Kat	2/snack size	9	170	48%
	1.5 oz	12	230	47%
Krackel Chocolate Bar	1.45 oz	12	220	49%
	1.65 oz	14	250	50%
Kudos, Nutty Fudge	1 oz	12	200	54%
Licorice-black	1 oz	< 1	100	5%
Life Savers-all flavors				
holes	1	–	2	–
lollipops				
assorted	1	–	45	–
Easter pastels	1	–	40	–
roll candy	1 piece	–	8	–
Lollipops (Estee)	1	–	25	–
M & M's				
Almond	1.3 oz	10	200	45%
Baking & decorating pack	1 oz	6	140	38%
Creamy Peanut	1 oz	7	140	45%
Mint	1 oz	6	140	39%
Peanut	1.6 oz	12	240	45%
Plain	1 oz	6	140	39%
Malt Balls-chocolate covered	2 pieces	4	50	72%
Marathon	1.38 oz	7	179	35%
Mars Bar	1.76 oz	11	240	41%
Mike & Ike	1 oz	–	109	–

Food and Description	Amount	Fat Grams	Total Calories	% Fat Calories
Milk Chocolate Bar				
(Hershey)	1.55 oz	14	240	53%
w/almonds	1.45 oz	14	230	55%
	1.75 oz	17	280	55%
(Nestle)	1.45 oz	13	220	53%
w/almonds	1.45 oz	14	230	55%
Milk Chocolate Stars	1 oz	8	160	45%
Milk Duds	1 oz	4	129	28%
Milk Shake	2 oz	8	250	29%
Milky Way (Mars)	3.63 oz	18	470	35%
	1.76 oz	11	240	41%
Dark	1.76 oz	8	220	33%
Fun Size	1 bar	4	110	33%
Mint Non Pariels	1 oz	9	150	54%
Mints (Kraft)				
Butter	1	–	8	–
Party	1	–	8	–
Mounds Bar (Hershey)	1.9 oz	14	260	48%
Mr. Goodbar	1.65 oz	16	260	55%
My Buddy	1.8 oz	13	250	47%
(Nestle) Chunky Bar	1.4 oz	12	210	51%
(Nestle) Crunch Bar	1.4 oz	10	210	43%
Snack Size Mini Bars	3 bars	8	160	45%
Nutcracker	1 oz	10	161	56%
Oh Henry! (Nestle)	2 oz	14	280	45%
PB Max	1.48 oz	16	240	60%
(Panda) Licorice	3.5 oz	< 1	340	1%
Raspberry-Flavored Chew	3.5 oz	< 1	340	1%
Pay Day	1.9 oz	12	250	43%
Park Avenue	1.8 oz	9	230	35%
Peanut Brittle				
(Estee)	¼ oz	1	35	26%
(Kraft)	1 oz	5	130	35%
Peanut Butter Cups				
(Estee)	1	3	40	68%
(Reese's)	1.8 oz/ 2 cups	17	280	55%
Miniatures	6 cups	14	230	55%
Snack Size	1 bar	6	100	54%
Peanuts-yogurt covered	1 oz	9	125	65%
(Pearson's) Carmel Nip	4 pieces	3	120	23%
Chocolate Parfait	4 pieces	3	120	23%
Coffee Nip	4 pieces	3	120	23%
Licorice Nip	4 pieces	3	120	23%

Food and Description	Amount	Fat Grams	Total Calories	% Fat Calories
Penuchi	1 oz	4	120	30%
Peppermint Patties				
(Nabisco)	1 oz	1	110	8%
(York)	1 oz	3	120	23%
(Planters)				
Old Fashioned Peanut Candy	1 piece	9	140	58%
Peanut Bar	1.6 oz	11	230	43%
Honey Roasted	1.6 oz	13	230	51%
Sweet'N Crunchy	1.6 oz	15	250	54%
Pom Poms	1 oz	3	100	27%
Power House	1 oz	5	130	35%
	2 oz	11	260	38%
Pralines	1 oz	3	90	30%
Raisinets (Nestle)				
milk chocolate covered	1.6 oz	7	200	32%
	1 oz	5	130	35%
Reese's Peanut Butter Cups/Crunchy	1.8 oz/ 2 cups	18	200	81%
Reese's Pieces (Hershey)	1.95 pkg	11	270	37%
Rolo chocolate caramels (Hershey)	9 pieces	12	270	40%
Skittles				
Fruit	1 oz	1	120	8%
Fruit Fun Bag	2.3 oz	2	270	7%
Skor Toffee Bar	1.4 oz	14	220	57%
Slo Poke	1 sucker	2	124	15%
Snickers (Mars)				
peanut butter	1.75 oz	18	280	58%
plain	Fun Size	5	110	41%
	2.07 oz	14	280	45%
	3.7 oz	24	500	43%
Sno Caps-sweet chocolate nonpareils				
(Nestle)	2.3 oz	13	320	37%
(Sorbee)				
sour lemon	1	–	12	–
wintergreen	1	–	12	–
Starbar	1 oz	7	140	45%
Starburst Fruit Chews	2 oz	5	240	19%
Sugar Babies	1 pkg	2	180	10%
Sugar Daddy	1	1	150	6%
Sugar Mama	¾ oz	3	90	30%
Summit	.76 oz	6	100	54%
Symphony (Hershey)				
milk chocolate	1.4 oz	13	220	53%
	1.75 oz	16	270	53%

Food and Description	Amount	Fat Grams	Total Calories	% Fat Calories
milk choc w/almonds & toffee chips	1.4 oz	14	220	57%
	1.75 oz	17	280	54%
Taffy	1 oz	1	100	9%
Thin Mint (Nabisco)	1	1	42	21%
Thousand Grand	1.5 oz	8	200	36%
3 Musketeers	1 oz	4	120	30%
	2.13 oz	9	260	31%
Toffee (Kraft)	1	1	30	30%
Tootsie Roll	1 small	–	28	–
	1 large	2.6	127	18%
Truffles (Home Recipe)	.5 oz	4	59	61%
Turtles (Demet's)	1 piece	3	82	33%
Twix				
Caramel	2 oz/2 bars	14	280	45%
Chocolate Fudge	1 bar	8	130	55%
Cookies-n-Creme	1 bar	7	120	52%
Peanut Butter	1.71 oz/ 2 bars	16	260	55%
Twizzlers-Strawberry (Y&S)	1 oz	< 1	100	5%
Vanilla Creams	1 oz	4.8	123	35%
Whatchamacallit	1.8 oz	13	260	45%
White Chocolate (Nestle)				
Alpine w/almonds	1.3 oz	13	200	59%
Zagnut	1 oz	4	131	28%
Zero	2 oz	8	250	29%
CANNELLINI BEAN (See KIDNEY BEAN, WHITE)				
CANTALOUPE				
~ 9.5 oz wt	½ fruit	.7	94	7%
pieces	1 cup	< 1	57	8%
CAPOCOLLO (See LUNCHEON MEAT)				
CAPON				
giblets-simmered	5 oz	7.8	238	30%
meat & skin-roasted	~1.5 lb	74	1457	46%
	3.5 oz	11.7	229	46%
meat only-roasted	3.5 oz	8.8	178	44%
CARAWAY SEEDS	1 tsp	–	8	–
CARDAMOM SEEDS	1 tsp	–	6	–
CARDOON				
cooked	3 oz	–	19	–
raw-shredded	1 cup	–	35	–
CARIBOU/raw-boneless	3 oz	5	159	28%
CARISSA (Natal Plum) raw	1	–	12	–
CAROB CHIPS	1 oz	7	140	45%
Mint	1 oz	7	140	45%

Food and Description	Amount	Fat Grams	Total Calories	% Fat Calories
CAROB POWDER				
(Chatfield's)	¼ cup/ 1 oz	–	96	–
(El Molino)	¼ cup	–	110	–
CARP				
cooked-dry heat	3 oz	6	138	39%
breaded & fried	3 oz	12	226	48%
raw	3 oz	4.76	108	40%
roe-raw	3 oz	1.7	111	14%
smoked	1 oz	1.8	50	32%
CARROT				
canned	½ cup	–	20	–
canned-fingerling				
(Thank You)	½ cup	–	30	–
canned-Julienne French Style				
Fancy (S&W)	½ cup	–	30	–
Whole Tiny Fancy (S&W)	½ cup	–	30	–
canned-sliced				
(Nutradiet)	½ cup	–	30	–
canned-sliced-Fancy				
(S&W)	½ cup	–	30	–
cooked-slices	½ cup	–	35	–
crinkle sliced				
(Freshlike)	½ cup	–	30	–
diced				
(S&W)	½ cup	–	30	–
diced, sliced, or whole				
(Del Monte)	½ cup	–	30	–
fresh-cooked	1	–	21	–
frozen-cooked	½ cup	–	26	–
Parisienne (C & W)	½ cup	–	37	–
raw	1	–	31	–
raw-shredded	½ cup	–	24	–
sliced				
(Pictsweet)	3.3 oz	–	40	–
(Pictsweet) Express Microwave	2.5 oz	–	30	–
whole baby				
(Birds Eye)	½ cup	–	40	–
(Pictsweet)	2.5 oz	–	30	–
CARROT DISHES				
Glazed Carrots, frozen				
(Birds Eye) Specialty Classics	5 oz	9	180	45%
CARROT JUICE /canned	6 oz	–	73	–
(Hain)	6 oz	–	60	–

Food and Description	Amount	Fat Grams	Total Calories	% Fat Calories
(Hollywood)	6 oz	–	60	–
CASABA MELON				
~ 6 oz wt	1/10 fruit	–	43	–
pieces	1 cup	< 1	45	10%
CASHEW				
dry roasted	1 oz	13	163	72%
(Guy's) whole salted	1 oz	14	170	74%
honey roasted				
(Eagle)	1 oz	12	170	64%
lightly salted	1 oz	14	170	74%
mixed w/peanuts	1 oz	13	170	69%
(Planters)	1 oz	12	170	64%
honey roasted/peanut cashew mix	1 oz	13	170	69%
(Planters)	1 oz	12	170	64%
oil roasted	1 oz	14	163	77%
(Planters)				
dry roasted	1 oz	13	160	73%
unsalted	1 oz	13	60	73%
oil roasted-fancy	1 oz	14	170	74%
oil roasted halves	1 oz	14	170	74%
unsalted	1 oz	14	170	74%
CASHEW BUTTER				
plain	1 oz	14	167	75%
	1 Tbs	8	94	77%
raw (Hain)				
regular	2 Tbs	15	190	71%
unsalted	2 Tbs	19	210	81%
toasted (Hain)	2 Tbs	17	210	73%
CATFISH (*See also* SEAFOOD ENTREE/DINNER)				
baked or broiled	3 oz	7	149	42%
cooked-breaded & fried	3 oz	11	194	51%
raw	3 oz	3.6	99	33%
CATSUP/Ketchup	1 cup	1	290	3%
	1 Tbs	–	15	–
(Del Monte) tomato	1/4 cup	–	60	–
(Hain) natural or no salt added	1 Tbs	–	16	–
(Heinz)				
Hot tomato	1 Tbs	–	18	–
Lite tomato	1 Tbs	–	8	–
Low Sodium tomato	1 Tbs	–	8	–
Regular tomato	1 Tbs	–	18	–
(Hunt's) tomato	1 Tbs	–	16	–
(Smucker's) tomato	1 tsp	–	8	–
(Weight Watchers) tomato	1 Tbs	–	15	–

Food and Description	Amount	Fat Grams	Total Calories	% Fat Calories
CAULIFLOWER				
fresh-cooked	½ cup	–	15	–
frozen-cooked	½ cup	–	17	–
frozen				
(Birds Eye)	½ cup	–	25	–
(Green Giant)	½ cup	–	12	–
(Freshlike)	3.3 oz	–	25	–
(Pictsweet)	3.3 oz	–	25	–
florets	3.2 oz	–	20	–
Hot & Spicy (Vlasic)	1 oz	–	4	–
raw	½ cup	–	12	–
sweet (Vlasic)	1 oz	–	35	–
CAULIFLOWER DISHES				
Cauliflower Crisp, frozen				
(Ore Ida)	3 oz	9	150	54%
Cauliflower in butter sauce				
(Green Giant)	½ cup	1	30	30%
Cauliflower in cheese flavored sauce				
frozen (Green Giant)	½ cup	2	60	30%
Cauliflower in cheese sauce, frozen				
(Birds Eye)	5 oz	6	110	49%
(Freshlike) Micro Quick	4.5 oz	3	70	39%
Cauliflower in cheese sauce				
one serving vegetables/frozen				
(Green Giant)	5.5 oz	2	80	23%
Cauliflower in cheese sauce Singles				
frozen (Stokely)	4 oz	3	70	39%
Cauliflower in White Cheddar cheese				
flavored sauce, frozen				
(Green Giant)	½ cup	2	50	36%
CAULIFLOWER SOUP (*See* SOUP)				
CAVIAR/ Black & Red				
granular	1 Tbs	3	40	68%
	1 oz	5	71	63%
pressed	1 Tbs	2.8	54	47%
	1 oz	4.7	90	47%
CELERIAC ROOT (wild celery) raw	4 or 5	–	40	–
	½ cup	–	31	–
CELERY				
cooked	½ cup	–	11	–
frozen (Freshlike)	3.5 oz	–	14	–
raw	1 stalk	–	6	–
	½ cup	–	9	–
CELERY SEED	1 tsp	.5	8	56%

Food and Description	Amount	Fat Grams	Total Calories	% Fat Calories

CELERY SOUP (*See* SOUP)
CEREAL

QUICK REFERENCE: MILK	Amount	Fat Grams	Total Calories	% Fat Calories
Skim	¼ cup	–	23	–
	½ cup	–	45	–
1% lowfat	¼ cup	.5	26	17%
	½ cup	1	55	16%
2% lowfat	¼ cup	1	31	29%
	½ cup	2.5	61	37%
Whole	¼ cup	2	38	47%
	½ cup	4	75	48%

■ **HOT/COOKED CEREAL**
(NOTE: All cereals are either dry or prepared with water per directions on packaging. If milk is used, calorie and fat content increase accordingly. Data on milk is shown in the Quick Reference above. For additional information on milk, see MILK.)

Food and Description	Amount	Fat Grams	Total Calories	% Fat Calories
Barley (*See* BARLEY)				
Bran (Health Valley)				
100% Natural Bran Cereal				
w/apples & cinnamon	¼ cup	1	100	9%
w/raisins	¼ cup	1	100	9%
100% Organic w/raisins	1 oz	< 1	90	5%
Bulgur (*See* BULGUR)				
Corn Grits (*See* CORN GRITS)				
Cream of Rice (Nabisco)				
Instant/dry	2½ Tbs	–	100	–
Cream of Rye (Roman Meal)	1 Serving	1	110	8%
(Cream of the West)				
Montana's 100% Roasted Wheat	¼ cup	< 1	106	4%
Cream of Wheat				
(Nabisco)				
Instant/dry	2½ Tbs	< 1	100	5%
Mix & Eat/prepared				
Apple cinnamon	1 serving	–	130	–
Brown sugar/cinnamon	1 serving	–	130	–
Cinnamon Toast	1 serving	–	130	–
Maple/brown sugar	1 serving	–	130	–

Food and Description	Amount	Fat Grams	Total Calories	% Fat Calories
Original	1 serving	–	100	–
Quick	2½ Tbs	< 1	100	5%
Regular	2½ Tbs	–	100	
Farina				
Generic	1 Tbs	–	40	–
Dry	1 oz	–	105	–
	1 cup	1	649	1%
Cooked	½ cup	–	57	–
	1 cup	–	116	–
(Krusteaz)	3 Tbs	–	100	–
(Pathmark) Enriched	1 oz	–	100	–
(Pillsbury)	1 serving	< 1	80	6%
(Quaker) Quick Creamy wheat	1 serving	–	100	–
Fiber Cereal-Hot (Golden Harvest)				
Maple/brown sugar	⅓ cup	2	100	18%
Hominy Grits (See CORN GRITS)				
Maltex	1 serving	1	180	5%
Malt-O-Meal				
Plain & chocolate	1 serving	–	122	–
Plus 40% Oat Bran	1 serving	1	120	8%
Wheat w/oat bran	1 serving	1	120	8%
(Maypo)				
30-second maple	1 serving	1	100	9%
Vermont Style	1 serving	1	105	9%
w/added oat bran	1 serving	2	130	14%
Oat Bran				
(Arrowhead Mills)	1 serving	2	110	16%
(Health Valley) 100% natural-hot				
Apple Cinnamon	1 serving	1	100	9%
Raisin spice	1 serving	1	100	9%
(Mother's)	1 serving	2	90	20%
(Nabisco) Wholesome'N Hearty	1 serving	2	90	20%
Instant				
Apple cinnamon	1 package	2	130	14%
Apple/spice	1 package	2	120	15%
Honey	1 package	2	110	16%
Oat	1 package	2	80	23%
Raisin/cinnamon	1 package	2	120	15%
Regular	1 package	2	80	23%
(Quaker)	1 serving	2	90	20%
Instant	1 serving	2	100	18%
(Roman Meal)	1 serving	2.5	94	20%
(Skinner's)	1 serving	2	110	16%
(Stone-Buhr)	1 serving	2	108	17%

Food and Description	Amount	Fat Grams	Total Calories	% Fat Calories
Oatmeal, Instant				
(General Mills)				
Oatmeal Swirlers				
Apple cinnamon/raspberry	1 package	2	160	11%
Cherry/strawberry	1 package	2	150	12%
Cinnamon spice/				
maple brown sugar	1 package	2	160	11%
Milk chocolate	1 package	2	170	11%
Undercover Bears				
Apple Cinnamon	1 package	3	170	16%
Fruit Punch	1 package	3	170	16%
Maple & Brown Sugar	1 package	3	170	16%
Strawberry	1 package	3	170	16%
(Quaker)				
Extra-fortified Instant				
Apples & Spice	1 package	2	130	17%
Raisins & Cinnamon	1 package	2	130	17%
Regular	1 package	2	100	18%
Honey Nut	1 package	3	130	21%
Regular	1 package	2	90	20%
w/apples & cinnamon	1 package	1	120	8%
w/bananas & cream	1 package	3	160	45%
w/blueberries & cream	1 package	3	160	45%
w/bran & raisins	1 package	1.9	158	11%
w/cinnamon & spice	1 package	2	160	11%
w/cinnamon/raisins/almonds	1 package	4	150	24%
w/honey & graham	1 package	1.7	136	11%
w/maple	1 package	2	150	12%
w/maple & brown sugar	1 package	2	150	12%
w/peaches & cream	1 package	2	130	14%
w/raisins & spice	1 package	2	150	12%
w/raisins/dates/walnuts	1 package	4	140	26%
w/strawberries & cream	1 package	2	130	14%
(Rogers)/Micro Quick				
Apples/cinnamon	1 package	2	142	13%
Maple/brown sugar	1 package	2	157	12%
Regular-unsweetened	1 package	2	120	15%
Sure Brunet d'Erable	1 package	2	157	12%
Tropical Fruit	1 package	3	164	17%
(Roman Meal)				
Oats/multi-bran/apple/cinnamon	1 serving	3	113	24%
Oats/wheat/dates/raisins/almonds	1 serving	3	140	19%
Oats/wheat/honey/coconut/almonds	1 serving	6	150	36%
Oats/wheat/rye/bran/flax	1 serving	2	120	15%

Food and Description	Amount	Fat Grams	Total Calories	% Fat Calories
(Total) Instant				
Apple cinnamon	1 package	2	130	14%
Cinnamon raisin	1 package	2	170	11%
Maple brown sugar	1 package	2	160	11%
Mixed nut	1 package	4	140	26%
Quick	1 serving	2	90	20%
Regular	1 package	2	100	18%
Oatmeal, Regular				
Generic				
Cooked	4 oz	1	70	13%
	1 cup	2	145	12%
Dry	1 oz	1.8	109	15%
	1 cup	5	311	14%
(Pritikin) Hearty Hot Cereal				
Apple Raisin Spice	1 package	2	160	11%
Multi grain	1 package	1	150	6%
(Quaker)				
Multi-Grain/dry	½ cup	1.5	130	10%
Plus Fiber/dry	½ cup	2.5	130	17%
Quick & Old Fashioned	1 serving	2	100	18%
(Ralston)				
High Fiber 100% Wheat Recipe	1 serving	1	90	10%
Plain	1 serving	.6	100	5%
(Roman Meal)				
Old fashioned oats	1 serving	2	100	18%
Plain	1 serving	.7	111	6%
Quick cooking	1 serving	2	100	18%
(Stone-Buhr)				
4 Grain Cereal Mates	1 serving	2	210	9%
Hot Apple Granola	1 serving	2	200	9%
7 Grain Cereal	1 serving	3	200	14%
Wheat Hearts				
(General Mills)	1 serving	1	110	8%
Wheat, Rye, Bran, Flax				
(Roman Meal)	1 serving	.5	80	6%
Wheatena	1 serving	1	100	9%
Whole Wheat Hot Natural Cereal				
(Mother's)	1 serving	1	100	9%
(Quaker's)	1 serving	1	90	10%
■ COLD/READY-TO-EAT CEREAL				
Almond Delight				
w/almonds/pecans/walnuts	1 oz/1 cup	1.6	110	13%
Alpen Muesli Raisins & Nuts	½ cup	3	220	12%
Alpha-Bits (Post)				
Original	1 cup	1	110	6%

Food and Description	Amount	Fat Grams	Total Calories	% Fat Calories
w/marshmallows	1 cup	1	110	8%
Amaranth Crunch				
w/raisins (Health Valley)	1 oz	1	100	9%
Amaranth Flakes (Health Valley)	1 oz	< 1	90	5%
Amaranth 100% Natural				
Sprouted w/bananas (Health Valley)	½ cup	2	110	16%
Apple Jacks (Kellogg's)	1 cup	–	110	–
Apple Raisin Crisp (Kellogg's)	⅔ cup	–	130	–
Arrowhead Crunch	1 oz	3	120	23%
Baby Cereal (See BABY FOOD)				
Basic 4 (General Mills)	¾ cup	2	130	14%
Batman Cereal (Ralston)	1 oz	1	110	8%
Benefit				
Regular	¼ cup	1	90	10%
w/raisins	1 cup	1	120	8%
Body Buddies (General Mills)				
Brown sugar and honey	1 cup	1	110	8%
Natural fruit flavor	1 cup	1	110	8%
Booberry (General Mills)	1 cup	1	110	8%
Bran (See also Oat Bran, in this listing)				
All Bran (Kellogg's)				
Original	⅓ cup	1	70	13%
Fruit & almonds	⅓ cup	2	100	18%
w/Extra Fiber	½ cup	–	50	–
Bran Buds (Kellogg's)	⅓ cup	1	70	13%
Bran Chex	⅔ cup	.7	90	7%
Bran Flakes				
(Arrowhead Mills)	1 oz	1	100	9%
(Kellogg's)	¾ cup	–	90	–
(Post)	⅔ cup	–	90	–
Bran Muffin Crisp	⅔ cup	1	130	7%
Bran News	1 oz	–	100	–
40+ Bran Flakes	⅔ cup	.5	90	5%
10% Bran Flakes	⅔ cup	1	106	9%
Fruitful Bran (Kellogg's)	⅔ cup	1	120	8%
Honey Bran	⅞ cup	.6	97	6%
(La Loma) Bran Cereal	1 oz	1	90	10%
Mueslix	½ cup	2	140	13%
100% Bran (Nabisco)				
plain	⅓ cup	1	70	13%
w/oat bran	1 oz	1	80	11%
Unprocessed Bran (Quaker)	2 Tbs	–	8	–
Breakfast O's w/oat bran				
(Barbara's)	1¼ cup	2	120	15%

Food and Description	Amount	Fat Grams	Total Calories	% Fat Calories
Breakfast w/Barbie	1 oz/1 cup	1	110	8%
Cap'n Crunch (Quaker)				
Regular	¾ cup	2	110	16%
Crunchberries	¾ cup	2	120	15%
Peanut butter	¾ cup	3	120	23%
Cheerios (General Mills)				
Apple Cinnamon	¾ cup	2	110	16%
Honey Nut				
Regular	¾ cup	1	110	8%
w/almonds	⅔ cup	3	120	23%
Multi-Grain	1 oz	–	100	–
Original	¾ cup	2	110	16%
Cheerios-To-Go (General Mills)				
Apple Cinnamon	1 oz pouch	2	110	16%
Cheerios	¾ oz pouch	2	80	23%
Honey Nut Cheerios	1 oz pouch	1	110	8%
Cinnamon Mini Buns (Kellogg's)	¾ cup	1	110	8%
Cinnamon Toast Crunch (General Mills)	¾ cup	3	120	23%
Circus Fun	1 oz/1 cup	1	110	8%
Clusters (General Mills)				
Regular	⅓ cup	2	110	16%
w/almonds/walnuts/pecans	½ cup	2	110	16%
Cocoa Flakes	⅔ cup	–	110	–
Cocoa Flakes Maizoro	1 oz	–	110	–
Cocoa Krispies (Kellogg's)	¾ cup	–	110	–
Cocoa Pebbles	⅞ cup	1	110	8%
Cocoa Puffs (General Mills)	1 oz/1 cup	1	110	8%
Common Sense Oat Bran (Kellogg's)				
Regular	¾ cup	1	100	9%
w/raisins	¾ cup	1	130	7%
Cookie Crisp				
Chocolate chip	1 cup	1	110	8%
Vanilla wafer	1 cup	1	110	8%
Corn Bran	⅔ cup	.9	109	7%
Corn Chex (Ralston)	⅔ cup	–	110	–
Corn Flakes				
(Arrowhead Mills)	1 oz	1	110	8%
(Barbara's) Blue Corn Flakes	1 cup	–	110	–
(Featherweight)	1 oz	–	110	–
(General Mills)				
Country	1 oz/1 cup	1	110	8%
Total	1 oz/1 cup	1	110	8%
(Health Valley) 100% Organic				
Blue	1 oz	< 1	90	5%

Food and Description	Amount	Fat Grams	Total Calories	% Fat Calories
Regular	1 oz	< 1	90	5%
(Kellogg's)	1 cup	–	100	–
(Krusteaz)	1 oz/1 cup	1	110	8%
(Post) Post Toasties	1 oz/1 cup	–	108	–
Corn Pops (Kellogg's)	1 cup	–	110	–
Count Chocula (General Mills)	1 cup	1	110	8%
Craklin Bran	⅓ cup	4	108	33%
Cracklin Oat Bran (Kellogg's)	½ cup	3	110	25%
Crispix (Kellogg's)	1 cup	–	110	–
Crispy Critters	1 cup	–	110	–
Crispy Oatmeal & Raisin Chex	¾ cup	.5	140	3%
Crispy Rice	1 oz/1 cup	–	112	–
(Grainfield's)	1 oz	< 1	100	5%
Crispy Wheats & Raisins				
(General Mills)	¾ cup	1	100	9%
Crunchy Bran (Quaker)	1 oz	1	90	10%
Crunchy Rice Bran (Quaker)	⅔ cup	1	100	9%
Crunchy Stars	1 cup	1	111	8%
Dinersaurs (Ralston)	1 oz/1 cup	1	110	8%
Dino Pebbles (Post)	1 oz/⅞ cup	1	110	8%
Double Chex (Ralston)	⅔ cup	–	110	–
Double Dip Crunch (Kellogg's)	⅔ cup	2	120	15%
Dunkin' Donuts (Ralston)	1 oz	1	120	8%
Fiber One	½ cup	1	60	15%
Fiber 7 Flakes, 100% Organic (Health Valley)				
Regular	1 oz/½ cup	< 1	90	5%
w/Raisins	1 oz/½ cup	< 1	90	5%
Fiberwise (Kellogg's)				
Flakes	1 oz	1	90	10%
Nuggets	1 oz	1	110	8%
Fortified Oat Flakes	⅔ cup	1	110	8%
Frankenberry (General Mills)	1 oz/1 cup	1	110	8%
Froot Loops (Kellogg's)	1 oz/1 cup	1	110	8%
Frosted Flakes (Kellogg's)	¾ cup	–	110	–
Frosted Krispies (Kellogg's)	⅔ cup	1	110	8%
Frosted Mini Wheats (Kellogg's)				
Bite size	½ cup	–	100	–
Regular	4 biscuits	–	100	–
Frosted Rice Chex Juniors (Ralston)	¾ cup	–	110	–
Frosted Rice Krinkles	⅞ cup	–	109	–
Frosted Wheat Squares	½ cup	–	100	–
Fruit & Fibre (Post)				
Dates/raisins/walnuts	⅔ cup	2	120	15%
Peaches/raisins/almonds	⅔ cup	2	120	15%

Food and Description	Amount	Fat Grams	Total Calories	% Fat Calories
Pineapple/banana/coconut	⅔ cup	3	120	23%
Fruit & Fitness (Health Valley)	2 oz	4	220	16%
Fruit Lites (Health Valley)	½ cup	–	45	–
Fruit'N Oat Bran Crunch (Kolln)	1 oz	1	110	8%
Fruit Wheats (Nabisco)				
Apple	½ cup	–	90	–
Blueberry	½ cup	–	90	–
Raisin	½ cup	–	100	–
Raspberry	½ cup	–	90	–
Strawberry	½ cup	–	90	–
Fruity Marshmallow Krispies				
(Kellogg's)	1¼ cups	–	140	–
Fruity Pebbles (Post)	⅞ cup	1	110	8%
Fruity Yummy Mummy				
(General Mills)	1 oz/1 cup	1	110	8%
Ghost Busters	1 oz/1 cup	1	110	8%
Golden Corn Lites (Health Valley)	½ cup	–	50	–
Golden Grahams (General Mills)	¾ cup	1	110	8%
Golden Wheat Lites(Health Valley)	½ cup	–	50	–
Graham Crackos	¾ cup	–	102	–
Granola				
(Arrowhead Mills)				
Maple nut	2 oz	11	260	38%
Bread Shop Granola Super Natural	⅓ cup	5	120	38%
(C. W. Post) Hearty Granola				
Plain	¼ cup	4	130	28%
w/raisins	¼ cup	4	123	29%
(Health Valley)				
Fat-free	1 oz	< 1	90	5%
(Kellogg's)				
Fat Free w/Raisins	⅓ cup	2	110	16%
Low-Fat	1.1 oz/			
	⅓ cup	2	120	15%
(Nature Valley)				
Cinnamon & raisin	⅓ cup	4	120	30%
Fruit & nut	⅓ cup	5	130	35%
(Nectar Sweet) Granola				
Blueberry'N Cream	⅓ cup	4	110	33%
Raspberry'N Cream	⅓ cup	4	110	33%
Strawberry'N Cream	⅓ cup	4	110	33%
Standard Home Recipe (USDA)	¼ cup	7.7	138	50%
(Sunbelt)				
Banana almond	1 oz	4	130	28%
Fruit & nut	1 oz	5	120	38%

Food and Description	Amount	Fat Grams	Total Calories	% Fat Calories
(Sun Country)				
w/almonds	¼ cup	5	130	35%
w/raisins	¼ cup	5	130	35%
w/raisins & dates	¼ cup	5	130	35%
Grape-Nuts (Post)				
Flakes	⅞ cup	< 1	100	5%
Original	¼ cup	–	110	–
Raisin	¼ cup	–	100	–
Great Grains (Post)				
Double Pecan	⅓ cup	3	120	23%
Raisin, date, & pecan	⅓ cup	3	130	21%
(Health Valley)				
Fat-free				
10 Bran Cereal	1 oz	< 1	90	5%
Almond Flavor	1 oz	< 1	90	5%
Apple Cinnamon	1 oz	< 1	90	5%
High Fiber	1 oz	< 1	90	5%
Healthy Crunch				
No Fat Added				
Almond Date	1 oz	1	90	10%
Apple Cinnamon	1 oz	1	90	10%
Healthy O's	1 oz	1	90	10%
Heartland Natural (Pet)				
Plain	¼ cup	4	130	28%
w/raisins	¼ cup	4	130	28%
Honey & Nut Corn Flakes	¾ cup	1.5	113	12%
Honey & Nut Toasty O's	¾ cup	1	110	8%
Honey Buc Wheat Crisp	¾ cup	1	110	8%
Honey Bunches of Oats				
Regular	⅔ cup	2	110	16%
w/almonds	⅔ cup	3	120	23%
Honey Graham Chex	⅔ cup	1	110	8%
Honey Nut Oat Chex	½ cup	1	110	8%
Honeycomb (Post)	1⅓ cups	–	110	–
Ice Cream Cones/all flavors	¾ cup	2	110	16%
Jetsons	¾ cup	1	110	8%
Just Right (Kellogg's)				
w/Fiber nuggets	⅔ cup	1	100	9%
w/Raisins, Dates & Nuts	¾ cup	1	140	6%
Kaboom (General Mills)	1 cup	1	110	8%
Kashi/puffed	1 cup	< 1	70	6%
(Kellogg's) Squares				
Apple Cinnamon	½ cup	–	90	–
Blueberry	½ cup	–	90	–

Food and Description	Amount	Fat Grams	Total Calories	% Fat Calories
Raisin	½ cup	–	90	–
Strawberry	½ cup	–	90	–
Kenmei Rice Bran (Kellogg's)	1 oz	1	110	8%
King Vitamin (Quaker)	1¼ cups	1	112	8%
Kix (General Mills)				
Berry Berry	1 cup	1	110	8%
Original	1½ cups	1	110	8%
Life (Quaker)				
Cinnamon	⅔ cup	1.6	110	13%
plain	⅔ cup	1.8	111	15%
w/raisins	⅔ cup	1.8	105	15%
Lites (Health Valley)				
Brown Rice	½ cup	–	50	–
Corn	½ cup	–	50	–
Wheat	½ cup	–	50	–
Lucky Charms (General Mills)	1 cup	1	110	8%
Morning Funnies	1 cup	1	110	8%
Most	⅔ cup	–	95	–
Multi-Bran Chex	⅔ cup	–	90	–
Muesli, Fruit (Ralston)				
Dates/almonds	1 oz	2	140	13%
Raisins/peaches/pecans	1 oz	3	150	18%
Raisins/walnuts/cranberries	½ cup	3	150	18%
Raspberry/almond	½ cup	3	150	18%
Walnuts/bananas	1 oz	3	150	18%
Mueslix (Kellogg's)				
Crispy Blend	⅔ cup	2	160	11%
Golden Crunch				
w/apples & almonds	½ cup	2	120	15%
Nature O's (Arrowhead Mills)	1 oz	1	110	8%
Nature Valley 100% Natural Cereals (General Mills)				
Cinnamon & Raisin	1 oz/⅓ cup	4	120	30%
Fruit & Nut	1 oz/⅓ cup	5	130	35%
Toasted Oat	1 oz/⅓ cup	5	130	35%
Nectar Sweet Crunch Oat Bran	⅓ cup	5	110	41%
Nintendo Cereal System	1 oz/1 cup	1	110	8%
Nut & Honey Crunch (Kellogg's)	⅔ cup	1	110	8%
Nut & Honey Crunch O's (Kellogg's)	⅔ cup	2	110	16%
Nutrific Oatmeal Flakes	1 oz	2	120	15%
Nutri-Grain (Kellogg's)				
Almond & Raisins	¾ cup	2	140	13%
Raisin Bran	1 cup	1	130	7%
Wheat	⅔ cup	–	90	–
Nutri-Grain Biscuits	1 oz	–	90	–

Food and Description	Amount	Fat Grams	Total Calories	% Fat Calories
Nutri-Grain Nuggets	¼ cup	–	110	–
Oatbake (Kellogg's)				
Honey Bran	1 oz	3	110	25%
Raisin Nut	1 oz	3	110	25%
Oat Bran				
(Health Valley)				
Flakes				
w/Almonds & Dates	1 oz	1	90	10%
100% Organic				
Plain	1 oz	< 1	90	5%
w/Raisins	1 oz	< 1	90	5%
No Fat Added Real				
Almond Flavor Crunch	1 oz	1	90	10%
Hawaiian Fruit	1 oz	1	100	9%
Raisin	1.2 oz	1	100	9%
O's				
Fruit & Nut-100% Organic	1 oz	< 1	90	5%
(Kolln) Krunch	1 oz	2	120	15%
Options (Ralston)	1.45 oz	–	130	–
(Quaker)	1 oz	2	100	18%
Raisin Fruit Wheats	½ cup	–	90	–
Oat Chex (Ralston)	1 oz	1	100	9%
Oat Flakes (Post)	⅔ cup	1	110	8%
Oat Squares (Quaker)				
Cinnamon	½ cup	1	100	9%
Original	1 oz	2	100	18%
Oatios				
Honey Almond	1.1 oz	2	120	15%
Oat Bran	1 oz	2	110	16%
Oatmeal Crisp (General Mills)				
Original	½ cup	2	110	16%
w/almonds	1 oz	3	120	23%
Oatmeal Raisin Crisp (General Mills)	½ cup	2	130	14%
Oh's				
Apple Cinnamon	1 cup	2	120	15%
Crunchy Nut	1 cup	4	130	28%
Honey Graham	1 cup	3	120	23%
Orangeola (Health Valley)				
No Fat Added				
Almonds & Dates	1 oz	1	90	10%
Bananas & Hawaiian Fruit	1 oz	1	90	10%
Outrageous Fruit & Grains	¼ cup	6	130	42%
Pac Man	1 cup	1	110	8%
Popeye Sweet Crunch Cereal (Quaker)	1 cup	2	120	15%

Food and Description	Amount	Fat Grams	Total Calories	% Fat Calories
Product 19 (Kellogg's)	1 cup	–	100	–
Puffed Corn (El Molino)	¾ cup	–	50	–
Puffed Millet (El Molino)	¾ cup	–	50	–
Puffed Rice				
(El Molino)	¾ cup	–	50	–
(Quaker)	1 cup	–	50	–
Puffed Wheat				
(El Molino)	¾ cup	–	50	–
(Quaker)	1 cup	–	50	–
(Quaker) 100% Natural				
low-fat	¼ cup	2	110	16%
plain	¼ cup	6	130	42%
w/apples & cinnamon	¼ cup	5	130	35%
w/raisins & dates	¼ cup	5	120	38%
Quisp	1 oz/1 cup	2	117	15%
Raisin Bran				
(Grainfield's)	1 oz	–	110	–
(Health Valley)				
100% Organic Flakes	1 oz	< 1	90	5%
(Kellogg's)	¾ cup	1	120	8%
(Krusteaz)	¾ cup	1	120	8%
(Post)	¾ cup	1	120	8%
(Ralston Purina)	¾ cup	–	120	–
(Skinner's)	½ cup	1	100	9%
Raisin Date Natural	1 oz	5	123	37%
Raisin Nut Bran (General Mills)	½ cup	3	110	25%
Raisin Squares (Kellogg's)	½ cup	–	90	–
Real 100% Natural				
Almond & Crunch	¼ cup	3	120	23%
Rice Bran				
(Health Valley) w/Almonds & Dates	1 oz	3	110	16%
(Quaker)				
Crunchy	⅔ cup	1	100	9%
Honey Crunch	¼ cup	5	100	45%
Rice Chex (Ralston)	1⅛ cups	–	110	–
Rice Krispies (Kellogg's)	1 oz/1 cup	–	110	–
Rice Toasties	¾ cup	–	108	–
Rocky Road	⅔ cup	2	120	15%
Ruskets Biscuits (La Loma)	~ 1 oz	–	110	–
7 Grain (La Loma)	1 oz	1	110	8%
Crunchy	1 oz	2	110	16%
(S. W. Graham)				
Cinnamon	½ cup	–	100	–
plain	½ cup	–	100	–

Food and Description	Amount	Fat Grams	Total Calories	% Fat Calories
Shredded Wheat				
(Kellogg's) Whole Grain	½ cup	–	90	–
(Nabisco)				
Original	1 biscuit	1	80	11%
Spoon Size	1 oz	1	90	10%
w/Oat Bran	1 oz	1	100	9%
(Quaker) Original	2 biscuits	1	130	7%
(Sunshine)				
Bite Size	⅔ cup	1	110	8%
Regular	1 biscuit	1	90	10%
Shredded Wheat'N Bran (Nabisco)	1 oz	–	90	–
Shredded Wheat Squares				
All flavors	½ cup	–	90	–
Smacks	¾ cup	1	110	8%
S'mores Crunch (General Mills)	¾ cup	2	120	15%
Smurf Berry Crunch (Post)	1 oz	1	110	8%
Smurf Magic Berries (Post)	1 oz/1 cup	1	120	8%
Special K (Kellogg's)	1 cup	–	110	–
Sprouts 7 (Health Valley)				
w/Bananas & Hawaiian Fruit	1 oz	< 1	90	5%
100% organic w/raisins	1 oz	< 1	90	5%
Stone Buhr 4 Grain Cereal Mates	2 oz	2	210	9%
Sugar Puffs	⅞ cup	1	110	8%
Sugar Sparkled Flakes	¾ cup	–	108	–
Sun Flakes				
Corn & Rice	1 oz/1 cup	.9	110	7%
Wheat & Rice	1 oz/1 cup	3	135	20%
Super Golden Crisp (Post)	1 oz	–	100	–
Super Sugar Crisp	⅞ cup	–	106	–
Swiss Breakfast (Health Valley)				
No fat added				
Raisin nut	1 oz	1	80	11%
Tropical fruit	1 oz	1	80	11%
Tasteeos	1¼ cups	.0	111	7%
Team Flakes (Nabisco)	1 oz/1 cup	1	110	8%
Teddy Grahams Breakfast Bears (Nabisco)				
Chocolate	⅓ cup	3	120	23%
Cinnamon	⅓ cup	3	120	23%
Honey	⅓ cup	3	120	23%
Teenage Mutant Ninja Turtles (Ralston)	1 oz	1	110	8%
Tiny Toon (Quaker)	1 oz	1	110	8%
Toasted Wheat and Raisins	1 oz	1	100	9%
Toasted Wheat Bran	⅓ cup	2	60	30%
Toasty O's	1¼ cups	2	110	16%

Food and Description	Amount	Fat Grams	Total Calories	% Fat Calories
Total (General Mills)				
Corn Flakes	1 oz/1 cup	< 1	110	4%
Raisin Bran	1.5 oz	1	140	6%
Whole Wheat	1 oz	1	100	9%
Triples (General Mills)	1 oz/¾ cup	1	110	8%
Trix (General Mills)	1.5 oz	1	119	8%
Uncle Sam	1 oz	2	110	16%
Urkel-os (Ralston)	1 oz/1 cup	1	110	8%
Waffelos	1.5 oz	1	115	8%
Weetabix Whole Wheat	2 biscuits	< 1	100	5%
Wheat Bran				
(Arrowhead Mills)	2 oz	2	200	9%
(Kretschmer) Toasted	⅓ cup	2	60	30%
Wheat'N Bran (Nabisco)	1 oz	&	90	–
Wheat'N Raisin Chex	¾ cup	–	130	–
Wheat Chex (Ralston)	⅔ cup	–	100	–
Wheat Germ				
(Arrowhead Mills)	2 oz	6	210	26%
(Kretschmer)				
Plain	¼ cup	3	100	27%
Honey crunch	¼ cup	3	110	25%
Toasted, w/brown sugar & honey	¼ cup	2	100	18%
Wheaties (General Mills)	1 oz/1 cup	1	100	9%
Honey Gold	¾ cup	< 1	100	5%
CHARD				
fresh-cooked	½ cup	–	18	–
raw-chopped	½ cup	–	3	–
CHARLOTTE RUSSE				
w/lady fingers & whipped cream filling	4 oz	16.6	326	46%
CHAYOTE				
tropical American perennial	1 medium	–	56	–
boiled	½ cup	–	19	–
CHEESE				
American				
(Alpine Lace)	1 oz	6	80	67%
Free 'N Lean	1 oz	–	40	–
(Borden) Processed Slices	1 oz	9	110	74%
Light 15% Milkfat	1 oz	5	70	64%
Processed Cheese Food				
Singles	1 oz	7	90	70%
(Harvest Moon)	1 oz	4	70	51%
(Nucoa) Heart Beat-Sandwich Slices	1 oz	2	50	36%
(Kraft)				
Cheese Food	1 oz	7	90	70%

Food and Description	Amount	Fat Grams	Total Calories	% Fat Calories
Deluxe-Loaf	1 oz	9	110	74%
Deluxe-Slices	1 oz	9	110	74%
Grated-Cheese Food	1 oz	7	130	49%
Light Singles	1 oz	4	70	51%
White-Cheese Food	1 oz	7	90	70%
(Land O'Lakes) Processed	1 oz	9	110	74%
Swiss-Processed	1 oz	8	100	72%
Sharp-Processed	1 oz	9	100	81%
(Light N'Lively) Cheese Food	1 oz	4	70	51%
(Lite-Line)	⅔ oz	2	35	51%
(Old English) Loaf	1 oz	9	110	74%
Slices	1 oz	9	110	74%
(Sargento) Hot Pepper	1 oz	9	110	74%
Pimento	1 oz	9	110	74%
Snack-Pasteurized/Process	1 oz	9	110	74%
(Weight Watchers)	1 oz	2	50	36%
Dijon	1 oz	2	50	36%
American-Swiss				
(Formagg)	¾ oz	5	70	64%
(Land O'Lakes)	1 oz	9	100	81%
Babybel (Fromageries Bel)	1 oz	7	91	69%
	8 oz	57	726	71%
mini	¾ oz	6	74	73%
Blue	1 oz	8	100	72%
	1 cup	38.8	477	73%
(Kraft)	1 oz	9	100	81%
(Sergento)	1 oz	8	100	72%
Bonbel (Fromageries Bel)	1 oz	8	100	72%
	8 oz	65	790	74%
Mini	¾ oz	6	74	73%
Bonbino (Fromageries Bel)	1 oz	9	103	79%
	8 oz	68	822	75%
Driok	1 oz	9	110	74%
(Kraft)	1 oz	9	110	74%
Natural (Land O'Lakes)	1 oz	8	110	66%
(Sargento)	1 oz	8	105	69%
Snack-Pasteurized Process	1 oz	9	100	81%
Brie	1 oz	7.85	95	74%
(Corneville) Soft Ripened	1 oz	7.5	90	75%
(Fromageries Bel)	1 oz	8	90	80%
(Sargento)	1 oz	8	95	76%
Burger Cheese (Sargento)	1 oz	8.86	106	75%
Cajun (Sargento)	1 oz	9	110	74%
Camembert	1 oz	6.9	85	73%

Food and Description	Amount	Fat Grams	Total Calories	% Fat Calories
(Corneville) Soft Ripened	1 oz	7.5	90	75%
(Fromageries)	1 oz	8	90	80%
(Sargento) Danish	1 oz	7	90	70%
Caraway	1 oz	8	107	67%
(Kraft) Natural	1 oz	8	100	72%
Cheddar				
Breaded/Frozen (Banquet)	3 oz	30	414	65%
Ched-R-Lo (Alpine Lace)	1 oz	5	80	56%
Extra Sharp (Land O'Lakes)				
Process	1 oz	9	100	81%
Imitation				
(Kraft) Golden Image-Mild	1 oz	9	110	74%
(Sargento)	1 oz	6	90	60%
(Weight Watchers)				
Shredded-Part Skim Milk	1 oz	5	80	56%
Mild	1 oz	9	114	71%
(Formagg) Cheese Food	1 oz	5	70	64%
(Fromageries Bel)	1 oz	9	110	74%
	8 oz	73	883	74%
Wedges-Process Cheese	1 oz	6	72	75%
Wedges Reduced Calorie	¾ oz	2	35	51%
Generic - Shredded	1 cup	37	455	73%
(Kraft) Healthy Favorites-Shredded	1 oz	4	70	51%
(Land O'Lakes) La Chedda				
Cheese Food	1 oz	7	90	70%
(Sargento)	1 oz	9	110	74%
Light Shredded	1 oz	5	90	50%
(Weight Watchers)	1 oz	5	80	56%
Natural				
(Cracker Barrel) Light-Reduced				
Fat Sharp-White	1 oz	5	80	53%
(Dorman's) Chedda Delite				
Deli Light	1 oz	7	90	70%
(Kraft)	1 oz	9	110	74%
Light Naturals Reduced Fat	1 oz	5	80	56%
(Land O'Lakes)	1 oz	9	110	74%
(Lifetime) Lite	1 oz	3	55	49%
(Weight Watchers)	1 oz	5	80	56%
New York (Sargento)	1 oz	9	110	74%
Sharp				
Cheese Ball w/Almonds	1 oz	6	90	60%
(Light N'Lively)	1 oz	4	70	51%
(Lite-Line) 8% Milkfat	1 oz	2	50	36%
(Sargento) Nut Log	1 oz	7	100	63%

Food and Description	Amount	Fat Grams	Total Calories	% Fat Calories
(Weight Watchers)	1 oz	2	50	36%
Sharp w/ Wine	1 oz	6.9	93	67%
Singles-Cheese Food				
(Kraft)	1 oz	8	100	72%
Smokey w/Almonds-Log	1 oz	6	90	60%
Cheddar Cheese Soup (See SOUP)				
Cheddarella				
(Land O'Lakes) Natural	1 oz	8	100	72%
(Lake to Lake)	1 oz	8	100	72%
Cheese Product Pasteurized Process Misc.				
Cheddar & Bacon (Land O'Lakes)	1 oz	9	110	74%
Jalapeno (Kraft)	1 oz	7	90	70%
Non-fat (See also Cream Cheese, in this listing)				
(Alpine Lace) Free 'N Lean				
American	1 oz	–	40	–
Cheddar	1 oz	–	40	–
Mozzarella	1 oz	–	40	–
Singles	1 oz	–	40	–
(Healthy Choice) Fat-free				
Slices				
Cheddar	1 oz	–	40	–
Mozzarella	1 oz	–	40	–
Snack Stix				
Mexican	1 oz	–	40	–
Mozzarella	1 oz	–	40	–
String-Pizza	1 oz	–	40	–
(Kraft) Free	1 oz	–	45	–
Port Wine (Wispride) Cold Pack	1 oz	7	100	63%
Sharp Cheddar (Wispride)				
Cold Pack	1 oz	7	100	63%
Slices (Land O'Lakes)	⅔ oz	4	60	60%
Cheese Sauce (See also SAUCE)				
Canned	2 oz	4	60	60%
Mix	1 oz	18	225	72%
Nacho (Kaukauna)	1 oz	6	80	68%
Cheese Souffle/Homemade (8" square)	~ 4 oz	18.8	240	71%
Collapsed	1 cup	16	207	70%
	1 oz	4.8	62	70%
Cheese Spreads				
(Alouette) Spreadable				
French Onion	1 oz	9	95	85%
Garlic & Spices	1 oz	9	95	85%
Zesty Pepper	1 oz	9	90	90%
American Pasteurized (Kraft)	1 oz	6	80	68%

Food and Description	Amount	Fat Grams	Total Calories	% Fat Calories
American Sharp Pasteurized Processed				
(Sargento)	1 oz	9	110	74%
(Cheez Whiz)				
Hot Mexican	1 oz	5.7	80	64%
Mild Mexican	1 oz	5.7	80	64%
Pimiento	1 oz	5.7	80	64%
Plain	1 oz	5.7	80	64%
w/Jalapeno Peppers	1 oz	5.7	80	64%
Country Crock (Shedds)				
Fresh Cheddar	1 oz	4	70	51%
Fresh Cheddar-Mexican style	1 oz	4	70	51%
Fresh French Onion	1 oz	7	70	90%
Fresh Garden Vegetable	1 oz	7	70	90%
Fresh Herb & Garlic	1 oz	7	70	90%
Crockery (Kraft)				
Classic Ranch	1 oz	7	70	90%
French Onion	1 oz	6	70	77%
Garden Vegetable	1 oz	6	70	77%
Garlic & Herb	1 oz	7	70	90%
Medium Cheddar	1 oz	4	70	51%
Port Wine	1 oz	4	70	51%
Easy Cheese (Nabisco)				
American	1 oz	6	80	68%
Cheddar	1 oz	6	80	68%
Cheddar'n Bacon	1 oz	6	80	68%
Nacho	1 oz	6	80	68%
Sharp Cheddar	1 oz	6	80	68%
(Fromageries Bel) Price's				
Pimiento Spread	1 oz	6	80	68%
(Fromageries Bel) The Laughing Cow				
Cheezbits	⅛ oz	1	13	69%
Lite Soft Cheese Spread	1 oz	2	45	40%
Regular Cheese Spread	1 oz	6	70	77%
Golden Velvet (Land O'Lakes)	1 oz	6	80	68%
(Imperial) Ala Mode Gourmet	1 Tbs	7	70	90%
Jalapeno Pasteurized-Loaf	1 oz	6	80	68%
Jalapeno Pepper (Kraft)	1 oz	5	70	64%
(Kaukauna) Microwave Spreadable Cheese				
Cheddar	1 oz	6	80	68%
Extra Sharp Cheddar	1 oz	7	90	70%
Jalapeno	1 oz	6	80	68%
Micro Melt-Real Cheddar-Processed				
Plastic Bottle Container	1 oz	6	80	68%
Nacho Cheese Sauce	1 oz	6	80	68%

Food and Description	Amount	Fat Grams	Total Calories	% Fat Calories
Neufchatel Spread				
Garlic & Herb	1 oz	7	80	79%
Garden Vegetable	1 oz	7	80	79%
Port Wine Cheddar	1 oz	7	90	70%
Sharp Cheddar	1 oz	6	90	60%
Lite Spread	1 oz	4	70	51%
Sharp Cheddar Log w/Almonds	1 oz	7	100	63%
Smoky Sharp Cheddar	1 oz	7	90	70%
Limburger (Mohawk Valley)	1 oz	6	70	77%
(Old English) Sharp	1 oz	7	80	79%
Olives & Pimiento (Kraft)	1 oz	5	60	75%
Pimiento (Kraft)	1 oz	5	70	64%
Pineapple (Kraft)	1 oz	5	70	64%
Roka Blue (Kraft)	1 oz	6	70	77%
Spreadery (Kraft) Cheese Snack				
Medium Cheddar Cold Pack	1 oz	4	70	51%
Mexican Cold Pack				
w/Jalapeno Peppers (Mild)	1 oz	4	70	51%
Nacho Cold Pack	1 oz	4	70	51%
Neufchatel Cheese				
w/Classic Ranch Flavor	1 oz	7	70	90%
w/French Onion	1 oz	6	70	77%
w/Garden Vegetables	1 oz	6	70	77%
w/Garlic & Herb	1 oz	6	70	77%
w/Strawberries	1 oz	5	70	64%
Port Wine Cold Pack	1 oz	4	70	51%
Sharp Cheddar Cold Pack	1 oz	4	70	51%
Vermont White Cold Pack	1 oz	4	70	51%
Squeeze-A-Snack (Kraft)				
Garlic	1 oz	7	80	79%
Hickory Smoke	1 oz	7	80	79%
Jalapeno Pepper	1 oz	6	80	68%
Sharp	1 oz	7	80	79%
w/Bacon	1 oz	7	90	79%
Velveeta Spread (Kraft)				
Light	1 oz	4	70	51%
Mexican Hot	1 oz	6	80	68%
Shredded	1 oz	7	100	63%
Light	1 oz	4	70	51%
Mexican Mild	1 oz	6	80	68%
Shredded	1 oz	7	100	63%
Original	1 oz	6	80	68%
Pimento	1 oz	6	80	68%
Slices	1 oz	6	90	60%

Food and Description	Amount	Fat Grams	Total Calories	% Fat Calories
w/Bacon	1 oz	6	80	68%
w/Garlic	1 oz	6	80	68%
Cheese & Sticks (Sargento)	1 oz	6	110	49%
Cheez'N Bacon Singles Cheese Food (Kraft)	1 oz	7	90	70%
Cheshire	1 oz	8.68	110	71%
Colby	1 oz	9	110	74%
(Alpine Lace) Colbi-Lo Cheese Alternative	1 oz	5	80	56%
(Dorman's) Lo-Chol	1 oz	6	90	60%
Golden Image-Imitation Colby(Kraft)	1 oz	9	110	74%
(Kraft)				
Light Natural	1 oz	5	80	56%
Natural	1 oz	9	110	74%
(Land O'Lakes) Natural	1 oz	9	110	74%
(Sargento)	1 oz	9	112	72%
(Weight Watchers) Natural	1 oz	5	80	56%
Colby-Jack (Sargento)	1 oz	9	109	74%
Colby Longhorn (Delcia) Imitation	1 oz	6	80	68%
Cold Packs				
Extra Sharp Cheddar	1 oz	7	90	70%
Port Wine Cheddar	1 oz	7	100	63%
Sharp Cheddar	1 oz	7	100	63%
w/Bacon	1 oz	7	90	70%
Cottage Cheese (*See* COTTAGE CHEESE)				
(Cracker Barrel)				
Cheese Ball				
Sharp Cheddar w/Almonds	1 oz	7	100	63%
Cheese Log-Port Wine Cheddar w/Almonds	1 oz	6	90	60%
Cheese Log-Sharp Cheddar w/Almonds	1 oz	6	90	60%
Cheese Log-Smokey Cheddar w/Almonds	1 oz	6	90	60%
Cream Cheese	1 oz	9.89	99	90%
(Alpine Lace) Fat-Free	1 oz	–	30	–
(Fleur De Lait) The Little Cheeserie Chunky Spreadables				
Bay Shrimp	1 oz	5	70	64%
Italian Garlic	1 oz	5	65	69%
Plump Strawberry	1 oz	5	80	56%
Zesty Salsa	1 oz	5	60	56%
(Healthy Choice) Fat-Free				
Plain	1 oz	–	30	–

Food and Description	Amount	Fat Grams	Total Calories	% Fat Calories
Strawberry	1 oz	–	30	–
(Kraft) Healthy Favorites	1 oz	5	60	90%
(Philadelphia Brand)				
Free (Fat-Free)	1 oz	–	25	–
Light Neufchatel	1 oz	7	80	79%
Light Pasteurized Process	1 oz	5	60	75%
Original				
Plain	1 oz	10	100	90%
w/Chives	1 oz	9	90	90%
w/Pimento	1 oz	9	90	90%
Soft				
Original	1 oz	10	100	90%
w/Chives & Onion	1 oz	9	100	81%
w/Herb & Garlic	1 oz	9	100	81%
w/Olives & Pimento	1 oz	8	90	80%
w/Pineapple	1 oz	8	90	80%
w/Smoked Salmon	1 oz	9	90	81%
w/Strawberries	1 oz	8	90	80%
Whipped				
Plain	1 oz	10	100	90%
w/Bacon & Horseradish	1 oz	9	90	90%
w/Bleu Cheese	1 oz	9	100	81%
w/Chives	1 ozs	8	90	80%
w/Onions	1 oz	8	90	80%
w/Smoked Salmon	1 oz	8	90	80%
(Weight Watchers)	1 oz	2	35	51%
w/Chives	1 oz	9	90	90%
w/Fruit-all flavors	1 oz	8	90	80%
w/Herb & Garlic	1 oz	9.9	103	87%
w/Honey	1 oz	8	100	72%
(Soft)	1 oz	8	100	72%
w/Olives & Pimento	1 oz	8	90	80%
w/Onions & Chives	1 oz	9	100	81%
w/Pimento	1 oz	9	90	90%
(Woody's)				
Chocolate Mint Fudge	1 oz	4	120	30%
Chocolate w/Walnuts	1 oz	4	120	30%
Maple Walnut Fudge	1 oz	4	120	30%
Diet Snack/(Weight Watchers)				
Sharp Cheddar Flavor	1 oz	3	70	39%
Port Wine Flavored	1 oz	3	70	39%
Edam	1 oz	7.88	101	70%
(Fromageries Bel)	1 oz	8	100	72%
	8 oz	66	800	74%

Food and Description	Amount	Fat Grams	Total Calories	% Fat Calories
(Kraft) Natural	1 oz	7	90	70%
(Land O'Lakes)-Natural	1 oz	8	100	72%
(May-Bud)	1 oz	8	100	72%
(Sargento)	1 oz	8	101	71%
Farmer's				
(May-Bud) Semisoft Part Skim	1 oz	7	90	70%
(Sargento)	1 oz	8	102	71%
Feta	1 oz	6	75	72%
(Churny) Natural	1 oz	6.5	75	78%
(Sargento)	1 oz	6	80	68%
Fontina				
(Sargento)	1 oz	8.8	110	72%
Gjetost	1 oz	8	132	55%
(Sargento)	1 oz	8	130	55%
(Ski Queen)	1 oz	9	130	62%
Gorgonzola (Sargento)	1 oz	8	100	72%
Gouda	1 oz	7.78	101	69%
(Fromageries Bel)	1 oz	9	110	66%
	8 oz	73	880	75%
Mini	¾ oz	6	80	68%
Mini-Reduced Calorie	¾ oz	2.5	45	50%
(Kraft)-Natural	1 oz	9	110	74%
(Land O'Lakes)-Natural	1 oz	8	100	72%
(May-Bud)	1 oz	8	100	72%
(Sargento)	1 oz	8	101	71%
Gruyere				
Wedges (Fromageries Bel)				
Process Cheese	1 oz	6	72	75%
Reduced Calorie	¾ oz	2	35	51%
Havarti	1 oz	10.6	121	79%
(Casino)-Natural	1 oz	11	120	83%
(Sargento)	1 oz	11	120	83%
(Heart Beat) Heart Smart				
Fat-Free Slices				
American Flavor	¾ oz	–	30	–
Sharp Cheddar Flavor	¾ oz	–	30	–
Swiss Flavor	¾ oz	–	30	–
(Hoffman's)				
American				
Pasteurized Process	1 oz	9	110	74%
Pasteurized-Colored	1 oz	7	100	63%
Cheddar				
Smokey Sharp-Pasteurized Process				
Hickory Smoked	1 oz	9	110	74%

Food and Description	Amount	Fat Grams	Total Calories	% Fat Calories
Cheese Food-Pasteurized Process				
Chees'N Bacon w/Bacon	1 oz	6	90	60%
Chees'N Onion w/Onion	1 oz	7	100	63%
Chees'N Salami w/Salami	1 oz	6	90	60%
Hot Pepper w/Jalapenos	1 oz	7	90	70%
Swiss on Rye w/Caraway	1 oz	7	90	70%
Smokey Swiss'N Cheddar				
Pasteurized Process	1 oz	8	110	66%
Super Sharp Cheddar				
Pasteurized Process	1 oz	8	110	66%
Hot Pepper (Alpine Lace)	1 oz	6	80	67%
Hot Pepper Montery Jack (Land O'Lakes)				
Natural	1 oz	9	110	74%
Italian Herb Cheese Food (Land O'Lakes)	1 oz	7	90	70%
Italian Style Grated Cheeses (Sargento)	1 oz	8	110	66%
Jalapeno Cheese Food (Land O'Lakes)	1 oz	7	90	70%
Jalapeno Jack (Land O'Lakes)-Process	1 oz	8	90	80%
Jarlsberg (Sargento)	1 oz	7	100	63%
Limburger	1 oz	7.7	93	75%
Little Gem Size				
(Mohawk Valley)	1 oz	8	90	80%
(Sargento)	1 oz	8	90	80%
Macaroni Cheese Loaf (Eckrich)	1 oz	6	75	72%
Monterey	1 oz	8.58	106	73%
Monterey Jack	1 oz	9	110	74%
(Alpine Lace) Monti-Jack-Lo	1 oz	5	80	56%
(Formagg) Cheese Food	1 oz	5	70	64%
Jalapeno Flavor	1 oz	5	70	64%
(Kraft)				
Cheese Food Singles	1 oz	7	90	70%
Light Naturals Reduced Fat	1 oz	5	90	50%
Natural				
Original	1 oz	9	110	74%
w/Caraway Oeeds	1 oz	8	100	72%
wJJalapeno Peppers	1 oz	9	110	74%
Lite (Lifetime)	1 oz	3	55	49%
(May-Bud)	1 oz	9	110	74%
Natural (Land O'Lakes)	1 oz	9	110	74%
(Sargento)	1 oz	9	110	74%
(Weight Watchers)	1 oz	5	80	56%
Monti-Jack-Lo (Alpine Lace)	1 oz	5	80	56%
Mozzarella				
(Banquet) Breaded-Frozen	2.6 oz	12	220	49%
(Formagg)	1 oz	5	70	64%

Food and Description	Amount	Fat Grams	Total Calories	% Fat Calories
Imitation (Sargento)	1 oz	6	80	68%
(Lite-Line) 8% Milkfat				
Pasteurized Process	1 oz	2	50	36%
Low Moisture	1 oz	7	90	70%
Natural				
(Alpine Lace) Free 'N Lean	1 oz	–	40	–
(Kraft) Light Naturals				
Healthy Favorites-Shredded	1 oz	3	60	45%
Reduced Fat	1 oz	4	80	45%
(Land O'Lakes) Low Moisture				
Part Skim	1 oz	5	80	56%
(Weight Watchers)	1 oz	4	70	51%
Shredded	1 oz	4	70	51%
Part Skim	1 oz	5	85	53%
(Alpine Lace)	1 oz	5	70	64%
Generic	1 oz	5	85	53%
Part Skim & Low Moisture				
(Sargento)	1 oz	5	80	56%
Light Shredded or Sliced	1 oz	3	60	45%
String	1 oz	5	80	56%
(Precious)	1 oz	6	88	61%
String w/Jalapeno Peppers (Kraft)	1 oz	5	80	56%
Strip (Arpin)				
Real Cheese Snacks	1 oz	6	85	64%
w/Pizza Spices (Sargento)	1 oz	5	80	56%
Whole Milk				
Generic	1 oz	6	80	68%
(Sargento)	1 oz	7	90	70%
Muenster	1 oz	8.5	104	74%
(Alpine Lace)	1 oz	9	100	81%
(Dorman's) Lo-Chol	1 oz	7	100	63%
(Kraft)	1 oz	9	110	74%
Natural (Land O'Lakes)	1 oz	9	100	81%
Red Rind (Sargento)	1 oz	9	100	81%
Nacho (Sargento)	1 oz	9	106	76%
Nacho Cheese Dip (*See also* Cheese Sauce in this listing)				
(Kraft) Premium	2 Tbs	4	50	72%
(New Holland)				
Caraway	1 oz	8	90	80%
Garlic & Herb	1 oz	8	90	80%
Hot Jalapeno	1 oz	8	90	80%
Natural-part-skim/semi-soft	1 oz	8	90	80%
Neufchatel	1 oz	7	80	79%
Nippy (Kraft)	1 oz	7	90	70%

Food and Description	Amount	Fat Grams	Total Calories	% Fat Calories
Norwegian Jarlsbery-Sliced				
(Sargento)	1 oz	7	100	63%
Nuggets-Breaded Cheese				
(Schwan's) Frozen	3.5 oz	19	360	48%
Onion (Land O'Lakes)				
Cheese Food	1 oz	7	90	70%
Parmesan				
Fresh (Sargento)	1 oz	7	111	57%
Grated	1 Tbs	1.5	23	59%
	1 oz	8.5	129	59%
(Sargento)	1 oz	9	130	55%
Hard	1 oz	7	111	57%
Natural (Kraft)	1 oz	7	110	57%
Parmesan & Romano (Sargento)				
Grated	1 oz	7	110	57%
Parmesan Wedge (Frigo)	1 oz	7	110	57%
Pepperoni (Land O'Lakes)				
Cheese Food	1 oz	7	90	70%
Pimiento				
Pasteurized	1 oz	8.8	106	75%
Pasteurized Process Slices (Kraft)	1 oz	8	100	72%
Singles Cheese Food (Kraft)	1 oz	7	90	70%
Snack (Sargento)				
Pasteurized Process	1 oz	9	110	74%
Pizza Double Cheese (Sargento)				
Light Shredded	1 oz	4	70	51%
Pizza Topper (Formagg)	1 oz	5	70	64%
Pizza Topping (Lunch Wagon)	1 oz	6	80	68%
Port du Salut	1 oz	8	100	72%
Port Wine Nut Log (Sargento)	1 oz	7	100	63%
Pot				
(Land O'Lakes)	4 oz	5	120	38%
(Sargento)	1 oz	–	25	–
Provolone	1 oz	7.55	100	68%
(Alpine Lace) Provo-Lo	1 oz	5	70	64%
(Formagg) Cheese Food	1 oz	5	70	64%
(Kraft)	1 oz	7	100	63%
(Land O'Lakes) Natural	1 oz	8	100	72%
(Sargento)	1 oz	8	100	72%
Pub Cheese -Soft w/Garlic & Herbs	1 oz	8	90	80%
Queso Blanco (Sargento)	1 oz	9	100	81%
Queso de Papa (Sargento)	1 oz	9	110	66%
Ricotta				
(Formagg) cheese food	1 oz	5	130	35%

Food and Description	Amount	Fat Grams	Total Calories	% Fat Calories
(Frigo)				
Low-Fat	1 oz	1	20	45%
Part Skim	1 oz	3	40	68%
Whole Milk	1 oz	5	60	75%
Generic				
Part Skim Milk	½ cup	9.8	171	52%
	1 oz	3	42	64%
Lite (Sargento)	1 oz	1	23	39%
(Sargento)				
Lite	1 oz	1	25	36%
Part Skim	1 oz	2	30	60%
Whole Milk				
Generic	½ cup	16	216	67%
	1 oz	4	40	90%
Romano	1 oz	7.6	110	62%
(Kraft) grated	1 oz	9	130	62%
(Sargento)	1 oz	8	110	66%
Romano-Flavored Spaghetti Topping				
Grated	1 oz	3	80	34%
(Rondele') Soft Spreadable Cheese				
Fine Herbs	1 oz	9	100	81%
Garlic & Herbs	1 oz	9	100	81%
Jardiniere-Garden Vegetables	1 oz	9	100	81%
Roquefort	1 oz	8.69	105	75%
Salami Cheese Food (Land O'Lakes)	1 oz	7	90	70%
Sandwich Slices (Lunch Wagon)	1 oz	7	90	70%
Smokelle (Kraft) Cheese Food	1 oz	7	90	70%
Smokestick (Sargento)	1 oz	7	100	63%
Spreads (See Cheese Spreads, in this listing)				
Squeeze Cheese				
Bacon	1 oz	6	82	66%
Jalapeno	1 oz	6	82	66%
Mild Cheddar	1 oz	6	82	66%
(Stella)				
Fontinella	1 oz	9	110	74%
Italian Sharp	1 oz	9	110	74%
Kasseri	1 oz	9	110	74%
Provolone	1 oz	7	100	63%
String Cheese				
(Sargento)				
Plain	1 oz	5	80	56%
Smoked	1 oz	5	80	56%
Swiss	1 oz	7.78	107	65%
Aged (Kraft)	1 oz	8	110	66%

Food and Description	Amount	Fat Grams	Total Calories	% Fat Calories
Almond Nut Log (Sargento)	1 oz	7	90	70%
(Alpine Lace) Swiss-Lo	1 oz	6	90	60%
(Borden)	1 oz	8	100	72%
(Cache Valley) Natural	1 oz	8	100	72%
(Cracker Barrel) Natural Baby Swiss	1 oz	9	110	65%
(Dorman's) Deli Light				
90% Less Salt	1 oz	8	100	72%
(Kraft)				
Deluxe Slices Cheese Food	1 oz	7	90	70%
Light Naturals-Reduced Fat	1 oz	5	90	50%
Very Low Sodium	1 oz	8	110	66%
(Land O'Lakes) Natural	1 oz	8	110	66%
(Lifetime) Lite	1 oz	3	55	49%
(Light N'Lively)	1 oz	4	70	51%
(Lite-Line)	1 oz	2	50	36%
Pasteurized	1 oz	7	95	66%
Processed	1 oz	7	95	66%
(Sargento)				
Cheese Food	1 oz	7	95	66%
Light Sliced or Shredded	1 oz	5	80	56%
Natural	1 oz	8	110	66%
Sliced Finland	1 oz	8	110	66%
Snack-Pasteurized Process	1 oz	7	100	63%
(Weight Watchers)	1 oz	2	50	36%
Natural	1 oz	5	80	56%
Taco				
(Kraft)				
Shredded	1 oz	9	110	74%
(Sargento)	1 oz	9	110	74%
Light Shredded	1 oz	5	80	56%
Tilsit	1 oz	7	96	66%
Tilsiter				
(Dorman's) Natural	1 oz	11	120	83%
(Sargento)	1 oz	7	100	63%
Tybo-Red Wax				
(Sargento)	1 oz	7	100	63%
(Velveeta) Spread (See Cheese Spreads in this listing)				
Welsh Rarebit (also Rabbit)				
Homemade	1 cup	32	415	69%
CHEESE SNACKS (See SNACKS)				
CHEESE SOUP (See SOUP)				
CHEESE SUBSTITUTE				
■ CHEESE-FLAVORED SPRINKLE PRODUCTS				
Best of Butter-cheddar cheese	½ tsp	< 1	6	75%
(Cheeztwin) singles	1 oz	6	90	60%

Food and Description	Amount	Fat Grams	Total Calories	% Fat Calories
(Delica)				
American pasteurized process	1 oz	6	80	68%
American & Caraway pasteurized process	1 oz	6	80	68%
American & Hot Pepper pasteurized process	1 oz	6	80	68%
American & Salami pasteurized process	1 oz	6	80	68%
American-Hickory Smoked pasteurized process	1 oz	6	80	68%
(Fisher Ched-O-Mate) Cheddar shredded	1 oz	7	90	70%
(Fisher Pizza-Mate) Mozzarella shredded	1 oz	7	90	70%
(Fisher Sandwich-Mate) singles	1 oz	6	90	60%
(Formagg) no lactose - lower in saturated fat - made w/canola oil				
American				
white	1 oz	5	70	64%
yellow	1 oz	5	70	64%
Cheddar	1 oz	5	70	64%
Cream Cheese Style	1 oz	5	70	64%
Cottage-flavored	1 oz	5	70	64%
Jalapeno	1 oz	5	70	64%
Mild Cheddar	1 oz	5	70	64%
Monterey Jack	1 oz	5	70	64%
Mozzarella-shredded	1 oz	5	70	64%
Parmesan-shredded	1 oz	5	70	64%
Pasta Topping-grated	1 oz	5	70	64%
Pizza Topper-shredded	1 oz	5	70	64%
Provolone	1 oz	5	70	64%
Ricotta	1 oz	.85	35	22%
Salad Topper-shredded	1 oz	5	70	64%
Sour Cream Style	1 oz	5	70	64%
Swiss	1 oz	5	70	64%
(Lite-Line) Low Cholesterol				
Singles	1 oz	7	90	70%
Molly McButter	½ tsp	–	4	–
CHERIMOYA				
raw–5" dia.	1	2	459	4%
CHERRY				
Maraschino	10 large	–	97	–
	1 large	–	10	–
w/liquid	1 oz	–	33	–

Food and Description	Amount	Fat Grams	Total Calories	% Fat Calories
Royal Anne				
canned (World Classic)	½ cup	–	90	–
Sour-Red	1 cup	< 1	51	9%
canned				
in water	1 cup	< 1	87	5%
in light syrup	1 cup	< 1	188	2%
in heavy syrup	1 cup	< 1	232	2%
in xtra heavy syrup	1 cup	< 1	296	2%
frozen				
no sugar	1 cup	.7	72	9%
	3.5 oz	<1	50	3%
sweetened	1 cup	.7	224	3%
Sweet	1 cup	1	104	9%
	10	.7	49	13%
candied				
whole	10	< 1	119	4%
	1 oz	< 1	96	5%
canned				
in water	1 cup	< 1	114	4%
in juice	1 cup	< 1	136	3%
in light syrup	1 cup	< 1	170	3%
in heavy syrup	1 cup	< 1	213	2%
in xtra heavy syrup	1 cup	< 1	266	2%
canned (Del Monte)				
dark sweet				
w/pits	½ cup	< 1	90	5%
w/o pits	½ cup	< 1	90	5%
light sweet				
w/pits	½ cup	< 1	100	5%
frozen				
sweetened	1 cup	< 1	232	2%
unsweetened	3.5 oz	< 1	60	8%
CHERRY DRINK (*See also* BLACK CHERRY DRINK)				
(Hi-C)	6 oz	–	100	–
	8.4 oz	–	141	–
(Juice Works)	6 oz	–	96	–
(Kool-Aid) Kooler	8.45 oz	–	140	–
(Kool-Aid) Mix				
Pre-sweetened	8 oz	–	70	–
Regular	8 oz	–	100	–
Squeezit (Betty Crocker)	6.75 oz	–	110	–
(Tang) Fruit Box	8.45 oz	–	120	–
CHERRY FRUIT JUICE COCKTAIL				
(Welch's)	6 oz	–	110	–

Food and Description	Amount	Fat Grams	Total Calories	% Fat Calories
frozen	6 oz	–	90	–
CHERRY JUICE (*See also* BLACK CHERRY JUICE)				
Juicy Juice				
(Libby's)	6 oz	–	90	–
Mountain				
(Dole) Pure & Light	6 oz	–	90	–
CHERRY NECTAR				
Cherry Delight Nectar	6 oz	–	80	–
CHERVIL				
dried	1 tsp	–	1	–
raw	4 oz	–	65	–
CHESTNUT				
Chinese				
boiled-steamed	1 oz	–	44	–
dried	1 oz	.5	103	4%
roasted	1 oz	–	68	–
European				
boiled-steamed	1 oz	–	37	–
dried	1 oz	1	106	8%
roasted	1 oz	.6	70	8%
Japanese				
boiled-steamed	1 oz	–	16	–
dried	1 oz	–	102	–
roasted	1 oz	–	57	–
CHESTNUT FLOUR	4 oz	4	410	9%
CHEWING GUM (*See* GUM)				
CHICKEN				
Chicken, broilers or fryers				
flesh, skin, giblets, & neck 1 chicken				
batter dipped/fried	~ 2¼ lb	180	2987	54%
flour coated/fried	~ 1½ lb	108	1928	50%
roasted	~ 1½ lb	90	1598	51%
stewed	~ 1½ lb	92.9	1625	52%
Chicken, broilers, or fryers-flesh & skin ½ chicken				
batter dipped/fried	~ 1 lb	80.8	1347	54%
flour coated/fried	~ ¾ lb	46.8	844	50%
roasted	~ ¾ lb	40.67	715	51%
stewed	~ ¾ lb	41.96	730	52%
Chicken, broilers, or fryers-flesh only				
fried	~ 5 oz	12.77	307	37%
roasted w/skin	~ 5 oz	10	266	34%
stewed w/skin	~ 5 oz	9	248	33%
Chicken-Dark Meat w/skin				
batter dipped/fried	~ 9.5 oz	51.8	828	56%

Food and Description	Amount	Fat Grams	Total Calories	% Fat Calories
flour coated/fried	~ 6.5 oz	31	523	53%
roasted	~ 6 oz	26	423	55%
stewed	~ 6.5 oz	26.97	428	57%
Chicken-Light Meat w/skin				
batter dipped/fried	~ 7 oz	29	520	50%
flour coated/fried	~ 5 oz	15.7	320	44%
roasted	~ 5 oz	14	293	43%
stewed	~ 5 oz	14.95	302	45%
Chicken-Dark Meat w/o skin				
fried	~ 5 oz	16	334	43%
roasted	~ 5 oz	13.6	286	43%
stewed	~ 5 oz	12.57	269	42%
Chicken-Light Meat w/o skin				
fried	~ 5 oz	7.76	268	26%
roasted	~ 5 oz	6	242	22%
stewed	~ 5 oz	5.58	223	23%
Chicken Giblets (chopped or diced)				
flour coated/fried	1 cup	19.5	402	44%
simmered	1 cup	6.9	228	27%
Chicken Gizzard/simmered	1 cup	5	222	20%
	1 oz	1	43	21%
Chicken Heart/simmered	3 oz	5	158	29%
Chicken Liver/simmered	~ 5 oz	7.6	219	31%
Individual Pieces of broilers or fryers				
Chicken Backs/meat & skin				
batter coated/fried	~ 4 oz	26	397	59%
flour-coated/fried	~ 2.5 oz	14.9	238	56%
roasted	~ 2 oz	11	159	62%
stewed	~ 2 oz	11	158	63%
Chicken Backs/meat only				
fried	~ 2 oz	8.88	167	48%
roasted	~ 1.5 oz	5	96	47%
stewed	~ 1.5 oz	4.7	88	48%
Chicken Breast/meat & skin				
batter dipped/fried	~ 5 oz	18.5	364	46%
flour-coated/fried	~ 3.5 oz	8.69	218	36%
roasted	~ 3.5 oz	7.6	193	35%
stewed	~ 4 oz	8	202	36%
Chicken Breast/meat only				
fried	~ 3 oz	4	161	22%
roasted	~ 3 oz	3	142	19%
stewed	~ 3 oz	2.88	144	18%
Chicken Breast/smoked				
(Butterball) 97% fat free	¾ oz	1	25	36%

Food and Description	Amount	Fat Grams	Total Calories	% Fat Calories
(Eckrich) Lite	1 oz	1	30	30%
Chicken Drumstick/meat & skin				
batter dipped/fried	~ 2.5 oz	11	193	51%
flour coated/fried	~ 2 oz	6.7	120	50%
roasted	~ 2 oz	5.8	112	47%
stewed	~ 2 oz	6	116	47%
Chicken Drumstick/meat only				
fried	~ 1.5 oz	3	82	33%
roasted	~ 1.5 oz	2	76	24%
stewed	~ 1.5 oz	2.6	78	30%
Chicken Leg/meat & skin				
batter dipped/fried	~ 5.5 oz	25.55	431	53%
flour coated/fried	~ 4 oz	16	285	51%
roasted	~ 4 oz	15	265	51%
stewed	~ 4 oz	16	275	52%
Chicken Leg/meat only				
fried	~ 3 oz	8.76	195	40%
roasted	~ 3 oz	8	182	40%
stewed	~ 3.5 oz	8	187	39%
Chicken Thigh/meat & skin				
batter dipped/fried	~ 3 oz	14	238	53%
flour coated/fried	~ 2 oz	9	162	50%
roasted	~ 2 oz	9.6	153	56%
stewed	~ 2 oz	10	158	57%
Chicken Thigh/meat only				
fried	~ 2 oz	5	113	40%
roasted	~ 2 oz	5.66	109	47%
stewed	~ 2 oz	5	107	42%
Chicken Wing/meat & skin				
batter dipped/fried	~ 2 oz	10.68	159	61%
flour coated/fried	~ 1 oz	7	103	61%
roasted	~ 1.5 oz	6.6	99	60%
stewed	~ 1.5 oz	6.7	100	60%
Chicken Wing/meat only				
fried	~ 1 oz	1.8	42	39%
roasted	~ 1 oz	1.7	43	36%
stewed	~ 1 oz	1.7	43	36%
Chicken, Roasting/roasted				
meat & skin	~ 5 oz	9	233	35%
light meat/meat only	~ 5 oz	5.7	214	34%
Chicken, Stewing				
meat, skin, & giblets				
stewed 1 chicken	~ 1¼ lb	106.9	1636	59%
meat & skin, no giblets	~ 9 oz	49	744	59%

Food and Description	Amount	Fat Grams	Total Calories	% Fat Calories
meat only	~5 oz	16.6	332	45%
light meat w/o skin	~5 oz	11	298	33%
dark meat w/o skin	~5 oz	21	361	52%
(Perdue)				
Cornish Game Hen/fresh-after roasting 1-oz uncooked portion				
dark meat w/skin	1 oz	3.3	49	61%
white meat w/skin	1 oz	2.3	41	50%
Oven Stuffer Roaster/fresh-after roasting 1-oz uncooked portion				
breast				
boneless	1 oz	.3	28	10%
whole	1 oz	2	40	45%
dark meat w/skin	1 oz	3.1	46	61%
drumsticks	1 oz	2.1	40	47%
thigh				
boneless cutlets	1 oz	1.9	37	46%
whole	1 oz	3.5	50	63%
white meat w/skin	1 oz	2.2	42	47%
wingettes	1 oz	3.3	50	59%
Perdue Done It!/cooked as packaged				
barbecued chicken wings	1 oz	4.1	65	57%
chicken breast cutlets	1 oz	4.3	70	55%
chicken breast nuggets				
cheese	1 oz	5.4	81	60%
fun-shaped	1 oz	4.5	74	55%
original	1 oz	4.3	70	55%
southern style batter	1 oz	4.2	71	53%
chicken breast tenders	1 oz	3.2	63	46%
garlic butter & herb chicken wings	1 oz	3.8	62	55%
roasted chicken	1 oz	2.2	46	43%
roasted cornish hen	1 oz	3	48	56%
Young Chicken/fresh-after roasting 1-oz uncooked portion				
breast				
boneless	1 oz	.6	30	18%
quarters	1 oz	2.2	42	47%
tenders	1 oz	.3	28	10%
whole	1 oz	2.3	43	48%
dark meat w/skin	1 oz	3.3	47	63%
drumstick	1 oz	1.9	38	45%
ground	1 oz	2.6	41	57%
leg				
quarters	1 oz	3	45	60%
whole	1 oz	3.5	50	63%
thigh	1 oz	4.2	55	69%
white meat w/skin	1 oz	2.4	42	51%

Food and Description	Amount	Fat Grams	Total Calories	% Fat Calories
wing drumettes	1 oz	3.1	48	58%
wings	1 oz	3.6	52	62%
CHICKEN ENTREE/DINNER (*See also* FROZEN ENTREE/DINNER)				
(Banquet) Frozen				
Boneless Chicken & Cheese Hot Bites				
Breast Tenders	2.25 oz	6	150	36%
Chicken Drum-Snackers	2.5 oz	14	210	60%
Chicken Nuggets	2.5 oz	13	200	59%
Chicken Nuggets w/Cheddar	2.5 oz	13	240	49%
Chicken Patties	2.5 oz	12	190	57%
Chicken Sticks	2.5 oz	14	210	60%
Hot'n Spicy Chicken Nuggets	2.5 oz	14	240	53%
Mozzarella Cheese Nuggets	2.5 oz	12	230	47%
Southern Fried				
Breast Tenders	2.25 oz	12	160	68%
Chicken Nuggets	2.5 oz	14	210	60%
Chicken Patties	2.5 oz	12	200	54%
Chicken Products				
Fried Chicken Breast Portions	5.75 oz	11	220	45%
Fried Chicken Thighs & Drumsticks	6.15 oz	14	250	50%
Hot'n Spicy Fried Chicken	6.4 oz	19	330	52%
Hot'n Spicy Snack'n Chicken	3.75 oz	9	140	58%
Original Fried Chicken	5.6 oz	17	290	53%
Southern Fried Chicken	5.6 oz	17	290	53%
Country Skillet				
Chicken Chunks	3 oz	16	260	55%
Chicken Nuggets	3 oz	15	250	54%
Chicken Patties	3 oz	15	230	59%
Southern Fried Chicken				
Chunks	3 oz	18	270	60%
Patties	3 oz	15	240	56%
Chicken A la king				
canned				
Generic	~ 5 oz	11.7	182	58%
(Swanson)	5.25 oz	12	190	57%
homemade	1 cup	34	468	65%
Chicken Almond w/rice				
(Van de Kamp's)	11 oz	15	440	31%
Chicken and Rice/box-mixes prepared				
Almond Chicken-Wild Rice				
(Savory Classics)	1 serving	4	140	26%
Chicken-Broccoli-Dijon				
(Savory Classics)	1 serving	5	160	28%
Chicken Flavor (Rice-A-Roni)	1 serving	1	130	7%

Food and Description	Amount	Fat Grams	Total Calories	% Fat Calories
Chicken Florentine				
(Savory Classics)	1 serving	.8	108	7%
Chicken Mushroom (Rice-A-Roni)	1 serving	1	129	7%
Chicken-Peas & Carrots				
(Minute Microwave)	½ cup	1	130	7%
Chicken Rice & Sauce (Lipton)	½ cup	4	150	24%
Chicken & Vegetables (Rice-A-Roni)	1 serving	3	140	19%
Chicken-Vermicelli				
(Rice-A-Roni)	1 serving	5	170	27%
Chicken and Vegetable Stew (Bounty)	7.5 oz	7	166	38%
Chicken Applause! Oven Bake Dinners (Kraft) Box				
Barbeque & scalloped potatoes	1 Serving	7	380	17%
Mushroom & rice	1 Serving	6	380	14%
Three Cheese & rice	1 Serving	15	430	31%
Chicken Cacciatore				
Homemade	1 cup	32	525	55%
(Lean Cuisine) frozen	~ 11 oz	10	280	32%
Chicken Cordon Bleu				
Homemade	8 oz	13	335	35%
(Swift) International Entree	6 oz	17	360	43%
Chicken (Country Pride) frozen				
Chicken Chunks	3 oz	15	238	57%
Chicken Patties	3 oz	16	245	59%
Chicken Sticks	3 oz	14	233	54%
Southern Fried Chicken Chunks	3 oz	20	276	65%
Southern Fried Chicken Patties	3 oz	15	232	58%
Chicken - creamed/homemade	½ cup	12	208	52%
Chicken Creole/no rice/homemade	~ 6.5 oz			
	(¾ cup)	3	137	20%
Chicken Croissant/frozen (Sara Lee)	1	17	340	45%
Chicken/Egg noodles w/chicken dinner				
(Kraft) box mix	¾ cup	9	240	34%
Chicken Fiesta (International Lites)				
microwaveable - box prepared	10 oz	3	220	12%
Chicken Fricassee				
Standard Home Recipe (USDA)	1 cup	22	386	51%
Chicken Glazed Breast of (Top Shelf)				
box prepared - microwaveable	10 oz	2	170	11%
Chicken Hash/homemade	1 cup	11	239	41%
Chicken Helper (Betty Crocker) Box mix - prepared				
Chicken Tetrazzini	1 serving	12	320	34%
Crispy Chicken & Biscuits	1 serving	42	710	53%
Crispy Chicken & Seasoned Rice	1 serving	38	690	50%
Mushroom Chicken	1 serving	25	470	48%

Food and Description	Amount	Fat Grams	Total Calories	% Fat Calories
Stuffing	1 serving	32	570	51%
Chicken (Hunt's Minute Gourmet) Box mix				
Barbeque Chicken	6.8 oz	4	320	11%
Chicken Cacciatore	~ 8 oz	6	280	19%
Chicken Italian Style				
(Weaver) frozen	3 oz	11	205	48%
Chicken Kiev (Swift)				
International Entree	6 oz	24	420	51%
Chicken Marsala, Breast of				
frozen (Lean Cuisine)	8.5 oz	5	190	24%
Chicken w/noodles/homemade	1 cup	18	365	44%
Chicken Pie/frozen (Stouffer's)	10 oz	33	530	56%
Chicken Pot Pies				
Frozen				
(Banquet)	7 oz	36	550	59%
(Morton)	7 oz	28	420	60%
(Swanson)	7 oz	22	380	52%
Homestyle Recipe	8 oz	21	410	46%
Hungry Man	16 oz	35	630	50%
(Tyson)				
Light & Dark Meat	9 oz	20	390	46%
White Meat	9 oz	20	400	45%
Standard Home Recipe				
USDA)-(9"dia)	⅓ serving/			
	~ 8 oz	31	545	51%
Chicken Salad				
Standard Home Recipe (USDA)	½ cup	8	121	60%
Chicken Stew				
canned				
(Chef Boyardee)	7 oz	5	140	32%
(Heinz) w/dumplings	7.5 oz	9	210	39%
(Swanson)	7⅝ oz	7	160	39%
Chicken Supreme-frozen				
(Lite Pockets)	1	5	240	19%
Chicken Tetrazzini-frozen	11.5 oz	14	320	39%
Chicken Tortellini Alfredo (International Lites)				
microwave box mix	10 oz	13	290	40%
Chunk Style Mixin' Chicken				
canned (Swanson)	2½ oz	8	130	55%
Great Beginnings (Hormel) Box mix				
w/chunky chicken	5 oz	8	147	49%
w/chunky turkey	5 oz	8	138	52%
(Hormel) Chicken By George Gourmet Entree-found in the grocery meat case				
Caribbean Grill	5 oz	6	200	27%

Food and Description	Amount	Fat Grams	Total Calories	% Fat Calories
Cajun	5 oz	8	180	40%
Country Mustard & Dill	5 oz	7	180	35%
for Fajitas	5 oz	4	170	21%
Italian Blue Cheese	5 oz	8	190	40%
Lemon Herb	5 oz	6	170	32%
Mesquite Barbeque	5 oz	6	170	32%
Mexican Style	5 oz	7	190	33%
Teriyaki	5 oz	5	180	25%
Tomato Herb w/Basil	5 oz	7	190	33%
(Lunch Bucket) Microwaveable Meals				
Light Balance				
Chicken Cacciatore	8.25 oz	1	100	9%
Chicken Fiesta	8.25 oz	3	210	13%
Original				
Dumplings'n Chicken	8.5 oz	3	170	16%
(Schwan's) chicken/frozen-partially or fully cooked, unless otherwise stated.				
BBQ Wings	3.5 oz	14	220	57%
Breaded Chicken	7.5 oz	14	250	50%
Breast Fillet-raw-unbreaded	3.25 oz	1	90	10%
Breast Patties	3 oz	14	210	60%
Breast Strips	3.5 oz	14	270	47%
Breast w/Asparagus & Cheese	6 oz	14	300	42%
Chicken Kiev	5 oz	24	360	60%
Chicken Marco Polo	5.3 oz	12	290	37%
Chicken Nuggets	3.5 oz	17	260	59%
Cordon Bleu	5 oz	14	290	43%
Diced Chicken Meat	3.5 oz	4	120	30%
Drummies	3.5 oz	15	260	52%
Golden Chicken Nuggets	3.5 oz/~ 7 nuggets	9	180	45%
Hot & Spicy Chicken Nuggets	3.5 oz/5-6 nuggets	19	320	53%
Hot Wings	3.5 oz	14	220	57%
(Swanson) frozen Plump & Juicy Chicken				
Chicken Dipsters	3 oz	14	220	57%
Chicken Drumlets	3 oz	14	220	57%
Chicken Nibbles	3¼ oz	20	300	60%
Chicken Nuggets	8¾ oz	25	460	49%
Fried Chicken-breast portion	4½ oz	22	360	55%
1 lb Take-Out pre-fried chicken	3¼ oz	17	270	57%
Take-Out fried chicken	3¼ oz	17	270	57%
Thighs and Drumsticks	3¼ oz	19	280	61%
(TastyBird Foods) chicken/frozen-raw-ready to cook				
Breast Fillet Pattie	3.5 oz	14	229	55%

Food and Description	Amount	Fat Grams	Total Calories	% Fat Calories
Breast Fillet Pattie				
hoagie shaped	3.5 oz	10.8	211	46%
Breast Strip	1 oz	2.8	54	47%
Breast Tenderloins	3.5 oz	8.7	189	41%
Chicken Delites	3.5 oz	19	252	68%
Chicken Nuggets	3.5 oz	13.8	215	58%
Hi-Pro Chicken Patties	3.5 oz	19	252	68%
Natural Breast Fillet	3.5 oz	8.6	187	41%
Spicy Breast Tenderloins	3.5 oz	7	170	37%
TastyBird Breaded Breast				
Quarters	3.5 oz	11	192	52%
TastyBird Breaded Leg Quarters	3.5 oz	11.7	199	53%
(Tyson)				
Frozen Boneless Portions				
Breast Chunks	3 oz	17	240	64%
Breast Fillets	3 oz	9	190	43%
Breast Fillets-southern fried	3 oz	11	220	45%
Breast Patties	2.6 oz	15	220	61%
Breast Patties-southern fried	2.6 oz	15	220	61%
Chick'n Cheddar	2.6 oz	15	220	61%
Chick'n Chunks	2.6 oz	15	220	61%
Chunk'n Chunks-southern fried	2.6 oz	15	220	61%
Cornish Game Hens	3.5 oz	14	240	57%
Diced Meat	3 oz	3	130	21%
Thick & Crispy Patties	2.6 oz	14	220	57%
Wings				
Barbecue	3.5 oz/6-7 wings	14	218	58%
Hot & Spicy	3.5 oz/6-7 wings	14	218	58%
Roasted	3.5 oz/6-7 wings	14	218	58%
Teriyaki	3.5 oz/6-7 wings	14	218	58%
Marinated				
Barbecue Chicken Breast	3.75	3	130	21%
Butter Garlic Chicken Breast	3.75	3	120	23%
Italian Chicken Breast	3.75 oz	3	120	23%
Lemon Pepper Chicken Breast	3.75 oz	3	130	21%
Microwave				
Breast Sandwich	1	14	328	39%
Chicken Corn Dogs	3.5 oz	14	280	45%
Chunks	3.5 oz	15	220	61%
Mini Sandwich	1	5	230	20%

Food and Description	Amount	Fat Grams	Total Calories	% Fat Calories
Nuggets	4 oz	15	220	61%
Tenders	3.5 oz	11	230	43%
Premium Dinners				
Francais	9.5 oz	14	280	45%
Glazed	9.25 oz	4	240	15%
Grilled	7.75 oz	3	220	12%
Grilled Italian	9 oz	4	220	16%
Honey Roasted	9 oz	4	220	16%
Kiev	9.25 oz	33	520	57%
Marsala	9 oz	4	200	18%
Mesquite	9.5 oz	8	320	23%
Parmigiana	11.25 oz	17	380	40%
Picante	9 oz	4	250	14%
Picatta	9 oz	10	240	38%
Roasted	9 oz	2	200	9%
Sweet & Sour	11 oz	8	440	16%
w/Gravy	9 oz	6	230	16%
Roasted (Fully Cooked)				
Breast Fillets	1 oz	2	50	36%
Breasts	1 oz	3	50	54%
Drumsticks	1 oz	3	50	54%
Half Chicken	1 oz	4	60	60%
Thighs	1 oz	5	70	64%
Whole Chicken	1 oz	4	60	60%
Wings	1 oz	5	70	64%
Wholesale Club Items				
Blanched Tenders	3.5 oz	8	200	8%
Boneless Breasts	3.5 oz	12	210	51%
Boneless Skinless Breasts	3.5 oz	2	130	8%
Boneless Skinless Thighs	3.5 oz	10	200	45%
Breast Halves	3.5 oz	13	230	51%
Breast Patties	3.5 oz	19	310	55%
Breast Tenders (breaded)	3.5 oz	11	240	41%
Breast Tenders (unbreaded)	3.5 oz	1	120	8%
Canned Chicken	3.5 oz	3	150	18%
Chicken Chili	3.5 oz	3	105	26%
Chicken Pattie Nuggets	3.5 oz	20	330	55%
Classic Colonial	3.5 oz	9	180	45%
Cordon Bleu	5 oz	16	340	42%
	7 oz	22	480	41%
Cordon Bleu Mini	each	4	90	40%
Cornish w/Wild Rice	3.5 oz	11	190	52%
Drums & Thighs	3.5 oz	17	270	57%
Fajita Kit	3.5 oz	5	150	30%

Food and Description	Amount	Fat Grams	Total Calories	% Fat Calories
Hors D'Oeuvres				
Barbecue Wings	3.5 oz	12	210	51%
Mesquite Chicken Chunks	3.5 oz	1	100	9%
Roaster Wings	3.5 oz	12	210	51%
Julienne Leg Meat	3.5 oz	6	160	34%
Mesquite B/S Breast Fillets	3.5 oz	2	110	16%
Mesquite Breast Pieces	3.5 oz	7	170	37%
Red Hot Wings	3.5 oz	19	280	61%
Roaster	3.5 oz	13	230	51%
Stir Fry Kit				
Chicken & Vegetables	4 oz	7	130	48%
Sauce Packet	.08 oz	1	50	18%
Wing Drumettes	3.5 oz	17	260	59%
Wings of Fire	3.5 oz	12	220	49%
(Weaver)				
Frozen Boneless Portions				
Batter Dipped				
Assorted	3.6 oz	18	290	56%
Breasts	4.4 oz	20	310	58%
Drums & Thighs	3 oz	14	210	60%
Wings	4 oz	28	400	63%
Breast Fillet Strips	3.3 oz	10	200	45%
Breast Fillets	4.5 oz	13	270	43%
Breast Patties	3 oz	11	205	48%
Chicken Nuggets	2.6 oz	12	190	57%
Crispy Dutch Frye				
Assorted	3.6 oz	18	290	56%
Breasts	4.5 oz	22	350	57%
Drums & Thighs	3.5 oz	19	290	59%
Wings	4 oz	28	400	63%
Crispy Light Skinless Chicken	2.9 oz	9	170	48%
Crispy Mini Drums	3 oz	12	210	51%
Croquettes	2 pieces	16	280	51%
Gravy	½ cup	2	26	69%
Herb & Spice Mini Drums	3 oz	11	200	50%
Honey Batter Tenders	3 oz	12	220	49%
Hot Wings	2.7 oz	11	170	48%
Premium Tenders	3 oz	9	170	48%
Rondelet				
Cheese	2.6 oz	11	190	52%
Italian	2.6 oz	11	190	52%
Original	3 oz	10	190	47%
CHICKEN PRODUCTS (*See also* LUNCHEON MEAT)				
Chicken/canned-boned w/broth	2.5 oz	5.6	117	43%

Food and Description	Amount	Fat Grams	Total Calories	% Fat Calories
(Hormel)				
Chunk Breast	6¾ oz	20	350	51%
Chunk Dark Meat	6¾ oz	18	327	50%
Chunk White & Dark	6¾ oz	20	340	53%
Chunk White & Dark no salt	6¾ oz	18	330	49%
(Swanson) Premium Chunk White	2½ oz	4	100	36%
(Swanson) Premium Chunk				
White & Dark	2½ oz	4	100	36%
Chicken Frankfurter	1 (1.5 oz)	8.8	116	68%
Chicken Liver-canned	1 oz	3.7	57	58%
Chicken Roll/light	2½ oz	4	90	40%
Chicken Spread/chunky/canned				
(Underwood)				
Light	2⅛ oz	5	100	45%
Original	2⅛ oz	9	150	66%
Smokey	2⅛ oz	8	150	48%
CHICKEN SALAD (See CHICKEN ENTREE/DINNER)				
CHICKEN SEASONING (See also SEASONINGS)				
(French's) Microwave Mixes				
Barbecue Chicken	¼ pkg	2	50	36%
Garlic Butter Chicken	¼ pkg	1	50	36%
Italian Parmesan Chicken	¼ pkg	2	50	36%
(Lipton) Microeasy Family Favorites - dry				
Barbeque Style Chicken	¼ pkg	.5	108	4%
Country Style Chicken	¼ pkg	.6	78	7%
(McCormick/Schilling)				
Bag'N Season - dry				
Chicken	1 pkg	1.5	177	8%
Italian Herb	1 pkg	–	94	–
Chicken Sauce Blends - dry				
Cacciatore	1 pkg	4.8	132	33%
Creole	1 pkg	4.8	140	31%
CHICKEN SOUP (See SOUP)				
CHICKPEA				
Boiled	½ cup	2	134	13%
Canned	½ cup	1	143	6%
(Del Monte) Salad Bar Vegetables				
Garbanzo Beans	2 oz	–	45	–
(Hain)	4 oz	2	80	23%
(Joan of Arc/Green Giant)	½ cup	2	90	20%
(Nutradiet)	½ cup	1	105	9%
(Progresso)	8 oz	4	200	18%
(S&W)				
lite-50% less salt	½ cup	1	110	8%

Food and Description	Amount	Fat Grams	Total Calories	% Fat Calories
marinaded	½ cup	1	120	8%
premium	½ cup	1	110	8%
Raw	½ cup	6	364	15%
CHICORY/ raw	8 oz	–	15	–
CHILI (*See* MEXICAN FOOD; SOUP)				
CHILI SAUCE (*See* SAUCE)				
CHINESE FOOD (*See* ORIENTAL FOOD)				
CHIVES				
freeze-dried	1 Tbs	–	1	–
raw	1 Tbs	–	1	–
	¼ cup	–	2	–
CHOCOLATE, BAKING				
(Baker's)				
Semi-sweet bar	1 oz	9	140	58%
Sweet German	1 oz	10	140	64%
Unsweetened	1 oz	15	140	96%
(Hershey's)				
Premium bar				
Semi-sweet	1 oz	8	140	51%
Unsweetened	1 oz	16	190	76%
(Nestles)				
Pre-melted-Unsweetened				
Choco Bake	1 oz	16	190	76%
Premier white	1 oz	5	80	56%
Semi-sweet	1 oz	9	160	51%
Unsweetened	1 oz	14	180	70%
CHOCOLATE CHIPS & CHUNKS				
(Baker's)				
Milk chocolate	1 oz	8	140	51%
Semi-sweet				
Big chips	¼ cup	13	220	53%
Flavored	½ cup	18	380	43%
Real	½ cup	24	400	54%
Chocolate-flavored	¼ cup	9	200	41%
(Hershey's)				
Milk chocolate				
Chips	1 oz	8	150	48%
	¼ cup	12	220	49%
Chunks	1 oz	9	160	51%
Mint	¼ cup	12	230	47%
Semi-sweet				
Chips	¼ cup	12	220	49%
Chunks	1 oz	8	140	51%
Vanilla Milk	¼ cup	14	240	53%

Food and Description	Amount	Fat Grams	Total Calories	% Fat Calories
CHOCOLATE MORSELS				
(Nestles)				
Butterscotch	1 oz	8	150	48%
Chocolate	1 oz	7	150	42%
Semi-sweet	1 oz	8	150	48%
CHOCOLATE NAPS (Champion)	1 oz	14	140	90%
CHOCOLATE SYRUP (Hershey's)	2 Tbs	< 1	110	4%
CHOCOLATE TREASURES				
(Nestles)				
Milk	1 oz	9	150	54%
Premier White	1 oz	10	160	56%
Semi-sweet chocolate	1 oz	8	150	48%
CHUB/raw	3 oz	7.5	124	54%
CINNAMON/ground	1 tsp	–	10	–
CITRON				
candied	1 oz	–	89	–
	3 oz	–	270	–
CLAM (*See also* SEAFOOD ENTREE/DINNER)				
breaded & fried	3 oz	9	171	47%
	20 Small	20.96	379	50%
canned	3 oz	1.65	126	12%
canned-chopped				
(Doxsee)				
liquid & solids	6.5 oz	.5	90	5%
(S&W)				
Fancy	2 oz	< 1	28	16%
canned-minced				
(Doxsee)				
liquid & solids	6.5 oz	.5	90	5%
(S&W)				
Fancy	2 oz	< 1	28	16%
canned-minced & chopped				
(Gorton's)	½ can	1	70	13%
canned-whole baby chowder				
(S&W)	2 oz	< 1	33	14%
raw	3 oz	.8	63	11%
steamed	3 oz	1.65	126	12%
	20 Small	1.75	133	12%
	1 cup	3	235	12%
CLAM CHOWDER (*See* SOUP)				
CLAM JUICE				
Clam (Doxsee)	3 oz	–	4	–
Clamato (Mott's)	6 oz	–	90	–
CLAM SAUCE (*See* SAUCE)				

Food and Description	Amount	Fat Grams	Total Calories	% Fat Calories
CLOVE/ground	1 tsp	–	7	–
CLUB SODA (*See* SOFT DRINKS)				
COBBLER (*See* PIE & COBBLER)				
COCKTAIL SAUCE (*See* SAUCE)				
COCKTAILS AND MIXERS (*See also* LIQUEUR)				
Alexander	2.5 fl oz	1.8	179	9%
Bacardi	2.5 fl oz	–	118	–
Black Russian	3 fl oz	–	255	–
Bloody Mary	5 fl oz	–	116	–
Bloody Mary Mix (Libby's)	6 fl oz	–	40	–
Bourbon & Soda	4 fl oz	–	105	–
Brandy	1 fl oz	–	75	–
Collins Mixer				
(Schweppes)	6 fl oz	–	70	–
(Shasta)	12 fl oz	–	118	–
Daiquiri	2 fl oz	–	111	–
Daiquiri Mixer (*See* Holland House)				
Gibson	2.5 fl oz	–	158	–
Gimlet	2.5 fl oz	–	132	–
Gin Rickey	7 fl oz	–	114	–
Gin & Tonic	7.5 fl oz	–	171	–
Gold Cadillac	4.5 fl oz	3.6	394	8%
Grasshopper	2.25 fl oz	3.6	164	20%
Grenadine Mixer (bottled)	1 fl oz	–	64	–
High Ball	8 fl oz	–	165	–
(Holland House) Mixers				
Bloody Mary (bottled)	1 fl oz	–	1	–
Daiquiri				
Plain				
(pouch)	1	–	4	–
(bottled)	1 fl oz	–	31	–
Strawberry (bottled)	1 fl oz	–	27	–
Mai Tai				
(bottled)	1 fl oz	–	29	–
(pouch)	1	–	4	–
Margarita (pouch)	1	–	4	–
Manhattan (bottle)	1 fl oz	–	27	–
Old Fashioned (bottle)	1 fl oz	–	33	–
Sweet & Sour Drink (bottle)	1 fl oz	–	29	–
Lemon Sour Mixer	6 fl oz	–	75	–
Mai Tai	4.5 fl oz	–	310	–
Manhattan	2.5 fl oz	–	128	–
Margarita	~3 fl oz	–	170	–
Martini	2.5 fl oz	–	156	–

Food and Description	Amount	Fat Grams	Total Calories	% Fat Calories
Mint Julep	10 fl oz	–	215	–
Old Fashioned	4 fl oz	–	180	–
Pina Colada				
Canned	4.5 fl oz	11	347	29%
Standard Home Recipe	4.5 fl oz	2.6	262	9%
Rum (hot-buttered)	~ 9 fl oz	11.9	317	34%
Screwdriver	7 fl oz	–	174	–
Singapore Sling	8 fl oz	–	228	–
Sloe Gin Fizz	8 fl oz	–	121	–
Sour Mixer				
(Canada Dry)	12 fl oz	–	135	–
(Schweppes)	12 fl oz	–	149	–
Stinger	3 fl oz	–	282	–
Tequila Sunrise	5.5 fl oz	–	189	–
Tom Collins	7.5 fl oz	–	121	–
	10 fl oz	–	180	–
Tom Collins Mix (bottled)	1 fl oz	–	42	–
Vodka Mixer				
(Schweppes)	12 fl oz	–	139	–
Whiskey Sour	3 fl oz	–	123	–
Whiskey Sour Mix				
(bottled)	2 fl oz	–	55	–
Prepared w/whiskey	3.5 fl oz	–	158	–
(powder)	1 packet	–	64	–
White Russian	3.5 fl oz	1	268	3%
COCOA (*See also* MILK MIXES)				
	⅓ cup	4	120	30%
	½ cup	5	173	26%
(Baker's)	3.5 oz	13	220	53%
(Hershey's)				
European	½ cup	3	90	30%
Original	⅓ cup	3	110	25%
(Nestles)	½ cup	6	180	30%
COCONUT				
(Baker's) Angel Flake				
Canned	⅓ cup	9	110	74%
Package	⅓ cup	8	120	60%
Premium Shred	⅓ cup	9	140	58%
Toasted	⅓ cup	17	200	77%
(Durkee) Shredded	1 cup	28	277	91%
Generic				
Dried-shredded				
sweetened	4 oz	40	570	63%
unsweetened	1 oz	18	187	87%

Food and Description	Amount	Fat Grams	Total Calories	% Fat Calories
Dried-canned-flakes sweetened	4 oz	36	505	64%
Dried-packaged flakes sweetened	4 oz	36.56	539	61%
	1 cup	23.8	351	61%
Raw-shredded	½ cup	13.39	141	86%
Toasted	1 oz	13	168	70%
COCONUT CREAM				
Canned, sweetened	1 Tbs	3	36	75%
	1 cup	52	568	82%
(Coco Lopez)	2 Tbs	5	120	38%
Raw	1 cup	83	792	94%
COCONUT MILK				
canned				
(A Taste of Thai) unsweetened	1 Tbs	2.5	25	90%
Generic	1 Tbs	3	30	90%
frozen	1 Tbs	3	30	90%
	1 cup	50	486	93%
raw	1 Tbs	3.58	35	92%
	1 cup	57	552	93%
COCONUT-PINEAPPLE NECTAR				
(Kern's)	6 oz	–	120	–
COCONUT WATER	1 cup	.5	46	10%
COD (*See also* SEAFOOD ENTREE/DINNER)				
Atlantic & Pacific				
breaded & fried	3 oz	9	175	46%
canned	3 oz	.7	89	7%
cooked-dry heat	3 oz	.7	89	7%
dried	3 oz	2	246	7%
frozen				
(Gorton's)	5 oz	1	110	8%
raw	3 oz	.57	70	7%
Roe	3 oz	1.7	111	14%
smoked	3 oz	< 1	87	5%
COFFEE & COFFEE-LIKE BEVERAGES				
Bottled				
(Maxwell House) Iced Cappucino				
Coffee Cappio	8 oz	3	120	23%
Cinnamon Cappio	8 oz	3	130	21%
Mocha Cappio	8 oz	3	130	21%
Brewed				
Decaf				
(Brim)	6 oz	–	2	–
Generic	6 oz	–	4	–

Food and Description	Amount	Fat Grams	Total Calories	% Fat Calories
(Maxwell House)	6 oz	–	2	–
(Sanka)	6 oz	–	2	–
(Yuban)	6 oz	–	2	–
Espresso	2 oz	–	1	–
Regular				
Generic	6 oz	–	4	–
(Yuban)	6 oz	–	2	–
Turkish	4 oz		45	–
Instant/flavored				
w/Cappuccino powder				
2 round tsp	6 oz	2	62	29%
w/Chicory powder				
1 round tsp	6 oz	–	6	–
w/French Flavor powder				
2 round tsp	6 oz	3	57	47%
(General Foods) International Coffees				
Cafe Amaretto powder	6 oz	2	50	36%
sugar-free	6 oz	2	35	51%
Cafe Francais	6 oz	3	60	45%
sugar-free	6 oz	2	35	51%
Cafe Irish Creme	6 oz	2	50	36%
sugar-free	6 oz	2	30	60%
Cafe Vienna	6 oz	2	60	30%
sugar-free	6 oz	2	30	60%
Double Chocolate Mint	6 oz	2	50	36%
Double Dutch Chocolate	6 oz	2	50	36%
Irish Mocha Mint	6 oz	2	50	36%
sugar-free	6 oz	2	25	72%
Orange Cappuccio	6 oz	2	60	30%
sugar-free	6 oz	2	30	60%
Suisse Mocha	6 oz	2	55	33%
sugar-free	6 oz	2	30	60%
(Hills Bros)				
Cafe Vienna	6 oz	2	60	30%
Dutch Chocolate	6 oz	2	60	30%
Orange Capri	6 oz	2	60	30%
Swiss Mocha	6 oz	2	60	30%
sugar free	6 oz	2	40	45%
(MJB)				
Banana Nut Mocha-sugar-free	6 oz	2	40	45%
Cafe Mocha	6 oz	1	50	18%
Cherry Mocha	6 oz	1	50	18%
Fudge Mocha-sugar-free	6 oz	2	40	45%
Mint Mocha	6 oz	1	50	18%

Food and Description	Amount	Fat Grams	Total Calories	% Fat Calories
sugar-free	6 oz	1	35	26%
Vanilla Mocha-sugar-free	6 oz	2	40	45%
Instant/regular	6 oz	–	4	–
(Brim)	6 oz	–	4	–
(KAVA)	1 tsp	–	2	–
(Maxwell House)	6 oz	–	2	–
(Nescafe)				
Brava	6 oz	–	4	–
Classic	6 oz	–	4	–
Decaf	6 oz	–	4	–
Silka	6 oz	–	4	–
(Sanka)	6 oz	–	2	–
(Taster's Choice)				
decaffeinated	6 oz	–	4	–
regular	6 oz	–	4	–
(Yuban)	6 oz	–	4	–
Kaffree Roma (Worthington)				
caffeine free	1tsp	–	6	–
(PERO) non-caffeinated Hot Beverage				
Drink w/malt & barley	6 oz	–	4	–
(Postum) coffee-flavored grain				
beverage	6 oz	–	12	–
w/whole milk + 1 tsp powder	6 oz	6	123	44%
coffee-flavored-no caffeine	6 oz	–	12	–
COLD CUTS (See LUNCHEON MEAT)				
COLLARDS				
canned-chopped, seasoned				
w/pork (Luck's)	7.5 oz	7	90	70%
fresh-cooked	½ cup	–	13	–
frozen				
Generic - cooked	½ cup	–	31	–
(Pictsweet)	3.3 oz	–	25	–
raw-chopped	½ cup	–	18	–
CONDIMENTS (See specific listings; SAUCE; SEASONINGS)				
COOKIE (See also BROWNIES, CRACKERS, SNACK CAKES)				
(NOTE: Homemade cookies were made with margarine.)				
Animal				
(Sunshine)	14 cookies	3	120	23%
Apple, Homestyle (Entenmann's)				
fat free	2 cookies	–	70	–
(Archway)				
Apple Filled Oatmeal	1 cookie	3	100	27%
Apple'N Raisin	1 cookie	3	120	23%
Chocolate Chip	1 cookie	5	110	41%

Food and Description	Amount	Fat Grams	Total Calories	% Fat Calories
Chocolate Chip & Toffee	1 cookie	7	150	42%
Cinnamon Snaps	1 cookie	2	40	45%
Coconut Macaroons	1 cookie	4	90	40%
Date Filled Oatmeal	1 cookie	3	100	27%
Dutch Cocoa	1 cookie	4	110	33%
Frosty Lemon	1 cookie	5	120	38%
Fruit & Honey Bar	1	3	100	27%
Ginger Snaps	1 cookie	1	35	28%
Iced Molasses	1 cookie	4	130	28%
Iced Oatmeal	1 cookie	5	140	32%
Lemon Snaps	2 cookies	2	35	51%
Molasses	1 cookie	3	120	23%
Old Fashion Windmill	1 cookie	3	90	30%
Oatmeal	1 cookie	3	110	25%
Oatmeal Raisin Bran	1 cookie	3	100	27%
Peanut Butter	1 cookie	6	110	49%
Rocky Road	1 cookie	5	130	35%
Ruth's Oatmeal	1 cookie	5	130	35%
Soft Sugar	1 cookie	3	90	30%
Vanilla Wafers	1 cookie	1	30	30%
Arrowroot	1 cookie	1	25	36%
(Austin)				
Chocolate Creme	1.8 oz pkg	7	230	27%
Lemon Ohs!	1.8 oz pkg	8	240	30%
Peanut Butter & Graham	1.8 oz pkg	9	240	34%
(Bakery Wagon)				
Apple Cinnamon	1 cookie	3	100	27%
Apple Filled Oatmeal	1 cookie	4	90	40%
Apple Walnut Raisin	1 cookie	3	100	27%
Date Filled Oatmeal	1 cookie	3	90	29%
Honey Fruit Bar	1 cookie	3	100	27%
Iced Molasses	1 cookie	4	100	36%
Oatmeal Chocolate Chunk	1 cookie	3	100	27%
Oatmeal Walnut Raisin	1 cookie	4	100	36%
Peanut Butter Oatmeal	1 cookie	7	110	57%
Raspberry Filled	1 cookie	3	90	30%
Soft Oatmeal	1 cookie	5	100	45%
(Barbara's)				
Fruit & Nut	2 cookies	2	125	14%
Fruit Bars				
Apricot	½ oz	1	50	18%
Cherry	½ oz	1	50	18%
Raspberry	½ oz	1	50	18%
Oatmeal Raisin	2 cookies	2	100	18%

Food and Description	Amount	Fat Grams	Total Calories	% Fat Calories
(Break Cake) Cookies				
Brownie Creme	1-2 oz	8	240	30%
Chips & Creme	1 cookie	6	140	39%
Chocolate Chip	1 oz	6	140	39%
Chocolate Sugar Wafer	4 wafers	9	200	41%
Coconut Macaroons	2-2 oz	14	270	47%
Devil's Food Creme	1 cookie	5	130	35%
Gingersnaps	5 cookies	5	130	42%
Hermit	1-2 oz	7	230	27%
Marshmallow Pie				
Banana	1-1.2 oz	5	150	30%
Chocolate	1-1.2 oz	5	150	30%
Devil's Food	1-1.2 oz	4	140	26%
Double Decker Chocolate	3 oz	11	360	28%
Oatmeal	5 cookies	6	140	39%
Peanut Butter (32 oz bag)	1 cookie	7	140	45%
Peanut Butter Wafer	1 wafer	9	180	45%
Raisin Creme	1 cookie	5	140	32%
Shortbread	5 cookies	6	140	39%
Strawberry Wafer	4 wafers	11	220	45%
Striper Wafer	1 wafer	10	190	47%
Vanilla Sugar Wafer	4 wafers	11	220	45%
Chocolate Chip				
box mix				
(Big Batch)	2 cookies	6	120	45%
(Duncan Hines)	2 cookies	5	130	35%
commercial (2¼"dia)	4 cookies	9	180	45%
(Entenmann's)	3 cookies	7	130	48%
homemade (2⅓" dia)	4 cookies	12	206	52%
refrigerated dough (2¼" dia)	4 cookies	11	225	44%
Chocolate Chip Cheese Cake				
(Formagg)	1 cookie	2	49	37%
Chocolate Creme-filled (Little Debbie)	1.8 oz	12	250	43%
Coconut Bars	1 cookie	5	110	41%
Coconut Macaroons (*See also* Macaroons in this listing)				
	2 cookies	5	100	45%
Date Bar-box mix (Classics Dessert)	2 bars	4	120	30%
Date Pecan Fancy Fruit (Health Valley)	2 cookies	2	70	26%
(Delicious)				
Almond Windmill	1 cookie	3	80	34%
Assorted Cookie Favorites				
Iced Oatmeal	2 cookies	6	130	42%
Macaroon	2 cookies	6	130	42%
Oatmeal	2 cookies	5	130	35%

Food and Description	Amount	Fat Grams	Total Calories	% Fat Calories
Sugar	2 cookies	6	130	42%
Chocolate Chip	2 cookies	8	140	51%
Coconut Bars	1 cookie	3	70	39%
Fig Bars	2 cookies	2	130	14%
Frosted Butter	1 cookie	5	88	51%
Ginger Snap	.5 oz	2	64	28%
Heath English Toffee Crunch	1 cookie	4	70	51%
Iced Oatmeal	2 cookies	6	130	42%
Jelly Top	.8 oz	5	112	40%
Land O'Lakes Butter	1 cookie	5	88	51%
Oatmeal	2 cookies	5	130	35%
Pecan	1 cookie	5	94	48%
Skippy Peanut Butter	1 cookie	6	80	68%
Sugar Cookies	2 cookies	6	130	42%
Sugar Wafers				
Assorted	¼ oz	2.5	40	56%
Chocolate	1 wafer	2	35	26%
Chocolate/Strawberry	1 wafer	2	35	26%
Lemon	1 wafer	2	35	26%
Mini Creme	1 wafer	1.5	25	54%
Strawberry	1 wafer	2	35	26%
Strawberry/Vanilla	1 wafer	2	35	26%
Vanilla	1 wafer	2	35	26%
	¼ oz	2.5	40	56%
Vanilla Wafers (bag)	.5 oz	2	70	26%
(Estee)				
Assorted Creme Filled Wafers	1 wafer	2	30	60%
Chocolate	1 wafer	1	20	45%
Vanilla	1 wafer	1	20	45%
Cookies	1 cookie	1	30	30%
Chocolate Chip	3 cookies	5	110	41%
Oatmeal Raisin	3 cookies	5	110	41%
Sandwich Cookies	1 cookie	2-3	45-50	50%-54%
Snack Wafers				
Chocolate, Vanilla, & Strawberry	1 wafer	4	80	45%
Snack Wafers/Chocolate coated	1 wafer	7	130	49%
(FFV)				
Animal	9 cookies	4	130	28%
Dinosaurs	10 cookies	5	130	35%
Ginger Boy	7 cookies	4	120	30%
Praline Pecan	1 cookie	2	40	45%
(Famous Amos)				
Chocolate Chip-no nuts				
extra chips	1 oz	8	147	49%

Food and Description	Amount	Fat Grams	Total Calories	% Fat Calories
Chocolate Chip w/Macadamias	1 oz	9	152	53%
Chocolate Chip w/Pecans	1 oz	8	151	48%
Oatmeal w/Cinnamon & Raisins	1 oz	6	133	41%
(Featherweight)				
Chocolate Chip	1 cookie	2	40	45%
Creme Wafers				
Chocolate	1 cookie	1	20	45%
Peanut Butter	1 cookie	1	25	36%
Strawberry	1 cookie	1	20	45%
Double Chocolate Chip	1 cookie	2	45	40%
Lemon	1 cookie	2	40	45%
Oatmeal Raisin	1 cookie	2	45	40%
Vanilla	1 cookie	2	40	45%
Vanilla Wafers	1 cookie	2	30	60%
Fig Bars	4 bars	4	210	17%
Figaroos (Little Debbie)	1.5 oz	4	160	23%
Fortune Cookies (Umeya)	4 cookied	< 1	120	4%
(Frookie)				
Apple Cinnamon Oat Bran	1 cookie	2	45	40%
Chocolate Chip	1 cookie	2	45	40%
Ginger Spice	1 cookie	2	45	40%
Mandarin Orange Chocolate Chip	1 cookie	2	45	40%
Oat Bran Muffin	1 cookie	2	45	40%
Oatmeal Raisin	1 cookie	2	45	40%
Fruit & Honey (Entenmann's)				
fat free	2 cookies	–	80	–
Grahamy Bears (Sunshine)	9 cookies	5	130	35%
(Grandma's)				
Candied Animal Cookies	1 oz	6	140	39%
Chocolate Chip Big Cookies	2 cookies	17	370	41%
Chocolate Sandwich Cookies	1.8 oz	12	260	42%
Fudge Choc Chip Big Cookies	2 cookies	13	350	33%
Glazed Gingerbread Soft Cookies	1 oz	3	120	23%
Oatmeal Apple Spice Big Cookies	2 cookies	12	330	33%
Old Time Molasses Big Cookies	2 cookies	9	320	25%
Peanut Butter Big Cookies	2 cookies	30	410	66%
Peanut Butter Sandwich Creme	1.8 oz	13	260	45%
Rich'N Chewey-Chocolate Chip	1 oz	6	140	39%
Soft Raisin Big Cookies	2 cookies	10	320	28%
Vanilla-Flavored Sandwich Creme	1.8 oz	12	260	42%
(Health Valley)				
Amaranth	2 cookies	4	120	30%
Amaranth Jumbo	1 cookie	3	70	39%
Crisp cinnamon Jumbo	1 cookie	2	70	26%

Food and Description	Amount	Fat Grams	Total Calories	% Fat Calories
Fancy Fruit Chunks				
Apricot Almond	2 cookies	3	90	30%
Date Pecan	2 cookies	3	90	30%
Raisin Oat Bran	2 cookies	3	90	30%
Tropical Fruit	2 cookies	3	90	30%
Fancy Peanut Chunks	2 cookies	3	90	30%
Fat-Free				
Apple Spice	3 cookies	< 1	75	6%
Apricot Delight	3 cookies	< 1	75	6%
Date Delight	3 cookies	< 1	75	6%
Hawaiian Fruit	3 cookies	< 1	75	6%
Raisin Oatmeal	3 cookies	< 1	75	6%
Fat-Free Fruit Bars				
Apple	1 bar	< 1	140	3%
Apricot	1 bar	< 1	140	3%
Date	1 bar	< 1	140	3%
Raisin	1 bar	< 1	140	3%
Fat-Free Jumbos				
Apple Raisin	1 cookie	< 1	70	6%
Raisin Raisin	1 cookie	< 1	70	6%
Raspberry	1 cookie	< 1	70	6%
Fat-Free w/Fruit Centers				
Apple	3 cookies	–	70	–
Apricot	3 cookies	–	70	–
Date	3 cookies	–	70	–
Raisin Apple	3 cookies	–	70	–
Raspberry	3 cookies	–	70	–
Tropical	3 cookies	–	70	–
Fruit Bars				
Apple Bakes	2 bars	4	164	22%
Raisin Bakes	2 bars	4	160	23%
Fruit & Fitness Cookies	2 oz	4	200	18%
Healthy Grahams				
Cinnamon	1 oz	3	110	25%
Ginger	1 oz	3	110	25%
Oat Bran & Honey	1 oz	3	110	25%
Honey Jumbos				
Cinnamon	2 cookies	3	100	27%
Oat Bran	2 cookies	3	120	23%
Peanut Butter	2 cookies	3	140	19%
Jumbos				
Fiber				
Blueberry Nut	1 cookie	3	100	27%
Chunky Pecan	1 cookie	3	100	27%

Food and Description	Amount	Fat Grams	Total Calories	% Fat Calories
Raisin Nut	1 cookie	3	100	27%
Fruit				
Almond Date	1 cookie	3	70	39%
Cinnamon	1 cookie	2	50	36%
Honey Peanut Butter	1 cookie	2	70	26%
Raisin Nut	1 cookie	3	70	39%
Tropical	1 cookie	3	70	39%
Fruit Bars				
Oat Bran-almond/date	1 bar	2	140	8%
Oat Bran-raisin/cinnamon	1 bar	1	140	6%
Rice Bran w/almond & date	1 bar	5	160	28%
Oat Bran Animal Cookies	1 oz	3	90	30%
Oat Bran Fruit Cookies	1 cookie	4	110	33%
Oat Bran Fruit Jumbos	2 cookies	3	120	23%
Oat Bran Fruit & Nut	1 oz	4	110	33%
Oat Jumbo	2 cookies	4	130	28%
Peanut Butter Jumbo	1 cookie	2	70	26%
The Great Tofu Cookie	2 cookies	3	90	30%
The Great Wheat-Free Cookie	2 cookies	3	80	34%
(Keebler)				
Baby Bear	3 cookies	3	70	39%
Bite Size				
Chips Deluxe	4 cookies	5	80	56%
Pecan Sandies	4 cookies	5	90	50%
Chips Deluxe	1 cookie	4	80	45%
Chocolate Fudge Sandwich	2 cookies	8	170	42%
Deluxe Grahams-Fudge Covered	1 cookie	2	40	45%
E.L. Fudge Sandwich	1 cookie	3	70	39%
Elfkins				
Butter w/fudge filling	4 cookies	3	70	39%
Chocolate Vanilla	4 cookies	3	70	39%
Fudge w/fudge filling	4 cookies	3	70	39%
Fudge Cremes	1 cookie	3	60	45%
Fudge Grasshoppers	2 cookies	6	140	39%
Fudge Stripes	1 cookie	3	50	54%
French Vanilla Creme	1 cookie	4	80	45%
Magic Middles/all flavors	1 cookie	5	80	56%
Mini Middles				
Chocolate Chip	4 cookies	4	80	45%
Oatmeal	4 cookies	5	80	56%
Shortbread	4 cookies	4	80	45%
Pecan Chips Deluxe	1 cookie	4	70	51%
Pecan Sandies	1 cookie	5	80	56%
Playland	3 cookies	2	60	30%

Food and Description	Amount	Fat Grams	Total Calories	% Fat Calories
Oatmeal Cremes	1 cookie	3	80	34%
Old Fashioned Oatmeal	1 cookie	3	80	34%
Pitter Patter	1 cookie	4	90	40%
Rainbow Chips Deluxe	2 cookies	8	140	51%
Rich'n Chips	1 cookie	4	80	45%
Soft Batch				
Chocolate Chip	1 cookie	4	80	45%
Peanut Butter Chocolate Chip	1 cookie	5	80	56%
Peanut Butter Nut	1 cookie	4	80	45%
Walnut Chocolate Chip	1 cookie	4	80	45%
Thin Bits				
Choc-Covered Graham Snacks	12 pieces	3	70	39%
Cinnamon Graham	12 pieces	3	70	39%
Honey Graham	14 pieces	3	70	39%
Vanilla Wafers	5 cookies	5	100	45%
Lady Fingers	1 cookie	–	40	–
	4 cookies	3	158	17%
(Lance) packaged				
Apple Cinnamon	1 pkg	5	120	38%
Apple Oatmeal Bar	1 pkg	7	190	33%
Blueberry	1 pkg	4	120	30%
Bonnie	1 pkg	4	100	36%
Chocolate Chip	1 pkg	7	135	47%
Chocolate Chip Fudge	1 pkg	5	130	35%
Fig Bar	1	1	71	13%
Malt	1	10	190	47%
Oatmeal	1 pkg	5	130	35%
Peanut Butter Creme Filled	1 pkg	10	240	38%
Strawberry	1 pkg	4	120	30%
Lemon Ohs! (Austin)	1.8 oz	9	240	34%
(Little Debbie) Cookie Caramel Bars	1 bar	8	170	42%
(LU)				
Chocolatiers	2 cookies	4	85	42%
Cream Wafer	3 cookies	7	110	57%
Crokine	2 cookies	–	35	–
Dipped Chocolatiers	2 cookies	6	105	51%
Little School Boy	1 cookie	4	70	51%
Marie Lu	1 cookie	2	50	36%
Marie Lu Whole Wheat & Cinnamon	1 cookie	1	45	20%
Petit Beurre	1 cookie	1	40	23%
Pims	2 cookies	2	95	19%
Macaroons				
homemade (2-¾" dia, ¼" thick)	2 cookies	8.8	181	44%

Food and Description	Amount	Fat Grams	Total Calories	% Fat Calories
Marshmallow Pies				
Banana (Little Debbie)	1 pkg/1.4 oz	6	170	32%
	1 pkg/3 oz	12	360	30%
Chocolate (Little Debbie)	1 pkg/1.38 oz	6	170	32%
	1 pkg/3 oz	13	370	32%
Milk Chocolate (Duncan Hines)	2 cookies	5	110	41%
(Mother's)				
Almond Shortbread	2 cookies	7	120	53%
Butter-Flavored	5 cookies	6	140	39%
Checkerboard Wafer	5 cookies	4	85	42%
Chocolate Chip	1 cookie	3	70	39%
(bag)	4 cookies	8	140	51%
Chocolate Chip Angel	2 cookies	8	120	60%
Circus Animal	4 cookies	6	110	49%
Cocadas Coconut	4 cookies	6	120	45%
Date Filled Oatmeal	1 cookie	3	94	29%
Dinosaur Grrrahams				
cinnamon	1 cookie	3	80	34%
original	1 cookie	2	70	25%
Double Fudge Sandwich	2 cookies	4	100	36
Duplex Sandwich	2 cookies	5	105	43%
English Tea Sandwich	1 cookie	4	100	36%
Fig Bars	2 bars	2	110	18%
Flaky Fix Fudge Wafer	2 cookies	9	130	62%
Flaky Fix Vanilla Wafer	2 cookies	5	115	39%
Fudge'N Chips	4 cookies	7	120	53%
Gaucho Peanut Butter Sandwich	1 cookie	5	90	50%
Iced Oatmeal	1 cookie	3	70	39%
Iced Raisin	1 cookie	4	80	45%
Macaroon	1 cookie	5	80	56%
Mini Dinosaur				
Cinnamon	7 cookies	2	70	26%
Original	7 cookies	1	60	15%
Oatmeal	1 cookie	3	60	45%
Oatmeal Chocolate Chip	1 cookie	3	70	45%
Oatmeal Raisin	4 cookies	7	130	48%
Oatmeal Walnut Chocolate Chip	1 cookie	3	70	39%
Royal Grahams	1 cookie	4	69	52%
Striped Shortbread	2 cookies	5	100	45%
Sugar	1 cookie	4	70	51%
Taffy Sandwich	1 cookie	6	100	54%
Vanilla Wafers	5 cookies	5	120	38%
Walnut Fudge	1 cookie	4	70	51%
Whole Wheat Fig Bars	2 bars	2	120	15%

Food and Description	Amount	Fat Grams	Total Calories	% Fat Calories
(Nabisco)				
Almost Home				
Fudge Chocolate Chip	1 cookie	3	70	39%
Oatmeal Raisin	1 cookie	3	70	39%
Old Fashioned Sugar	1 cookie	3	70	39%
Real Chocolate Chip	1 cookie	3	60	45%
Bakers Bonus Oatmeal	1 cookie	3	80	34%
Bakers Own				
Apple filled	1 cookie	2	70	26%
Blueberry filled	1 cookie	2	70	26%
Raspberry filled	1 cookie	2	70	26%
Barnum's Animal Crackers	5 cookies	2	60	30%
Biscos Sugar Wafers	4 wafers	3	70	39%
Biscos Waffle Cremes	2 pieces	4	70	51%
Brown Edge Wafers	2½ wafers	3	70	39%
Bugs Bunny Graham Cookies	5 cookies	2	60	30%
Cameo Creme Sandwich	1 cookie	3	70	39%
Chips Ahoy				
Chewy Chocolate Chip	1 cookie	3	60	45%
Mini Chocolate Chip	6 cookies	3	70	39%
Pure Chocolate Chip	1 cookie	2	50	36%
Rockers	1 cookie	3	60	45%
Sprinkled	1 cookie	3	60	45%
Striped	1 cookie	5	90	50%
Chips Ahoy-Selections				
Chocolate Chocolate Chunk	1 cookie	5	90	50%
Chocolate Chocolate Walnut	1 cookie	6	95	57%
Chocolate Chunk Pecan	1 cookie	6	100	54%
Chunky Chocolate Chip	1 cookie	5	90	50%
Health Toffee Chunk	1 cookie	5	90	50%
Oatmeal Chocolate Chunk	1 cookie	5	95	47%
White Fudge Chunk	1 cookie	5	90	50%
Chocolate Chip Snaps	3 cookies	2	70	26%
Chocolate Grahams	1 piece	3	60	30%
Chocolate Snaps	4 cookies	2	70	26%
Cookie Break				
Vanilla Creme Sandwich	1 cookie	2	50	36%
Cookies'N Fudge				
Party Grahams	1 cookie	2	45	40%
Striped Chocolate Chip	1 cookie	3	60	30%
Striped Peanut Butter Nut	3 cookies	8	150	48%
Striped Shortbread	3 cookies	7	150	42%
Striped Wafers	1 wafer	4	70	51%
Devil's Food Cakes	1 cake	1	70	13%

Food and Description	Amount	Fat Grams	Total Calories	% Fat Calories
Famous Chocolate Wafers	5 wafers	4	130	28%
	2½ wafers	2	70	26%
Famous Cookie Assortment				
Baronet Creme Sandwich	3 cookies	6	140	39%
Biscos Sugar Wafers	3 wafers	7	150	42%
Butter-Flavored	6 cookies	5	130	35%
Cameo Creme Sandwich	2 cookies	5	140	31%
Kettle Cookies	4 cookies	5	130	35%
Lorna Doone Shortbread	4 cookies	7	140	45%
Oreo Chocolate Sandwich	3 cookies	6	140	39%
Giggles Sandwich				
chocolate	1 cookie	3	60	45%
vanilla	1 cookie	3	60	45%
Heyday Bars				
fudge, caramel & peanut	1 bar	6	110	49%
Ideal Bars /chocolate peanut	1 bar	5	90	50%
Lorna Doone Shortbread	3 cookies	4	70	51%
Mallomars Chocolate Cakes	1 piece	3	60	45%
Marshmallow Puffs	1 piece	4	90	40%
Marshmallow Twirls Cakes	1 piece	6	140	39%
Mystic Mint Sandwich	1 cookie	5	90	50%
National Arrowroot Biscuit	1 biscuit	1	20	45%
Newtons Fruit Chewy Cookies				
Apple	1 cookie	2	70	26%
Cinnamon Raisin Nut	1 cookie	2	60	30%
Fat Free				
Apple	1 cookie	–	70	–
Plain	1 cookie	–	70	–
Strawberry	1 cookie	–	70	–
Fig Newtons	1 cookie	1	60	15%
Raspberry	1 cookie	2	70	26%
Strawberry	1 cookie	2	70	26%
Variety Pack/all flavors	1 cookie	3	120	23%
Nilla Wafers				
Cinnamon	3½ cookies	2	60	30%
Original	3½ cookies	2	60	30%
Nutter Butter				
Bites	4.5 cookies	3	70	39%
Peanut Butter Sandwich	1 cookie	3	70	39%
Peanut Butter Creme Patties	2 cookies	4	80	45%
Old Fashion Ginger Snaps	1 cookie	1	30	30%
Oreo Big Stuf Chocolate Sand	1 cookie	12	250	43%
Oreo Chocolate Sand	1 cookie	2	50	36%
Oreo Double Stuf Chocolate Sand	1 cookie	4	70	51%

Food and Description	Amount	Fat Grams	Total Calories	% Fat Calories
Oreo White Fudge Covered				
Chocolate Sand	1 cookie	6	110	49%
Pantry Molasses cookies	1 cookie	3	80	34%
Pecan Shortbread	1 cookie	5	80	56%
Pecan Supremes	1 cookie	5	80	56%
Pinwheels Choc & Marshmallow cakes	1 cake	5	130	35%
Pure Chocolate Middles	1 cookie	5	80	56%
Snack Wells				
Chocolate Chip	6 cookies	1	60	15%
Cinnamon Graham	9 cookies	–	50	–
Oatmeal Raisin	1 cookie	1	60	15%
Social Tea Biscuits	1 biscuit	1	20	45%
Suddenly S'Mores	1 cookie	4	100	36%
Oatmeal				
Homemade	1 cookie	3	65	42%
Packaged (Little Debbie)	2.75 oz	12	340	32%
Oatmeal Chocolate Chip/homemade	1 cookie	3	60	45%
Oatmeal Creme Pies (Little Debbie)	1.35 oz	8	170	42%
	3 oz	18	390	42%
Oatmeal w/raisins (2⅝" dia ¼" thick)	4 cookies	10	245	37%
box mix (Duncan Hines)	2 cookies	6	130	42%
homemade	4 cookies	10	245	37%
packaged				
(Duncan Hines)	2 cookies	5	110	41%
(Entenmann's) Fat Free	2 cookies	–	80	–
(Peak Frean)				
Fruit Cream	2 cookies	5	130	35%
Petit Bere	4 cookies	4	130	28%
Shortcake Sable	2 cookies	7	150	42%
Peanut Butter				
box mix (Duncan Hines)	2 cookies	7	140	45%
homemade (2⅝" dia)	4 cookies	14	245	51%
Peanut Butter Bars (Little Debbie)	2.5 oz	18	370	44%
	1.83 oz	13	260	45%
(Pepperidge Farm)				
American Collection Cookies				
Beacon Hill Brownie Nut	1 cookie	7	120	52%
Chesapeake Chocolate Chunk				
Pecan	1 cookie	7	120	53%
Cheyenne Peanut Butter				
Milk Chocolate Chunk	1 cookie	6	110	49%
Dakota Milk Chocolate Oatmeal	1 cookie	6	110	49%
Nantucket Chocolate Chunk	1 cookie	6	120	45%
Sante Fe Oatmeal Raisin	1 cookie	4	100	36%

Food and Description	Amount	Fat Grams	Total Calories	% Fat Calories
Sausalito Milk Choc Macadamia	1 cookie	7	120	53%
Distinctive Box Cookies				
Champagne	3 cookies	5	95	47%
Chocolate Laced Pirouettes	2 cookies	4	70	51%
Monte Carlo	2 cookies	5	90	50%
Original Pirouettes	2 cookies	4	70	51%
Paris	2 cookies	5	100	45%
Seville	2 cookies	5	100	45%
Southport	2 cookies	8	150	48%
Distinctive Cookies				
Bordeaux	2 cookies	3	70	39%
Brussels	2 cookies	5	110	41%
Brussels Mint	2 cookies	7	130	48%
Cappucino	1 cookie	3	50	54%
Capri	1 cookie	5	80	56%
Chantilly	1 cookie	2	80	23%
Chessmen	2 cookies	4	90	40%
Geneva	2 cookies	6	130	42%
Lido	1 cookie	5	90	50%
Linzer	1 cookie	4	120	30%
Milano	2 cookies	6	120	45%
Mint Milano	2 cookies	7	150	42%
Nassau	1 cookies	5	80	56%
Orange Milano	2 cookies	7	150	42%
Orleans	3 cookies	6	90	60%
Orleans Sandwich	2 cookies	8	120	60%
Tahiti	1 cookie	6	90	60%
Zurich	1 cookie	2	60	30%
Fruit Cookies				
Apricot-Raspberry	2 cookies	4	100	36%
Strawberry	2 cookies	5	100	45%
Kitchen Hearth Cookies				
Date Pecan	2 cookies	5	110	41%
Raisin Bran	2 cookies	5	110	41%
Old Fashioned Cookies				
Brownie Chocolate Nut	2 cookies	7	110	57%
Chocolate Chip	2 cookies	5	100	45%
Chocolate Toffee Chip	2 cookies	5	100	45%
Gingerman	2 cookies	3	70	39%
Hazelnut	2 cookies	6	110	49%
Irish Oatmeal	2 cookies	5	90	50%
Lemon Nut Crunch	2 cookies	7	110	57%
Molasses Crisps	2 cookies	3	70	39%
Oatmeal Raisin	2 cookies	5	110	41%

Food and Description	Amount	Fat Grams	Total Calories	% Fat Calories
Pecan Shortbread	1 cookie	8	150	48%
Shortbread	1 cookie	5	70	64%
Sugar	2 cookies	5	100	45%
Special Collection				
Chocolate Chunk Pecan	1 cookie	4	70	51%
Milk Chocolate Macadamia	1 cookie	4	70	51%
Wholesome choice				
Apple Oatmeal Tart	1 cookie	2	0	25%
Carrot Walnut	1 cookie	1	60	15%
Cranberry Honey	1 cookie	2	60	30%
Date Walnut	1 cookie	2	60	30%
Raspberry Tart	1 cookie	2	70	25%
Pumpkin Bar-homemade	1.5 oz	11	190	52%
Raisin (Entenmann's)				
fat free	2 cookies	–	70	–
Ready-To-Bake (Nestle Toll House)				
Chocolate Chip	2 cookies	7	150	42%
Chocolate Chip w/nuts	2 cookies	8	160	45%
Double Chocolate Chip	2 cookies	7	150	42%
Oatmeal Raisin	2 cookies	5	130	35%
Refrigerated (Pillsbury)				
Chocolate Chip	1 cookie	3	70	39%
Chocolate Chocolate Chip	1 cookie	3	70	39%
Oatmeal Rasin	1 cookie	3	70	39%
Peanut Butter	1 cookie	3	70	39%
Sugar	1 cookie	3	70	39%
(Rippin' Good)				
Assorted Creme	2 cookies	4	100	36%
Chocolate Chip Creme	2 cookies	6	160	34%
Cookie Jar	3 cookies	6	150	36%
Duplex Creme	2 cookies	4	100	36%
Fudge Stripe Oatmeal	2 cookies	8	140	51%
Granola & Peanut Butter Sandwich	2 cookies	6	140	39%
Iced Oatmeal	2 cookies	2	90	30%
Macaroon Cremes	2 cookies	8	160	45%
Marshmallow Blossoms	2 cookies	2	90	30%
Marshmallow Daisies	2 cookies	2	90	30%
Marshmallow Fudge Stripes	2 cookies	4	100	36%
Peanut Butter	2 cookies	4	100	36%
Striped Dainties	1 cookie	3	50	54%
Vanilla Creme	2 cookies	4	100	36%
Sandwich (Estee)	1 cookie	2	45	40%
Sandwich type				
choc or vanilla (1¾" dia)	4 cookies	8	195	37%

Food and Description	Amount	Fat Grams	Total Calories	% Fat Calories
(Savoir Faire)				
Galettes Butter	1 oz	7	180	35%
Petit Butter Biscuit	1 oz	5	170	26%
Shortbread				
commercial-small	4 cookies	8	155	47%
homemade-large	2 cookies	8	145	50%
(Stella D'Oro)				
Almond Toast	1 piece	1	58	16%
Angel Bars	1 cookie	4.7	74	57%
Angel Puffs	1 cookie	–	13	–
Angel Wings	1 cookie	4.7	74	57%
Angelica Goodies	1 cookie	4	104	35%
Anginetti	1 cookie	1	31	29%
Anisette Sponge	1 cookie	.8	51	14%
Anisette Toast	1 cookie	.6	46	12%
Anisette Toast-Jumbo	1 cookie	1	109	8%
Apple Pastry	2 pieces	7	180	35%
Breakfast Treats	1 piece	3.6	101	32%
Castelets				
chocolate	1 piece	2.8	64	39%
vanilla	1 piece	3	72	38%
Chinese Dessert	1 cookie	8.9	169	47%
Coconut Macaroons	1 cookie	3	60	45%
Coconut, Dietetic	1 cookie	2	50	36%
Como Delight	1 cookie	7	145	43%
Dietetic Egg Biscuits	1 piece	1	43	21%
Dutch Apple Bars	1 piece	3	112	24%
Egg Jumbo	1 piece	.7	47	13%
Fruit Slices	1 cookie	2	60	30%
Golden Bars	1 cookie	4	109	33%
Holiday Trinkets	1 cookie	1.9	38	45%
Hostess Assortment	1 cookie	2	42	43%
Lady Stella Assortment	1 cookie	2	42	43%
Love, Dietetic	1 cookie	5	106	42%
Margherite, chocolate	1 cookie	3	72	38%
Margherite, vanilla	1 cookie	2.8	72	35%
Peach Apricot Pastry	2 pieces	8	180	40%
Pfeffernusse	3 cookies	2	110	16%
Roman Egg Biscuits	1 piece	5	137	33%
Royal Nuggets	1 piece	–	1	–
Sesame	1 piece	2	48	38%
Sesame, Dietetic	1 piece	2	43	42%
Sugared Egg Biscuits	1 piece	1	75	12%
Swiss Fudge	1 piece	3	68	40%

Food and Description	Amount	Fat Grams	Total Calories	% Fat Calories
Sugar				
homemade	1 cookie	3	90	30%
refrigerated dough				
(2½"dia, ¼"thick)	4 cookies	12	235	46%
Sugar, Golden-box mix				
(Duncan Hines)	2 cookies	6	130	42%
(Sunshine)				
Butter Flavored	2 cookies	2	60	30%
Chip-A-Roos	2 cookies	7	130	49%
Chip-o-lotomus	2 cookies	7	120	53%
Chips'n Middles	2 cookies	6	140	39%
Chocolate Fudge Sandwich	2 cookies	7	150	42%
Cup Custard	2 cookies	6	130	42%
Family Bears				
Chocolate	2 cookies	7	140	45%
Peanut butter	2 cookies	6	140	39%
Vanilla	2 cookies	6	130	42%
Fig Bars	2 cookies	2	90	20%
Ginger Snaps	5 cookies	3	90	30%
Golden Fruit Cookie	2 cookies	3	150	18%
Hydrox				
Original	1 cookie	2	50	36%
Peanut Butter	1 cookie	3	60	45%
Lemon Coolers	2 cookies	2	60	30%
Mallowpuffs	2 cookies	4	140	26%
Oat Bran w/nuts & raisins	2 ookies	6	120	45%
Oatmeal	2 cookies	5	110	41%
Oatmeal Peanut Sandwich	2 cookies	6	140	39%
Peanut Butter Wafers	3 wafers	6	120	45%
School House	15 pieces	4	120	30%
Sprinkles	2 cookies	3	130	42%
Sugar Wafers	3 wafers	6	130	42%
Super Mario Bros.				
Chocolate	5 cookies	3	70	39%
Cinnamon	5 cookies	3	70	39%
Honey	5 cookies	3	70	39%
Vanilla Wafers	6 wafers	6	130	42%
Vienna Fingers	2 cookies	6	140	39%
(Sweet Pretenders)				
Chocolate Flavored Chip	1 cookie	2	45	40%
Lemon	1 cookie	2	45	40%
Oatmeal Raisin	1 cookie	2	45	40%
Vanilla	1 cookie	2	45	40%
Peanut Butter	1 cookie	2	40	45%

Food and Description	Amount	Fat Grams	Total Calories	% Fat Calories
(Twookies)				
Creamy Chocolate	1 oz	6	130	42%
Creamy Peanut Butter	1 oz	5	130	35%
Strawberry	1 oz	6	140	39%
Vanilla Creme	1 oz	6	140	39%
Vanilla Wafers (1¾" dia)	10 cookies	7	185	34%
(Weight Watchers)				
Apple Raisin Bar	1 cookie	3	100	27%
Chocolate	3 cookies	3	80	34%
Chocolate Chip	2 cookies	2	90	20%
Chocolate Sandwich	2 cookies	3	90	30%
Fruit Filled				
Apple	1 bar	< 1	80	6%
Raspberry	1 bar	< 1	80	6%
Oatmeal Spice	3 cookies	2	80	23%
Shortbread	3 cookies	2	80	34%
Vanilla Sandwich	2 cookies	3	90	30%
COOKING SPRAY				
(Mazola)	2 second spray	.8	6	100%
(Pam)				
Butter Flavor	⅓ of 10" Skillet	1	2	100%
Olive Oil	⅓ of 10" Skillet	1	2	100%
Original	¼ second spray	1	7	100%
(Weight Watchers)				
Butter	.64 gram	< 1	2	100%
Cooking	1 gram	< 1	2	100%
Olive Oil	1 gram	< 1	2	100%
(Wesson)	.27 gram	< 1	< 1	100%
CORIANDER/raw	¼ cup	–	1	–
CORIANDER LEAF/dried	1 tsp	–	2	–
CORIANDER SEED	1 tsp	–	5	–
CORN				
Sweet-white or yellow				
cooked	½ cup	1	89	10%
	1 ear	1	89	10%
Canned				
Baby Corn On Cob				
(Bristol)	4 ears/ ½ oz	–	12	–
Cream Style	½ cup	.5	93	5%

Food and Description	Amount	Fat Grams	Total Calories	% Fat Calories
(Green Giant)	½ cup	1	100	9%
(Nutradiet)	½ cup	1	100	9%
(S&W) Cream Premium Homestyle	½ cup	1	120	8%
Cream-Golden				
(Del Monte)	½ cup	1	90	10%
Cream-White				
(Del Monte)	½ cup	–	90	–
Golden Whole Kernels				
(Del Monte)	½ cup	1	70	13%
Kernels Golden Vacuum Packed				
(Del Monte)	½ cup	1	90	10%
Kernels				
(Green Giant)	½ cup	–	80	–
50%Less Salt	½ cup	–	70	–
(Niblets)	½ cup	–	80	–
(Nutradiet)	½ cup	1	80	11%
Kernels in Brine (Festal)	½ cup	1	90	10%
Kernels w/Peppers				
(Freshlike)	½ cup	1	90	10%
(Mexicorn)	½ cup	1	80	11%
Young, Tender Whole Kernel				
Premium (S&W)	½ cup	1	90	10%
Whole Kernels (Del Monte)				
Salad Bar Vegetables	2 oz	–	22	–
Whole White Kernels (Del Monte)	½ cup	–	70	–
Frozen				
Cob Corn				
(Ore Ida)	1 ear	1	150	6%
cream style	½ cup	.6	120	5%
cut (Pictsweet)	3.2 oz	1	80	11%
kernels				
(Birds Eye)	3.3 oz	1	80	11%
(Health Valley)	5.8 oz	–	134	–
frozen-On-The-Cob,				
Big Ears (Birds Eye)	1 ear	1	160	6%
frozen-On-The-Cob,				
Little Ears (Birds Eye)	2 ears	1	130	7%
frozen-on-the-cob	1 ear	1	150	6%
(Pictsweet)				
3"	1 ear	–	50	–
6"	1 ear	1	110	8%
(Pictsweet)				
Express microwave	1 ear	–	50	–
frozen (Niblets)	½ cup	1	80	11%

Food and Description	Amount	Fat Grams	Total Calories	% Fat Calories
frozen (Niblets)				
Corn-on-the-Cob (pkg of 4)	1 ear	1	150	6%
Corn-on-the-Cob (pkg of 6)	2 ears	1	150	6%
White Shoepeg				
canned				
(Green Giant)	½ cup	–	90	–
frozen	½ cup	1	70	13%
frozen				
(Harvest Fresh)	½ cup	1	90	10%
(Green Giant) microwaveable				
Pantry Express	½ cup	1	80	11%
CORN CAKES (*See* RICE CAKES)				
CORN CHIPS (*See* TORTILLA CHIPS)				
CORN CHOWDER (*See* SOUP)				
CORN DISHES				
Corn on the Cob in butter sauce				
frozen				
(Green Giant)	1 ear/ 2 half ears	2	150	12%
Corn Pudding				
homemade	½ cup	6.6	136	44%
Delicorn				
canned				
(Green Giant)	½ cup	1	80	11%
Fritters				
homemade	1 oz	2	62	29%
frozen				
(Mrs. Paul's)	2	9	240	34%
Mexican Style Corn in Mild Red Chile Sauce				
microwave Vegetable Classics				
(Del Monte)	½ cup	4	90	40%
Micro Quick				
(Freshlike)				
frozen corn in butter sauce	5 oz	2	130	14%
(Niblets) in butter sauce	½ cup	2	100	18%
(Niblets) in butter sauce				
one serving vegetables,frozen	4.5 oz	2	110	16%
Scalloped/homemade	½ cup	7	250	25%
White Shoepeg Corn in butter sauce				
(Green Giant)	½ cup	2	100	18%
CORN FLAKE CRUMBS (Kellogg's)	¼ cup	–	110	–
CORN GRITS				
(Albers)	1 serving	–	150	–
Instant/White Hominy	1 serving	–	82	–

Food and Description	Amount	Fat Grams	Total Calories	% Fat Calories
Quick/yellow Hominy				
dry	3 Tbs	–	101	–
Regular and quick	1 serving	.5	146	3%
w/cheddar cheese flavor	1 serving	1	104	9%
w/cheese flavor	1 serving	.9	107	8%
w/imitation bacon bits	1 serving	.5	104	4%
w/imitation ham bits	1 serving	–	103	–
(Arrowhead Mills)				
White	2 oz	1	200	5%
Yellow	2 oz	1	200	5%
Generic				
Cooked	4 oz	–	68	–
	1 cup	.5	146	3%
Dry	1 oz	–	105	–
	1 Tbs	–	36	–
	1 cup	1.8	579	3%
(Quaker)				
Instant				
Real Butter Flavor	1 packet	1	100	9%
White Hominy	1 pkt	–	80	–
w/Imitation Bacon Bits	1 pkg	< 1	100	4%
w/Imitation Ham Bits	1 pkg	< 1	100	4%
w/Real Cheddar Cheese	1 pkg	1	100	9%
Quick/Dry				
White Hominy	3 Tbs	< 1	100	4%
Regular/Dry				
White Hominy	3 Tbs	< 1	100	4%
CORN MEAL				
(Albers) yellow or white	1 oz	–	100	–
(Aunt Jemima) yellow or white				
Enriched/unenriched	3 Tbs	1	100	9%
(Quaker/Aunt Jemima)				
Self-rising				
Whole ground yellow or white	1 cup	4	465	8%
Degermed	1 cup	1.6	491	3%
Whole-ground				
Bolted	1 cup	4	442	8%
Unbolted	1 cup	4.8	433	10%
CORN MEAL MIX				
(Aunt Jemima)				
Bolted white	3 Tbs	1	100	9%
Self-rising				
Buttermilk or white	3 Tbs	1	100	9%
White enriched bolted	3 Tbs	1	100	9%

Food and Description	Amount	Fat Grams	Total Calories	% Fat Calories
Yellow	3 Tbs	1	100	9%
CORN PONE				
w/whole ground cornmeal (9" dia)	⅛ pone	3	122	22%
CORN PUDDING (See PUDDING & MOUSSE)				
CORN STARCH	1 Tbs	–	30	–
	1 cup	–	463	–
CORNBREAD				
Box Mix				
(Aunt Jemima)				
Easy Mix	⅙ pkg	7	210	30%
(Ballard)	⅛ pkg	3	140	19%
(Dromedary)	2"x2" sq.	5	130	35%
(Krusteaz) Honey Cornbread	1⁄16 pkg	3	120	23%
(Martha White)				
Cotton Pickin	¼ pan	3	170	16%
Yellow, Light Crust	2 oz mix	4	140	26%
Homemade				
Southern Style w/Degermed				
Cornmeal	~ 3 oz	5	186	24%
3" sq.	1 piece	3	122	22%
w/whole-Ground Cornmeal	~3 oz	6	161	34%
Pouch Mix (Robin Hood/Gold Medal)				
White or Yellow	⅙ mixture	5	50	30%
CORNED BEEF (See also LUNCHEON MEAT)				
Brisket	3 oz	16	213	68%
Canned	1 oz	4	71	51%
(Hormel) 12 oz	2 oz	8	130	55%
Jellied loaf	1 oz	1.9	46	37%
CORNED BEEF HASH				
Canned				
(Armour) Premium				
Lite	7.5 oz	21	350	54%
Original	7.5 oz	27	390	62%
Generic				
w/Potatoes	7.8 oz	24.9	399	56%
(Libby's)	7.5 oz	27	400	61%
	8 oz	28	420	60%
(Mary Kitchen)	7.5 oz	24	360	60%
	8⅓ oz	27	400	61%
Standard Home Recipe (USDA)	1 cup	21.5	344	56%
CORNISH GAME HEN (See CHICKEN)				
COTTAGE CHEESE				
(Borden)				
4% milk fat	4 oz	5	120	38%

Food and Description	Amount	Fat Grams	Total Calories	% Fat Calories
Dry Curd .5% milk fat	4 oz	1	80	11%
(Carnation) Slender 1½% milk fat	4 oz	2	90	20%
Generic - creamed	4 oz	5	117	39%
(Kemps)				
dry curd	4 oz	1	80	11%
nonfat	4 oz	< .5	80	3%
1% lite	4 oz	1	90	10%
2% lowfat	4 oz	2	100	18%
whole milk	4 oz	5	120	38%
(Knudsen) 4% milk fat	4 oz	5	120	38%
(Land O'Lakes) 2%	4 oz	2	100	18%
(Light N' Lively)	4 oz	1	80	11%
fat free	4 oz	–	80	–
1% lowfat	4 oz	1	82	11%
2% lowfat	4 oz	2	101	18%
(Lite-Line) 1½% lowfat	4 oz	2	90	20%
(Weight Watchers)				
1%	4 oz	1	90	10%
2%	4 oz	2	100	18%
COTTAGE CHEESE FRUIT SALAD				
(Lucerne)	4 oz	4	130	28%
COUSCOUS (See PASTA, SOUP/DEHYDRATED)				
COWPEA (See BLACK-EYED PEA)				
CRAB (See also SEAFOOD ENTRÉE/DINNER)				
Alaska King				
cooked-moist heat	3 oz	1	82	11%
	1 Leg	2	129	14%
raw	3 oz	1	71	13%
	1 Leg	1	145	6%
Blue				
canned	3 oz	1	84	11%
raw	3 oz	.9	74	11%
Dungeness				
canned				
(S&W)	3.25 oz	2	01	£2%
Imitation				
(from surimi)	3 oz	1	87	10%
(Louis Kemp) Crab Delights				
chunk style	2 oz	< 1	50	9%
flake style	2 oz	< 1	50	9%
leg style	2 oz	< 1	50	9%
salad style	2 oz	< 1	60	8%
Queen				
raw	3 oz	1	76	12%

Food and Description	Amount	Fat Grams	Total Calories	% Fat Calories
Soft Shell				
fried	1	13	213	55%
CRAB SALAD				
homemade	5.5 oz	10.7	205	47%
CRAB SOUP (*See* SOUP)				
CRACKER CRUMBS-GRAHAM				
(Nabisco)				
Original	2 Tbs	1	60	15%
Premium Fat-Free	2 Tbs	–	50	–
(Sunshine)	½ cup	7	275	23%
CRACKER MEAL (*See also* MATZO MEAL)				
(Golden Dipt)	1 oz	–	100	–
(Nabisco)	2 Tbs	–	50	–
CRACKERS (*See also* CRISPBREAD, MATZO)				
(A1-MAK) Sesame Crackers				
100% Stone-Ground Whole Wheat	½ oz	< 1	23	30%
(Austin)				
Cheese on Cheese	1.4 oz pkg	10	180	50%
Cheese and Peanut Butter	1.4 oz pkg	10	200	45%
Rye Cheese w/Zesty Cheese	1.4 oz pkg	10	200	45%
Toasty Peanut Butter	1.4 oz pkg	10	200	45%
Wheat'N Cheddar	1.4 oz pkg	9	190	43%
Cheddar Cheese Lights (Old Brussels)	1 oz	10	167	54%
Cheese (Ritz)	10 crackers	6	140	39%
Cheese & Peanut Butter (Ritz)	6 crackers	10	210	43%
Chowder and Oyster (O.T.C.)	1 cracker	1	25	36%
Cracker Bread				
Armenian (Venus)	5 pieces	< 1	60	8%
Extra Crisp (Wasa)	1 piece	1	25	33%
100% Stoneground Armenian (AK-MAK)	1 piece	1	117	8%
Crisp Bakes, Dutch (Hans Boersma)	1 cracker	–	29	–
Crispbread (*See* CRISPBREAD)				
(Dare) Breton				
50% Less Salt	4 crackers	3.9	83	42%
Original	4 crackers	3.9	83	42%
Sesame	4 crackers	4.4	86	46%
Thin Wheat	4 crackers	3.8	84	41%
(Delicious)				
CrocoDiles	13 crackers	3	70	39%
Hearty Wheat	5 crackers	3	70	39%
Real Cheddar Cheese	½ oz	4	70	51%
Snackers	4 crackers	3	70	39%
Wholesome Wheat	7 crackers	3	70	39%
Wholesome Sesame	6 crackers	3	70	39%

Food and Description	Amount	Fat Grams	Total Calories	% Fat Calories
(Eagle) Snack Crackers				
Bacon Flavor Cheese	1 oz	6	140	39%
Cheese Flavor	1 oz	6	130	42%
Honey Roasted Peanut Butter	1.8 oz	16	280	51%
(Estee)				
6-Calorie Wafer	1 piece	–	6	–
Cheddar Crackers	½ oz	4	70	51%
Party Crackers	½ oz	4	70	51%
Sesame	½ oz	4	70	51%
Fiber bread				
(Bran-A-Crisp)	1 piece	–	22	–
Flat Bread				
Extra Thin (Wasa)	3 slices	–	48	–
Fiber w/sesame seeds (Ideal)	2 slices	–	40	–
Whole Grain, No Salt (Ideal)	2 slices	–	43	–
Graham Crackers				
(Health Valley)				
Amaranth	1.2 oz	2	120	15%
Fancy Honey Graham	1 oz	5	130	35%
Oat Bran Graham	1.16 oz	3	120	23%
(Honey Maid)				
Cinnamon	2 crackers	1	60	15%
Honeycomb Graham Bites				
Apple Cinnamon	11 crackers	2	60	30%
Brown Sugar'N Spice	11 crackers	2	60	30%
Honey'N Oat Bran	11 crackers	2	60	30%
Plain	2 crackers	1	60	15%
Raisin	2 crackers	1	60	15%
(Keebler)				
Cinnamon Crisp	1 cracker	2	70	26%
Grahams	4 crackers	2	60	30%
Honey Grahams	4 crackers	3	80	34%
Thin Bits				
Cinnamon	12 crackers	3	70	39%
Chocolate	12 crackers	3	70	39%
(Nabisco)	2 crackers	1	60	15%
(Sunshine)				
Cinnamon	1 cracker	3	70	39%
Grahamy Bears	8 crackers	4	120	30%
Honey	1 cracker	2	60	30%
(Hain)				
Cheese Crackers	6 crackers	3	70	39%
Crackerbread				
Hearts	2 crackers	–	28	–

Food and Description	Amount	Fat Grams	Total Calories	% Fat Calories
Rounds				
Hors d'oeuvre size	1 cracker	1	28	32%
Luncheon size (5")	1 cracker	1	70	13%
Small	1 cracker	1	28	32%
Whole Wheat (5")	1 cracker	.8	66	11%
Onion				
No Salt Added	6 crackers	3	70	39%
Salted	6 crackers	3	70	39%
Rich				
No Salt Added	6 crackers	3	70	39%
Salted	6 crackers	3	70	39%
Rye				
No Salt Added	6 crackers	2	60	30%
Salted	6 crackers	3	70	39%
Sesame				
No Salt Added	6 crackers	3	70	39%
Salted	6 crackers	3	70	39%
Sourdough				
Low Salt	6 crackers	3	70	39%
Regular	6 crackers	3	70	39%
Vegetable				
No Salt Added	6 crackers	3	70	39%
Salted	6 crackers	3	60	30%
(Health Valley)				
Cheese Wheels	1 oz	9	140	48%
Fat-Free Wheat				
Cheese	½ oz	< 1	40	11%
Herbs	½ oz	< 1	40	11%
Onions	½ oz	< 1	40	11%
Vegetables	½ oz	< 1	40	11%
Whole Wheat	½ oz	< 1	40	11%
Garden Vegetable	1 oz	5	120	38%
Herb	1 oz	6	120	45%
Herb Stoned Wheat				
no salt	½ oz	2	55	33%
7 Grain Vegetable	1 oz	5	130	35%
Rice Bran	1 oz	3	100	27%
Sesame	1 oz	6	130	42%
Sesame Stoned Wheat-no salt	½ oz	2	55	33%
7 Grain & Vegetable				
Stoned Wheat-no salt	½ oz	2	55	33%
Stoned Wheat	½ oz	2	55	33%
Hi-Ho (Sunshine)				
Original Deluxe	4 crackers	5	80	56%

Food and Description	Amount	Fat Grams	Total Calories	% Fat Calories
Whole Wheat	4 crackers	3	65	42%
Honey Bran (El Molino)	2 crackers	1	40	23%
(Keebler)				
Cheddar Cracker Chips	18 crackers	3	70	39%
Club				
Original & Low Salt	4 crackers	3	60	45%
Whole Wheat	4 crackers	3	70	39%
Clubettes				
Cheddar	20 crackers	3	60	45%
Original	22 crackers	4	70	51%
Cracker Sandwiches				
Cheese & Peanut Butter	2 sandwiches	3	70	39%
Club & Cheddar	1 sandwich	4	70	51%
Harvest Wheat & Cheddar	1 sandwich	4	70	51%
Toast & Peanut Butter	2 sandwiches	3	70	39%
Town House & Cheddar	1 sandwich	4	70	51%
Harvest Wheats	3 crackers	4	70	51%
Munch ems				
Cheddar	13 crackers	3	60	45%
Nacho	14 crackers	2	60	30%
Original	14 crackers	3	60	45%
Ranch	14 crackers	3	90	30%
Sour Cream & Onion	13 crackers	3	60	45%
Onion Toast	5 crackers	3	60	45%
Sun Toasted Wheats	10 crackers	4	70	51%
Toasted Buttercrisp	4 crackers	3	60	45%
Toasted Poppy Seed	5 crackers	3	60	45%
Toasted Rye	4 crackers	3	60	45%
Toasted Sesame	4 crackers	3	60	45%
Toasted Wheat	4 crackers	3	60	45%
Town House				
original	5 crackers	5	80	56%
whole wheat	4 crackers	3	70	39%
Town House Jrs. Cheddar Cheese	8 crackers	4	80	45%
TUC	3 crackers	4	70	51%
Wheat & American Cheese				
Cracker Snack	1 cracker	4	70	51%
Wheatables				
French Onion	12 crackers	3	70	39%
Low Salt	12 crackers	3	70	39%
Original	12 crackers	3	70	39%
Ranch	11 crackers	3	70	39%
White Cheddar	11 crackers	4	70	51%
Whole Wheat	12 crackers	3	70	39%

Food and Description	Amount	Fat Grams	Total Calories	% Fat Calories
Zesta Saltines				
Low Salt	5 crackers	2	60	30%
Original	5 crackers	2	60	30%
Soup	39 crackers	2	60	30%
Unsalted Tops	5 crackers	2	60	30%
Wheat	5 crackers	2	60	30%
(Lance)				
Bonnie	1 5/16 oz	6	160	34%
Captain's Wafers	2 wafers	1	30	30%
Captain's Wafers w/cream cheese	1 5/8 oz	9	170	48%
Cheese On Wheat	1 5/16 oz	9	180	45%
Gold-N-Chee, Spicy	15 crackers	3	70	39%
Lanchee	1 1/4 oz	10	180	50%
Nip-Chee	1 5/16 oz	9	180	45%
Oyster	1/2 oz	2	70	11%
Peanut Butter Wheat	1 5/8 oz	10	190	47%
Rye Twins	2 crackers	1	30	30%
Rye-Chee	1 7/16 oz	9	190	43%
Saltines	2 crackers	1	25	36%
Sesame Twins	2 crackers	1	40	23%
Thin Wheat Snacks	7 crackers	4	80	45%
Toastchee	1 3/8 oz	10	190	47%
Toasty	1 1/4 oz	10	180	50%
Wheat Twins	2 crackers	1	30	30%
Wheatswafer	4 crackers	2	60	30%
Matzo Cracker (See MATZO)				
Melba Toast (See MELBA TOAST)				
(Nabisco)				
American Classic Crackers				
Cracked Wheat	4 crackers	4	70	51%
Dairy Butter, Golden Sesame,				
Minced Onion, & Toasted Poppy	4 crackers	3	70	39%
Bacon Flavored Thins	7 crackers	4	70	51%
Better Cheddars'N Bacon	10 crackers	4	70	51%
Better Cheddars'N Onion	10 crackers	3	70	39%
Better Cheddars	10 crackers	4	70	51%
Cheddar Wedges	31 pieces	3	70	39%
Cheese Peanut Butter Sandwich	2 sandwiches	3	70	39%
Cheese Tid-Bits	16 crackers	4	70	51%
Chicken In a Biskit	7 crackers	5	80	56%
Chocolate Grahams	1 piece	3	60	45%
Crown Pilot Crackers	1 cracker	2	70	26%
Dandy Soup & Oyster	20 crackers	2	60	30%
Escort	3 crackers	4	70	51%

Food and Description	Amount	Fat Grams	Total Calories	% Fat Calories
Garden Crisps/Vegetable	7 pieces	2	60	30%
Grahams	2 pieces	1	60	15%
Harvest Crisps				
5-Grain	6 crackers	2	60	30%
Oat	6 crackers	2	60	30%
Malted Milk Peanut Butter	2 sandwiches	3	70	39%
Meal Mates Sesame Bread Wafers	3 wafers	3	70	39%
Nips Cheese Snack	13 crackers	3	70	39%
Oat Thins	8 crackers	3	70	39%
Oysterettes Soup & Oyster	18 crackers	1	60	15%
Premium Bits	16 crackers	3	70	39%
Premium Saltine	5 crackers	2	60	30%
Fat Free	5 crackers	–	50	–
Original Unsalted Tops	5 crackers	2	60	30%
Whole Wheat Premium Plus				
Saltines	5 crackers	2	60	30%
Ritz				
Regular & Low-Salt	4 crackers	4	70	51%
Whole Wheat	5 crackers	2	60	30%
Ritz Bits				
Cheese	22 crackers	4	70	51%
Original Mini	22 crackers	4	70	51%
Sandwiches				
Cheese Pizza	5 sandwiches	5	80	56%
Nacho Cheese	6 sandwiches	5	80	56%
Peanut Butter	6 sandwiches	4	80	45%
w/Real Cheese	6 sandwiches	5	80	56%
Royal Lunch Milk Crackers	1 cracker	2	60	30%
Sea Round	1 cracker	2	60	30%
SnackWells				
Wheat	5 crackers	–	50	–
Sociable	6 crackers	3	70	39%
Swiss Cheese Snack	7½ crackers	3	70	39%
Teddy Grahams Whole Wheat	26 crackers	3	70	39%
Bearwich's				
Chocolate w/vanilla creme	4 pieces	3	70	39%
Cinnamon w/vanilla creme	4 pieces	3	70	39%
Vanilla w/chocolate creme	4 pieces	3	70	39%
Chocolate Graham Snacks	11 pieces	2	60	30%
Cinnamon Graham Snacks	11 pieces	2	60	30%
Honey Graham Snacks	11 pieces	2	60	30%
Vanilla Graham Snacks	11 pieces	2	60	30%
Toasted Bran Thins	7 crackers	3	60	45%
Toasted Peanut Butter Sandwich	2 sandwiches	4	70	51%

Food and Description	Amount	Fat Grams	Total Calories	% Fat Calories
Triscuit Wafers				
Deli Style Rye	3 wafers	2	60	30%
Regular & Low-Salt	3 crackers	2	60	30%
Triscuit Bits	8 crackers	2	60	30%
Wheat'n Bran Triscuit	3 crackers	2	60	30%
Twigs - sesame & cheese	5 pieces	4	70	51%
Uneeda Biscuits-unsalted tops	2 biscuits	2	60	30%
Vegetable Thins	6 crackers	4	70	51%
Waverly (regular & low-salt)	4 crackers	3	70	39%
Wheat Thins				
Cheese	8 crackers	3	70	39%
Low-salt	8 crackers	3	70	39%
Multi-grain	8 crackers	2	60	30%
Regular	8 crackers	3	70	39%
Nutty	8 crackers	4	70	51%
Wheatsworth Stone-ground Wheat	4 crackers	3	70	39%
Zings				
Cheddar	15 pieces	3	70	39%
Original	15 pieces	3	70	39%
Ranch	15 pieces	3	70	39%
Zwieback Teething Toast	2 pieces	1	60	15%
Oat Bran Krisp	2 crackers	3	60	45%
Oyster	10 crackers	1	44	21%
Peanut Butter Cheese (Little Debbie)	.93 oz	6	130	42%
Peanut Butter Toasty (Little Debbie)	.93 oz	7	140	45%
	1.4 oz	12	200	54%
(Pepperidge Farm)				
Butter Thins	4 crackers	3	70	39%
Cracked Wheat	4 crackers	4	100	36%
English Water Biscuits	4 biscuits	1	70	13%
Flutters				
Garden Herb	¾ oz	4	100	36%
Golden Sesame	¾ oz	5	110	41%
Original Butter	¾ oz	4	100	36%
Toasted Wheat	¾ oz	5	110	41%
Goldfish Cheese Thins	4 crackers	2	50	36%
Goldfish-Tiny				
Cheddar Cheese	1 oz	4	120	30%
Low Salt Cheddar Cheese	1 oz	4	120	30%
Original	1 oz	5	130	35%
Parmesan Cheese	1 oz	4	120	30%
Pizza Flavored	1 oz	5	130	35%
Pretzel	1 oz	3	110	25%
Hearty Wheat	4 crackers	4	100	36%

Food and Description	Amount	Fat Grams	Total Calories	% Fat Calories
Sesame	4 crackers	3	80	34%
Toasted Wheat	4 crackers	3	80	34%
(Planters)				
Round Toast Crackers	4 sandwiches	7	140	45%
Square Cheese Crackers	4 sandwiches	7	140	45%
Rice Crunch Crackers (KA-ME)				
Unsalted Wafers	.44 oz	< 1	50	9%
Rusk (See CRISPBREAD)				
(Ry Krisp)				
Natural	2 crackers	–	40	–
Seasoned	2 crackers	1	45	20%
Sesame	2 crackers	2	50	36%
Saltines-regular	4 crackers	1	50	18%
(Sea Rounds)	½ oz	2	60	30%
(Sesmark) Deli Style				
Cheddar Sesame Thins	4 crackers	3	80	34%
Original Sesame Thins	4 crackers	3	71	38%
Unsalted Sesame Thins	4 crackers	3	71	38%
(Sunshine)				
Cheddar American Heritage	5 crackers	4	80	45%
Cheez-it	12 crackers	4	70	51%
Krispy saltines				
mild cheddar	5 crackers	2	60	30%
regular & unsalted tops	5 crackers	1	60	15%
whole wheat	5 crackers	2	60	30%
Oyster	16 crackers	1	60	15%
Oyster & Soup	16 crackers	1	60	15%
Parmesan American Heritage	4 crackers	4	70	51%
Sesame American Heritage	4 crackers	4	70	51%
Wheat American Heritage	4 crackers	3	60	45%
Wheat Snack	8 crackers	4	70	51%
Wheat Wafers	8 wafers	4	80	45%
Tam Tams (Manischewitz)				
Garlic	10 pieces	8	153	47%
no salt	10 pieces	7	138	46%
Onion	10 pieces	8	150	48%
regular	10 pieces	8	147	49%
Wheat	10 pieces	8	150	48%
(Valley Lahvosh)				
Cracker Bread				
Hors d'oeuvre size	1 piece	.5	28	26%
Rounds white 5"	1 piece	1	70	13%
Small Wheat Lahvosh	1 piece	< 1	28	23%
Small White Lahvosh	1 piece	1	28	32%

Food and Description	Amount	Fat Grams	Total Calories	% Fat Calories
Wheat Crackers w/Cheese				
(Little Debbie)	~ 1 oz	7	140	39%
(Wheat-Krisp) Whole Wheat	2 pieces	1	50	18%
Wheat Wafers (Venus)	8 wafers	2	100	18%
Whole Wheat (Manischewitz)	10 crackers	1	90	10%
CRANBERRY/fresh				
chopped	1 cup	–	54	–
whole	1 cup	–	46	–
CRANBERRY JUICE				
(Hain) Concentrate	1 oz	–	40	–
(Knudsen) Just Cranberry Juice	8 oz	–	40	–
(Smucker's)	8 oz	–	130	–
CRANBERRY JUICE COCKTAIL	8 oz	–	147	–
Bottled				
(Ocean Spray)	6 oz	–	100	–
low cal	6 oz	–	40	–
(Seneca)	6 oz	–	110	–
Frozen				
(Birds Eye)	6 oz	–	100	–
(Seneca)	6 oz	–	110	–
(Sunkist)	6 oz	–	110	–
CRANBERRY JUICE DRINK				
(Welch's)	6 oz	–	100	–
CRANBERRY NECTAR				
Cranberry Delight Nectar	6 oz	–	80	–
Cranberry Nectar (Knudsen)	8 oz	–	110	–
CRANBERRY SAUCE				
Canned				
Generic	1 cup	–	419	–
(Ocean Spray)				
Jellied	2 oz	–	90	–
Whole	2 oz	–	90	–
(S&W)				
Jellied	¼ cup	–	90	–
Old Fashioned-Whole Berry	¼ cup	–	90	–
CRANBERRY-APPLE JUICE DRINK				
Cranapple Drink				
(Ocean Spray)	6 oz	–	130	–
low-cal	6 oz	–	40	–
(Welch's)	6 oz	–	120	–
Cranberry-Apple	6 oz	–	123	–
(Seneca)	6 oz	–	110	–
frozen	6 oz	–	110	–
(Tropical Sno) mix	6 oz	–	110	–

Food and Description	Amount	Fat Grams	Total Calories	% Fat Calories
Cranberry-Apple Cooler				
(Health Valley)	13 oz	1	144	6%
CRANBERRY-APRICOT JUICE DRINK	6 oz	–	118	–
Cranicot Drink (Ocean Spray)	6 oz	–	110	–
CRANBERRY-BLUEBERRY JUICE DRINK				
(Ocean Spray)	6 oz	–	120	–
CRANBERRY-GRAPE JUICE DRINK	6 oz	–	130	–
Crangrape (Ocean Spray)	6 oz	–	130	–
CRANBERRY-ORANGE JUICE DRINK				
(Ocean Spray)	6 oz	–	100	–
(Tropicana) Single Serve	10 oz	–	159	–
CRANBERRY-ORANGE RELISH				
canned	½ cup	–	246	–
uncooked	½ cup	–	245	–
CRANBERRY-RASPBERRY JUICE DRINK				
(Ocean Spray)	6 oz	–	110	–
low-cal	6 oz	–	40	–
CRAN-ORANGE SAUCE (Ocean Spray)	2 oz	–	100	–
CRAN-RASPBERRY SAUCE				
(Ocean Spray)	2 oz	–	90	–
CRAN-TASTIC BLENDED (Ocean Spray)	6 oz	–	110	–
CRAYFISH/mixed				
cooked-moist heat	3 oz	1	97	9%
raw	3 oz	.9	76	11%
	8 fish	< 1	24	19%
CREAM (*See also* ICE CREAM TOPPING, SOUR CREAM, SOUR CREAM SUBSTITUTES, WHIPPED TOPPING)				
Coffee/Table light cream	1 Tbs	3	30	90%
	1 cup	46	469	90%
Coffee Lightener-non-dairy/frozen				
(Kemps)	1 Tbs	2	22	82%
(Rich's)				
Coffee Rich	1 Tbs	2	18	100%
Farm Rich				
Light	1 Tbs	< 1	10	45%
Original	1 Tbs	2	18	100%
Poly Rich	½ oz	1	20	45%
Coffee Lightener-non-dairy/liquid				
(Carnation) Coffee Mate				
Amaretto	1 Tbs	2	40	45%
Hazelnut	1 Tbs	2	40	45%
Irish Creme	1 Tbs	2	40	45%
Light	1 Tbs	< 1	10	45%
Original	1 Tbs	1	16	56%

Food and Description	Amount	Fat Grams	Total Calories	% Fat Calories
(Coffee Delight)	1 Tbs	2	20	90%
(Coffee Rich)	1 Tbs	1.6	22	66%
(Half & Half)	1 Tbs	1.7	20	77%
	½ cup	13	150	78%
(International Delight)				
Amaretto	1 Tbs	2	45	40%
Hazelnut	1 Tbs	2	45	40%
Irish Creme	1 Tbs	2	45	40%
(Maxwell House)	1 Tbs	1	12	75%
(Mocha Mix)				
Amaretto	1 Tbs	1	35	20%
Irish Creme	1 Tbs	1	35	20%
Lite	1 Tbs	< 1	10	45%
	1 cup	12	150	72%
Original	1 Tbs	2	20	90%
Coffee Lightener-non-dairy/powdered				
(Carnation) Coffee Mate				
Lite	1 tsp	< 1	8	56%
Original	1 tsp	1	10	90%
	1 pkt	1	16	56%
(Cremora)				
Lite	1 tsp	< 1	8	56%
Original	1 tsp	1	12	75%
(Maxwell House)	1 pkt	1	14	64%
(N-Rich)	1 tsp	< 1	10	45%
(Weight Watchers)	1 pkt	–	10	–
Whipping Cream/fluid				
heavy	1 cup	88	820	100%
	1 Tbs	6	50	100%
heavy-whipped	2 cups	88	820	100%
(Land O'Lakes)				
Gourmet heavy	1 Tbs	6	60	100%
light	1 cup	73.88	704	100%
	1 Tbs	5	45	100%
light-whipped	2 cups	73.88	704	100%
(Land O'Lakes) light	1 Tbs	5	45	100%
CREAM CHEESE (See CHEESE)				
CREAM OF TARTAR	1 Tbs	–	23	–
	1 tsp	–	7	–
CREPE				
Frozen				
(Chief Francois)	1 crepe	3	80	34%
Mix				
(Krusteaz)	2 (7")	1	80	11%

Food and Description	Amount	Fat Grams	Total Calories	% Fat Calories
Ready to use				
(Table de France)	1 (9")	1	45	20%
CRISPBREAD (See also CRACKERS)				
(Ideal)				
Extra Thin Crispbread	3 slices	–	48	–
Whole Grain Crispbread	2 slices	–	43	–
w/sesame seeds	2 slices	–	40	–
(LU) Crokine Crispbread	2 slices	o	37	–
(Kavli) Norwegian				
Crispy Thin	1 slice	< 1	15	10%
Hearty Thick	1 slice	< 1	40	11%
Rye-bran	2 slices	–	30	–
(Ryvita)				
Dark	2 slices	–	38	–
Dark Rye	1 piece	–	26	–
Dark Rye w/caraway seeds	2 pieces	–	38	–
High Fiber	1 piece	–	25	–
Light Rye Hi-Fiber	1 piece	–	35	–
Original Wheat	1 piece	–	20	–
Toasted Sesame Rye	1 piece	–	31	–
(Wasa)				
Breakfast	1 slice	1	50	18%
Extra Crisp	1 slice	–	25	–
Fiber Plus	1 slice	1	35	26%
Golden Rye	1 slice	–	35	–
Hearty Rye	1 slice	–	50	–
Lite Rye	1 slice	–	25	–
Sesame Wheat	1 slice	–	25	–
(Weight Watchers) all flavors	2 wafers	–	30	–
Rusk (Sweet hard crisp bread)				
(3⅜" dia ½" thick)	1 piece	.8	38	19%
CROAKER				
breaded & fried	3 oz	10	188	48%
raw	3 oz	2.69	89	27%
CROISSANT				
Croissant (recipe)	1/~ 2 oz	12	235	46%
(Pepperidge Farm) frozen				
all butter	1	14	240	53%
all butter-petite	1	8	140	51%
(Pepperidge Farm) ready-to-serve	1	7	170	37%
(Rainbo) Wheat	1	19	300	57%
(Sara Lee) frozen				
all butter	1	9	170	48%
all butter-petite	1	6	120	45%

Food and Description	Amount	Fat Grams	Total Calories	% Fat Calories
CROUTON				
(Kellogg) Croutettes	1 cup	–	144	–
(Pepperidge Farm)				
Cheddar & Romano Cheese	½ oz	2	60	30%
Cheese & Garlic	½ oz	3	70	39%
Onion & Garlic	½ oz	3	70	39%
Seasoned	½ oz	3	70	39%
Sour Cream & Chive	½ oz	3	70	39%
(Progresso) Italian Style	½ oz	1	30	30%
CROWDER PEA/canned				
Seasoned w/pork (Luck's)	7.5 oz	7	200	32%
CRUMPETS				
(Wolferman's)				
Brown Sugar Cinnamon	1	2	110	16%
Original	1	< 1	90	5%
Raspberry	1	< 1	90	5%
CUCUMBER (*See also* PICKLE)				
Raw				
slices	½ cup	–	7	–
whole	1	–	29	–
CUMIN SEED	1 tsp	.5	8	56%
CUPCAKE (*See* CAKE AND CAKE PASTRY, SNACK CAKES)				
CURRANT				
Black				
dried	½ cup	–	204	–
raw	½ lb	–	120	–
	½ cup	–	36	–
Red or White				
raw	½ lb	–	110	–
	½ cup	–	31	–
Zante				
(Del Monte) dried	½ cup	–	200	–
(Sun Maid)	½ cup	–	210	–
CURRANT JUICE				
Black	8 oz	–	138	–
CURRY POWDER	1 tsp	–	6	–
CURRY SAUCE (*See* SAUCE)				
CUSK				
raw	3 oz	1	74	12%
steamed	1 lb	3	481	6%
	1 oz	< 1	30	15%
CUSTARD (*See also* PUDDING & MOUSSE)				
homemade				
baked	1 cup	14.6	305	43%

Food and Description	Amount	Fat Grams	Total Calories	% Fat Calories
boiled	½ cup	7	164	38%
mix				
(Jell-O)				
Americana Golden Egg				
prepared w/whole milk	½ cup	5	160	28%
Flan-Spanish Style				
prepared w/whole milk	½ cup	4	148	24%
Zabaglione/sauce topping for fruit				
homemade	¼ cup	4	80	45%
CUTTLEFISH/raw	3 oz	.6	67	8%

D

Food and Description	Amount	Fat Grams	Total Calories	% Fat Calories
DANDELION GREENS				
fresh-cooked	½ cup	–	17	–
raw-chopped	½ cup	–	13	–
DANISH (See CAKE AND CAKE PASTRY)				
DATE				
chopped	1 cup	.8	489	2%
(Dole)	½ cup	< 1	280	2%
(Dromedary)				
chopped	¼ cup	–	130	–
no pits	5 dates	–	100	–
	1 oz	–	100	–
natural & dry	10	–	228	–
(Sun Giant)				
chopped	1 cup	1	490	2%
pitted	10 dates	1	220	4%
DESSERT TOPPINGS (See CREAM; ICE CREAM TOPPING)				
DIETING AIDS (See BREAKFAST BARS; BREAKFAST DRINK; NUTRITIONAL SUPPLEMENTS)				
DILL SAUCE (See SAUCE)				
DILL SEED	1 tsp	–	6	–
dried	1 tsp	–	3	–
DINNER (See FAST FOOD, FROZEN ENTREE/DINNER)				

Food and Description	Amount	Fat Grams	Total Calories	% Fat Calories
DIPS				
■ MIX				
(Casbah)				
Humus Bean Dip	2 oz	10	220	41%
(Hidden Valley) Party Dip				
Original Ranch-Reduced Calorie				
Prepared	1 Tbs	2	20	90%
■ READY-TO-SERVE				
(Dean's)				
French Onion Dip				
Extra Light	1 oz	2	30	60%
Original	1 oz	4	50	72%
w/Bacon Bits	1 oz	4	50	72%
Ranch	1 oz	4	50	72%
(Hain)				
Hot Bean	2 Tbs	1	40	23%
Mexican Bean	2 Tbs	1	35	26%
Onion Bean Dip	2 Tbs	1	35	26%
(Kemps)				
Lite Healthy Vegetable Dip	1 oz	2	30	60%
Party Dips	1 oz	4	50	72%
(Kraft)				
Avocado (Guacamole)	2 Tbs	4	50	72%
Bacon & Horseradish	2 Tbs	5	60	75%
Clam	2 Tbs	4	60	60%
French Onion	2 Tbs	4	60	60%
Green Onion	2 Tbs	4	60	60%
Jalapeno Pepper	2 Tbs	4	50	72%
Premium Bacon & Horseradish	2 Tbs	5	50	72%
Premium Bacon & Onion	2 Tbs	5	60	60%
Premium Blue Cheese	2 Tbs	4	50	72%
Premium Clam	2 Tbs	4	45	80%
Premium Creamy Cucumber	2 Tbs	4	50	72%
Premium Creamy Onion	2 Tbs	4	45	80%
Premium French Onion	2 Tbs	4	45	80%
Premium Jalapeno Pepper	2 Tbs	4	50	72%
Premium Nacho Cheese	2 Tbs	4	55	65%
(Marzetti)				
Apple				
Caramel	1 Tbs	4	317	11%
Peanut Butter	1 Tbs	17	367	42%
Veggie				
Blue Cheese	1 Tbs	11	100	99%
Dill	1 Tbs	7	68	93%
Ranch	1 Tbs	7	67	94%

Food and Description	Amount	Fat Grams	Total Calories	% Fat Calories
Spinach	1 Tbs	7	70	90%
(Slender Choice)				
French Onion	1 Tbs	1	14	64%
Green Onion	1 Tbs	1	16	56%
Jalapeno	1 Tbs	1	16	56%
Ranch Style	1 Tbs	1	16	56%
(Sonora Valley)				
Bean & Cheese	1 oz	3	50	54%
DISTILLED LIQUOR (*See* LIQUOR, DISTILLED)				
DOCK				
cooked	3 oz	–	17	–
raw-chopped	3 oz	–	15	–
DOGFISH/raw	3 oz	6.5	135	43%
DOLPHIN FISH	3 oz	.6	73	7%
DONUT (*See also* SNACK CAKES)				
(Break Cake)				
Chocolate	1-1 oz	8	130	55%
Cinnamon	1-1 oz	6	115	47%
Powdered	1-1 oz	5	115	39%
Cake Type Donuts				
(3¼"dia 1"high)	1	7.8	164	43%
(1½"dia 1"high)	1	2.6	155	15%
(Drake's)				
Old Fashioned	1 pkg	8	180	40%
Powdered Sugar	1 pkg	15	300	45%
(Dunkin' Donuts)				
Apple Filled				
w/Cinnamon Sugar	1	11	250	40%
Bavarian Filled				
w/Chocolate Frosting	1	14	226	56%
Blueberry Filled	1	11	240	34%
Chocolate Frosted Yeast Ring	1	8	210	34%
Cookies				
Chocolate Chunk	1	10	200	45%
Chocolate Chunk w/Nuts	1	11	210	47%
Oatmeal Bran Raisin	1	9	200	41%
Croissants				
Almond	1	29	420	62%
Chocolate	1	29	440	59%
Plain	1	19	310	55%
Glazed				
Buttermilk Ring	1	14	290	43%
Chocolate Ring	1	21	324	58%
Coffee Roll	1	12	280	39%

Food and Description	Amount	Fat Grams	Total Calories	% Fat Calories
French Cruller	1	8	140	51%
Whole Wheat Ring	1	18	330	49%
Yeast Ring	1	9	200	41%
Jelly Filled	1	9	220	37%
Lemon Filled	1	12	260	42%
Munchkin				
Cake w/Powdered Sugar	1	4	69	52%
Chocolate w/Glaze	1	5	88	51%
Yeast w/Glaze	1	2	43	42%
Plain Cake Ring	1	17	270	57%
(Earth Grains)				
Cinnamon Apple	1	17	310	49%
Devil's Food	1	21	330	57%
Glazed (Old Fashioned)	1	18	310	52%
Powdered (Old Fashioned)	1	19	290	59%
(Entenmann's)				
Crumb Topped	1	12	260	42%
Devil's Food	1	12	250	43%
Rich Frosted	1	18	280	58%
(Hostess) Breakfast Bake Shop				
Cinnamon				
8 Pack	1	6	140	39%
Donette Gems	1	3	60	45%
Donette Gems, Apple Filled	1	3	70	39%
Family Pack	1	6	120	34%
Pantry (assorted)	1	10	190	47%
Crumb				
Donette Gems				
Frosted	1	5	80	56%
Frosted, Strawberry Filled	1	4	80	45%
Plain	1	5	80	56%
Frosted	1.25 oz	10	160	56%
	1.4 oz	11	180	55%
	1.5 oz	12	190	57%
Donette Gems, Plain	1	3	60	45%
Family Pack, Plain	1	6	120	45%
Glazed Whirl	1	7	190	33%
Honey Wheat	1	12	250	43%
Hostess O's				
Frosted	1	14	260	48%
Plain	1	10	230	39%
Old Fashioned				
Glazed	1	12	250	43%
Plain	1	9	170	48%

Food and Description	Amount	Fat Grams	Total Calories	% Fat Calories
Plain				
8 Pack	1	7	130	48%
Pantry				
(assorted)	1	11	190	52%
Powdered Sugar				
8 Pack	1	7	140	45%
Donette Gems	1	3	60	45%
Donette Gems, Strawberry Filled	1	3	70	39%
Family Pack	1	6	120	45%
Pantry (assorted)	1	10	190	47%
(Little Debbie)				
Donut Sticks	1 pkg/2.5 oz	18	330	49%
	1 pkg/			
	1.67 oz	13	230	51%
(Tastykake)				
Assorted (9 count)				
Cinnamon	1	8	180	40%
Plain	1	10	190	47%
Powdered Sugar	1	9	180	45%
Honey Wheat	1	8	210	34%
Mini				
Cinnamon	1	2	50	36%
Honey Wheat	1	1	40	23%
Powdered Sugar	1	1	40	23%
Rich Frosted	1	3	60	45%
Orange Glazed	1	9	220	37%
Rich Frosted	1	16	260	55%
(Winchell's)				
Apple Fritter	1	37	580	57%
Cinnamon Crumb	1	11	240	41%
Cinnamon Roll	1	21	360	53%
Glazed Jelly	1	13	300	39%
Glazed Round	1	12	210	51%
Glazed Twist	1	11	210	47%
Iced Chocolate Bar	1	11	220	45%
Iced Chocolate Cake	1	10	230	39%
Iced Chocolate Devil's	1	12	240	45%
Iced Chocolate French	1	13	220	53%
Iced Chocolate Raised	1	10	210	43%
Plain	1	11	200	50%
Plain Donut Hole	1	3	50	54%
Yeast-Leavened-Glazed Donuts				
(3¾" dia. 1¼" high)	1	13	235	50%
Yeast-Leavened-Jelly Filled Donuts	1	9	225	36%

Food and Description	Amount	Fat Grams	Total Calories	% Fat Calories
DRUM/raw (freshwater)	3 oz	4	100	36%
DUCK				
Domestic				
liver-raw	1.5 oz	2	60	30%
meat & skin-roasted	~ ¾ lb	108	1287	76%
meat only-roasted	8 oz	24.75	445	50%
Wild				
breast meat only-raw	3 oz	35	102	31%
meat & skin-raw	9.5 oz	41	571	65%

E

Food and Description	Amount	Fat Grams	Total Calories	% Fat Calories
ECLAIR (See CAKE AND CAKE PASTRY)				
EEL				
cooked-dry heat	3 oz	12.7	200	57%
raw	3 oz	9.9	156	57%
smoked	~2 oz	16	188	77%
EGG (See also EGG SUBSTITUTE, MEAT SUBSTITUTES, VEGETARIAN FOOD)				
Chicken-large				
boiled, hard/soft	1 egg	5.6	79	64%
fried in butter	1 egg	7	95	66%
hard boiled	1 egg	5.6	79	64%
pickled	1 egg	5	80	56%
poached	1 egg	5.6	79	64%
raw	1 egg	5.6	79	64%
raw, yolk & white	1 egg	5.6	79	64%
raw, white only	1 egg	–	16	–
raw, yolk only	1 egg	5.6	63	64%
white	1 egg	–	16	–
	1 cup	–	120	–
yolk	1 egg	5.6	63	64%
Duck/raw	1 egg	9.6	130	67%
Goose/raw	1 egg	19	276	62%
Quail/raw	1 egg	1	14	64%
Turkey/raw	1 egg	9	135	60%

Food and Description	Amount	Fat Grams	Total Calories	% Fat Calories
EGG MEALS (*See also* BREAKFAST SANDWICH; EGG; EGG SUBSTITUTE; FRENCH TOAST)				
Deviled	1 egg	13	145	81%
Egg Breakfast Sandwiches-frozen				
(Schwan's)				
Muffin				
w/ham steak	1	17	340	45%
(Swanson-Great Starts)				
Biscuit				
w/Canadian bacon & cheese	5¼ oz	22	420	47%
w/sausage	4.7 oz	22	410	48%
w/sausage & cheese	5½ oz	28	460	55%
Muffin				
w/beefsteak & cheese	4.9 oz	20	360	50%
w/Canadian bacon & cheese	4.1 oz	15	290	47%
(Weight Watchers)				
Muffin				
w/ham & cheese	4 oz	8	230	31%
Egg Foo Young-homemade	~ 5 oz	10	150	60%
Omelette				
Standard Home Recipe (USDA)				
w/whole milk, cooked in butter	1 egg	7	95	66%
(Swanson-Great Starts) frozen				
Spanish Style	7¾ oz	16	240	60%
(Weight Watchers) frozen				
Garden Vegetable Omelet				
Sandwich	3.6 oz	6	210	26%
Ham & Cheese Handy Omelet	4 oz	5	180	25%
w/Cheese Sauce and Ham	7 oz	29	390	67%
Quiche				
Lorraine/8" diameter				
Standard Home Recipe (USDA)	⅛ quiche	48	600	72%
Spinach	5 oz	26	337	69%
Scrambled Eggs				
Frozen				
(Aunt Jemima)				
& Sausage				
w/Hash Browns	5.7 oz	20	290	62%
w/Pancakes	5.2 oz	14	270	47%
w/Cheddar Cheese & Fried				
Potatoes	5.9 oz	13	250	45%
(Downyflake)				
w/Ham & Hash Browns	6¼ oz	26	350	67%
w/Ham & Pecan Twirls	6¼ oz	28	470	54%

Food and Description	Amount	Fat Grams	Total Calories	% Fat Calories
(Swanson-Great Starts)				
w/Bacon & Home Fries	5¼ oz	26	340	69%
w/Cheese & Cinnamon Pancakes	3.4 oz	23	290	71%
w/Home Fries	4⅜ oz	19	260	66%
w/Mini Oat Bran Muffins	4¾ oz	12	250	43%
w/Sausage & Hash Browns	6½ oz	34	430	71%
Standard home recipe (USDA)				
w/whole milk/cooked in butter	1 egg	7	95	66%
EGG ROLL (*See* FROZEN ENTREE/DINNER, ORIENTAL FOOD, SEAFOOD ENTREE/DINNER)				
EGG SALAD-homemade	⅓ cup	19	205	83%
EGG SUBSTITUTE				
frozen	¼ cup	6.7	96	64%
liquid	1½ oz	1.6	39	37%
powder	.35 oz	1	44	21%
■ BY BRAND NAME				
(Country Morning)	½ cup	12	173	62%
(Crystal Farms) Simply Eggs	¼ cup	5	70	64%
(Egg Watchers)	2 oz =			
	1 egg	2	50	36%
(Featherweight) Egg Magic	1 pkg			
	2 eggs	8	120	60%
(Fleischmann's) Egg Beaters				
Plain	¼ cup	–	25	–
Cheese Omelette Mix	½ cup	5	110	41%
Vegetable Omelette Mix	½ pkg	–	50	–
(Healthy Choice)	¼ cup	< 1	30	15%
(Morning Star Farms) Scramblers	¼ cup	3	60	45%
(Second Nature)	2 oz =			
	1 egg	2	60	30%
EGGNOG				
Canned				
(Borden)	4 oz	9	160	51%
Commercial				
(Carnation) Lite	8 oz	8	320	23%
(Farm Rich) Non-Dairy	8 oz	18	380	43%
Generic	8 oz	19	342	50%
(Kemps)				
Holly Nog	4 oz	2	110	16%
Lite Egg Nog	4 oz	3	120	23%
Original	4 oz	9	175	46%
Premium	4 oz	9	180	45%
(Land O'Lakes)				
Original	8 oz	7	380	17%
TLC Light	4 oz	3	130	21%

Food and Description	Amount	Fat Grams	Total Calories	% Fat Calories
Mix				
dry	2 tsp	–	110	–
(2 heaping tsp) + whole milk	8 oz	8	260	28%
(PDQ) ⅔ tsp + whole milk	8 oz	5	230	20%
EGGPLANT				
fresh-boiled	½ cup	–	13	–
raw-sliced	½ cup	–	11	–
EGGPLANT DISHES (*See also* FROZEN ENTREE/DINNER)				
Eggplant Parmigiana				
frozen				
(Celentano)	8 oz	15	280	48%
(Mrs. Paul's)	5 oz	16	240	60%
Eggplant Sticks				
fried				
frozen				
(Pepperidge Farm)	3½ oz	12	240	45%
ELDERBERRY/raw	½ lb	1	154	6%
	1 cup	.8	105	7%
ENCHILADA (*See* MEXICAN FOOD)				
ENCHILADA SAUCE (*See* MEXICAN FOOD, SAUCE)				
ENDIVE/raw	½ cup	–	4	–
ESCAROLE/raw	4 oz	–	20	–
ESCAROLE SOUP (*See* SOUP)				
EXTRACTS & FLAVORINGS				
(Durkee)				
Almond pure extract	1 tsp	–	13	–
Anise extract	1 tsp	–	16	–
Banana flavor	1 tsp	–	15	–
Butter flavor	1 tsp	–	3	–
Brandy flavor	1 tsp	–	15	–
Black Walnut flavor	1 tsp	–	4	–
Cherry extract	1 tsp	–	3	–
Chocolate flavor	1 tsp	–	7	–
Coconut flavor	1 tsp	–	8	–
Creme De Menthe extract	1 tsp	–	9	–
Lemon extract	1 tsp	–	17	–
Malt extract-dried	1 oz	–	104	–
Maple extract	1 tsp	–	6	–
Orange extract	1 tsp	–	14	–
Peppermint extract	1 tsp	–	15	–
Pineapple flavor	1 tsp	–	6	–
Raspberry extract	1 tsp	–	10	–
Rum flavor	1 tsp	–	14	–
Strawberry extract	1 tsp	–	12	–

Food and Description	Amount	Fat Grams	Total Calories	% Fat Calories
Vanilla-pure extract	1 tsp	–	8	–
Vanilla flavor	1 tsp	–	3	–
Vanilla Butter & Nut extract (McCormick/Schilling)	1 tsp	–	5	–
Almond extract	1 tsp	–	10	–
Anise-pure extract	1 tsp	–	23	–
Banana-imitation extract	1 tsp	–	11	–
Black Walnut extract				
Cold	1 tsp	–	12	–
Heated	1 tsp	–	< 1	–
Brandy-imitation extract	1 tsp	–	20	–
Butter Flavor	1 tsp	–	< 1	–
Chocolate extract				
Cold	1 tsp	–	8	–
Heated	1 tsp	–	2	–
Coconut-imitation extract	1 tsp	–	7	–
Lemon-extract				
Cold	1 tsp	–	35	–
Heated	1 tsp	–	< 1	–
Maple-imitation flavor	1 tsp	–	8	–
Mint & Peppermint pure extract	1 tsp	–	20	–
Orange-pure extract	1 tsp	–	23	–
Pineapple-imitation extract	1 tsp	–	12	–
Root Beer concentrate	1 tsp	–	13	–
Rum-imitation extract	1 tsp	–	19	–
Sherry-pure extract	1 tsp	–	14	–
Strawberry-imitation extract	1 tsp	–	7	–
Vanilla				
Cold	1 tsp	–	12	–
Heated	1 tsp	–	< 1	–

F

Food and Description	Amount	Fat Grams	Total Calories	% Fat Calories
FALAFEL				
homemade-pattied or balled	1 oz	6	115	47%
mix (Casbah)	1.33 oz	2	134	13%
FAST FOODS (*See* separate section at end of book)				

Food and Description	Amount	Fat Grams	Total Calories	% Fat Calories
FAT (*See also* LARD, OILS, SHORTENING)				
Bacon fat	1 Tbs	14	126	100%
Beef fat/separable/raw	1 Tbs	12	108	100%
Chicken fat	1 Tbs	12	115	100%
Duck fat	1 Tbs	12	115	100%
Pork back fat/raw	2 oz	50	464	100%
FAT, COOKING (*See* SHORTENING)				
FAVA BEANS/canned				
(Progresso)	8 oz	1	180	5%
FENNEL LEAVES/raw	2 oz	–	15	–
FENNEL SEED	1 tsp	–	7	–
FENUGREEK SEED	1 tsp	–	12	–
FIG				
canned	1 cup	–	228	–
(Del Monte) whole	½ cup	–	100	–
(S&W) fancy, whole kadota	½ cup	–	100	–
dried				
cooked	½ cup	–	140	–
	1 large	–	55	–
(Mariani) Calimyma	½ cup	2	250	7%
(Sun Maid)				
Calimyma	½ cup	2	250	7%
Mission	½ cup	1	210	4%
fresh	1 large	–	47	–
FILBERT OR HAZELNUT (*See also* HAZELNUT SPREAD)				
dried				
blanched	1 oz	17.8	179	90%
unblanched	1 oz	18.5	190	88%
dry roasted	1 oz	18.8	188	90%
oil roasted	1 oz	18	187	87%
FISH (*See* SEAFOOD ENTREE/DINNER and individual listings)				
FISH CHOWDER (*See* SOUP)				
FISH SEASONINGS (*See* SEASONINGS)				
FLAN (*See* CUSTARD)				
FLATBREAD (*See* CRACKERS)				
FLATFISH				
cooked	3 oz	1	100	9%
raw	3 oz	1	80	11%
FLAVORINGS (*See* EXTRACTS & FLAVORINGS)				
FLOUNDER (*See also* SEAFOOD ENTREE/DINNER)				
baked w/butter	3 oz	7	171	37%
baked w/o butter	3 oz	1	80	11%
frozen-breaded	5 oz	15	300	45%
frozen-raw (Van de Kamp's)	4 oz	1	100	9%

Food and Description	Amount	Fat Grams	Total Calories	% Fat Calories
FLOUR				
Amaranth	2 oz	1	190	5%
	1 cup	2	698	3%
Arrowroot	1 Tbs	–	29	–
Barley	1 Tbs	< 1	28	16%
Bread				
(Gold Medal) high protein	1 cup	1	400	2%
(Pillsbury's Best)	1 cup	2	400	5%
Brown Rice	2 oz	1	200	5%
Buckwheat, dark	1 cup	2	326	6%
Buckwheat, light	1 cup	1	340	3%
Buckwheat, whole grain	1 cup	2	335	5%
Cake or Pastry	4 oz	1	413	2%
Carob				
(St. John's Bread)	4 oz	3	420	6%
Corn	1 cup	3	430	6%
	1 oz	1	102	9%
Cottonseed				
Low-fat	1 oz	–	95	–
Partially defatted	2 Tbs	–	40	–
	1 cup	6	335	16%
Cracked Wheat				
(Krusteaz)	1 cup	2	320	6%
Drifted Snow				
(Pillsbury)	4 oz	1	400	2%
Garbanzo (Arrowhead Mills)				
Toasted	2 oz	4	210	18%
Graham (Krusteaz)	1 cup	2	320	6%
Gluten	1 cup	3	530	5%
La Pina	1 cup	1	400	2%
Millet (Arrowhead Mills)	2 oz	2	185	10%
Oat (Arrowhead Mills)	2 oz	1	200	5%
Oat Flour Blend (Gold Medal)	4 oz/1 cup	3	390	7%
Peanut				
Defatted	1 oz	–	92	–
	2 Tbs	–	30	–
	1 cup	–	200	–
Low-fat	1 oz	6	120	45%
	1 cup	13	260	45%
Potato	1 cup	1.5	632	2%
Rice	2 oz	1	200	5%
	1 cup	1	398	2%
Rye (Fisher)	1 cup	2	450	4%
Rye, dark	1 cup	3	419	6%

Food and Description	Amount	Fat Grams	Total Calories	% Fat Calories
Rye, light	1 cup	1	364	3%
Rye, medium				
(Pillsbury)	1 cup	2	400	5%
Rye & Wheat, Bohemian Style				
(Pillsbury)	1 cup	1	400	2%
Sesame-low-fat	1 cup	–	95	–
Shake & Blend				
(Pillsbury)	2 Tbs	–	50	–
Softasilk	¼ cup	–	100	–
Soy				
Gluten free	½ cup	< 1	180	3%
Whole grain				
(Arrowhead Mills)	2 oz	11	250	40%
Soybean, full fat				
Not stirred	1 cup	17.6	358	44%
Stirred	1 cup	14	295	43%
Soybean, defatted	1 cup	1	327	3%
Soybean, low-fat	1 cup	6	326	17%
Triticale	2 oz	1	200	5%
Wheat & Gluten	1 cup	3	530	5%
White, all purpose	1 cup	1	401	2%
(Ballard & Pillsbury)	1 cup	1	400	2%
(Gold Medal)	1 cup	1	400	2%
(Mrs. Wright)	1 cup	1	400	2%
(Pillsbury's Best)	1 cup	1	400	2%
(Red Band)	1 cup	1	390	2%
Unbleached	1 cup	2	401	5%
(Pillsbury)	1 cup	1	400	2%
White, bread	1 cup	3	401	7%
White, cake	1 cup	1	430	2%
White, self-rising	1 cup	1	440	2%
(Gold Medal)	1 cup	1	380	2%
(Pillsbury & Ballard)	1 cup	1	380	2%
Whole Wheat	1 cup	2	400	5%
(Arrowhead Mills)	2 oz	1	200	5%
(Gold Medal)	1 cup	2	350	5%
(Krusteaz)	1 cup	2	450	4%
Self rising	1 cup	1	440	2%
Whole Wheat Blend				
(Gold Medal)	1 cup	2	370	5%
(Red Band)	1 cup	2	400	5%
Whole Wheat				
stoneground	2 oz	1	200	5%
(Wondra)	1 cup	1	400	2%

Food and Description	Amount	Fat Grams	Total Calories	% Fat Calories
FRANKFURTER				
(Armour)				
Beef & Turkey	2 oz	6	90	60%
(Ball Park)				
Lite	1	12	140	77%
Weiners				
Beef	1	16	175	82%
Regular	1	16	167	86%
(Best's)				
Kosher Lower Fat	1	8	110	66%
(Butterball)				
Turkey	1	11	130	76%
(Eckrich)				
Bunsize				
Lite	1	12	150	72%
Regular	1	17	190	81%
Cheese	1	16	180	80%
Jumbo				
Beef	2 oz	17	190	81%
Cheese	2 oz	17	190	81%
Lite	1	10	120	75%
Pork, Turkey & Beef	2 oz	17	180	85%
Regular	1	14	150	84%
(Giant)				
All-meat				
Great 8	2 oz	17	180	85%
Regular	1.6 oz	13	150	78%
Beef				
Great 8	2 oz	17	180	85%
(Health Valley)				
Chicken Weiners	1	8	96	75%
Turkey Weiners	1	8	96	75%
(Healthy Choice)				
Jumbo	1	2	70	26%
Regular	1	1	50	18%
(Hebrew National)				
Beef	1.7 oz	14	150	84%
Knocks-Beef	3 oz	25	260	87%
Lite	1.7 oz	10	120	75%
Natural Casing	2 oz	18	178	91%
(Hillshire Farm)				
Bun Size				
Cheese	2 oz	16	180	80%
Wieners	2 oz	16	180	80%

Food and Description	Amount	Fat Grams	Total Calories	% Fat Calories
Hot				
Beef	2 oz	17	190	81%
Meat	2 oz	16	190	76%
(Hormel)				
Beef				
One Pound Package	1	13	140	84%
Quarter Pounder	1	34	360	85%
12 Ounce Package	1	10	100	90%
Beef & Pork				
One Pound Package	1	13	140	84%
12 Ounce Package	1	10	110	82%
Chili-Frank'n Stuff	1	15	175	82%
Cocktail				
Smokie Cheezers	1 oz	8	90	80%
Smokies	1 oz	7	83	76%
Wieners	1 oz	7	80	79%
Corn Dogs				
frozen	1	12	220	49%
Light & Lean	1	1	45	20%
Mexicali Dogs	5 oz	21	400	47%
Tater Dogs				
frozen	1	14	210	60%
(Kahn's)				
Beef Jumbo	2 oz	16	190	76%
Beef'n Cheddar	1	16	180	80%
Bun Size				
Beef	1	17	190	81%
Franks	1	17	190	81%
Wieners	2 oz	16	180	80%
Cheese Wiener	1	13	150	78%
Jumbo Pork & Beef	2 oz	16	180	80%
Smokey				
Big Red	1	14	170	74%
Bun Size	1	15	180	75%
Wieners	1	13	140	84%
(La Loma) Meatless				
canned				
Big Franks	1.8 oz	6	110	49%
Linketts	2.5 oz	8	140	51%
Sizzle Franks	2.4 oz	13	170	69%
(Louis Rich)				
Bun Length	2 oz	11	130	76%
Cheese Franks	1.5 oz	9	110	74%
Franks	1.6 oz	8	100	72%

Food and Description	Amount	Fat Grams	Total Calories	% Fat Calories
(Oscar Meyer)				
Bun Length				
Beef Franks	2 oz	17	180	85%
Wieners-pork & turkey	2 oz	17	190	81%
Cheese				
Bacon & Cheese	1	13	140	84%
Original	1	13	140	84%
Jumbo	2 oz	17	185	83%
Light	1	11	130	76%
Little	9 grams	3	30	90%
Pork & Turkey	1	14	150	84%
(Perdue) Chicken	1 oz	5.7	71	72%
(Tyson)				
Cheese Franks	1	11	145	68%
Chicken Corn Dogs	1	14	280	45%
Chicken Franks	1	10	115	78%
(Weaver) Chicken Cheese	1	11	145	68%
(Worthington)				
Vegetarian				
Dixie Dogs/frozen				
on a stick	2.5 oz	10	200	45%
Super-Links/canned	1.7 oz	7	100	63%
Veja-Links/canned	2.2 oz	10	140	64%
Leanies/frozen	1.4 oz	6	100	54%
(Wranglers) Cheese Smoked	1	16	180	80%
FRANKFURTER WRAP				
(Wiener Wrap) refrigerated	1 wrap	2	60	30%
FRENCH FRIES (See POTATO; individual FAST FOOD listings)				
FRENCH ONION SOUP (See SOUP)				
FRENCH TOAST				
Frozen				
(Aunt Jemima)				
Cinnamon Swirl	2 slices	4	170	21%
Original	2 slices	4	166	22%
Sticks w/Syrup	5.2 oz	20	400	45%
Wedges & 2 Sausages	5.3 oz	17	360	43%
(Downyflake)				
Cinnamon	2 slices	7	210	30%
Extra Thick	1 slice	9	150	54%
Plain	2 slices	12	270	40%
Texas Style & Sausage	4.25 oz	24	400	54%
(Farm Rich)				
Sticks				
Apple Cinnamon	1 serving	15	310	44%

Food and Description	Amount	Fat Grams	Total Calories	% Fat Calories
Blueberry	1 serving	14	310	41%
Original	1 serving	15	300	45%
(Krusteaz)				
Cinnamon Swirl	2 slices	5	270	17%
Classic Style	2 slices	6	250	22%
Oat Bran	2 slices	3	210	13%
(Morningstar Farms)				
Vegetarian, Cinnamon Swirl w/Patties	6.5 oz	15	380	36%
(Swanson-Great Starts)				
Cinnamon Swirl w/Sausages	5½ oz	21	390	48%
Mini w/Sausage	2.5 oz	9	190	43%
Regular w/Sausage	5.5 oz	21	380	50%
Oatmeal w/Lite Links	4.65 oz	13	310	38%
(Weight Watchers)				
Cinnamon	3 oz	4	160	23%
w/Links	4.5 oz	11	270	37%
Standard Home Recipe (USDA)	1 slice	7	155	41%
FRITTER				
(Mrs. Paul's)/Frozen				
apple	2	9	240	34%
corn	2	9	240	34%
Standard Homemade Recipe (USDA)	1	7.5	132	51%
FROG LEGS				
fried-floured	1 oz	5	70	64%
	3 oz	17	250	61%
raw	3 oz	< 1	63	7%
FROSTING (See CAKE ICING)				
FROZEN DAIRY DESSERT (See also FROZEN NON-DAIRY DESSERT; ICE CREAM; ICE MILK)				
(Diet Count) Dietetic				
Chocolate	½ cup	6	120	45%
Strawberry	½ cup	5	140	32%
Vanilla	½ cup	7	120	53%
(Dreyer's)				
American Dream Frozen Dairy Desert				
Chocolate Chip	3 oz	1	100	9%
Mocha Almond Fudge	3 oz	1	110	8%
Rocky Road	3 oz	1	110	9%
Vanilla	3 oz	< 1	80	6%
Vanilla, Chocolate, Strawberry	3 oz	1	80	11%

Food and Description	Amount	Fat Grams	Total Calories	% Fat Calories
Frozen Dietary Dessert				
Chocolate	4 oz	7	140	45%
Chocolate Fudge	4 oz	9	160	51%
Strawberry	4 oz	6	120	45%
Vanilla	4 oz	7	130	49%
Light Dairy Desert				
Bananapolitan	½ cup	4	110	33%
Candy Bar	½ cup	5	140	32%
Chocolate Fudge Mousse	½ cup	5	130	35%
Malt Ball'N Fudge	½ cup	5	140	32%
Rocky Road	½ cup	5	130	35%
(Edy's)				
Chocolate	½ cup	7	140	45%
Marble Fudge	½ cup	9	160	51%
Strawberry	½ cup	6	120	45%
Vanilla	½ cup	7	130	49%
(Fudgesicle) Fat-Free Fudge Pop	1 bar	–	70	–
(Healthy Choice)				
Bordeau Cherry	4 oz	2	120	15%
Chocolate	4 oz	2	130	14%
Cookies'N Cream	4 oz	2	130	14%
Neapolitan	4 oz	2	120	15%
Old Fashioned Vanilla	4 oz	2	120	15%
Praline & Caramel	4 oz	2	130	14%
Rocky Road	4 oz	2	160	11%
Strawberry	4 oz	2	120	15%
Vanilla	4 oz	2	120	15%
Wild Berry Swirl	4 oz	2	120	15%
(Klondike) Lite	1 bar	6	110	49%
(Knudsen) Free Frozen Dessert				
Chocolate	½ cup	–	100	–
Vanilla	½ cup	–	100	–
Vanilla Flavored				
Strawberry Royal	½ cup	–	100	–
(Knudsen) Free Frozen Dessert Bars				
Chocolate Fudge	1 bar	–	90	–
Vanilla Fudge	1 bar	–	80	–
Vanilla Strawberry	1 bar	–	80	–
(Simplesse)				
Simple Pleasures				
Light				
Chocolate	4 oz	< 1	80	5%
Chocolate Caramel Sundae	4 oz	< 1	90	5%
Vanilla	4 oz	< 1	80	6%

Food and Description	Amount	Fat Grams	Total Calories	% Fat Calories
Vanilla Fudge	4 oz	< 1	90	5%
Original				
Chocolate	½ cup	< 1	140	3%
Chocolate Chip	½ cup	3	150	18%
Coffee	½ cup	< 1	120	4%
Cookies'N Cream	½ cup	2	150	12%
Mint Chocolate Chip	½ cup	2	150	12%
Peach	½ cup	< 1	120	4%
Pecan Praline	½ cup	2	140	13%
Rum Raisin	½ cup	< 1	130	3%
Strawberry	½ cup	< 1	120	4%
Toffee Crunch	½ cup	< 1	130	3%
Vanilla	½ cup	< 1	120	4%
Sugar Freedom Eskimo Pie				
Bars				
Vanilla w/Chocolate-Flavored Coating	1 bar	11	140	71%
Vanilla w/Chocolate-Flavored Coating & Crisped Rice	1 bar	11	150	66%
Cones				
Caramel	1 cone	16	260	55%
w/Chocolate Coating & Peanuts	1 cone	12	230	47%
Fudge Ripple	4 oz	6	130	42%
Sandwich	1	6	170	32%
Fat Freedom	1	–	130	–
Vanilla	4 oz	7	130	37%
(Slimmery) Skinny Dip Bars	1 Bar	7	110	57%
(Sweet'N Low)				
Butter Pecan	4 oz	6	120	45%
Chocolate	4 oz	2	90	20%
Strawberry	4 oz	1	80	11%
Vanilla	4 oz	2	80	23%
(Thrifty) Light Frozen Dairy Dessert				
Chocolate Chocolate Chip	4 oz	6	130	42%
Swiss Mocha	4 oz	5	120	38%
Vanilla	4 oz	5	120	38%
Wild Berry	4 oz	4	110	33%
(Weight Watchers)				
Chocolate Mousse				
Sugar Free	1 bar	.8	35	21%
Double Fudge	1 bar	1	60	15%
Fat Free				
Chocolate	½ cup	–	80	–
Chocolate Swirl	½ cup	–	90	–

Food and Description	Amount	Fat Grams	Total Calories	% Fat Calories
Chocolate Treat	1 bar	–	90	–
Neopolitan	½ cup	–	80	–
Orange-Vanilla Treat	1 bar	–	30	–
Vanilla	½ cup	–	80	–

FROZEN ENTREE/DINNER (*See also* CHICKEN ENTREE/DINNER; MEXICAN FOOD; MICROWAVEABLE NONFROZEN MEALS; POTATO DISHES; VEGETARIAN FOOD)

(Armour) Dinners

Classics

Chicken & Noodles	11 oz	7	230	27%
Chicken Fettucini	11 oz	9	260	31%
Chicken Mesquite	9.5 oz	16	370	39%
Chicken Parmigiana	11.5 oz	19	370	46%
Chicken w/wine & mushroom sauce	10.75 oz	11	280	35%
Glazed Chicken	10.75 oz	16	300	48%
Meat Loaf	11.25 oz	17	360	43%
Salisbury Parmigiana	11.5 oz	21	410	46%
Salisbury Steak	11.25 oz	17	350	44%
Swedish Meatballs	11.25 oz	18	330	49%
Turkey & Dressing & Gravy	11.5 oz	12	320	34%
Veal Parmigiana	11.25 oz	22	400	50%

Classics-Lite

Beef Pepper Steak	11.25 oz	6	250	22%
Beef Stroganoff	11.25 oz	6	250	22%
Chicken Ala King	11.25 oz	7	290	22%
Chicken Burgundy	10 oz	2	210	9%
Chicken Marsala	10.5 oz	7	250	22%
Chicken Oriental	10 oz	1	180	5%
Salisbury Steak	11.5 oz	11	300	33%
Shrimp Creole	11.25 oz	2	260	7%
Sweet & Sour Chicken	11 oz	2	240	8%

(Banquet)

Casseroles & Pot Pies

Macaroni & Cheese	6.5 oz	14	290	43%
Vegetable Pie w/Beef	7 oz	33	510	58%
Vegetable Pie w/Chicken	7 oz	36	550	59%
Vegetable Pie w/Turkey	7 oz	31	510	55%

Cookin' Bags

Chicken & Vegetables Primavera	4 oz	2	100	18%
Chicken Ala King	4 oz	5	110	41%
Creamed Chipped Beef	4 oz	4	100	36%
Gravy & Salisbury Steak	5 oz	14	190	66%

Food and Description	Amount	Fat Grams	Total Calories	% Fat Calories
Gravy & Sliced Beef	4 oz	5	100	45%
Gravy & Sliced Turkey	5 oz	6	100	54%
Turkey Chili	4 oz	2	80	23%
Entree Express				
Beef Patties & Mushroom Gravy	7 oz	26	350	67%
Chicken Noodles	8.5 oz	10	240	38%
Gravy & Turkey w/Dressing	7 oz	8	220	33%
Meatloaf w/Tomato Sauce	7 oz	22	330	60%
Salisbury Steak & Gravy	7 oz	21	300	63%
Spaghetti w/Meat Sauce	8.5 oz	4	220	16%
Extra Helping Dinners				
Beef	15.5 oz	13	430	27%
Chicken Nuggets				
w/BBQ sauce	10 oz	19	540	32%
w/sweet & sour sauce	10 oz	19	540	32%
Fried Chicken	14.25 oz	43	790	49%
All White Meat	14.25 oz	38	760	45%
Meat Loaf	16.25 oz	34	640	48%
Mexican Style	19 oz	25	680	33%
Salisbury Steak	16.25 oz	28	590	43%
Southern Fried Chicken	13.25 oz	39	790	44%
Turkey	17 oz	12	460	23%
Family Entrees				
Beef Stew	7 oz	5	140	32%
Chicken & Dumplings	7 oz	14	280	45%
Chicken & Vegetables				
Primavera	7 oz	3	140	19%
Gravy & Salisbury Steak	7 oz	19	260	66%
Gravy & Sliced Beef	7 oz	5	140	32%
Gravy & Sliced Turkey	6 oz	6	120	45%
Lasagna w/meat sauce	7 oz	10	270	33%
Macaroni & Cheese	7 oz	11	260	38%
Mostaccioli & Meat Sauce	7 oz	3	170	16%
Mushroom Gravy & Charbroiled				
Beef Patties	7 oz	10	260	62%
Noodles & Beef w/gravy	7 oz	6	180	30%
Onion Gravy & Beef Patties	7 oz	19	260	66%
Stroganoff Sauce w/Beef				
& Noodles	7 oz	6	190	28%
Veal Parmagian Patties	7 oz	16	320	45%
Family Favorites Dinners				
Chicken & Dumplings	10 oz	24	420	51%
Macaroni & Cheese	10 oz	20	415	43%
Noodles & Chicken	10 oz	15	340	40%

Food and Description	Amount	Fat Grams	Total Calories	% Fat Calories
Spaghetti & Meatballs	10 oz	9	290	28%
Healthy Balance				
Baked Boneless Chicken				
Breast Nuggets	2.25 oz	4	120	30%
Breast Patties	2.25 oz	4	120	30%
Breast Tenders	2.25 oz	4	120	30%
Chicken Enchilada	11 oz	4	300	12%
Chicken Mesquite	10.5 oz	9	310	26%
Chicken Parmesan	10.8 oz	9	300	27%
Homestyle Barbecue	10.25 oz	5	270	17%
Meat Loaf	11 oz	7	270	23%
Salisbury Steak	10.5 oz	8	260	24%
Sweet & Sour Chicken	10.25 oz	4	270	13%
Turkey & Gravy w/Dressing	11.25 oz	5	270	20%
Meals & Platters				
Beans & Frankfurters	10 oz	14	350	36%
Beef & Bean Burrito	9.5 oz	12	390	28%
Beef Enchilada	11 oz	12	370	29%
Beef Platter	9 oz	6	230	23%
Beef Tamale	11 oz	18	420	39%
Boneless Chicken				
Drumsnacker Platter	7 oz	12	290	37%
Nugget Platter	6 oz	16	340	42%
Pattie Platter	6.75 oz	15	310	44%
Cheese Enchilada	11 oz	9	340	24%
Chicken & Dumplings	10 oz	10	270	33%
Chicken Enchilada	11 oz	9	340	24%
Chimichanga	9.5 oz	21	480	39%
Fish Platter	8 oz	7	270	23%
Fried Chicken	9 oz	29	520	50%
Gravy & Beef Pattie	9 oz	14	250	50%
Ham Platter	8.25 oz	5	200	23%
Italian Style	9 oz	2	180	10%
Macaroni & Cheese	9 oz	8	240	30%
Meat Loaf	9.5 oz	19	340	50%
Mexican Style	11 oz	17	410	37%
Mexican Style Combination	11 oz	12	360	30%
Noodles & Chicken	10 oz	4	170	21%
Salisbury Steak	9 oz	13	280	42%
Spaghetti & Meat Sauce	8.75 oz	4	160	23%
Southern Fried Chicken	8.75 oz	16	400	36%
Turkey & Gravy w/Dressing	9.25 oz	8	260	28%
Veal Parmigiana	9.25 oz	16	330	44%
Western Style	9 oz	16	300	48%

Food and Description	Amount	Fat Grams	Total Calories	% Fat Calories
White Meat Fried Chicken	8.75 oz	13	390	30%
White Meat Hot'n Spicy Fried Chicken	9 oz	15	440	31%
(Budget Gourmet)				
Light & Healthy Dinners				
Chicken Breast Parmigiana	11 oz	8	260	28%
Herbed Chicken Breast w/Fettucine	11 oz	7	240	26%
Italian Style Meat Loaf	11 oz	10	270	33%
Sirloin Salisbury Steak	11 oz	9	260	31%
Special Recipe Sirloin Beef	11 oz	10	250	36%
Stuffed Turkey Breast	11 oz	6	230	23%
Teriyaki Beef	10.75 oz	6	270	20%
Teriyaki Chicken Breast	11 oz	6	270	20%
Light Entrees				
Beef Stroganoff	8.75 oz	12	290	37%
Cheese Ravioli	9.5 oz	10	290	31%
Chicken Au Gratin	9.1 oz	11	250	40%
Chicken Enchilada Suiza	8.75 oz	12	290	37%
French Recipe Chicken & Vegetables	10 oz	9	240	38%
Glazed Turkey	9 oz	5	270	17%
Lasagna w/meat sauce	9.4 oz	13	300	39%
Mandarin Chicken	10 oz	7	300	21%
Oriental Beef	10 oz	9	290	28%
Sirloin Beef in Herb Sauce	9.5 oz	10	270	33%
Sirloin Salisbury Steak	8.5 oz	13	260	45%
Light & Healthy Dinners				
Beef Pot Roast	10.5 oz	8	210	34%
Chicken Breast Parmigiana	11 oz	8	260	28%
Herbed Chicken	11 oz	7	240	26%
Italian Style Meatloaf	11 oz	10	270	30%
Sirloin Salisbury Steak	11 oz	9	260	31%
Clipped Sirloin in Wine	11 oz	8	270	26%
Special Recipe Sirloin Beef	11 oz	10	250	36%
Stuffed Turkey Breast	11 oz	6	230	23%
Teriyaki Chicken Breast	11 oz	6	270	13%
Regular Entrees				
Cheese Manicotti w/meat Sauce	10 oz	25	450	50%
Chicken & Egg Noodles w/broccoli	10 oz	26	450	52%
Chicken Marsala	10 oz	5	500	9%
Chicken w/Fettucini	10 oz	21	400	47%
Italian Sausage Lasagna	10 oz	20	420	43%
Italian Style Meatballs w/noodles & peppers	10 oz	12	310	35%

Food and Description	Amount	Fat Grams	Total Calories	% Fat Calories
Linguini w/shrimp	10 oz	15	330	41%
Pasta Shells & Beef	10 oz	14	340	37%
Pepper Steak w/rice	10 oz	9	300	27%
Roast Sirloin	9.5 oz	14	560	23%
Seafood Newberg	10 oz	12	350	31%
Shrimp Fettucini	9.5 oz	20	630	29%
Sirloin Tips w/countrystyle vegetables	10 oz	18	310	52%
Spaghetti w/Italian sausage	10 oz	19	400	43%
Swedish Meatballs w/Noodles	10 oz	39	600	59%
Sweet & Sour Chicken w/rice	10 oz	7	350	18%
Three Cheese Lasagna	10 oz	17	400	38%
Turkey A La King w/rice	10 oz	18	390	42%
Side Dishes				
Cauliflower in cheddar cheese sauce	5 oz	5	110	41%
Cheddared Potatoes	5.5 oz	13	230	51%
Cheddared Potatoes & Broccoli	5 oz	4	130	28%
Cheese Tortellini	5.5 oz	6	180	30%
Country Style Corn	5.75 oz	5	140	32%
Glazed Apples in Raspberry Sauce	5 oz	3	110	25%
Macaroni & Cheese	5.3 oz	8	210	34%
Nacho Potatoes	5 oz	10	180	50%
New England Recipe Vegetables	5.5 oz	10	210	43%
New Potatoes in Sour Cream Sauce	5 oz	6	120	45%
Oriental Rice & Vegetables	5.75 oz	10	210	43%
Pasta Alfredo w/broccoli	5.5 oz	8	200	36%
Peas & Cauliflower in Cream Sauce	5.75 oz	7	170	37%
Peas & Water Chestnuts Oriental	5 oz	3	120	23%
Rice Pilaf w/green beans	5.5 oz	9	240	34%
Spinach Au Gratin	6 oz	5	120	38%
Spring Vegetables in cheese sauce	5 oz	3	90	30%
Sweet Corn in butter sauce	5.5 oz	6	190	28%
Three Cheese Potatoes	5.75 oz	11	230	43%
Ziti in Marinara Sauce	6.25 oz	9	220	37%
Slim Selects				
Beef Stroganoff	8.75 oz	12	290	37%
Cheese Ravioli	10 oz	10	290	31%
Chicken Au Gratin	9.1 oz	11	250	40%
Chicken Enchilada Suiza	8.8 oz	12	290	37%
Fettucini w/meat sauce	10 oz	10	290	31%
French Recipe Chicken	10 oz	10	260	35%
Glazed Turkey	9 oz	5	270	17%
Ham & Asparagus Au Gratin	9 oz	12	290	37%
Lasagna w/meat sauce	10 oz	10	290	31%
Linguini w/scallops & clams	9.5 oz	11	290	34%

Food and Description	Amount	Fat Grams	Total Calories	% Fat Calories
Mandarin Chicken	10 oz	6	300	18%
Oriental Beef	10 oz	9	290	28%
Sirloin of Beef in herb sauce	9.5 oz	10	270	33%
Sirloin Enchilada Ranchero	8.75 oz	9	270	30%
Sirloin Salisbury Steak	9 oz	13	260	45%
Three Dish Dinners				
Beef Mexicana	12.8 oz	15	510	27%
Chicken Cacciatore	11 oz	13	300	39%
Chicken Mexicana	12.8 oz	15	510	27%
Roast Chicken	11.2 oz	7	280	23%
Scallops & Shrimp Mariner	11.5 oz	9	320	25%
Sirloin Salisbury Steak	11.5 oz	22	410	48%
Sirloin Tips in burgundy sauce	11 oz	11	310	32%
Sliced Turkey Breast	11.1 oz	9	290	28%
Swiss Steak	11.2 oz	22	450	44%
Teriyaki Chicken	12 oz	12	360	30%
Turkey Breast Dijon	11.2 oz	12	340	32%
Veal Parmigiana	12 oz	20	440	41%
Yankee Pot Roast	11 oz	21	380	50%
(Campbell's)				
Food Service-Meat Lasagna	8 oz	15	360	38%
(Celentano) Entrees				
Baked Pasta & Cheese	6 oz	7	280	23%
Broccoli Stuffed Shells	6.75 oz	14	270	47%
Cannelloni Florentine	12 oz	8	350	21%
Cavatelli	3.2 oz	1	250	4%
Chicken Parmigiana	9 oz	21	400	47%
Chicken Primavera	11.5 oz	7	260	24%
Eggplant Parmigiana				
(10 oz)	10 oz	19	350	49%
(16 oz)	8 oz	15	280	48%
(25 oz)	6.25 oz	10	260	35%
Eggplant Rollettes	11 oz	14	320	39%
Lasagna				
(10 oz)	10 oz	24	460	47%
(16 oz)	8 oz	19	370	46%
(25 oz)	6.25 oz	16	300	48%
Lasagna Primavera	11 oz	14	330	38%
Manicotti				
(10 oz)	10 oz	14	380	37%
(14 oz)	7 oz	16	360	40%
(16 oz)	8 oz	11	300	33%
Pizza				
9-Slice	2.7 oz	4	150	24%

Food and Description	Amount	Fat Grams	Total Calories	% Fat Calories
Thick Crust	4.3 oz	11	290	34%
Ravioli	6.5 oz	11	380	26%
Ravioli-Mini	4 oz	5	250	18%
Stuffed Shells				
(10 oz)	10 oz	14	410	31%
(12.5 oz)	6.25 oz	16	340	42%
(16 oz)	8 oz	11	330	30%
(Dining Light)				
Cheese Cannelloni	9 oz	9	310	26%
Cheese Lasagna	9 oz	6	260	21%
Chicken Ala King	9 oz	7	250	26%
Chicken Chow Mein	9 oz	2	180	10%
Chicken w/Noodles	9 oz	7	240	23%
Fettucini	9 oz	12	290	37%
Lasagna	9 oz	5	240	23%
Salisbury Steak	9 oz	8	200	36%
Sauce & Swedish Meatballs	9 oz	10	280	32%
Spaghetti	9 oz	8	220	33%
(Freezer Queen) Frozen Family Supper				
Gravy & 6 Salisbury Steaks	7 oz	13	200	59%
Gravy & Sliced Turkey	7 oz	5	110	41%
Mushroom Gravy & 6				
Charbroiled Beef Patties	7 oz	11	180	55%
Onion Gravy & Beef Patties	7 oz	12	200	54%
Onion Gravy & Salisbury Steak	8 oz	16	240	60%
Salisbury Steak	7 oz	13	200	59%
Tomato Sauce & Meatloaf	7 oz	13	230	51%
(Golden) Entrees				
Apple-Raisin Blintz	2	3	160	17%
Blueberry Blintz	2	2	180	10%
Cheese Blintz	2	2	160	11%
Cherry Blintz	2	3	190	14%
Potato Blintz	2	9	210	39%
Potato Cheese Pierogie	3	8	250	29%
Potato Onion Pierogie	3	6	210	17%
Potato Pancakes				
Mexican	1	2	70	26%
Regular	1	3	80	34%
(Growing Healthy Baby Food) (See BABY FOOD)				
(Healthy Choice)				
Dinners				
Beef Enchilada	13.4 oz	5	370	12%
Beef Pepper Steak	11 oz	6	290	19%
Beef Sirloin Tips	11.25 oz	7	270	23%

Food and Description	Amount	Fat Grams	Total Calories	% Fat Calories
Breast of Turkey	10.5 oz	5	290	16%
Chicken & Pasta Divan	11.5 oz	4	310	12%
Chicken Dijon	11 oz	3	260	10%
Chicken Enchilada	13.4 oz	5	340	13%
Chicken Oriental	11.25 oz	1	230	4%
Chicken Parmigiana	11.5 oz	3	270	10%
Chicken w/Barbecue Sauce	12.75 oz	6	410	13%
Herb Roasted Chicken	12.3 oz	4	290	12%
Lemon Pepper Fish	10.7 oz	5	300	15%
Meatloaf	12 oz	8	340	21%
Mesquite Chicken	10.5 oz	1	340	3%
Pasta Primavera	11 oz	3	280	10%
Salisbury Steak	11.5 oz	7	300	21%
Salsa Chicken	11.25 oz	2	240	8%
Shrimp Creole	11.25 oz	2	230	8%
Shrimp Marinara	10.5 oz	1	260	3%
Sirloin Beef w/Barbecue Sauce	11 oz	6	300	18%
Sirloin Tips	11.75 oz	6	290	19%
Sole Au Gratin	11 oz	5	270	17%
Southwestern Style Chicken	12.5 oz	5	340	13%
Sweet & Sour Chicken	11.5 oz	2	280	6%
Teriyaki Chicken	12.25 oz	4	290	12%
Turkey Tetrazzini	12.6 oz	6	340	16%
Yankee Pot Roast	11 oz	4	260	14%
Entrees				
Baked Cheese Ravioli	9 oz	2	250	7%
Beef Fajitas	7 oz	4	210	17%
Beef Pepper Steak	9.5 oz	4	250	14%
Broccoli & Cheese Sauce w/Baked Potato Wedges	9.5 oz	5	240	23%
Cheese Manicotti	9.25 oz	3	220	12%
Chicken A L 'Orange	9 oz	2	240	8%
Chicken & Vegetables	11.5 oz	1	210	4%
Chicken Chow Mein	8.5 oz	3	220	12%
Chicken Enchiladas	9.5 oz	9	310	20%
Chicken Fajitas	7 oz	3	200	14%
Chicken Fettucini	8.5 oz	4	240	15%
Fettucini Alfredo	8 oz	7	240	26%
Glazed Chicken	8.5 oz	3	220	12%
Lasagna w/meat sauce	10 oz	5	260	17%
Linguini w/Shrimp	9.5 oz	2	230	8%
Macaroni & Cheese	9 oz	6	280	19%
(17 oz)	8.5 oz	5	260	21%
Mandarin Chicken	11 oz	2	260	7%

Food and Description	Amount	Fat Grams	Total Calories	% Fat Calories
Rigatoni in Meat Sauce	9.5 oz	6	260	21%
Roasted Turkey & Mushroom Gravy	8.5 oz	3	200	14%
Seafood Newburg	8 oz	3	200	14%
Sole w/Lemon Butter Sauce	8.25 oz	4	230	16%
Spaghetti w/meat sauce	10 oz	6	280	19%
Zucchini Lasagna	11.5 oz	3	250	11%
Homestyle and Pasta Classics				
Barbecue Beef Ribs	11 oz	6	330	16%
Cacciatore Chicken	12.5 oz	3	310	9%
Pasta w/Shrimp	12.5 oz	4	270	13%
Rigatoni w/Chicken	12.5 oz	4	360	10%
Salisbury Steak w/Mushroom Gravy	11 oz	6	280	19%
Sliced Turkey w/Gravy & Dressing	10 oz	4	270	13%
Stuffed Pasta Shells in Tomato Sauce	12 oz	3	330	8%
Teriyaki Pasta w/Chicken	12.6 oz	3	350	8%
Turkey Breast Madallions & Vegetables	12.5 oz	6	350	15%
Zesty Tomato Sauce Over Ziti Pasta	12 oz	5	350	13%
(Hormel's)				
Frozen				
Mrs. Paterson's Aussie Pie				
Chicken	5.5 oz	24	440	49%
Steak & Mushroom	5.5 oz	20	410	44%
Supreme Pizza	5.5 oz	27	470	52%
Turkey & Broccoli	5.5 oz	26	460	51%
New Traditions				
Frozen Microwaveable Sandwiches (*See also* BREAKFAST SANDWICH)				
Bacon Cheeseburger	5 oz	24	440	49%
BBQ Beef	4.3 oz	17	370	41%
BBQ Pork	4.3 oz	14	350	36%
Cheeseburger	4.8 oz	20	400	45%
Chicken	4.3 oz	11	320	31%
Chili Dog w/Cheese				
Hot	4.5 oz	20	340	53%
Regular	4.5 oz	20	340	53%
Fish Fillet	5.2 oz	16	430	33%
Hamburger	4.8 oz	20	400	45%
(Kibun Gold)				
Entrees				
Chicken Oriental	8 oz	3	230	12%

Food and Description	Amount	Fat Grams	Total Calories	% Fat Calories
Ellen's Homestyle Chicken	10 oz	4	300	12%
Honey Garlic Chicken	10 oz	4	290	12%
Lemon Ginger Beef	8 oz	4	230	16%
Pasta & Chicken				
w/dressing	½ package	9	220	37%
w/o dressing	½ package	2	150	12%
Pasta & Turkey Ham				
w/dressing	½ package	12	250	43%
w/o dressing	½ package	2	140	13%
Sweet & Sour Chicken	10 oz	1	310	3%
(Kid's Cuisine)				
Entrees				
Cheese Beef Patty Sandwich	6.25 oz	22	430	46%
Cheese Pizza	6.85 oz	12	380	28%
Chunky Chicken Supreme	10 oz	23	430	48%
Fish Nuggets	7 oz	15	320	42%
Fried Chicken	7.5 oz	23	425	49%
Macaroni & Cheese				
w/mini franks	9 oz	15	360	38%
Mini Cheese Ravioli	8.75 oz	8	290	25%
Spaghetti w/meat sauce	9.25 oz	8	310	23%
Mega Meal				
Cheese Pizza	9.7 oz	7	430	15%
Chicken Nuggets	8.4 oz	20	470	38%
Double Beef Patty Sandwich				
w/Cheese	9.1 oz	20	480	38%
Fried Chicken	20.8 oz	41	720	51%
Hot Dog w/Bun	8.25 oz	25	500	45%
Macaroni & Cheese	12.45 oz	13	470	25%
(Kraft)				
Entrees				
Barbecue Beef w/corn	9 oz	12	340	32%
Beef Stew	10 oz	12	250	43%
Cheese Enchilada	9.8 oz	20	390	46%
Chicken A La King	10 oz	14	350	36%
Chicken & Egg Noodles	10 oz	20	420	43%
Chili w/Beef & Beans	9.7 oz	22	380	52%
Creamed Chipped Beef	9 oz	27	380	64%
Fettucini Alfredo	10 oz	30	465	58%
Lasagna w/meat sauce	10 oz	16	390	37%
Macaroni & Beef	11.5 oz	16	370	39%
Macaroni & Cheese	12 oz	30	610	44%
Ravioli	10 oz	11	320	31%
Salisbury Steak & Fries	9 oz	20	360	50%

Food and Description	Amount	Fat Grams	Total Calories	% Fat Calories
Sirloin Chili w/Steak Fries	9 oz	23	390	53%
Spaghetti & Meatballs	9.7 oz	15	340	40%
Tuna Noodle Casserole	10.2 oz	20	370	47%
Turkey & Dressing	9 oz	10	300	30%
Microwave				
Beef Stew	10 oz	4	230	16%
Beef Stroganoff	9 oz	13	330	35%
Cheese Tortellini	10 oz	8	320	23%
Chicken Cacciatore	10 oz	6	260	21%
Chicken Fettuccine	9 oz	12	270	40%
Lasagna	10.2 oz	14	370	34%
Salisbury Steak	9 oz	13	300	39%
Spaghetti & Meatballs	10 oz	12	360	25%
Sweet & Sour Chicken	9 oz	1	290	3%
(Le Menu)				
Dinners				
Beef Sirloin Tips	11.5 oz	18	400	41%
Beef Stroganoff	10 oz	24	430	50%
Chicken A La King	10.25 oz	13	330	35%
Chicken Cordon Bleu	11 oz	20	460	39%
Chicken in Wine Sauce	10 oz	7	280	23%
Chicken Parmigiana	11.25 oz	20	410	44%
Chopped Sirloin Beef	12.25 oz	24	430	50%
Ham Steak	10 oz	11	300	33%
Manicotti w/Three Cheeses	11.75 oz	15	390	35%
Pepper Steak	11.5 oz	13	370	32%
Salisbury Steak	10.5 oz	20	370	49%
Sliced Breast of Turkey w/Mushroom Gravy	10.5 oz	7	300	21%
Sweet & Sour Chicken	11.25 oz	18	400	41%
Veal Parmigiana	11.5 oz	17	390	39%
Yankee Pot Roast	10 oz	13	330	35%
Healthy Dinners (Light Style)				
Cheese Tortellini	10 oz	6	230	23%
Glazed Chicken Breast	10 oz	3	230	12%
Herb Roasted Chicken	9.25 oz	7	240	26%
Salisbury Steak	10 oz	9	280	29%
Sliced Turkey	10 oz	5	210	21%
3-Cheese Stuffed Shells	10 oz	8	280	26%
Turkey Divan	10 oz	7	260	24%
Veal Marsala	10 oz	3	230	12%
Healthy Entrees (Light Style)				
Chicken Dijon	8 oz	7	240	26%
Chicken Enchiladas	8 oz	8	280	26%

Food and Description	Amount	Fat Grams	Total Calories	% Fat Calories
Chicken A La King	8.25 oz	5	240	19%
Empress Chicken	8 oz	5	210	21%
Garden Vegetables Lasagna	10.5 oz	8	260	28%
Glazed Turkey	8.25 oz	6	260	21%
Herb Roasted Chicken	7.75 oz	6	260	14%
Lasagna w/meat sauce	10 oz	8	290	25%
Meat Sauce & Cheese Tortellini	8 oz	8	250	29%
Spaghetti w/Beef Sauce & Mushrooms	9 oz	6	280	19%
Swedish Meatballs	8 oz	8	260	28%
Traditional Turkey	8 oz	5	200	23%
Lean Cuisine (Stouffer's)				
Baked Cheese Ravioli w/Tomato Sauce	8.5 oz	8	240	30%
Beef & Bean Enchanadas	9¼ oz	6	240	23%
Beef Cannelloni w/Tomato Sauce	9⅝ oz	4	210	17%
Breaded Breast of Chicken (w/Ribmeat) Parmesan	10⅞ oz	9	270	30%
Breast of Chicken Marsala	8⅛ oz	5	190	24%
Broccoli & Cheddar Baked Potato	10⅜ oz	9	290	28%
Cheese Cannelloni w/Tomato Sauce	9⅛ oz	8	270	27%
Chicken a l'Orange w/Almond Rice	8 oz	4	280	13%
Chicken & Vegetables w/Vermicelli	11¾ oz	6	250	22%
Chicken Cacciatore	10⅞ oz	7	280	23%
Chicken Chow Mein w/Rice	9 oz	5	240	19%
Chicken Enchanadas	9⅞ oz	9	290	28%
Chicken in Barbecue Sauce	8¾ oz	6	260	21%
Chicken Fettucini	9 oz	8	280	26%
Chicken Italiano w/Fettuccini	9 oz	8	290	25%
Chicken Oriental w/Vegetables	9 oz	7	280	23%
Chicken Tenderloins in Herb Cream Sauce	9.5 oz	5	240	19%
Chicken Tenderloins in Peanut Sauce	9 oz	7	290	22%
Fiesta Chicken	8.5 oz	5	240	19%
Filet of Fish Divan	10⅜ oz	5	210	21%
Filet of Fish Florentine	9⅝ oz	7	220	29%
Glazed Chicken w/Vegetable Rice	8.5 oz	8	260	28%
Homestyle Turkey w/Vegetables & Pasta	9⅜ oz	5	230	20%
Lasagna w/Meat Sauce	10¼ oz	6	260	21%
Linguini w/Clam Sauce	9⅝ oz	8	280	26%
Macaroni & Beef in Tomato Sauce	10 oz	6	240	23%
Macaroni & Cheese	9 oz	9	290	28%

Food and Description	Amount	Fat Grams	Total Calories	% Fat Calories
Oriental Beef w/Vegetables	8⅝ oz	9	290	28%
Rigatoni Bake w/Meat Sauce	9¾ oz	8	250	26%
Salisbury Steak w/Gravy & Scalloped Potatoes	9.5 oz	7	240	26%
Sliced Turkey Breast in Mushroom Sauce w/Rice Pilaf	8 oz	6	220	25%
Sliced Turkey Breast w/Dressing	7⅛ oz	5	200	23%
Spaghetti & Meat Sauce	11.5 oz	6	290	19%
Spaghetti w/Meatballs & Sauce	9.5 oz	7	280	23%
Stuffed Cabbage w/Meat in Tomato Sauce	10¾ oz	6	210	26%
Swedish Meatballs in Gravy w/Pasta	9⅛ oz	8	290	25%
Tuna Lasagna w/Spinach Noodles & Vegetables	9¾ oz	7	240	26%
Turkey Dijon	9.5 oz	5	230	20%
Zucchini Lasagna	11 oz	5	260	17%
Lean Pockets (Chef America)				
Beef & Broccoli	1 pocket	8	250	29%
Chicken Parmesan	1 pocket	6	250	22%
Chicken Supreme	1 pocket	4	210	17%
Pizza Deluxe	1 pocket	10	280	32%
Looney Tunes (See Tyson)				
(Morton)				
Casserole and Pot Pies				
Macaroni & Cheese	6.5 oz	14	290	43%
Vegetable Pie w/Beef	7 oz	31	430	65%
Vegetable Pie w/Chicken	7 oz	28	420	60%
Vegetable Pie w/Turkey	7 oz	28	420	60%
Entrees				
Beans & Franks w/Sauce	8.5 oz	11	300	33%
Chili Gravy w/Beef Enchilada & Tamale	10 oz	10	300	30%
Fish w/Mashed Potatoes & Carrots	9.25 oz	12	350	31%
Glazed Ham	8 oz	3	230	12%
Gravy & Charboiled Beef Patty	9 oz	12	270	40%
Gravy & Salisbury Steak	9 oz	16	270	53%
Spaghetti & Meat Sauce	8.5 oz	2	170	11%
Tomato Sauce & Meatloaf	9 oz	16	280	51%
Veal Parmigiana	8.75 oz	7	230	27%
(Pitaria) Pita Stuffs				
Gyros	6 oz	29	520	50%
Ham'N Swiss	6 oz	17	420	36%

Food and Description	Amount	Fat Grams	Total Calories	% Fat Calories
Pizza	6 oz	18	430	38%
Taco	6 oz	16	390	37%
(Prego)				
Beef Marsala w/noodles	11.3 oz	15	384	35%
(Quaker) Ovenstuffs				
Beef/Cheddar Deli Melt	1	22	390	51%
Chicken Turnover	1	16	350	41%
Ham/Turkey Deli Melt	1	15	360	38%
Italian Sausage French Roll	1	22	390	51%
Pepperoni French Roll	1	20	370	49%
Turkey Turnover	1	16	350	41%
(Schwan's) Frozen				
BBQ Beef	3.5 oz	8	180	40%
BBQ Beef Brisket				
Chopped	3.5 oz	12	210	51%
Sliced	3.5 oz	5	150	30%
BBQ Ribs	3.5 oz	15	260	52%
Ball Tip Steaks	6 oz	10	240	38%
Beef Patties	4 oz	24	300	72%
Beef Patty Melt	4 oz	28	330	76%
Big Sam Steaks	6 oz	18	300	54%
Breaded Beef Steak Fingers	3.5 oz	7	220	29%
Chopped Beef Steak	5.33 oz	31	390	72%
Cross Cut Tenderloin Steak	6 oz	41	500	74%
Floured Cubed Beef Steak	4 oz	20	290	62%
Haugin's Pride Dinner Steaks	7 oz	45	560	72%
Pizza Patties	3.5 oz	22	270	73%
Ribeye Steak	8 oz	64	730	79%
Sirloin Fillet of Beef Steak	4 oz	12	200	54%
Strip Steak				
Lean & fat	10 oz	65	790	74%
Lean only	10 oz	20	430	42%
(Schwan's) Frozen Entrees & Sandwiches				
Bagel Dogs	4.5 oz	21	410	46%
Beef Casserole	3.5 oz	9	160	51%
Beef Lasagna	3.5 oz	6	150	34%
Beef Teriyaki	11 oz	14	430	29%
Beef Tortellini	3.5 oz	8	270	27%
Cheese Tortellini	3.5 oz	5	220	21%
Chicken a la Orange	9.5 oz	8	300	24%
Chicken Casserole	3.5 oz	8	150	48%
Chicken Oriental	10.25 oz	7	270	23%
Club Croissant Sandwich	1	22	400	50%
Grandma's Chicken Casserole	3.5 oz	9	160	51%

Food and Description	Amount	Fat Grams	Total Calories	% Fat Calories
Jumbo Beef Ravioli	3.5 oz	4	180	20%
Macaroni & Cheese	3.5 oz	10	160	56%
Ranchero Sandwich	1	19	450	38%
Roast Beef & Swiss Croissant	1	20	370	49%
Round Cheese Ravioli	3.5 oz	8	200	36%
Shrimp Oriental	10 oz	3	190	14%
Sweet & Sour Chicken-bag	11 oz	15	530	26%
Sweet & Sour Chicken-plate	11 oz	15	420	32%
Vegetable Lasagna (Shanghai)	3.5 oz	3	130	21%
Stir Fry Shrimp & Oriental Vegetables	10.3 oz	2	140	13%
(Simplot) Micro Magic Sandwiches				
Bacon Cheeseburger	1	20	396	45%
Cheeseburger	1	25	450	50%
Chicken	1	16	390	37%
Hamburger	1	18	350	46%
(Stouffer's)				
Entrees				
Beef Pie	10 oz	32	500	58%
Beef Stroganoff w/Parsley Noodles	9.75 oz	20	390	46%
Cashew Chicken in Sauce w/rice	9.5 oz	16	380	38%
Cheese Enchiladas	10⅛ oz	40	590	61%
Chicken a la King w/rice	9.5 oz	9	290	28%
Chicken Chow Mein w/o noodles	8 oz	4	130	28%
Chicken Divan	8.5 oz	20	320	56%
Chicken Enchiladas	10 oz	29	490	53%
Chicken Pie	10 oz	33	530	56%
Creamed Chicken	6.5 oz	21	300	63%
Creamed Chipped Beef	5.5 oz	16	230	63%
Escalloped Chicken & Noodles	10 oz	25	420	54%
Green Pepper Steak w/rice	10.5 oz	11	330	30%
Ham & Asparagus Bake	9.5 oz	35	510	62%
Homestyle Chicken & Noodles	10 oz	13	290	40%
Lasagna				
21 oz	10.5 oz	13	360	33%
96 oz	9.6 oz	15	370	36%
Lasagna, Single Serving	10.5 oz	13	360	33%
Macaroni & Beef w/tomatoes				
11.5 oz	5.75 oz	6	170	32%
76 oz	9.5 oz	11	280	35%
Macaroni & Cheese				
12 oz	6 oz	13	250	47%

Food and Description	Amount	Fat Grams	Total Calories	% Fat Calories
20 oz	5 oz	11	210	47%
76 oz	9.5 oz	23	440	47%
Pasta Shells, Cheese				
w/Tomato Sauce	9¼ oz	15	330	41%
Spaghetti w/meat sauce	12⅞ oz	11	370	27%
Spaghetti w/meatballs	12⅝ oz	15	380	36%
19.5 oz	9¾ oz	11	300	33%
Stuffed Green Peppers w/beef				
in tomato sauce-15.5 oz	7.75 oz	9	200	41%
Stuffed Pepper				
Single Serving	10 oz	11	230	43%
Swedish Meatballs in Gravy				
w/parsley noodles	11 oz	26	480	49%
Tortellini				
Cheese in Alfredo Sauce	8⅞ oz	40	600	60%
Cheese w/tomato sauce	9⅝ oz	16	360	40%
Tuna Noodle Casserole	10 oz	13	310	38%
Turkey Pie	10 oz	33	530	56%
Turkey Tetrazzini	10 oz	20	380	47%
Vegetable Lasagna	10.5 oz	24	420	51%
Welsh Rarebit-10 oz	5 oz	30	350	77%
Food Service				
Lasagna w/Meat & Sauce	8 oz	12	300	36%
Homestyle				
Baked Chicken Breast				
in Gravy w/Whipped				
Potatoes	8⅞ oz	9	230	35%
Beef & Noodles w/Gravy				
& Vegetable Medley	8⅜ oz	7	230	27%
Beef Pot Roast & Browned				
Potatoes	8⅞ oz	11	280	35%
Breaded Chicken Breast Tenders				
& O'Brien Potatoes	8⅜ oz	18	430	38%
Chicken & Noodles	10 oz	13	290	51%
Chicken Fettucini &				
Vegetable Medley	9.5 oz	17	350	44%
Chicken Parmigiana &				
Pasta Alfredo	9⅞ oz	15	360	38%
Fried Chicken Breast &				
Whipped Potatoes	7⅛ oz	18	350	46%
Grilled Chicken Breast				
in Barbecue Sauce	7⅝ oz	7	210	30%
Meatloaf in Gravy &				
Whipped Potatoes	9⅞ oz	20	360	50%

Food and Description	Amount	Fat Grams	Total Calories	% Fat Calories
Rigatoni w/Meat Sauce & Italian-Style Green Beans	9 oz	10	250	36%
Roast Turkey Breast w/Gravy & Homestyle Stuffing	7⅞ oz	13	300	39%
Salisbury Steak in Gravy & Macaroni & Cheese	9⅝ oz	17	350	44%
Spaghetti Parmesan w/Italian-Style Green Beans	10¼ oz	9	240	34%
Veal Parmigiana & Pasta Alfredo	9¼ oz	15	350	39%
Side Dishes				
Corn Souffle-12 oz	4 oz	7	160	39%
Creamed Spinach-9 oz	4.5 oz	14	170	74%
Escalloped Apples-12 oz	4 oz	2	130	14%
Fettucini Alfredo-10 oz	5 oz	19	270	63%
Green Bean Mushroom Casserole-9.5 oz	4.75 oz	11	160	62%
Noodles Romanoff-12 oz	4 oz	9	170	48%
Potatoes au Gratin-11.5 oz	~4 oz	6	110	49%
Scalloped Potatoes-11.5 oz	~4 oz	4	90	40%
Spinach Soufle-12 oz	4 oz	9	140	58%
(Swanson)				
Chicken				
Chicken Nibbles	3.25 oz	19	300	57%
Chicken Nuggets	3 oz	14	230	55%
Fried Chicken Breast	4.5 oz	20	360	50%
1 Lb Pre-Fried Chicken Parts	3.25 oz	16	270	53%
Thighs & Drumsticks	3.25 oz	18	290	56%
Dinners-3 Compartment				
Beans & Franks	10.5 oz	19	440	39%
Macaroni & Beef	12 oz	15	370	37%
Macaroni & Cheese	12.25 oz	15	380	36%
Noodles & Chicken	10.5 oz	8	280	26%
Spaghetti & Meatballs	12.5 oz	17	390	39%
Dinners-4 Compartment				
Beef	11.25 oz	6	310	17%
Beef Enchiladas	13.75 oz	21	480	39%
Beef in Barbecue Sauce	11 oz	17	460	33%
Chicken Nuggets	8.75 oz	23	470	44%
Chopped Sirloin Beef	10.75 oz	16	340	42%
Fish'n'Chips	10 oz	21	500	38%
Fried Chicken, BBQ flavored edible portion	10 oz	22	540	37%
Fried Chicken, White Meat edible portion	10.25 oz	25	550	41%

Food and Description	Amount	Fat Grams	Total Calories	% Fat Calories
Fried Chicken, Dark Meat				
edible portion	9.75 oz	28	560	45%
Loin of Pork	10.75 oz	12	280	39%
Meatloaf	10.75 oz	15	360	38%
Mexican Style Combination	14.25 oz	18	490	33%
Salisbury Steak	10.75 oz	17	400	38%
Swiss Steak	10 oz	11	350	28%
Turkey	11.5 oz	11	350	28%
Veal Parmigiana	12.25 oz	20	430	42%
Western Style	11.5 oz	19	430	40%
Homestyle Recipe Entrees				
Chicken Cacciatore	11 oz	8	260	28%
Chicken Nibbles edible portion	4.25 oz	20	340	53%
Chicken Pie	8 oz	21	410	46%
Chili Con Carne	8.25 oz	10	270	33%
Fish'n'Fries	6.5 oz	16	340	42%
Fried Chicken edible portion	7 oz	21	390	48%
Lasagna w/meat sauce	10.5 oz	15	400	34%
Macaroni & Cheese	10 oz	19	390	44%
Salisbury Steak	10 oz	16	320	45%
Scalloped Potatoes & Ham	9 oz	13	300	39%
Seafood Creole w/Rice	9 oz	6	240	23%
Sirloin Tips in Burgundy Sauce	7 oz	5	160	28%
Spaghetti w/Italian Style				
Meatballs	13 oz	18	490	33%
Swedish Meatballs	8.5 oz	20	360	52%
Turkey w/Dressing & Potatoes	9 oz	11	290	34%
Veal Parmigiana	10 oz	13	330	36%
Hungry Man Dinners				
Boneless Chicken	17.75 oz	28	700	36%
Chopped Beef Steak	16.75 oz	37	640	52%
Fried Chicken, White Meat				
edible portion	14.25 oz	46	870	48%
Fried Chicken-Dark Meat				
edible portion	14.25 oz	45	000	17%
Mexican	10.25 oz	41	820	45%
Pot Pies				
Beef	16 oz	31	610	46%
Chicken	16 oz	35	630	50%
Turkey	16 oz	36	650	50%
Salisbury Steak	18.25 oz	41	680	54%
Sliced Beef	15.25 oz	12	450	24%
Turkey	17 oz	18	550	30%
Veal Parmigiana	18.25 oz	26	590	40%

Food and Description	Amount	Fat Grams	Total Calories	% Fat Calories
Pot Pies				
Beef	7 oz	19	370	46%
Chicken	7 oz	22	380	52%
Macaroni & Cheese	7 oz	8	200	36%
Turkey	7 oz	21	380	50%
(Tyson) (*See also* CHICKEN ENTREE/DINNER)				
Healthy Portion Meals				
BBQ Chicken Meal	12.5 oz	8	470	15%
Chicken Marinara	13.75 oz	7	330	19%
Herb Chicken	13.75 oz	4	340	11%
Honey Mustard	13.75 oz	5	380	12%
Italian Style	13.75 oz	4	320	11%
Mesquite Chicken	13.25 oz	5	330	14%
Salsa Chicken Meal	13.75 oz	6	370	15%
Sesame Chicken	13.5 oz	5	390	12%
Looney Tunes				
Bugs Bunny Chicken Chunks	1 serving	11	290	34%
Daffy Duck Spaghetti & Meatballs	1 serving	10	340	26%
Elmer Fudd Turkey & Dressing	1 serving	7	260	24%
Foghorn Leghorn Pepperoni Pizza	1 serving	13	400	29%
Henry Hawk Hot Dog	1 serving	12	350	31%
Porky Pig Pattie Deluxe	1 serving	14	370	34%
Road Runner Chicken Sandwich	1 serving	11	300	33%
Sylvester Fish Sticks	1 serving	11	290	34%
Tasmanian Devil Chicken Drummettes	1 serving	14	310	41%
Tweety Macaroni & Cheese	1 serving	10	340	26%
Yosemite Sam BBQ Glazed Chicken	1 serving	8	230	31%
Wile E Coyote Hamburger Pizza	1 serving	11	310	32%
Premium Dinners				
Beef Champignon	10.5 oz	15	370	37%
Short Ribs	11 oz	24	470	46%
Resolutions				
Chicken Pasta Salad Kit Italian Style	1 serving	2	110	16%
Chicken Vegetable Salad Kit Russian Dressing	1 serving	3	110	25%
(Ultra Slim Fast)				
Beef Pepper Steak & Parsleyed Rice	12 oz	4	270	13%
Chicken & Vegetables	12 oz	3	290	9%
Chicken Fettucini	12 oz	12	390	28%
Country Style Vegetables & Beef Tips	12 oz	5	230	23%

Food and Description	Amount	Fat Grams	Total Calories	% Fat Calories
Cheese Ravioli	12 oz	3	330	8%
Chicken Chow Mein	12 oz	6	320	17%
Glazed Turkey w/Dressing	10.5 oz	5	340	16%
Lasagna w/Meat Sauce	12 oz	9	330	25%
Mesquite Chicken	12 oz	1	360	3%
Mushroom Gravy over Salisbury Steak	10.5 oz	5	290	19%
Roasted Chicken w/mushrooms	12 oz	6	280	15%
Shrimp Marinara	12 oz	3	290	9%
Shrimp Creole	12 oz	4	240	15%
Spaghetti w/beef & mushrooms	12 oz	10	370	24%
Sweet & Sour Chicken	12 oz	2	330	5%
Tomato Sauce over Meatloaf	10.5 oz	9	340	24%
Turkey Medallions	12 oz	6	280	19%
Vegetable Lasagna	12 oz	4	240	15%
(Weight Watchers)				
Entrees				
Angel Hair Pasta	10 oz	4	200	18%
Baked Cheese Ravioli	9 oz	6	240	23%
Baked Potatoes				
Broccoli & Cheese	10.5 oz	6	270	20%
Chicken Divan	11.25 oz	7	280	23%
Ham Lorraine	11.5 oz	5	240	19%
Homestyle Turkey	11.25 oz	7	230	27%
Vegetable Primavera	11.15 oz	9	320	23%
Beef Cantonese w/Rice	9 oz	4	200	18%
Beef Stroganoff	8.5 oz	9	280	29%
Cheese Enchiladas Ranchero	8.87 oz	10	260	35%
Cheese Manicotti	9.25 oz	8	260	28%
Cheese Tortellini	9.25 oz	8	260	28%
Chicken Ala King	9 oz	4	230	16%
Chicken Divan Baked Potato	11.25 oz	7	280	23%
Chicken Enchilada Suiza	9 oz	7	230	27%
Chicken Fajitas	6.75 oz	5	210	21%
Chicken Fettucini	8.25 oz	9	280	29%
Chicken Nuggets	5.9 oz	7	220	29%
Chicken Polynesian	9 oz	1	190	5%
Fettucini Alfredo	8 oz	7	230	27%
Garden Lasagna	11 oz	7	260	24%
Homestyle Chicken & Noodles	9 oz	7	240	26%
Italian Cheese Lasagna	11 oz	7	290	22%
Jade Garden Beef	9 oz	3	150	18%
Lasagna	10.25 oz	6	270	20%
Orange Glazed Chicken w/Rice	9 oz	2	170	11%

Food and Description	Amount	Fat Grams	Total Calories	% Fat Calories
Sesame Chicken				
w/Lo Mein Noodles	9 oz	4	200	18%
Spaghetti w/meat sauce	10 oz	7	240	26%
Spring Vegetables				
w/Teriyaki Chicken	9 oz	3	140	19%
Stuffed Turkey Breast	8.5 oz	8	270	27%
Vegetable Hunan &				
Ginger Chicken	9 oz	2	160	11%
Smart Ones				
Fiesta Chicken	8 oz	1	210	4%
Lasagna Florentine	11 oz	1	220	4%
Lemon Herb Chicken Picatta	7.5 oz	< 1	160	3%
Pasta Portafino	9.5 oz	1	160	6%
Roast Turkey Medallions				
& Mushrooms	8.5 oz	1	200	5%
Shrimp Marinara w/Linguini	8 oz	1	150	6%
Stir Fry				
Beef Cantonese	9 oz	4	200	18%
Chicken Polynesian	9 oz	1	190	5%
Jade Garden Beef	9 oz	3	150	18%
Sesame Chicken	9 oz	4	200	18%
Spring Vegetables				
w/Teriyaki Chicken	9 oz	3	140	19%
Ultimate 200				
Barbecue Glazed chicken	7 oz	6	200	27%
Beef Enchiladas Ranchero	9.12 oz	5	190	24%
Beef Sirloin Tips	7.5 oz	6	200	27%
Chicken Cordon Bleu	7.7 oz	5	170	26%
Chicken Kiev	7 oz	5	190	24%
Deluxe Pizza Pocket Sandwich	4 oz	5	200	23%
Grilled Chicken Sandwich	4 oz	5	200	23%
Grilled Glazed Chicken	7.5 oz	2	150	12%
Ham & Cheese Pocket	4 oz	6	200	27%
Imperial Chicken	8.5 oz	3	200	14%
London Broil	7.5 oz	3	110	25%
Oven Baked Fish	6.64 oz	2	120	15%
Pasta Italiano	8 oz	2	160	11%
Southern Baked Chicken	6.3 oz	7	170	37%
Teriyaki Chicken	7.6 oz	4	150	24%
Veal Patty Parmigiana	8.2 oz	4	150	24%
FROZEN NON-DAIRY DESSERT				
(Carnation) Lite Wonder				
Chocolate	½ cup	3	110	25%
Mocha Fudge	½ cup	3	120	23%

Food and Description	Amount	Fat Grams	Total Calories	% Fat Calories
Neapolitan	½ cup	3	110	25%
Strawberry	½ cup	3	110	25%
Vanilla	½ cup	3	100	27%
Vanilla Praline	½ cup	5	130	35%
(Costello's) Mellorine				
Fudge Revel	½ cup	6	130	42%
Vanilla	½ cup	7	130	49%
(Hood Free)				
Boston Brownie Sundae	4 oz	1	120	8%
Heavenly Mash	4 oz	1	110	8%
Mississippi Mud Pie	4 oz	2	120	15%
Praline Pecan Delight	4 oz	1	120	8%
Super Strawberry Swirl	4 oz	–	90	–
Very Vanilla	4 oz	–	90	–
(Mocha Mix) lower in saturated fat				
Chocolate Chip	4 oz	9	180	45%
Dutch Chocolate	4 oz	8	130	55%
Mocha Almond Fudge	4 oz	8	150	48%
Neapolitan	4 oz	7	130	49%
Strawberry Swirl	4 oz	7	140	45%
Toasted Almond	4 oz	9	150	54%
Vanilla	4 oz	7	140	45%
Vanilla-Chocolate-Chocolate Almond	4 oz	9	150	54%
Vanilla-Chocolate Covered Bars	1 bar	21	300	63%
(Sealtest) Free				
Chocolate	½ cup	–	100	–
Chocolate Vanilla Strawberry	½ cup	–	100	–
Vanilla	½ cup	–	100	–
Vanilla Fudge Royale	½ cup	–	100	–
FRUIT (See individual listings)				
FRUIT BITS/dried				
(Sun Maid)	2 oz	.5	160	3%
FRUIT COCKTAIL				
canned				
in water	½ cup		40	–
in juice	½ cup	–	56	–
in heavy syrup	½ cup	–	93	–
in extra heavy syrup	½ cup	–	115	–
(Del Monte)	½ cup	–	80	–
Lite	½ cup	–	50	–
(Nutradiet)	½ cup	–	40	–
(S&W)				
Heavy syrup	½ cup	–	90	–
Natural style	½ cup	–	90	–

Food and Description	Amount	Fat Grams	Total Calories	% Fat Calories
FRUIT CUP				
(Hunt's) Snack Pack	5 oz	< 1	120	4%
FRUIT DRINK (*See also* individual listings; FRUIT PUNCH; SOFT DRINKS)				
Caribbean Cooler				
(Crystal Light) mix	8 oz	–	3	–
Citrus Blend (Crystal Light)mix-diet	8 oz	–	4	–
Citrus Fruit Juice Drink	8 oz	–	113	–
Fruit Medley (Libby's)	8 oz	–	80	–
(Hi-C)				
Double Fruit Cooler	6 oz	–	93	–
Ecto Cooler	6 oz	–	95	–
Hula	6 oz	–	97	–
Juice Medley	6 oz	–	80	–
(Kool-Aid) Flavored Drinks				
all flavors	8 oz	–	2	–
sugar added	8 oz	–	100	–
pre-sweetened	8 oz	–	70	–
sugar-free	8 oz	–	4	–
(Tang) Fruit Juice Box				
mixed	8.45 oz	–	140	–
FRUIT ICES				
Berry Blend Pops (Crystal Light)	1	–	14	–
Chilly Things-Light/all flavors	1	–	12	–
(Dole)				
Fresh Lites				
Cherry	1	–	25	–
Lemon	1	–	25	–
Pineapple Orange	1	–	25	–
Raspberry	1	–	25	–
Fruit And Cream Bars				
Blueberry	1 bar	1	90	10%
Chocolate/Banana	1 bar	9	175	46%
Chocolate/Strawberry	1 bar	8	140	51%
Peach	1 bar	1	90	10%
Raspberry	1 bar	1	90	10%
Strawberry	1 bar	1	90	10%
Fruit & Yogurt Bars				
Cherry	1 bar	.5	80	6%
Raspberry	1 bar	.5	70	6%
Strawberry	1 bar	.5	70	6%
Fruit'N Juice Bars				
Pina Colada	1 bar	3	90	30%
Pineapple	1 bar	< 1	70	6%
Raspberry	1 bar	< 1	70	6%

Food and Description	Amount	Fat Grams	Total Calories	% Fat Calories
Strawberry	1 bar	< 1	70	6%
Fruit Sorbet				
Peach	4 oz	< 1	110	4%
Pineapple	4 oz	< 1	100	5%
Strawberry	4 oz	< 1	120	4%
Sorbet				
Mandarin Orange	4 oz	–	110	–
Peach	4 oz	–	120	–
Pineapple	4 oz	–	120	–
Raspberry	4 oz	–	110	–
Strawberry	4 oz	–	110	–
SunTops				
Fruit Punch	1 bar	–	40	–
Grape	1 bar	–	40	–
Lemonade	1 bar	–	40	–
Tropical Orange	1 bar	–	40	–
(Eskimo) Rainbow Twin Pops	1	–	60	–
Frozfruit-On A Stick-all flavors	1	–	70	–
Fruit Bars (Jell-O)				
all flavors-averaged data	1 bar	–	45	–
Fruit Ice (Haagen Dazs)				
Boysenberry	½ cup	–	90	–
Lemon	½ cup	–	140	–
Lime	½ cup	–	123	–
Orange	½ cup	–	140	–
Raspberry	½ cup	–	100	–
Fruit Juice Bars (Minute Maid)				
cherry	1 bar	–	60	–
fruit punch	1 bar	–	60	–
grape	1 bar	–	60	–
orange	1 bar	–	60	–
strawberry	1 bar	–	60	–
Fruit Juice Bars (Welch's)				
Grape	1 bar	–	45	–
Raspberry	1 bar	–	45	–
Strawberry	1 bar	–	45	–
no sugar added				
Grape	1 bar	–	25	–
Raspberry	1 bar	–	25	–
Strawberry	1 bar	–	25	–
Fruit Punch Pops (Crystal Light)	1 bar	–	14	–
Fruit Slush (Wyler's) Freeze & Eat				
Cherry	4 oz	–	157	–
Fruit Punch	4 oz	–	157	–

Food and Description	Amount	Fat Grams	Total Calories	% Fat Calories
Grape	4 oz	–	157	–
Orange	4 oz	–	157	–
Pink Lemonade	4 oz	–	157	–
Strawberry	4 oz	–	157	–
Tropical Punch Fruit	4 oz	–	157	–
Gelatin Pops (Jell-O)				
all flavors-averaged data	1 bar	–	35	–
(Good Humor)				
Calippo				
Cherry	1 bar	–	140	–
Lemon	1 bar	–	112	–
Orange	1 bar	–	110	–
Cherry Italian Ice	1 bar	–	138	–
Cool Shark Bar	1 bar	–	70	–
Ice Stripes				
Cherry/orange	1 bar	–	35	–
Grape/Lemon	1 bar	–	35	–
Jumbo Jet Star	1 bar	< 1	85	5%
Strawberry Finger	1 bar	–	50	–
Stripes	1 bar	–	35	–
(Koolaid) Kool-pops/all flavors	1 bar	–	40	–
Life Saver Pops (Nabisco)				
all flavors	1 bar	–	40	–
(Natural Nectar)				
Lemony-Lime	1 bar	< 1	70	6%
Tropical Delite	1 bar	< 1	70	6%
Pink Lemonade Pops (Crystal Light)	1 bar	–	13	–
(Popsicle) Ice Pops				
sugar-free/all flavors	1 bar	–	18	–
regular/all flavors	1 bar	–	50	–
Snowburst (Jell-O)				
Lemon	1 bar	–	45	–
Spot Pops				
Diet 7-up	1 pop	–	15	–
Diet Cherry 7-up	1 pop	–	15	–
(Sunkist)				
Coconut Bar	4 oz	8	138	52%
Lemonade Bar	4 oz	–	68	–
Orange Juice Bar	4 oz	–	72	–
Orange & Cream	4 oz	.5	84	16%
Wild Berry Fruit & Juice	4 oz	.5	103	4%
(Trix) Pops/all flavors	1 bar	–	40	–
FRUIT JUICE (*See also* individual listings)				
Juicy Juice (Libby's)	6 oz	–	100	–

Food and Description	Amount	Fat Grams	Total Calories	% Fat Calories
Paradise Punch/from frozen conc.	8 oz	1	100	9%
Tropical-Juicy Juice (Libby's)	6 oz	–	100	–
Tropical Nectar				
(Kern's)	6 oz	–	112	–
Tropical Squeeze				
(Chiquita)	6 oz	< 1	90	5%
FRUIT JUICE COCKTAIL (*See also* individual listings)				
(Welch's)				
Orchard Harvest Blend				
Bottled	6 oz	–	110	–
Cocktails-In-A-Box	8.45 oz	–	150	–
Frozen	6 oz	–	110	–
FRUIT JUICE PUNCH (*See also* FRUIT PUNCH DRINK; PUNCH)				
Bottled, Boxed, or Canned				
(Minute Maid)	8.45 oz	–	128	–
Concord	8.45 oz	–	131	–
Juices to Go	9.6 oz	–	145	–
Concord	9.6 oz	–	148	–
Tropical	9.6 oz	–	147	–
On the Go	10 oz	–	152	–
Concord	10 oz	–	156	–
(Libby's) Juicy Juice	6 oz	–	100	–
	8.45 oz	–	140	–
Paradise punch				
from frozen concentrate	8 oz	1	100	9%
(Tropical)	8.45 oz	–	130	–
FRUIT MEDLEY				
(Mariani)				
dried	¼ cup	1	150	5%
dried Tropical	1 oz	1	90	10%
FRUIT, MIXED				
canned heavy syrup	1 cup	–	184	–
(Del Monte)				
chunky	½ cup	–	80	–
chunky lite	½ cup	–	50	–
cup	5 oz	–	100	–
(Nutradiet) natural in water	½ cup	–	40	–
(S&W) natural style juice	½ cup	–	90	–
dried	4 oz	.6	278	2%
(Del Monte)	2 oz	–	130	–
(Mariani) Fancy	¼ cup	–	140	–
frozen				
sweetened	1 cup	.5	245	2%
unsweetened	3.5 oz	< 1	45	10%

Food and Description	Amount	Fat Grams	Total Calories	% Fat Calories
frozen syrup (Birds Eye)	5 oz	–	120	–
FRUIT'N NUT MIX (Planters)	1 oz	9	150	54%
FRUIT PECTIN				
Certo	1 Tbs	–	2	–
Sure Jell				
light	¼ pkg	–	36	–
sweetened	¼ pkg	–	40	–
FRUIT PUNCH DRINK (See also FRUIT JUICE PUNCH; PUNCH; individual listings)				
Bottled, Boxed, or Canned				
(Bama)	6 oz	–	87	–
(Betty Crocker) Squeezeit				
Billy B Wild	6.75 oz	–	90	–
Chucklin Cherry	6.75 oz	–	90	–
Mean Green Puncher	6.75 oz	–	110	–
Red Punch	6.75 oz	–	110	–
Smarty Arty Orange	6.75 oz	–	90	–
(Hawaiian Punch)				
Fruit Juicy Red-Lite	6 oz	–	60	–
Island Fruit Cocktail	6 oz	–	90	–
Regular	6 oz	–	90	–
Regular-From Concentrate	6 oz	–	90	–
Tropical	6 oz	–	90	–
Very Berry	6 oz	–	90	–
Wild Fruit	6 oz	–	90	–
(Hi-C)				
Hula Punch	6 oz	–	87	–
Regular	6 oz	–	96	–
(Kern's)				
Islander Punch	8 oz	–	120	–
(Kool-Aid) KoolBursts				
Cherry	6.75 oz	–	130	–
Grape	6.75 oz	–	130	–
Great Bluedini	6.75 oz	–	110	–
Orange	6.75 oz	–	130	–
Rock-A-Dile Red	6.75 oz	–	110	–
Tropical Puncch	6.75 oz	–	130	–
(Mott's)	9.5 oz	–	150	–
	10 oz	–	170	–
(Tropicana)				
Single Serve	10 oz	–	170	–
From Frozen Concentrate	8 oz	–	113	–
(Birds Eye)	6 oz	–	80	–
Mix				
(Country Time) Lemonade Punch	8 oz	–	80	–

Food and Description	Amount	Fat Grams	Total Calories	% Fat Calories
(Crystal Lite)				
Fruit-Diet	8 oz	–	4	–
Paradise Punch	8 oz	–	3	–
(Kool-Aid)				
Sugar-Free				
Mountain Berry	8 oz	–	4	–
Surfin' Berry	8 oz	–	4	–
Tropical	8 oz	–	4	–
Sugar-Sweetened				
Mountain Berry	8 oz	–	70	–
Rainbow	8 oz	–	70	–
Unsweetened				
Mountain Berry	1 pkg	–	2	–
Prepared w/Sugar	8 oz	–	100	–
Surfin' Berry	1 pkg	–.	2	–
Prepared w/Sugar	8 oz	–	100	–
Tropical	1 pkg	–	2	–
Prepared w/Sugar	8 oz	–	100	–
(Tropicana) 2 tsp.	8 oz		97	
(Wyler's) All Flavors				
Sugar-Sweetened	8 oz	–	90	–
w/o Sugar	8 oz	–	2	–
FRUIT SALAD				
Canned				
(Del Monte)				
For Fruit Salad	½ cup	–	90	–
Tropical	½ cup	–	90	–
Generic				
in water	½ cup	< 1	37	12%
in juice	½ cup	< 1	62	7%
in heavy syrup	½ cup	< 1	94	15%
tropical	½ cup	–	110	–
in extra heavy syrup	½ cup	< 1	114	4%
(Kraft)	½ cup	–	50	–
FRUIT SNACKS				
Candied Fruit (*See* individual fruit listings)				
(Del Monte)				
Sierra Trail Mix	.9 oz	7	130	49%
Tropical Fruit Punch	.9 oz	1	90	10%
Yogurt Raisins	.9 oz	< 1	120	38%
(Estee)				
Fruit & Nut Mix	4 pieces	2	35	51%
Tropi Mix				
assorted sugar-free	2 pieces	–	25	–

Food and Description	Amount	Fat Grams	Total Calories	% Fat Calories
(Featherweight) Sweet Pretenders				
Berry Patch Blend	1 piece	–	12	–
Orange Blend	1 piece	–	12	–
Tropical Blend	1 piece	–	12	–
(Flavor Tree)				
Fruit Bears				
assorted	1.05 oz	1.6	117	12%
Fruit Circus				
assorted	1.05 oz	1.6	117	12%
Fruit Roll				
Apple	1 roll	–	80	–
Apricot	1 roll	.5	80	6%
Cherry	1 roll	–	80	–
Fruit Punch	1 roll	–	70	–
Grape	1 roll	–	80	–
Raspberry	1 roll	–	80	–
Strawberry	1 roll	–	80	–
(Fruit Corners)				
Berry Bears				
Assorted Fruit	1 pouch	.5	100	5%
Fruit Punch	1 pouch	.5	100	5%
Shark Bites				
Assorted Fruit	1 pouch	.5	100	5%
Fruit Punch	1 pouch	.5	100	5%
(Fruit Roll-Ups) all flavors	1 roll	.5	50	9%
Peel-Outs-all flavors	1 roll	.5	50	9%
(Fruit Snackers) Peter Pan	1 pouch	1	90	10%
(Fruit Wrinkles) all flavors	1 pouch	1	100	9%
(Nintendo)				
Link	1 pouch	–	100	–
Super Mario Bros	1 pouch	–	100	–
(Sunkist)				
Flippits chocolate covered fruit				
snacks/all flavors	1 pouch	4	110	33%
Fun Fruits				
all shapes/all flavors	1 pouch	1	100	9%
Fun Fruits Creme Supremes				
Strawberry/yogurt covered	.9 oz	3.6	114	28%
2-T Fruit all flavors	1 pouch	1	90	10%
(Weight Watchers) fruit snacks				
apple	½ oz	< 1	50	9%
cinnamon	.5 oz	< 1	50	9%
peach	.5 oz	< 1	50	9%
strawberry	.5 oz	< 1	50	9%

G

Food and Description	Amount	Fat Grams	Total Calories	% Fat Calories
GARBANZO BEAN (See CHICKPEA)				
GARLIC/raw, minced	1 clove	–	4	–
GARLIC CLOVE/raw	1 clove	–	5	–
GARLIC POWDER	1 tsp	–	9	–
GAZPACHO (See SOUP)				
GEFILTE FISH				
commercial				
sweet	1 piece ~ 1.5 oz	.7	35	18%
(Manischewitz)				
homestyle	3.5 oz	3.89	111	32%
sweet	3.5 oz	4	132	27%
(Mother's) Old Fashioned				
sweetened	1 fishball	1	70	13%
w/o sugar	1 fishball	1	54	17%
(Rokeach)				
w/Natural Broth	2 oz	1	46	20%
Old Vienna	2.6 oz	2	68	27%
GELATIN				
Drinking Powder				
1 packet + water	4 oz	–	67	–
(Knox) w/Nutrasweet	1 env	–	39	–
Dry	1 pkt	–	23	–
Mix				
(D-Zerta) Low-Calorie/all flavors				
averaged data	½ cup	–	8	–
(Estee) Low-Cal Gelatin Desserts	½ cup	–	8	–
(Jell-O) 1-2-3				
Cherry	⅔ cup	2	130	14%
Orange	⅔ cup	2	130	14%
Strawberry	⅔ cup	2	130	14%
Triple Fruit Rainbow	⅔ cup	2	130	14%
(Jell-O) regular				
Apricot	½ cup	–	80	–
Black Cherry	½ cup	–	80	–

Food and Description	Amount	Fat Grams	Total Calories	% Fat Calories
Black Raspberry	½ cup	–	80	–
Blackberry	½ cup	–	80	–
Cherry	½ cup	–	80	–
Concord Grape	½ cup	–	80	–
Lemon	½ cup	–	80	–
Lime	½ cup	–	80	–
Mixed Fruit	½ cup	–	80	–
Orange	½ cup	–	80	–
Orange Pineapple	½ cup	–	80	–
Peach	½ cup	–	80	–
Raspberry	½ cup	–	80	–
Strawberry	½ cup	–	80	–
Strawberry Banana	½ cup	–	80	–
Wild Strawberry	½ cup	–	80	–
(Jell-O) sugar-free				
Hawaiian Pineapple	½ cup	–	8	–
Lemon	½ cup	–	8	–
Lime	½ cup	–	8	–
Mixed Fruit	½ cup	–	8	–
Orange	½ cup	–	8	–
Peach	½ cup	–	8	–
Raspberry	½ cup	–	8	–
Strawberry	½ cup	–	8	–
Strawberry Banana	½ cup	–	8	–
Triple Berry	½ cup	–	8	–
(Jell-O) unflavored	½ cup	–	6	–
(Jell-Well) regular				
Cherry	½ cup	–	80	–
Lemon	½ cup	–	80	–
Lime	½ cup	–	80	–
Mixed Fruit	½ cup	–	80	–
Orange	½ cup	–	80	–
Raspberry	½ cup	–	80	–
Strawberry	½ cup	–	80	–
Strawberry Banana	½ cup	–	80	–
(Jell-Well) sugar-free				
Orange	½ cup	–	8	–
Raspberry	½ cup	–	8	–
Strawberry	½ cup	–	8	–
Strawberry Banana	½ cup	–	8	–
(Royal) regular				
Apple	½ cup	–	80	–
Blackberry	½ cup	–	80	–
Cherry	½ cup	–	80	–

Food and Description	Amount	Fat Grams	Total Calories	% Fat Calories
Concord Grape	½ cup	–	80	–
Lemon	½ cup	–	80	–
Lemon-Lime	½ cup	–	80	–
Lime	½ cup	–	80	–
Mixed Berry	½ cup	–	80	–
Orange	½ cup	–	80	–
Peach	½ cup	–	80	–
Pineapple	½ cup	–	80	–
Raspberry	½ cup	–	80	–
Strawberry	½ cup	–	80	–
Strawberry Banana	½ cup	–	80	–
Tropical Fruit	½ cup	–	80	–
(Royal) sugar-free				
Cherry	½ cup	–	6	–
Lime	½ cup	–	6	–
Orange	½ cup	–	6	–
Raspberry	½ cup	–	6	–
Strawberry	½ cup	–	6	–
GIN (*See* LIQUOR, DISTILLED)				
GINGER/ground	1 tsp	–	6	–
GINGER ROOT/raw	¼ cup	–	17	–
	5 Slices	–	8	–
GINKGO				
canned	1 oz	.5	32	14%
dried	1 oz	.57	99	5%
raw	1 oz	–	52	–
GOAT/raw-boneless	1 oz	6.6	177	34%
GOOSE/domestic				
meat & skin-roasted	~ 2 lb	69.69	2362	65%
meat only-roasted	1¼ lb	74.86	1406	48%
Goose Gizzard/raw	3 oz	4.5	119	34%
Goose Liver				
pate-smoked, canned	1 oz	12	131	82%
raw	3 oz	3.6	114	28%
GOOSEBERRY				
canned in light syrup	½ cup	–	93	–
raw	1 cup	.87	67	12%
GOULASH (*See* BEEF DISHES, FROZEN ENTREE/DINNER)				
GRANDILLA (*See* PASSION FRUIT)				
GRANOLA (*See* CEREAL)				
GRANOLA/GRANOLA-TYPE BARS (*See also* BREAKFAST BARS)				
(Betty Crocker) IncrediBites				
Chocolate	1 pouch	7	170	37%
Vanilla	1 pouch	7	170	37%

Food and Description	Amount	Fat Grams	Total Calories	% Fat Calories
(Health Valley)				
Bakes				
Apple	1 bar	3	100	27%
Date	1 bar	3	100	27%
Oat	1 bar	3	100	27%
Raisin	1 bar	3	100	27%
Fat-Free Fruit				
Apple	1 bar	<1	140	3%
Apricot	1 bar	<1	140	3%
Date	1 bar	<1	140	3%
Fat-Free Granola				
Blueberry Apple	1 bar	<1	140	3%
Date Almond	1 bar	<1	140	3%
	1 oz	<1	90	5%
Raisin Cinnamon	1 oz	<1	90	5%
Raspberry	1 bar	<1	140	3%
Tropical Fruit	1 oz	<1	90	5%
Fruit & Fitness Bars	2 bars	5	200	23%
No Fat Added Oat Bran Jumbo				
Fruit Bars				
Date & Almond	1 bar	2	140	13%
Fruit & Nut	1 bar	2	140	13%
Raisin & Cinnamon	1 bar	1	140	6%
Rice Bran Jumbo Fruit Bars				
w/Almonds & Nuts	1 bar	5	160	28%
(Jack LaLane) Chewey Fruit & Nut				
Apple Nut	1 bar	2	90	20%
Banana Nut	1 bar	2	90	20%
Date Nut	1 bar	2	90	20%
Orange Nut	1 bar	3	100	27%
(Kudos)				
Butter Almond	1 bar	10	180	50%
Chocolate Chip	1 bar	10	180	50%
Cookies & Creme	1 bar	10	180	50%
Crunchy Nut	1 bar	11	180	55%
Nutty Fudge	1 bar	12	200	54%
Peanut Butter	1 bar	12	190	57%
Raisin	1 bar	9	170	48%
(Natural Nectar) Fi-Bar Snack Bars				
Chewy & Nutty				
Cocoa Almond	1 bar	4	130	28%
Cocoa Peanut	1 bar	4	130	28%
Vanilla Almond	1 bar	4	130	28%
Vanilla Peanut Butter	1 bar	4	130	28%

Food and Description	Amount	Fat Grams	Total Calories	% Fat Calories
Granola				
Coconut	1 bar	4	120	30%
Peanut Butter	1 bar	4	130	28%
Nectar Nuggets				
Almond Butter Crunch	1 cup	7	120	53%
Almond Cappuccino Crunch	1 cup	5	110	41%
Coconut Almond Crunch	1 cup	5	110	41%
Peanut Butter Crunch	1 cup	7	120	53%
Original Fruit				
Apple w/Vanilla Yogurt Coating	1 bar	2	100	18%
Cranberry & Wild Berries	1 bar	2	120	15%
Lemon	1 bar	3	100	27%
Mandarin Orange w/Chocolate Yogurt Coating	1 bar	3	100	27%
Raspberry	1 bar	2	120	15%
Strawberry	1 bar	2	120	15%
(Nature Valley)				
Chocolate Chip	1 bar	4	110	33%
Cinnamon	1 bar	5	120	38%
Oat Bran-Honey Graham	1 bar	4	110	33%
Oats'N Honey	1 bar	5	120	38%
Peanut Butter	1 bar	6	120	45%
Rice Bran-Cinnamon Graham	1 bar	4	90	40%
(Nature's Choice)				
Carob Chip	1 bar	3	90	30%
Cinnamon & Raisin	1 bar	3	90	30%
Oats & Honey	1 bar	3	90	30%
Peanut Butter	1 bar	3	90	30%
(New Trail) Chocolate Covered				
Chocolate Chip	1 bar	11	200	50%
Cocoa Creme	1 bar	9	190	43%
Cookies & Creme	1 bar	11	200	50%
Peanut Butter	1 bar	11	200	50%
(Quaker)				
Chewy				
Chocolate Chip	1 bar	5	130	35%
Chunky Nut	1 bar	6	130	42%
Honey & Oats	1 bar	4	125	29%
Maple Oatmeal	1 bar	4	130	28%
Nut & Raisin	1 bar	6	130	42%
Peanut Butter	1 bar	5	130	35%
Peanut Butter Chocolate Chip	1 bar	6	130	42%
Raisin Cinnamon	1 bar	5	128	35%
S'mores	1 bar	4	130	28%

Food and Description	Amount	Fat Grams	Total Calories	% Fat Calories
Dipps				
Caramel Nut	1 bar	6	150	36%
Chocolate Chip	1 bar	6	140	39%
Chocolate Fudge	1 bar	8	160	45%
Peanut Butter	1 bar	9	170	48%
Peanut Butter Chocolate Chip	1 bar	10	170	53%
Fudge Dipped Chewy				
Chocolate Chip	1.63 oz bar	11	220	45%
Oats & Honey	1.38 oz bar	10	190	47%
w/Peanuts	1.38 oz bar	12	200	54%
	2.25 oz bar	18	300	54%
w/Raisins	1.5 oz bar	12	200	54%
(Sunbelt)				
Chewy				
Chocolate Chip	1.25 oz bar	7	150	42%
	1.75 oz bar	9	220	37%
Oats & Honey	1 oz bar	5	130	35%
w/Almonds	1 oz bar	6	120	45%
w/Raisins	1.25 oz bar	6	150	36%
Fudge Dipped				
Chocolate Chip	1.5 oz bar	10	210	43%
Macaroo	1.4 oz bar	11	200	50%
w/Peanuts	1.5 oz bar	12	200	54%
Granola Cereal				
Banana Almond	1.06 oz bar	4	130	28%
Fruit & NUt	1 oz bar	5	120	38%
(Ultra Slim Fast)				
Nutrition				
Dutch Chocolate Flavored	1 bar	4	140	26%
Peanut Butter w/Chocolate				
Flavored Coating	1 bar	4	140	26%
Snack				
Chocolate Chip Crunch	1 bar	4	120	30%
Cocoa Almond Crunch	1 bar	4	120	30%
Vanilla Almond	1 bar	4	120	30%
(Worthington) Natural Touch				
Caroby Almond Bar	1 bar	10	150	60%
Caroby Milk Bar	1 bar	13	150	78%
Caroby Mint Bar	1 bar	9	150	54%
GRAPE				
Concord				
fresh	½ cup	.75	33	21%
(S&W)				
heavy syrup	½ cup	–	100	–

Food and Description	Amount	Fat Grams	Total Calories	% Fat Calories
Thompson				
seedless-fresh	½ cup	–	48	–
canned in heavy syrup	½ cup	–	94	–
GRAPE JUICE				
Blend-Juicy Juice (Libby's)	6 oz	–	100	–
Grape, Concord				
(Ocean Spray) liquid concentrate				
sweetened-reconstituted	6 oz	–	200	–
(S&W) unsweetened	6 oz	–	100	–
Grape-from frozen concentrate	8 oz	–	128	–
frozen-undiluted	6 oz	–	385	–
Grape, Purple				
bottled	6 oz	–	120	–
frozen				
(Birds Eye)	6 oz	–	90	–
(Seneca)	6 oz	–	115	–
(Welch's)	6 oz	–	100	–
Juice Bowl-Grape				
(Campbell's)	6 oz	–	110	–
(Kraft) Pure 100%	6 oz	–	104	–
(Seneca) Natural	6 oz	–	100	–
(Sippin' Pak) from concentrate	8.45 oz	–	130	–
(Sunglo)	8.45 oz	–	169	–
(Tree Top)	6 oz	–	120	–
(Welch's)	6 oz	–	120	–
Grape, Red (Welch's) sparkling	6 oz	–	128	–
Grape, White/bottled	6 oz	–	110	–
(Welch's)	6 oz	–	120	–
sparkling	6 oz	–	120	–
GRAPE JUICE DRINK				
(Bama)	8.45 oz	–	120	–
(Betty Crocker) Grape-Squeezit	6.75 oz	–	110	–
Generic Grape Juice Drink/canned	6 oz	–	94	–
(Hawaiian Punch)	6 oz	–	90	–
(Juice Works)	6 oz	–	98	–
(Kool-Aid Kooler)	8.45 oz	–	140	–
(Libby's) Grape Medley	6 oz	–	90	–
(Ocean Spray)				
Concord Liquid Concentrate				
Sweetened-Reconstituted	6 oz	–	100	–
(Tang) Fruit Box	8.45 oz	–	130	–
GRAPE-APPLE DRINK				
(Mott's)	10 oz	–	167	–
	9.5 oz	–	158	–

Food and Description	Amount	Fat Grams	Total Calories	% Fat Calories
GRAPE-CRANBERRY JUICE COCKTAIL				
(Seneca)	6 oz	–	110	–
GRAPEFRUIT				
Pink, White, & Red	½ fruit	–	38	–
canned				
in water	½ cup	–	44	–
in juice	½ cup	–	46	–
in light syrup	½ cup	–	76	–
sections				
(Kraft)	½ cup	–	50	–
(Nutradiet)	½ cup	–	40	–
(S&W)				
light syrup	½ cup	–	80	–
natural	½ cup	–	40	–
GRAPEFRUIT JUICE				
Boxed, Bottled, or Canned				
(Campbell's) Juice Bowl	6 oz	–	80	–
(Del Monte) Unsweetened	6 oz	–	70	–
Generic Sweetened	8 oz	–	116	–
Generic Unsweetened	8 oz	–	95	–
(Kraft) Pure 100%	6 oz	–	70	–
(Libby's)	6 oz	–	70	–
(Mott's) unsweetened	10 oz	–	124	–
(Ocean Spray) white grapefruit	6 oz	–	60	–
(S&W) Unsweetened	6 oz	–	80	–
(Sunglo)	8.45 oz	–	94	–
(Sunkist) fresh squeezed	8 oz	–	96	–
	6 oz	–	56	–
(Tropicana)	8 oz	–	101	–
Fresh	8 oz	–	96	–
From Frozen Concentrate	8 oz	–	102	–
Frozen				
(Birds Eye)	6 oz	–	70	–
GRAPEFRUIT JUICE COCKTAIL, PINK				
(Minute Maid)	6 oz	–	80	–
(Ocean Spray)	6 oz	–	80	–
GRAPEFRUIT JUICE DRINK				
Pink Grapefruit Drink				
(Citrus Hill) Plus Calcium	6 oz	<1	70	6%
(Tropicana) Twister	8 oz	–	112	–
GRAPEFRUIT-ORANGE JUICE				
canned				
sweetened	8 oz	–	125	–
unsweetened	8 oz	–	108	–

Food and Description	Amount	Fat Grams	Total Calories	% Fat Calories
frozen	8 oz	–	110	–
GRAPEFRUIT PEEL				
candied	1 oz	–	90	–
GRAVY (*See also* SAUCE, SEASONINGS)				
Canned & Jars				
Au jus	1 cup	.5	38	12%
	1 can	.6	201	3%
(Franco-American)	2 oz	–	10	–
(Heinz)	2 oz	–	10	–
Beef	1 cup	5.5	124	40%
	1 can	6.8	156	39%
(Pepperidge Farm) Hearty	2 oz	1	25	36%
Brown	4 oz	6	94	57%
(Franco-American)	2 oz	1	25	36%
w/onions				
(Franco-American)	4 oz	1	25	36%
(Heinz)	2 oz	1	25	36%
Chicken	1 cup	13.6	189	65%
	1 can	17	236	65%
(Franco-American)	2 oz	4	45	80%
(Heinz)	2 oz	1	25	36%
(Pepperidge Farm) Golden	2 oz	1	25	36%
Chicken Giblet				
(Franco-American)	2 oz	2	30	60%
Mushroom	1 cup	6.5	120	49%
	1 can	8	150	48%
(Franco-American)	2 oz	1	25	36%
(Heinz)	2 oz	–	16	–
(Pepperidge Farm) Mushroom				
& Wine	2 oz	1	30	36%
Pork	4 oz	5	76	59%
(Franco American)	2 oz	3	40	68%
(Heinz)	2 oz	–	18	–
Turkey	1 cup	5	122	37%
	1 can	6	152	36%
(Franco American)	2 oz	2	30	60%
(Heinz)	2 oz	1	25	36%
homestyle	4 oz	4	58	62%
(Pepperidge Farm) Seasoned	2 oz	1	25	36%
■ **GRAVY/DEHYDRATED MIXES: Prepared as Directed**				
Au jus	1 cup	.8	19	38%
(Durkee)	2 cups	–	62	–
Roastin' Bag w/gravy	1 pkg	1	64	14%
(French's)	¼ cup	–	10	–
(Knorr)	1 pkg	< 1	8	56%

Food and Description	Amount	Fat Grams	Total Calories	% Fat Calories
Beef	1 cup	–	9	–
Brown				
(Durkee)	1 cup	–	59	–
(Estee)	¼ cup	–	14	–
(French's)	¼ cup	< 1	20	23%
(Hain)	¼ pkg	–	16	–
(Knorr) Classic				
As packaged	1 serving	1	25	36%
Prepared w/Water	2 oz	1	25	36%
(McCormick/Schilling)				
Au Jus	¼ cup	< 1	20	23%
Brown, Lite	¼ cup	1	10	90%
Country				
Regular	¼ cup	2	40	45%
Sausage	¼ cup	2	41	44%
Herb	¼ cup	< 1	20	23%
Homestyle	¼ cup	< 1	24	23%
Original	¼ cup	.8	23	31%
Pork	¼ cup	< 1	20	23%
(Pillsbury)	¼ cup	–	15	–
Brown w/Mushrooms				
(Durkee)	1 cup	.5	59	8%
Brown w/Onions				
(Durkee)	1 cup	.5	66	7%
Chicken	1 cup	1.9	83	21%
(Durkee)	1 cup	1	92	10%
Roastin' Bag w/gravy	1 pkg	1	122	7%
(French's)	¼ cup	< 1	25	36%
(McCormick/Schilling)				
Lite	¼ cup	1	10	90%
Original	¼ cup	< 1	22	20%
(Pillsbury)	¼ cup	1	25	36%
Chicken & Herb				
(Estee)	¼ cup	–	20	–
Chicken, Creamy				
(Durkee)	1 cup	9	156	52%
Roastin' Bag w/gravy	1 pkg	12	242	45%
Chicken-Italian Style				
(Durkee)				
Roastin'Bag w/gravy	1 pkg	1	144	6%
Homestyle				
(Durkee)	1 cup	2	70	26%
(French's)	¼ cup	1	20	45%
(Pillsbury)	¼ cup	–	15	–

Food and Description	Amount	Fat Grams	Total Calories	% Fat Calories
(La Loma) Prepared				
Quik				
Brown	2 Tbs	4	45	80%
Chicken	2 Tbs	4	45	80%
Country	2 Tbs	< 1	10	45%
Mushroom	2 Tbs	< 1	10	45%
Onion	2 Tbs	< 1	10	45%
Mushroom	1 cup	.9	70	12%
(Durkee)	1 cup	1	60	15%
(French's)	¼ cup	< 1	20	23%
(McCormick/Schilling)	¼ cup	.5	19	24%
Onion				
(Durkee)	1 cup	.5	84	5%
(French's)	¼ cup	< 1	25	18%
Generic (contains beef fat & coconut oil)	1 cup	.7	80	8%
(McCormick/Schilling)	¼ cup	.6	22	25%
Onion Pot Roast				
(Durkee)				
Roastin' Bag w/gravy	1 pkg	–	124	–
Pork	1 cup	1.9	76	23%
(Durkee)	1 cup	.5	70	6%
Roastin' Bag w/gravy	1 pkg	1	130	7%
(French's)	¼ cup	< 1	20	23%
Pot Roast & Stew				
(Durkee)				
Roastin'Bag w/gravy	1 pkg	1	125	7%
(French's) Roastin' Bag	⅛ pkg	< 1	18	25%
Swiss Steak				
(Durkee)	1½ cups	–	68	–
Roastin' Bag w/gravy	1 pkg	.9	115	7%
Turkey	1 cup	1.9	87	20%
(Durkee)	1 cup	–	87	–
(French's)	¼ cup	< 1	25	18%
(McCormick/Schilling)	¼ cup	.5	22	21%
GREAT NORTHERN BEANS				
boiled	½ cup	–	104	–
canned	½ cup	.5	150	3%
(Hain)	4 oz	1	80	11%
(Joan of Arc/Green Giant)	½ cup	1	80	11%
w/liquid	8 oz	1	300	3%
canned-Seasoned w/Pork				
(Luck's)	7.25 oz	5	220	21%
	7.5 oz	6	230	24%

Food and Description	Amount	Fat Grams	Total Calories	% Fat Calories
dry-cooked	½ cup	.5	105	4%
GREEK SOUP (See SOUP)				
GREEN (SNAP) BEAN				
boiled	½ cup	–	22	–
canned	½ cup	–	13	–
(Del Monte)				
cut	½ cup	–	20	–
French style	½cup	–	20	–
Italian Cut	½ cup	–	25	–
Seasoned	½ cup	–	20	–
Whole	½ cup	–	20	–
(Festal)				
cut	½ cup	–	20	–
French Style	½ cup	–	20	–
(Green Giant)				
50% Less Salt	½ cup	–	20	–
1-½" cut	½ cup	< 1	20	23%
French style	½ cup	–	20	–
Kitchen Cut	½ cup	–	20	–
(Joan of Arc)	½ cup	< 1	25	18%
(Libby) cut	½ cup	–	20	–
(Nutradiet) cut	½ cup	–	20	–
(S&W)				
cut	½ cup	–	20	–
dilled	½ cup	–	60	–
Fancy stringless whole	½ cup	–	20	–
Premium Blue Lake				
Cut	½ cup	–	20	–
Premium Blue Lake				
French style	½ cup	–	20	–
Vertical Pack whole	½ cup	–	20	–
(Luck's) cut & shelled				
Seasoned w/Pork	8 oz	8	200	36%
frozen	½ cup	–	25	–
French style	½ cup	–	26	–
(Freshlike)	3 oz	–	25	–
(Health Valley)	4.5 oz	–	36	–
(Green Giant)	½ cup	–	14	–
(Freshlike)				
cut	3 oz	–	25	–
(Harvest Fresh)	½ cup	–	16	–
Italian				
(Birds Eye)	3.3 oz	–	30	–
(Freshlike)	3 oz	–	30	–

Food and Description	Amount	Fat Grams	Total Calories	% Fat Calories
whole				
(Freshlike)	3 oz	–	25	–
microwaveable				
(Green Giant) Pantry Express	½ cup	–	12	–
raw	½ cup	–	17	–
GREEN BEAN DISHES				
Bavarian Style Recipe (Birds Eye)	3.3 oz	6	110	49%
Blue Lake Green Beans, Potatoes, & Julienne Carrots in Grey Poupon Dijon Mustard Sauce Vegetable Classics (Del Monte)				
microwave	3⅓ oz	4	70	51%
Cut Green Beans in Butter Sauce				
frozen (Green Giant)	½ cup	1	30	30%
Cut Green Beans & Cut Wax Beans				
canned (S&W)	½ cup	–	20	–
French Style W/Almonds				
frozen (Birds Eye)	½ cup	1.6	52	28%
French Style Green Beans in Butter Sauce				
(Green Giant)	½ cup	1	35	26%
German Style Green Bean Salad				
canned (Read)	1 cup	7	180	35%
Green Beans w/Mushrooms Casserole				
frozen (Birds Eye)	5 oz	5	90	50%
GRITS (*See* CORN GRITS)				
GROUNDCHERRY				
raw	½ cup	.5	37	12%
GROUPER				
cooked-dry heat	3 oz	1	100	9%
raw	3 oz	.9	78	10%
GUAVA				
fresh	1 med	.5	45	10%
GUAVA BUTTER	1 Tbs	–	39	–
GUAVA FRUIT DRINK				
(Ocean Spray)				
Mauna Lai Hawaiian Guava	6 oz	–	100	–
Mauna Lai Hawaiian Guava Passion	6 oz	–	100	–
GUAVA JUICE				
Guava Juice/canned	1 cup	–	172	–
GUAVA NECTAR				
Bottled (Kern's)	6 oz	–	110	–
From Frozen Conc.	6 oz	–	90	–
Ripe Nectar (Libby's)	8 oz	–	140	–

Food and Description	Amount	Fat Grams	Total Calories	% Fat Calories
GUAVA SAUCE				
cooked	½ cup	–	43	–
GUAVA STRAWBERRY-raw	1 cup	1.5	169	8%
	1 med	–	4	–
GUINEA HEN-meat & skin				
raw-meat only	3.5 oz	2.5	110	20%
raw-ready to cook	1 lb	23	568	36%
GUINEA PIG-raw	3 oz	1.7	82	19%
GUM				
Big Red	1 stick	–	10	–
Bubble Yum				
regular	1 piece	–	25	–
sugar-free	1 piece	–	20	–
Candy-Coated Pieces	12 pieces	–	63	–
Diet				
(Carefree)	1 stick	–	8	–
(Carefree) bubble gum	1 piece	–	10	–
(Extra) sugarfree				
bubble gum	1 piece	–	7	–
cinnamon	1 piece	–	8	–
peppermint	1 piece	–	8	–
spearmint	1 piece	–	8	–
winter fresh	1 piece	–	8	–
Doublemint (Wrigley's)	1 stick	–	10	–
(Freedent)				
Cinnamon	1 stick	–	10	–
Peppermint	1 stick	–	10	–
Spearmint	1 stick	–	10	–
Fruit Stripes-all flavors	1 stick	–	10	–
(Hubba Bubba)				
Blueberry	1 piece	–	23	–
Cola	1 piece	–	23	–
Grape	1 piece	–	23	–
Original	1 piece	–	23	–
Raspberry	1 piece	–	23	–
Strawberry	1 piece	–	23	–
(Hubba Bubba) sugar free				
Grape	1 piece	–	13	–
Original	1 piece	–	14	–
(Juicy Fruit)	1 stick	–	10	–
Spearmint (Wrigley's)	1 stick	–	10	–

H

Food and Description	Amount	Fat Grams	Total Calories	% Fat Calories
HADDOCK (*See also* SEAFOOD DINNER/ENTREE)				
breaded & fried	3 oz	9.7	194	45%
cooked-dry heat	3 oz	.79	95	8%
raw	3 oz	.6	74	7%
smoked	3 oz	.8	99	7%
HALIBUT (*See also* SEAFOOD DINNER/ENTREE)				
Atlantic & Pacific				
batter-fried	3 oz	6	153	35%
broiled w/butter	3 oz	6	140	39%
cooked-dry heat	3 oz	2.49	119	19%
raw	3 oz	1.95	93	19%
smoked	3 oz	12.7	190	60%
Greenland				
raw	3 oz	12	160	68%
HAM (*See also* LUNCHEON MEAT)				
Bits (Hormel)	2 Tbs	5	103	44%
Bone-In (Hormel)	4 oz	15	210	64%
Boneless				
Canned-Black Label				
(Hormel)				
1½ lb	4 oz	7	150	42%
3 lb	4 oz	7	140	45%
5 lb	4 oz	7	140	45%
Chopped	1 oz	4.89	65	68%
canned	1 oz	5	68	66%
(Hormel)				
12 oz	2 oz	9	120	68%
8 lb	3 oz	21	240	79%
Chunk (Hormel)	6¾ oz	20	310	58%
Country Style-Center Slice-lean				
& fat-cold	1 oz	3.66	57	58%
Cured				
regular	3 oz	11	163	61%
roasted	3 oz	13	194	60%
Cured-lean	3 oz	4	103	35%

Food and Description	Amount	Fat Grams	Total Calories	% Fat Calories
Curemaster				
(Hormel)	4 oz	5	140	32%
Deviled-canned	1 Tbs	4	46	78%
	1 oz	9	100	81%
	1 cup	72.7	790	83%
Extra Lean (5%fat)				
cold	1 oz	1	37	24%
roasted	3 oz	4.7	123	34%
(Wilson) Masterpiece				
95% fat-free	3 oz	4	110	33%
Extra Lean (4% fat)				
cold	1 oz	1	34	27%
roasted	3 oz	4	116	31%
(Wilson)				
96% fat-free	1 oz	1	30	30%
Extra Lean Deli-10 lb	4 oz	6	130	42%
Holiday Glaze Ham-3 lb	4 oz	4	130	28%
(Hormel) Extra Lean	4 oz	6	120	45%
Light & Lean (Hormel)				
BBQ	2 slices	2	50	36%
boneless	2 oz	2	60	30%
chopped	2 slices	4	70	51%
cooked	2 slices	2	50	36%
glazed	2 slices	2	50	36%
red peppered	2 slices	2	50	36%
smoked cooked	2 slices	2	50	36%
Minced	1 oz	5.86	75	70%
(Oscar Meyer) Boneless-Jubilee	1 oz	3	45	60%
Breakfast, Honey	1 slice	2	50	36%
Canned-Jubilee w/natural				
juices	1 oz	1	30	30%
Slice-Jubilee-95% fat-free	1 oz	1	30	30%
Steaks-Jubilee-95% fat-free	2 oz	2	60	30%
Patties-grilled	1 pattie	18	203	80%
unheated	1 pattie	18	206	79%
(Hormel) canned	1 pattie	16	180	80%
(Swift) Premium brown'n				
serve ham patties	1 pattie	13	130	90%
Premium sugarplum	1 oz	1	30	30%
Regular/cooked				
cold	1 oz	2	46	39%
roasted	3 oz	6.5	140	42%
Regular (11% fat)				
cold	1 oz	3	52	52%

Food and Description	Amount	Fat Grams	Total Calories	% Fat Calories
roasted	3 oz	7.66	151	46%
Roasted	3 oz	4	117	31%
Sliced/frozen (Schwan's)	3.5 oz	5	130	35%
Steak, Extra Lean (Boneless)				
cold	2 oz	2	69	26%
(Swift) Premium Hostess	1 oz	1	30	30%
(Underwood) Deviled Ham Spread				
Light	2⅛ oz	8	120	60%
Original	2⅛ oz	19	220	78%
Smoked	2⅛ oz	18	190	85%
Whole				
cold-lean only	1 oz	1.6	42	34%
roasted-lean & fat	3 oz	14	207	61%
roasted-lean only	3 oz	4.67	133	32%
HAM AND CHEESE				
Loaf or Roll	1 oz	5.7	73	70%
Roll (Hormel)	4 oz	10	170	53%
Spread	1 Tbs	2.78	37	68%
HAM SALAD	1 Tbs	2	32	56%
	1 oz	4	61	59%

HAMBURGER (*See* BEEF, GROUND; BEEF DISHES; individual FAST FOOD listings; FROZEN ENTREE/DINNER)

HAMBURGER HELPER

(Betty Crocker) Box Mix, Prepared

Food and Description	Amount	Fat Grams	Total Calories	% Fat Calories
Beef Noodle	1 serving	15	330	41%
Beef Romanoff	1 serving	16	350	41%
Beef Taco	1 serving	14	330	38%
Cheddar'n Bacon	1 serving	19	380	45%
Cheeseburger Macaroni	1 serving	19	370	46%
Cheesy Italian	1 serving	18	370	44%
Chili Tomato	1 serving	14	330	38%
Hamburger Hash	1 serving	15	320	42%
Hamburger Pizza Dish	1 serving	14	360	35%
Hamburger Stew	1 serving	14	300	42%
Lasagna	1 serving	14	340	37%
Meat Loaf	1 serving	22	360	55%
Nacho Cheese	1 serving	15	360	38%
Pizzabake	1 serving	14	320	39%
Potatoes Au Gratin	1 serving	18	350	46%
Potato Stroganoff	1 serving	16	330	44%
Rice Oriental	1 serving	14	340	37%
Sloppy Joe Bake	1 serving	15	340	40%
Spaghetti	1 serving	14	340	37%
Stroganoff	1 serving	20	390	46%

Food and Description	Amount	Fat Grams	Total Calories	% Fat Calories
Tacobake	1 serving	15	320	42%
Zesty Italian	1 serving	13	340	34%
12 Minute Microwave (Betty Crocker)				
Box Mix				
Beefy Noodle	1 serving	20	370	49%
Cheeseburger Spiral	1 serving	19	380	45%
Lasagna	1 serving	19	400	32%
Mushroom w/Wild Rice	1 serving	20	400	45%
HASH (See CORNED BEEF HASH, ROAST BEEF HASH)				
HAZELNUT (See FILBERT)				
HAZELNUT SPREAD				
(Nutella) Chocolaty	1 Tbs	5	85	53%
HERRING				
Atlantic				
breaded & fried	3 oz	18	279	58%
canned-tomato sauce	2 oz	6	100	54%
cooked-dry heat	3 oz	9.85	172	52%
dried	1 oz	5	72	63%
kippered	1 piece/			
	~ 1.5 oz	4.95	87	51%
pickled	1 piece/			
	~ ½ oz	2.7	39	62%
	3 oz	13	190	62%
raw	3 oz	7.68	134	52%
roe-raw	3 oz	1.7	111	14%
Pacific				
raw	3 oz	11.8	166	64%
HICKORY NUT				
dried	1 oz	18	187	87%
HOKI				
raw	3.5 oz	.8	74	10%
HOLLANDAISE SAUCE (See SAUCE)				
HOMINY				
white/canned				
(Van Camp's)	1 cup	.7	138	5%
yellow/canned				
(Van Camp's)	1 cup	.6	128	4%
HOMINY GRITS (See CORN GRITS)				
HONEY	1 Tbs	–	64	–
	½ cup	–	512	–
HONEY BUTTER				
(Downey's)				
Cinnamon	1 Tbs	1	50	18%
Original	1 Tbs	1	50	18%

Food and Description	Amount	Fat Grams	Total Calories	% Fat Calories
HONEYDEW				
~ 4.5 oz	1/10 fruit	< 1	47	10%
	1 cup	< 1	50	9%
HORSERADISH (See also SAUCE)				
prepared	1 oz	–	11	–
(Kraft)				
cream style	1 Tbs	1	12	75%
mustard	1 Tbs	1	14	64%
regular	1 Tbs	–	10	–
raw	1 oz	–	18	–
HOT CROSS BUNS (See CAKE AND CAKE PASTRY)				
HOT DOGS (See FRANKFURTER)				
HUMMUS				
homemade	1 cup	21	420	45%
mix (Casbah)	1 oz	5	110	41%
mix-bean dip w/sesame tahini (Casbah)	2 oz	10	220	41%
HUNTER'S SOUP (See SOUP)				
HUSHPUPPY (See BREAD)				
HYACINTH BEAN				
boiled	1/2 cup	.56	114	4%
raw	1/2 cup	2	350	5%

I

Food and Description	Amount	Fat Grams	Total Calories	% Fat Calories
ICE CREAM (See also FROZEN DAIRY DESSERT, FROZEN NON-DAIRY DESSERT, ICE MILK)				
(Baskin-Robbins)				
Chocolate	4 oz	13	264	44%
Chocolate Mousse Royale	4 oz	14	293	43%
Chocolate Raspberry Truffle	4 oz	17	310	49%
French Vanilla	4 oz	19	290	59%
Pralines'N Cream	4 oz	13	283	41%
Rocky Road	4 oz	11	291	34%
Strawberry	4 oz	10	226	40%
Vanilla	4 oz	14	240	53%

Food and Description	Amount	Fat Grams	Total Calories	% Fat Calories
Very Berry Strawberry	4 oz	10	220	41%
World Class Chocolate	4 oz	14	280	45%
(Baskin-Robbins) Fat Free				
Chocolate Vanilla Twist	4 oz	–	100	–
Just Peachy	4 oz	–	100	–
(Baskin-Robbins) Light				
Praline Dream	4 oz	6	130	42%
Strawberry Royal	4 oz	3	110	25%
(Baskin-Robbins) Sugar Free				
Jamoca Swiss Almond	4 oz	2	90	20%
Strawberry	4 oz	1	80	11%
(Borden)				
Chocolate Swirl	½ cup	6	130	42%
Strawberry	½ cup	6	130	42%
Olde Fashioned Recipe				
Dutch Chocolate	½ cup	6	130	42%
Strawberries'N Cream	½ cup	5	130	35%
Vanilla Flavored	½ cup	7	130	49%
(Breyers) Original				
Butter Almond	½ cup	10	170	53%
Butter Pecan	½ cup	12	180	60%
Cherry	½ cup	7	140	45%
Cherry-Vanilla	½ cup	7	140	45%
Chocolate	½ cup	8	160	45%
Chocolate Chocolate Chip	½ cup	10	180	50%
Mint Chocolate Chip	½ cup	10	170	53%
Peach	½ cup	6	140	39%
Strawberry	½ cup	6	130	42%
Vanilla	½ cup	8	150	48%
Vanilla w/Chocolate Almonds	½ cup	10	170	53%
Vanilla Fudge Swirl	½ cup	8	160	45%
(Breyers) Light				
Chocolate	½ cup	4	120	30%
Chocolate Fudge Swirl	½ cup	4	130	28%
Praline Almond Crunch	½ cup	5	130	35%
Strawberry	½ cup	3	110	25%
Vanilla Raspberry Parfait	½ cup	3	130	21%
(Carnation) Ice Cream Nuggets				
Bon Bon				
Vanilla				
w/dark chocolate coating	5 nuggets	11	170	58%
w/milk chocolate coating	5 nuggets	11	165	60%
(Dreyer's) Grand				
Chocolate Chip	½ cup	9	150	54%

Food and Description	Amount	Fat Grams	Total Calories	% Fat Calories
Cookies'N Cream	½ cup	9	160	51%
Marble Fudge	½ cup	8	150	48%
Rocky Road	½ cup	10	170	53%
Vanilla	½ cup	10	160	56%
Other Flavors (listed below)	½ cup	7-10	130-180	49%-50%
Almond Praline				
Butter Pecan				
Chocolate				
Chocolate Chocolate Chip				
Chocolate Fudge Mousse				
Coffee				
Creamy Caramel Nut				
Dark Dutch Chocolate				
French Vanilla				
International Stripes				
Mocha Almond Fudge				
Mocha Mania				
Mom's Lemon Cream Pie				
New York Blueberry Cheesecake				
Strawberry				
Toasted Almond				
Vanilla-Chocolate-Strawberry				
Very Vanilla				
(Dreyer's) Grand Light				
Almond Roca Crunch	½ cup	5	120	38%
Almond Praline	½ cup	4	110	33%
Ameretto Fudge	½ cup	4	120	30%
Banana Politan	½ cup	4	110	33%
Berry Wonderful	½ cup	4	110	33%
Cafe Au Lait	½ cup	4	110	33%
Chocolate Chip	½ cup	5	120	38%
Chocolate Fudge Mousse	½ cup	5	130	35%
Cookies'N Cream	½ cup	5	120	38%
Dreamy Caramel Cream	½ cup	5	120	38%
Fudgescotch Swirls	½ cup	4	110	33%
Malt Ball'N Fudge	½ cup	5	110	41%
Marble Fudge	½ cup	4	120	30%
Mocha Fudge	½ cup	4	110	33%
Raspberry Truffle	½ cup	4	110	33%
Rocky Road	½ cup	5	130	35%
Strawberries'N Cream	½ cup	4	110	33%
Strawberry Cheesecake	½ cup	4	110	33%
Vanilla	½ cup	4	100	36%
Vanilla-Chocolate-Strawberry	½ cup	4	110	33%

Food and Description	Amount	Fat Grams	Total Calories	% Fat Calories
Very Vanilla	½ cup	4	100	36%
(Dreyer's & Edy's) Limited Editions				
Candy Bar	½ cup	5	120	38%
Chocolate Chocolate Chip	½ cup	5	120	38%
English Toffee	½ cup	5	110	41%
Malted Milk Ball	½ cup	5	110	41%
Mandarin Orange Chip	½ cup	5	110	41%
(Eagle Brand)				
Homestyle Vanilla-All Natural	½ cup	9	150	54%
(Haagen-Dazs)				
Butter Pecan	½ cup	17	290	53%
Carob	½ cup	17	260	59%
Cherry-Vanilla	½ cup	17	260	59%
Chocolate	½ cup	17	270	57%
Chocolate Chip	½ cup	18	290	56%
Chocolate Swiss Almond	½ cup	17	250	61%
Coffee	½ cup	15	260	52%
Cookies & Cream	½ cup	17	270	57%
Alberta Peach	½ cup	16	250	58%
Honey Vanilla	½ cup	16	250	58%
Macadamia Nut	½ cup	24	330	66%
Maple Walnut	½ cup	19	290	59%
Mocha Chip	½ cup	18	270	60%
Pralines'N Cream	½ cup	16	260	55%
Rum Raisin	½ cup	17	260	59%
Strawberry	½ cup	15	250	54%
Vanilla	½ cup	17	260	59%
Vanilla Chip	½ cup	17	280	55%
Vanilla Swiss Almond	½ cup	19	290	59%
(Haagen-Dazs) Special Additions				
Chocolate Chocolate Mint	½ cup	20	300	60%
Deep Chocolate Fudge	½ cup	15	300	45%
Deep Chocolate Peanut Butter	½ cup	19	330	52%
Macadamia Brittle	½ cup	18	280	58%
Mocha Double Nut	½ cup	20	290	62%
(Lady Borden)				
Buttered Pecan	½ cup	12	180	60%
(Kemps) Vanilla				
Old Fashioned				
Round	4 oz	7	140	45%
Square	4 oz	7	130	48%
(Lucerne)				
Chocolate Chip	½ cup	8	150	48%
Coffee Ice Cream	½ cup	7	140	45%

Food and Description	Amount	Fat Grams	Total Calories	% Fat Calories
French Vanilla	½ cup	8	150	48%
Light-Dairy				
Chocolate	½ cup	4	115	31%
Cookie Cream	½ cup	5	130	35%
Mocha Almond	½ cup	4	125	29%
Rocky Road	½ cup	4	130	28%
Strawberry Cream	½ cup	3	105	26%
Mint Chocolate Chip	½ cup	8	150	48%
Neapolitan	½ cup	7	140	45%
Ranch Pecan	½ cup	9	160	51%
Rocky Road	½ cup	8	150	48%
Strawberry Cheesecake	½ cup	6	140	39%
Vanilla	½ cup	8	140	39%
(Pet)				
Black Sweet Cherry	½ cup	6	120	45%
Butter Pecan	½ cup	9	140	58%
Chocolate	½ cup	7	130	49%
Chocolate Chip	½ cup	7	120	53%
Cookies'N Cream	½ cup	7	140	45%
Heavenly Hash	½ cup	7	140	45%
Neapolitan	½ cup	6	130	42%
Strawberry Cheesecake	½ cup	5	130	35%
Vanilla	½ cup	7	130	49%
Vanilla Fudge Swirl	½ cup	6	130	42%
(Schwan's) Ice Cream & Ice Milk				
Black Raspberry	½ cup	7	140	45%
Butter Brickle	½ cup	7	150	42%
Butter Pecan	½ cup	9	150	54%
Butterscotch Ripple	½ cup	7	140	45%
Cherry Nut	½ cup	7	140	45%
Cherry Vanilla	½ cup	7	140	45%
Chip & Mint	½ cup	8	150	48%
Chocolate	½ cup	7	140	45%
Chocolate Almond	½ cup	8	150	48%
Chocolate Chip	½ cup	8	150	48%
Chocolate French Silk	½ cup	7	150	42%
Chocolate Fudge Ripple	½ cup	7	140	45%
Chocolate Marshmallow Ripple	½ cup	6	140	39%
Coffee	½ cup	7	140	45%
Cookies & Cream	½ cup	8	160	45%
Dark Sweet Cherry	½ cup	6	140	39%
French Vanilla	½ cup	8	150	48%
Holiday Special	½ cup	6	140	39%
Maple Nut	½ cup	9	150	54%

Food and Description	Amount	Fat Grams	Total Calories	% Fat Calories
Neapolitan	½ cup	7	140	45%
Peach	½ cup	6	130	42%
Peanut Butter Fudge Ripple	½ cup	7	150	42%
Pecan Praline	½ cup	7	150	42%
Pink Divinity	½ cup	7	150	42%
Raspberry Delight	½ cup	5	130	35%
Raspberry Ripple	½ cup	7	140	45%
Rocky Road	½ cup	6	150	36%
Strawberry	½ cup	7	140	45%
Strawberry Ripple	½ cup	7	140	45%
Summer's Dream	½ cup	5	130	35%
Tin Roof Sundae	½ cup	7	150	42%
Vanilla	½ cup	7	140	45%
(Sealtest)				
Butter Pecan	½ cup	10	160	56%
Chocolate	½ cup	6	140	39%
Cubic Scoops	½ cup	4	130	28%
French Vanilla	½ cup	7	140	45%
Fudge Royale	½ cup	7	140	45%
Heavenly Hash	½ cup	7	150	42%
Strawberry	½ cup	5	130	35%
Strawberry-Chocolate-Vanilla	½ cup	6	140	39%
(Thrifty)				
Apple Cinnamon	½ cup	7	150	42%
Black Cherry	½ cup	6	130	42%
Butter Pecan	½ cup	9	150	54%
Chocolate	½ cup	7	140	45%
Chocolate Almond Amaretto	½ cup	9	160	51%
Chocolate Brownie	½ cup	9	170	48%
Chocolate Chip	½ cup	8	150	48%
Chocolate Malted Krunch	½ cup	8	160	45%
Coconut Pineapple	½ cup	6	130	42%
Cookies'N Cream	½ cup	7	150	42%
French Vanilla	½ cup	8	150	48%
½ & ½ (Vanilla Ice Cream & Orange Sherbet)	½ cup	4	130	28%
Marble Fudge	½ cup	6	140	39%
Mint'N Chip	½ cup	8	150	48%
Pecan Praline	½ cup	8	160	45%
Pistachio Nut	½ cup	8	150	48%
Raspberry Fudge Torte	½ cup	7	160	39%
Rocky Road	½ cup	8	160	45%
Strawberry	½ cup	6	130	42%
Vanilla	½ cup	7	140	45%

Food and Description	Amount	Fat Grams	Total Calories	% Fat Calories
(Weight Watchers) Grand Collection				
Chocolate Swirl, Pralines				
& Cream	½ cup	3	120	23%
Neopolitan	½ cup	3	110	25%
Strawberries'N Creme	½ cup	3	120	23%
Vanilla	½ cup	3	100	27%
Ice Cream & Frozen Custard				
Chocolate	1 cup	16	295	49%
French Vanilla-Soft Serve	1 cup	22.5	377	54%
Strawberry	1 cup	12	250	43%
Vanilla (10% fat)	1 cup	14.3	269	48%
Vanilla (16% fat)	1 cup	24	350	62%
Ice Cream mixed w/Sorbet-(Haagen-Dazs)				
Key Lime Sorbet & Vanilla Ice Cream	½ cup	7	190	33%
Orange Sorbet & Vanilla Ice Cream	½ cup	8	190	38%
Raspberry Sorbet & Vanilla Ice Cream	½ cup	7	180	35%
ICE CREAM BAR & SANDWICH				
(A & P) Vanilla w/Chocolate Coating	1	10	151	60%
(Baskin-Robbins)				
Chilly Burgers	1	11	240	41%
Sundae Bar				
Light/Chocolate w/Caramel Ribbon	1	5	150	30%
Pralines 'N Cream	1	13	310	38%
Tiny Toon Adventures				
Bars				
Mint Chocolate Chip	1	15	230	59%
Vanilla	1	14	210	60%
Toonwiches				
Chocolate	1	14	330	38%
Vanilla	1	16	340	42%
Vanilla w/Dark Chocolate Coating	1 bar	21	310	61%
(Betty Crocker)				
Brownie Sundaes				
Vanilla Fudge Swirl	1	10	240	38%
Gold Rush Bar				
Peanut Butter	1	16	233	62%
Vanilla	1	13	208	56%
(Creamsicle)	1	3	103	26%
Sugar-Free Cream Pops	1	1	25	36%
(Dolly Madison)				
Vanilla-Chocolate Coating	1	12	197	55%
(Dove Bar)				
Almond Bar	1	23	350	59%
Chocolate-Dark Chocolate Coating	1	22	350	57%

Food and Description	Amount	Fat Grams	Total Calories	% Fat Calories
Chocolate-Milk Chocolate Coating	1	21	340	56%
Crunchy Cookies	1	20	330	55%
Vanilla-Milk Chocolate Coating	1	21	340	56%
Vanilla-Dark Chocolate Coating	1	22	340	58%
(Dove Light)				
Vanilla w/Milk Chocolate Coating	1	12	230	47%
Vanilla w/Dark Chocolate Coating	1	12	230	47%
(Dreyer's) Vanilla-Dark Chocolate				
Coating	1	20	295	61%
(Drumstick) Sundae Cone				
Caramel Surprise	1	19	352	49%
Vanilla	1	19	332	52%
(Eskimo Pie)				
Original Dark Chocolate Coating	1	12	140	71%
Dark Chocolate Coating	1	15	209	65%
Fudge Bars-Sugar Free	1	1	60	15%
Light-Sugar Free	1	9	140	58%
Sandwich-Sugar Free	1	6	170	32%
w/Crispy Rice-Sugar Free	1	11	150	66%
(Freezer Pleezer) Vanilla-Chocolate				
Coating	1	10	147	61%
(Fudgetastics) Sundaes on a Stick				
Crunchy	1	14	230	55%
Plain	1	15	220	61%
(Good Humor)				
Almond Supreme	1	23	350	59%
Bubble o Bill	1	8	149	48%
Chip Candy Crunch	1	17.9	255	63%
Chocolate Eclair	1	10	188	48%
Chocolate Fudge Cake	1	15	214	63%
Fat Frog	1	9	154	53%
Fudge Bar	1	< 1	127	4%
Fudge Cake	1	15	214	63%
Halo Bar	1	13.7	230	54%
King Cone	5.5 oz	12	290	37%
Boysenberry	5 oz	13	340	34%
Laser Blazer	1	3	131	21%
Milk Supreme	1	16.8	278	54%
Chocolate Chip Cookie				
Chocolate	1	8	204	35%
Vanilla	1	10.5	246	38%
Vanilla Ice Cream Sandw	2.5 oz	4.9	165	27%
	3 oz	5.7	191	27%
Milky Pop	3 oz	.8	47	15%

Food and Description	Amount	Fat Grams	Total Calories	% Fat Calories
Sandwich	1	5	162	28%
Strawberries & Cream	4 oz	1	94	10%
Strawberry Shortcake	3 oz	8	176	41%
Supreme	1	25	375	60%
Toasted Almond	3 oz	11.8	212	50%
Vanilla Cup	3 oz	5	98	46%
Vanilla-Chocolate Combo Cup	6 oz	9	201	40%
Vanilla w/Chocolate Coating	1 bar	13.7	198	62%
Whammy	1 bar	7	95	66%
(Haagen-Dazs)				
Caramel Almond Crunch	1 bar	18	240	68%
Chocolate-Dark Chocolate Coating	1 bar	27	390	62%
Coffee & Almond Crunch	1 bar	26	360	65%
Vanilla Crisp Crunch	1 bar	11	160	62%
Vanilla-Dark Chocolate Coating	1 bar	27	360	68%
Vanilla-Milk Chocolate Coating	1 bar	27	360	68%
Vanilla-Milk Choc Coating w/Almonds	1 bar	27	370	66%
(Heath) Toffee Bars	1 bar	11	160	62%
(Kemps)				
Bar	1	12	160	68%
Sandwich				
Cookies'N Cream	1	7	120	53%
Original	1	6	160	34%
Toffee Bar	1	8	110	65%
(Klondike)				
Chocolate-Milk Chocolate Coating	1 bar	20	287	63%
Krispy	1 bar	19	290	59%
Vanilla-Milk Chocolate Coating	1 bar	20	294	61%
(Milky Way Bars) Chocolate	1 bar	11	190	52%
(Natural Nectar)				
Cream Freezes				
Banana Cream	1 bar	8	170	42%
Cocoa-Fudge'N Cream	1 bar	8	170	42%
Raspberries'N Cream	1 bar	5	120	38%
WildBerry Cream	1 bar	3	120	23%
Ice Cream Rounds				
Mocha Pie	1 round	14	300	42%
Nectar Pie	1 round	15	300	45%
(Nestle)				
Butterfinger	1	12	130	83%
Crunch/Vanilla-Milk Chocolate Coating				
Light	1 bar	10	150	60%
Original	1 bar	12	180	66%
Milk Chocolate w/Almonds	1 bar	23	350	59%

Food and Description	Amount	Fat Grams	Total Calories	% Fat Calories
Premium				
Alpine White	1 bar	25	350	64%
Milk Chocolate Premium	1 bar	20	300	60%
Quik/Chocolate				
Milk Chocolate Coating	1 bar	14	210	60%
Semi-Sweet	1 bar	21	310	61%
Vanilla				
Milk Chocolate Coating	1 bar	18.5	286	58%
(Oreo)				
Cookies Cream on a Stick	1 bar	15	220	61%
Sandwich	1	11	240	41%
(Pathmark) Vanilla				
Chocolate Coating	1 bar	10	151	60%
(Polar Bar) Vanilla				
Milk Chocolate Coating	1 bar	17.5	234	67%
(Rondos)				
Chicago Cherry	.75 oz	4	60	60%
Classic Vanilla	1 bar	4	60	60%
French Vanilla	1 bar	4	60	60%
Original Chocolate	1 bar	4	60	60%
(Schwan's)				
Chocolate Scooter Crunch	1 bar	9	170	48%
English Toffee	1 bar	12	190	57%
Gold'N Nugit	1 bar	16	260	55%
Peaches & Cream Bar	1 bar	1	80	11%
Pecan Sundae Cone	1 cone	12	270	40%
Peanut Stick Bars	1 bar	13	190	62%
Raspberry Cordial Bar	1 bar	13	210	56%
Rootbeer Float	1 bar	2	90	21%
Sandwich	1	6	160	34%
Schwan bar	1 bar	12	190	57%
Silver Mint Bar	1 bar	10	160	56%
Strawberries & Cream	1 bar	2	80	23%
Sundae Cones	1 bar	11	210	47%
Swiss Chocolate Almond				
Sundae Cone	1 bar	13	260	45%
Tin Roof Sundae Bar	1 bar	16	250	58%
(Snickers)	1 bar	14	220	57%
(Steve's) Vanilla				
Milk Chocolate Coating	1 bar	29	439	60%
(3 Musketeers)				
Chocolate	1 bar	10	170	53%
Sugar Free Vanilla	1 bar	4	50	72%
Vanilla	1 bar	10	170	53%

Food and Description	Amount	Fat Grams	Total Calories	% Fat Calories
ICE CREAM CONE				
Cones only				
(Baskin-Robbins)				
Sugar	1 cone	1	57	16%
Waffle	1 cone	2	140	13%
(Colosso)				
Bowl	1	1	73	12%
Cone	1	1.5	98	14%
(Comet)				
Cones	1 cone	–	40	–
Cups	1 cup	–	40	–
(Country Inn)	1 cone	–	18	–
(Disney) Cakes	1 cone	–	17	–
(Disney) Sugar Cones	1 cone	–	53	–
(Disney) Waffle Cones	1 cone	< 1	59	8%
(Keebler)				
Ice Cream Cups	1 cup	< 1	15	30%
Sugar Cups	1 cone	–	45	–
(Little Debbie) Ice Cream Cups	1 cup	–	15	–
ICE CREAM SANDWICH (*See* ICE CREAM BAR AND SANDWICH)				
ICE CREAM TOPPING				
Butterscotch				
(Kraft)	1 Tbs	1	60	15%
(Smucker's)	2 Tbs	1	140	6%
Caramel				
(Kraft)	1 Tbs	–	60	–
(Smucker's)	2 Tbs	1	140	6 %
Cherry				
(Smucker's)	1 Tbs	–	53	–
Chocolate				
(Kraft)	1 Tbs	–	50	–
(Smucker's)	2 Tbs	2	130	14%
Chocolate Fudge				
(Hershey)	2 Tbs	4	100	36%
(Smucker's)	2 Tbs	1	130	7%
Chocolate Sauce-homemade	1 Tbs	2	55	33%
Chocolate Syrup				
(Estee)	1 Tbs	–	6	–
(Hershey)	1 Tbs	–	36	–
(Nestle)	1.22 oz	1	100	9%
(Smucker's)	2 Tbs	–	130	–
Hard Sauce-homemade	1.22 oz	6	95	57%
Hot Caramel				
(Smucker's)	2 Tbs	4	150	24%

Food and Description	Amount	Fat Grams	Total Calories	% Fat Calories
Hot Fudge				
(Kraft)	1 Tbs	2	70	26%
(Mrs. Richardson's) Lite	2 Tbs	1	90	10%
(Smucker's)				
Light	2 Tbs	–	70	–
Original	2 Tbs	4	110	33%
Hot Toffee Fudge				
(Smucker's)	2 Tbs	4	110	33%
Lemon Sauce				
homemade	2 Tbs	1.5	60	23%
Magic Shell (Smucker's)				
Chocolate	2 Tbs	15	190	71%
Chocolate Fudge	2 Tbs	15	190	71%
Chocolate Nut	1.22 oz	16	200	72%
Marshmallow				
(Baker's)	2 Tbs	–	120	–
(Smucker's)	2 Tbs	–	120	–
Peanut Butter Caramel				
(Smucker's)	2 Tbs	2	150	12%
Pecans in Syrup				
(Smucker's)	2 Tbs	1	130	7%
Pineapple				
(Kraft)	1 Tbs	–	50	–
(Smucker's)	2 Tbs	–	130	–
(Planter's) Nut Topping	1 oz	16	180	80%
Special Recipe (Smucker's)				
Butterscotch Caramel-Flavored	2 Tbs	3	160	17%
Dark Chocolate	2 Tbs	1	130	7%
Hot Fudge	2 Tbs	5	150	30%
Strawberry				
(Kraft)	1 Tbs	–	50	–
(Smucker's)	2 Tbs	–	120	–
Swiss Milk Chocolate Fudge				
(Smucker's)	2 Tbs	1	140	6%
Walnuts in Syrup				
(Smucker's)	2 Tbs	1	130	7%
Whipped Toppings (See also CREAM; WHIPPED TOPPING)				
Frozen				
(Birds Eye)				
Cool Whip Extra Creamy	1 Tbs	1	16	56%
Cool Whip Non-Dairy	1 Tbs	1	12	75%
Lite	1 Tbs	< 1	8	56%
(Rich Whip)	1 Tbs	1	12	75%
(Kemps) Dairy Aerosol	2 oz	3	30	90%

Food and Description	Amount	Fat Grams	Total Calories	% Fat Calories
(Kraft)				
Original	¼ cup	3	35	77%
Real Whipped Cream Topping	¼ cup	2	30	60%
Mix				
(Dream Whip) prepared w/				
whole milk	2 Tbs	1	10	90%
(D-Zerta) reduced calorie	1 Tbs	< 1	8	90%
(Estee)	1 Tbs	< 1	4	90%
(Featherweight)	1 Tbs	–	4	–
Pressurized				
cream	1 Tbs	< 1	8	90%
	½ cup	7	75	84%
non dairy	1 Tbs	1	10	90%
	½ cup	8	95	76%
(Reddi Whip) Lite	1 Tbs	< .5	6	45%
Zabaglione (*See* CUSTARD)				
ICE MILK (*See also* ICE CREAM)				
(Carnation) Smooth'N Lite				
96% Fat Free				
Cherry Vanilla	½ cup	3	100	27%
Chocolate	½ cup	2	90	20%
Chocolate Chip	½ cup	4	110	33%
Cookies 'N Cream	½ cup	3	120	23%
Double Dutch Fudge	½ cup	3	150	18%
Marble Fudge	½ cup	4	150	24%
Neapolitan	½ cup	3	100	27%
Praline Pecan	½ cup	6	180	30%
Rocky Road	½ cup	4	120	30%
Strawberry	½ cup	2	90	20%
Vanilla	½ cup	2	90	20%
Vanilla Bean	½ cup	4	140	26%
(Light N'Lively)				
Caramel Nut	½ cup	4	120	30%
Chocolate Chip	½ cup	4	120	30%
Cookies'N Cream	½ cup	3	120	23%
Heavenly Hash	½ cup	3	120	23%
Vanilla	½ cup	3	100	27%
Vanilla, Chocolate, Strawberry	½ cup	3	110	25%
Vanilla Flavored & Chocolate Covered				
Almonds	½ cup	4	120	30%
Vanilla, Fudge Twirl	½ cup	3	110	25%
(Natural Nectar) Incredible Edibles				
Raspberry Swirl	1	8	220	33%
Strawberry Swirl	1	8	220	33%

Food and Description	Amount	Fat Grams	Total Calories	% Fat Calories
(Schwan's) (See ICE CREAM)				
(Steve's) Light Ice Milk				
Butter Pecan	4 oz	8	190	38%
Cherry Chocolate Chunk	4 oz	8	190	38%
Deep Chocolate Peanut Butter	4 oz	8	200	36%
Fudge Nut Fantasy	4 oz	8	200	36%
Heath Bar Crunch	4 oz	8	210	34%
Vanilla	4 oz	8	190	38%
Strawberry (Borden)	½ cup	2	90	20%
Vanilla	1 cup	5.6	184	27%
(Borden)	½ cup	2	90	20%
Soft Serve (3%)	1 cup	5	225	20%
(Weight Watchers)	½ cup	3	100	27%
(Weight Watchers)				
Grand Collection				
Chocolate Chip	½ cup	4	120	30%
Pecan Pralines'N Creme	½ cup	4	120	30%
One-Ders				
Brownies'N Cream	4 oz	4	130	28%
Chocolate Chip	4 oz	4	120	30%
Heavenly Hash	4 oz	3	130	21%
Pecan Pralines'N Creme	4 oz	4	130	28%
Strawberry	4 oz	3	110	25%
Sundaes				
Hot Caramel Fudge	4 oz	4	160	23%
Hot Chocolate Fudge	4 oz	4	160	23%
Hot Mocha Fudge	4 oz	5	160	28%
ICE MILK BAR				
(Crystal Light) Cool'N Creamy				
Bavarian Bar	1 bar	2	50	36%
Chocolate Amaretto	1 bar	2	60	30%
Double Chocolate Fudge	1 bar	2	50	36%
Orange	1 bar	1	50	18%
(Kemps) Lite	1 bar	3	130	21%
(Sweet'N Low) Vanilla				
w/Chocolate Coating	1 bar	6	90	60%
(3 Musketeers)	1 bar	4	50	72%
(Weight Watchers)				
Caramel Nut	1 bar	7	120	53%
Chocolate Crispy Treat	1 bar	7	110	57%
Chocolate Dip	1 bar	7	110	57%
English Toffee Crunch bar	1 bar	8	120	60%

ICES (See FRUIT ICES)
INDIAN PUDDING (See PUDDING & MOUSSE)

J

Food and Description	Amount	Fat Grams	Total Calories	% Fat Calories
JACKFRUIT/raw	1 medium	–	107	–
JAM/JELLY/PRESERVES				
(Bama)				
Apple jelly	2 tsp	–	30	–
Grape jelly	2 tsp	–	30	–
Peach preserves	2 tsp	–	30	–
Red Plum Jam	2 tsp	–	30	–
Strawberry preserves	2 tsp	–	30	–
(Country Pure) Jam				
Apricot	2 tsp	–	35	–
Blackberry	2 tsp	–	35	–
Red Cherry	2 tsp	–	35	–
Red Raspberry	2 tsp	–	35	–
Strawberry	2 tsp	–	35	–
(Empress)				
Apple Jelly	2 tsp	–	35	–
Apricot Pineapple Preserves	2 tsp	–	35	–
Apricot Preserves	2 tsp	–	35	–
Black Cherry Preserves	2 tsp	–	35	–
Black Raspberry Preserves	2 tsp	–	35	–
Blackberry Jelly	2 tsp	–	35	–
Boysenberry Preserves	2 tsp	–	35	–
California Orange Marmalade	2 tsp	–	35	–
Concord Grape Jam	2 tsp	–	35	–
Grape Jam	2 tsp	–	35	–
Mixed Fruit Jelly	2 tsp	–	35	–
Peach Pineapple Preserves	2 tsp	–	35	–
Peach Preserves	2 tsp	–	35	–
Plum Preserves	2 tsp	–	35	–
Red Cherry Preserves	2 tsp	–	35	–
Red Currant Jelly	2 tsp	–	35	–
Red Raspberry Preserves	2 tsp	–	35	–
Seedless Blackberry Preserves	2 tsp	–	35	–
Strawberry Preserves	2 tsp	–	35	–
(Estee) Preserves & Jelly-all flavors	1 tsp	–	2	–

Food and Description	Amount	Fat Grams	Total Calories	% Fat Calories
(Featherweight) Fruit Spreads-all flavors	1 tsp	–	4	–
(Kraft)				
Jam-all flavors	1 tsp	–	17	–
Jelly-all flavors	1 tsp	–	17	–
reduced calorie-grape	1 tsp	–	8	–
Preserves-all flavors	1 tsp	–	17	–
reduced calorie-strawberry	1 tsp	–	8	–
(Mary Ellen)				
Apricot Jam	2 tsp	–	35	–
Grape Jam	2 tsp	–	35	–
Grape Jelly	2 tsp	–	35	–
Red Raspberry Jam	2 tsp	–	35	–
Seedless Blackberry Jam	2 tsp	–	35	–
Strawberry Jam	2 tsp	–	35	–
Strawberry Jelly	2 tsp	–	35	–
(Nutradiet) sugar-free				
Jam				
Blackberry	1 tsp	–	4	–
Red Raspberry	1 tsp	–	4	–
Strawberry	1 tsp	–	4	–
Jelly				
Concord Grape	1 tsp	–	4	–
Marmalade				
Orange	1 tsp	–	4	–
Preserves				
Apricot-Pineapple	1 tsp	–	4	–
Boysenberry	1 tsp	–	4	–
Red Tart Cherry	1 tsp	–	4	–
(Poiret) 100% Pure Fruit Spreads				
Apple	½ tsp	–	17	–
Pear,apricot,apple	½ tsp	–	17	–
Pear, black cherry	½ oz	–	35	–
Pear, strawberry	½ oz	–	35	–
Pear,strawberry,apple	½ tsp	–	17	–
(Polaner) All Fruit Spread				
Apricot	1 tsp	–	14	–
Black cherry	1 tsp	–	14	–
Blackberry	1 tsp	–	14	–
Blueberry	1 tsp	–	14	'
Raspberry	1 tsp	–	14	–
Strawberry	1 tsp	–	14	–
(Pritikin) Fruit Spread-all flavors	1 tsp	–	14	–
(R W Knudsen) All Fruit Spread				
Blackberry	2 tsp	–	35	–

Food and Description	Amount	Fat Grams	Total Calories	% Fat Calories
Red Raspberry	2 tsp	–	35	–
Strawberry	2 tsp	–	35	–
(Smucker's)				
Imitation Grape Jelly & Strawberry Jam (artificially sweetned)	1 tsp	–	2	–
Jam-all flavors	1 tsp	–	18	–
Low-Sugar Spreads-all flavors	1 tsp	–	8	–
Mint Apple Jelly	1 tsp	–	18	–
Natural, Cider, Simply Fruit & Autumn Harvest	1 tsp	–	12	–
Orange Marmalade	1 tsp	–	18	–
Preserves-all flavors	1 tsp	–	18	–
Simply Fruit Spread-all flavors	1 tsp	–	16	–
Slenderella-low-cal imitation jams and jellies	1 tsp	–	8	–
(Weight Watchers) Spreads all flavors	2 tsp	–	16	–
(Welch's)				
Jams-all flavors	2 tsp	–	35	–
Jelly-all flavors	2 tsp	–	35	–
Preserves	2 tsp	–	35	–
Squeezables	2 tsp	–	35	–
Totally Fruit-all flavors	1 tsp	–	14	–
JAPANESE FOOD (See ORIENTAL FOOD)				
JELLO (See GELATIN)				
JELLY (See JAM/JELLY/PRESERVES)				
JICAMA				
cooked	½ cup	< 1	46	10%
raw-sliced	1 cup	< 1	50	9%
JUICE (See individual flavors)				
JUJUBE				
dried	3 oz	.9	246	3%
raw	3 oz	–	68	–

K

Food and Description	Amount	Fat Grams	Total Calories	% Fat Calories
KALE				
fresh-cooked	½ cup	–	21	–
frozen-cooked	½ cup	–	20	–
raw	½ cup	–	17	–
KANPYO (Dried Gourd Strips)	3 strips	–	49	–
KASHA (See BUCKWHEAT KERNELS)				
KETCHUP (See CATSUP)				
KIDNEY BEAN				
Dark Red				
canned				
(Hain)	4 oz	–	60	–
(Van Camp's)	1 cup	1	180	5%
canned dry				
(Joan of Arc/Green Giant)	½ cup	< 1	90	5%
(Ranch Style)	7.5 oz	1	170	5%
(S&W) 50% Less Salt	½ cup	1	120	8%
Generic				
boiled	½ cup	< 1	112	4%
canned	½ cup	< 1	104	4%
dried	½ cup	.5	130	4%
raw	½ cup	1	300	3%
Light Red				
canned dry				
(Joan of Arc/Green Giant)	½ cup	< 1	90	5%
(Van Camp's)	1 cup	1	180	5%
Red				
boiled	½ cup	< 1	112	4%
canned	½ cup	< 1	108	4%
(B&M) baked	~ 1 cup	7	290	22%
(Del Monte) Salad Bar Vegetables	2 oz	–	50	–
(Luck's)				
Seasoned w/Pork	7.5 oz	6	220	25%
Special Cook	7.5 oz	4	190	19%
(Nutradiet)	½ cup	1	90	10%
(Progresso)	8 oz	1	190	5%

Food and Description	Amount	Fat Grams	Total Calories	% Fat Calories
(Van Camp's) New Orleans Style White	1 cup	1	180	5%
canned (Progresso)	8 oz	1	180	5%
KIELBASA (*See* LUNCHEON MEAT)				
KINGFISH				
cooked-dry heat	3 oz	11	219	45%
raw	3 oz	2.57	90	26%
KIWI JUICE DRINK	6 oz	–	98	–
KIWI-BANANA JUICE DRINK	3 oz	–	98	–
KIWI-PEACH DRINK	6 oz	–	98	–
KIWI-STRAWBERRY DRINK	6 oz	–	98	–
KIWIFRUIT/raw	1 medium	< 1	46	10%
	1 large	< 1	55	8%
KNOCKWURST (*See* LUNCHEON MEAT)				
KOHLRABI				
fresh-cooked	½ cup	–	24	–
raw	½ cup	–	19	–
KRAUT JUICE (*See* SAUERKRAUT JUICE)				
KUMQUAT/raw	1	–	12	–

L

Food and Description	Amount	Fat Grams	Total Calories	% Fat Calories
LAMB				
(NOTE: All portions are cooked, unless otherwise stated. Lean = all separable fat has been trimmed. Lean & fat = untrimmed and cooked as purchased.)				
Chop, arm/lean-braised	3 oz	14	270	47%
Chop, arm/lean & fat-braised	2.2 oz	15	220	61%
Chop, loin				
lean-broiled	3 oz	8	182	40%
lean & fat-broiled	4 oz	23	336	62%
Chop, rib				
lean-broiled	2 oz	7	130	49%
lean & fat-broiled	2.5 oz	25	289	79%
Chop, shoulder/lean-raw	7 oz	9	185	39%

Food and Description	Amount	Fat Grams	Total Calories	% Fat Calories
Chop, shoulder/lean & fat-raw	7 oz	34	427	72%
Ground-cooked-1.7 oz meat-raw	4 oz	22.5	275	74%
Heart-braised	½ cup	10	189	48%
Hocks	4 oz	16	236	61%
Leg, roast/lean-roasted	3 oz	7	162	39%
Leg, roast/lean & fat-roasted	3 oz	16	237	61%
Liver/broiled	1.6 oz slice	5.6	117	43%
Ribs/cooked-3 oz meat-raw	6 oz	8.9	178	45%
Shoulder				
lean-roasted	3 oz	8.5	174	44%
lean & fat-roasted	3 oz	23	287	72%
Sweetbreads-cooked	3 oz	5	149	30%
Tongue/braised	2 oz	10	144	63%
lamb/sheep	2 oz	14	183	69%
LAMB DISHES				
Lamb Curry/homemade	1 cup	23	460	45%
Lamb Stew/homemade	1 cup	7	165	38%
LAMB'S-QUARTERS				
fresh-cooked	1 cup	.6	29	19%
LARD (See also FAT, OILS, SHORTENING)				
	1 Tbs	12.8	115	100%
	1 cup	205	1850	100%
	8 oz	227	2046	100%
LASAGNA (See also BEEF DISHES; FROZEN ENTREE/DINNER; PASTA DINNER)				
Frozen-w/meat sauce				
(Banquet)	7 oz	10	270	33%
(Swanson's)	10.5 oz	16	400	36%
Standard Home Recipe (USDA) (~2-½"x4" piece)				
with meat	~ 7 oz	12	325	33%
without meat	8 oz	9.5	317	27%
(Van de Kamp's) w/mushrooms	11 oz	25	430	52%
Vegetable Lasagna				
(Impromptu Lite)	10.6 oz	11	270	37%
(Weight Watchers)				
Italian Cheese Lasagna-frozen	11 oz	14	380	33%
w/Meat Sauce (Weight Watchers)	11 oz	13	330	36%
LEEK				
cooked	¼ cup	–	8	–
freeze-dried	¼ cup	–	3	–
raw	¼ cup	–	16	–
	1 leek	–	17	–
LEMON	1 medium	–	17	–
	1 large	–	25	–

Food and Description	Amount	Fat Grams	Total Calories	% Fat Calories
LEMON JUICE				
bottled	1/3 cup	–	17	–
	1 Tbs	–	5	–
(Realemon)	1 oz	–	6	–
fresh	1/3 cup	–	20	–
	1 Tbs	–	4	–
frozen	1 Tbs	–	3	–
(Sunkist)	1 oz	–	7	–
LEMON PEEL				
candied	1 oz	–	90	–
grated	1 Tbs	–	–	–
LEMONADE (*See also* SOFT DRINK MIX)				
Bottled or Canned				
(Hi-C)	8.45 oz	–	109	–
(Shasta)	12 oz	–	146	–
(Sunkist)	8 oz	–	141	–
(Tropicana) Single-Serve	8 oz	–	120	–
Frozen				
(Birds Eye)	6 oz	–	70	–
Generic concentrate	8 oz	–	100	–
(Minute Maid)	6 oz	–	77	–
(Sunkist)	8 oz	–	92	–
Mix				
(Country Time)				
Pink				
Sugar-Free	8 oz	–	4	–
Sweetened	8 oz	–	80	–
Regular				
Sugar-Free	8 oz	–	4	–
Sweetened	8 oz	–	80	–
(Crystal Light)				
Sugar-Free	8 oz	–	4	–
Lemonade-flavored drink mix	2 Tbs + 8 oz water	–	113	–
Lemonade powder mix	1 Tbs + 4 oz water	–	102	–
LEMON-LIME DRINK (*See also* SOFT DRINKS)				
Mix				
(Country Time)				
Regular	8 oz	–	80	–
Sugar-Free	8 oz	–	4	–
(Crystal Light) Diet Soft Drink	8 oz	–	4	–
LENTIL				
boiled	1/2 cup	–	115	–

Food and Description	Amount	Fat Grams	Total Calories	% Fat Calories
canned	½ cup	–	130	–
cooked	½ cup	–	103	–
dry	½ cup	1	374	2%
green (Arrowhead Mills)	2 oz	1	190	5%
red (Arrowhead Mills)	2 oz	1	190	5%
split/dry	½ cup	1	379	2%
sprouts	½ cup	–	40	–
LENTIL PILAF-Zesty				
(Health Valley)	4 oz	2.75	110	23%
LENTIL SOUP (*See* SOUP)				
LETTUCE				
Butterhead	1 head	–	21	–
Iceburg	1 head	1	70	13%
Looseleaf or Simpson	½ cup	–	5	–
Romaine/shredded	½ cup	–	4	–
LICHEE (LYCHEE) NUTS				
dried/shelled	3 oz	.9	237	3%
raw	~6 nuts	–	45	–
raw/shelled	4 oz	1	314	3%
	1 cup	.8	125	6%
LIMA BEAN				
Baby				
boiled	½ cup	–	115	–
frozen	½ cup	–	94	–
(Birds Eye)	3.3 oz	–	130	–
(Freshlike)	3.3 oz	–	130	–
raw	½ cup	1	330	3%
Canned				
(Dennison's) w/ham	7.5 oz	7	250	25%
(Libby)	½ cup	–	80	–
Frozen				
(Green Giant)	½ cup	–	100	–
(Harvest Fresh)	½ cup	–	60	–
(Health Valley) thin	6 oz	.5	188	2%
Giant				
canned-Seasoned w/Pork				
(Luck's)	7.5 oz	7	230	27%
Green				
canned (Del Monte)	½ cup	–	70	–
Large				
boiled	½ cup	–	108	–
canned	½ cup	–	95	–
frozen	½ cup	–	85	–
raw	½ cup	.5	300	2%

Food and Description	Amount	Fat Grams	Total Calories	% Fat Calories
Small green				
canned-Seasoned w/Pork (Luck's)	7.5 oz	7	220	29%
fancy (S&W)	12 cup	–	80	–
LIMA BEAN DISHES				
In butter sauce				
frozen				
(Green Giant)	½ cup	2	100	18%
w/ ham				
canned (Dennison's)	7.5 oz	7	250	25%
LIME	1	–	20	–
LIME JUICE				
fresh	⅓ cup	–	22	–
bottled	⅓ cup	–	17	–
	1 Tbs	–	3	–
(Realime)	1 oz	–	6	–
LIMEADE				
from frozen concentrate	8 oz	–	102	–
LINGCOD/raw	3 oz	1	70	13%
LIQUEUR				
Anisette	¾ fl oz	–	74	–
B & B	1 fl oz	–	94	–
Benedictine	¾ fl oz	–	69	–
Brandy-fruit flavored	1.5 fl oz	–	129	–
Brandy-coffee	1.5 fl oz	–	132	–
Cherry Hering	1.5 fl oz	–	120	–
Coffee	1.5 fl oz	–	174	–
Coffee w/ cream	1.5 fl oz	7	154	41%
Creme de Almonde	1.5 fl oz	–	151	–
Creme de Banana	1.5 fl oz	–	144	–
Creme de Cacao	1.5 fl oz	–	150	–
Creme de Cassis	1.5 fl oz	–	122	–
Creme de Menthe	1.5 fl oz	–	186	–
Curacao	3/4 fl oz	–	54	–
Drambuie	1.5 fl oz	–	165	–
Gin-Citrus	1.5 fl oz	–	114	–
Kirsch	1.5 fl oz	–	124	–
Maraschino	1.5 fl oz	–	112	–
Peppermint Schnapps	1.5 fl oz	–	124	–
Pernod	1.5 fl oz	–	117	–
Rock & Rye	1.5 fl oz	–	140	–
Sloe Gin	1.5 fl oz	–	124	–
Southern Comfort	1.5 fl oz	–	180	–
Tia Maria	1.5 fl oz	–	138	–
Triple Sec	1.5 fl oz	–	121	–

Food and Description	Amount	Fat Grams	Total Calories	% Fat Calories
Vodka-Citrus	1.5 fl oz	–	150	–
LIQUOR, DISTILLED				
(NOTE: In all cases, the higher the proof [the % of alcohol], the higher the calories.)				
80 proof	1 fl oz	–	67	–
84 proof	1 fl oz	–	70	–
86 proof	1 fl oz	–	72	–
86.8 proof	1 fl oz	–	· 72	–
90 proof	1 fl oz	–	75	–
90.4 proof	1 fl oz	–	75	–
94 proof	1 fl oz	–	78	–
94.6 proof	1 fl oz	–	79	–
97 proof	1 fl oz	–	81	–
100 proof	1 fl oz	–	83	–
LIVER (See BEEF, CHICKEN, GOOSE, LAMB, PORK)				
LIVER LOAF (See LUNCHEON MEAT)				
LIVERWURST (See LUNCHEON MEAT)				
LOAF, LUNCHEON (See LUNCHEON MEAT)				
LOBSTER (See also SEAFOOD ENTREE/DINNER)				
Northern				
boiled	3 oz	.5	83	5%
	1 cup	.86	142	6%
raw -1 lobster	~ 5 oz	1	140	6%
Spiny-raw	3 oz	1	95	10%
LOBSTER BISQUE (See SOUP)				
LOBSTER PASTE	1 Tbs	2	39	46%
LOBSTER SALAD				
homemade-includes mayonnaise, tomato,				
celery, carrots, onion, & egg	3 oz	5.5	94	53%
LOGANBERRY				
canned				
in water	½ cup	–	40	–
in heavy syrup	½ cup	–	89	–
frozen	1 cup	.5	80	56%
raw	½ lb	–	45	–
LOGANBERRY JUICE	8 oz	–	100	–
LOQUAT	1	–	5	–
	½ lb	–	84	–
LOTUS ROOT				
cooked	1 root	–	50	–
raw	1 root	–	64	–
LOTUS SEED				
dried	1 oz	.6	94	6%
	1 cup	.6	106	5%
raw	1 oz	–	25	–

Food and Description	Amount	Fat Grams	Total Calories	% Fat Calories
LOX (*See* SALMON, SMOKED)				
LUNCHEON MEAT (*See also* BACON, HAM, SAUSAGE)				
(Armour/Armour Star)				
Canned				
Beef Tripe	6 oz	4	180	20%
Deviled Ham	1.5 oz	9	110	74%
Potted Meat	1.5 oz	6	80	68%
Sliced Dried Beef	1 oz	2	60	30%
Treet				
low salt	2 oz	16	190	76%
regular	2 oz	17	200	77%
Vienna Sausage				
Chicken Premium-Lite	2 oz	13	150	78%
Hot 'n Spicy	2.5 oz	17	190	81%
In BBQ Sauce	2.5 oz	17	190	81%
In Beef Stock	2 oz	17	200	77%
Smoked	2.5 oz	17	180	85%
Cold Cuts				
Barbecue Loaf	1 oz	3	50	54%
Bologna				
Beef	1 oz	9	100	81%
Lower Salt	1 oz	8	90	80%
Liverwurst	1 oz	8	90	80%
Old Fashioned Loaf	1 oz	7	80	90%
Pepperoni				
Italian	1 oz	11	130	76%
Sliced	1 oz	11	130	76%
Salami				
Genoa	1 oz	10	110	82%
Hard	1 oz	10	120	75%
Italian Hard	1 oz	10	120	75%
Lower salt	1 oz	7	80	79%
Sliced	1 oz	10	120	75%
Spiced Luncheon Meat				
w/chicken	3 oz	24	280	77%
regular	3 oz	25	280	80%
Summer Sausage Cheese	1 oz	8	100	72%
Turkey Bologna	2 oz	8	110	66%
Turkey Cotto Salami	2 oz	5.5	90	55%
Turkey Ham	2 oz	2	70	26%
Sausages				
links/raw	1 oz	11	110	90%
lower salt	1 oz	11	110	90%
patties/raw	1.5 oz	16	160	90%

Food and Description	Amount	Fat Grams	Total Calories	% Fat Calories
lower salt	1.5 oz	16	160	90%
rolls/raw	1 oz	11	110	90%
lower salt	1 oz	11	110	90%
Barbeque Loaf-pork and beef	~1 oz	2.5	49	46%
(Eckrich)	1 slice/1 oz	2	35	51%
Beef				
Slender sliced (Eckrich)	1 oz	1	35	26%
Thin sliced (Carl Buddig)	1 oz	2	40	45%
Beef Loaf-jellied (Hormel)	2 slices	4	90	40%
Beef Sausage Sticks (Red Baron)				
smoked	1 oz	10	120	75%
Beerwurst, Beer Salami/Beef	1 slice/1 oz	6.76	75	81%
Beef & Pork (Eckrich)	1 oz	6	70	77%
Beer Salami	1 slice/			
	2¾" dia	1	14	64%
	1 oz	4	55	66%
Pork	1 oz	4	55	66%
Berliner-Beef/Pork	1 oz	4.88	65	68%
Blood Sausage	1 oz	9.78	107	82%
Bockwurst	1 link/~2 oz	18	200	81%
Bologna-Beef	1 oz	8	89	81%
(Eckrich)				
plain	1 slice/1 oz	8	90	80%
thick sliced	1.5 oz	12	130	83%
	1.8 oz	15	170	79%
(Health Valley)	3.5 oz	30	310	87%
(Hebrew National) Original				
Deli style	1 oz	3	90	30%
(Hormel)	2 slices	16	170	85%
coarse ground	2 oz	14	160	79%
(Oscar Meyer)	1 oz	8	90	80%
Garlic Beef	1 oz	8	90	80%
Lebanon	1 oz	3	50	54%
Bologna-Beef & Pork	1 oz	8	89	81%
(Eckrich) w/ cheese	1 slice/1 oz	9	90	90%
garlic	1 oz	9	90	90%
German Brand	1 oz	7	80	79%
Lite	1 oz	6	70	77%
plain	1 oz	9	100	81%
Sandwich	1 oz	9	100	81%
thick sliced	1 slice/			
	1.7 oz	15	160	84%
(Hormel) coarse ground	2 oz	14	160	79%
fine ground	2 oz	16	170	85%

ood and Description	Amount	Fat Grams	Total Calories	% Fat Calories
plain	2 slices	16	180	80%
Bologna-Chicken				
(Health Valley)	3.5 oz	30	310	87%
(Perdue)	1 oz	5.7	71	72%
(Weaver)	1 slice	3.7	44	76%
Bologna-Pork	1 oz	5.6	70	72%
Bologna-Turkey	2 slices/2 oz	8.6	113	69%
(Butterball)	1 slice/1 oz	6	70	77%
Deli	1 oz	6	70	77%
Slice'N Serve	1 oz	6	70	77%
variety pak	¾ oz	4	50	72%
Bratwurst/cooked-Pork	1 link/3 oz	22	256	77%
	1 oz	7	85	74%
(Eckrich)	1 link	30	310	87%
fresh (Schwan's)	1 link/4 oz	34	370	83%
Braunschweiger (Liverwurst)-Pork	1 oz	9	102	79%
(Hormel)	1 oz	7	80	79%
(Oscar Meyer)				
German Brand-tube	1 oz	8	95	76%
Liver Sausage	1 oz	9	100	81%
Brotwurst/Pork, Beef				
(w/nonfat dry milk)	1 oz	7.88	92	77%
	1 link/			
	~2.5 oz	19.5	226	78%
(Butterball) Fresh Deli				
Honey Roasted Turkey Breast	1 slice	< 1	20	23%
Oven Roasted Turkey Breast	1 slice	< 1	20	23%
Smoked Chicken Breast	1 slice	< 1	20	23%
Smoked Turkey Breast	1 slice	< 1	20	23%
Turkey Ham	1 slice	< 1	20	23%
Capocollo (Hormel)-dry	1 oz	6	80	68%
Cervalat-Viking/dry (Hormel)-chub	1 oz	8	90	80%
Cheesefurter	1/1.5 oz	12.5	141	80%
Chicken-Thin sliced (Carl Buddig)	1 oz	4	60	60%
Chicken Hickory Breast (Weaver)	1 slice	.8	26	28%
Chicken Oven Roasted Breast (Weaver)	1 slice	.8	25	29%
Chicken Roll-Light Meat	3 oz	6	135	40%
(Weaver)	1 slice	1.4	26	49%
Chicken Sandwich Makin's (Hormel)				
canned	½ oz	2	25	72%
Chorizo Sausage	1 link/~2 oz	23	273	76%
Corned Beef				
Slender sliced (Eckrich)	1 oz	1	40	23%
Thin sliced (Carl Buddig)	1 oz	2	40	45%

Food and Description	Amount	Fat Grams	Total Calories	% Fat Calories
Corned Beef Loaf-canned (Libby's)	2.3 oz	9	160	51%
Cotto Salami				
(Eckrich)	1 slice/1 oz	6	70	77%
Beef	1 slice/1 oz	8	100	72%
(Hormel)	2 slices	7	105	60%
dried chub	1 oz	9	100	81%
Dutch Brand Loaf	1 oz	5	68	66%
(Gallo Salame) 96% fat free				
Deli Style				
Ham-Smoked	1 slice	< 1	10	45%
Italian Dry Salame	1 slice	1	14	64%
Pastrami	1 slice	< 1	12	38%
Turkey Breast	1 slice	< 1	10	45%
Genoa Salami-dry (Hormel)	1 oz	10	110	82%
Di Lusso	1 oz	8	100	72%
Gran Valore	1 oz	10	110	82%
San Remo Brand	1 oz	10	118	76%
Gourmet Loaf (Eckrich)	1 slice/1 oz	1	30	30%
Ham-Pork				
Boiled	3/4 oz	1	25	36%
Boneless-Prosciutto (Hormel)/dry	1 oz	7	90	70%
Chopped				
(Eckrich)	1 slice/1 oz	2	45	40%
(Hormel)	2 slices	5	88	51%
Chopped-canned	1.5 oz	5	68	66%
(Hormel) 12 oz can	2 oz	9	120	68%
Chopped-spiced/canned	1.5 oz	5	68	66%
Cooked				
(Eckrich) Lite	1 oz	1	25	36%
(Hormel)	1 oz	1	30	30%
Danish (Danola)				
sliced (98% fat free)	2 slices	.5	45	10%
Deviled/canned	3.5 oz	32	348	83%
(Libby's)	1.5 oz	11	130	76%
(Hormel)	1 Tbs	3	35	77%
(Underwood)				
Light	2⅛ oz	8	120	60%
Original	2⅛ oz	19	220	78%
Hostess (Swift Premiium)	1 oz	1	30	30%
Loaf (Eckrich)	1 slice/1 oz	4	50	72%
Minced	1 oz	5.86	75	70%
Patties (Hormel)	1 patty	16	180	80%
Slender sliced (Eckrich)	1 oz	2	40	45%
Sliced (extra lean 5% fat)	1 oz	1.5	37	37%

Food and Description	Amount	Fat Grams	Total Calories	% Fat Calories
Sliced (regular 11% fat)	1 oz	3	52	52%
Sliced w/black cracked pepper/pkg	¾ oz	.9	24	34%
Smoked (97% fat free)	2 slices/			
	~.5 oz	1.5	20	68%
Spiced (Hormel)	3 oz	21	240	79%
Thin sliced (Carl Buddig)	1 oz	3	50	54%
Ham & Cheese Loaf or Roll	1 oz	5.7	73	70%
(Eckrich)	1 oz	4	50	72%
(Hormel)	3 oz	22	260	76%
	2 slices	7	110	57%
Ham & Cheese Patties (Hormel)	1 patty	18	190	85%
Ham & Cheese Spread	1 Tbs	2.78	37	68%
Ham Salad Spread	1 oz	4	61	59%
	1 Tbs	2	32	56%
Headcheese/Pork	1 oz	4	60	60%
(Healthy Choice)				
Cold Cuts				
Baked Cooked Ham	2 oz	2	60	30%
Bologna	2 oz	2	60	30%
Cooked Ham	2 oz	2	60	30%
Honey Ham	2 oz	2	60	30%
Honey Roasted Smoked Turkey	2 oz	1	60	15%
Oven Roasted Chicken	2 oz	1	60	15%
Oven Roasted Turkey	2 oz	2	60	30%
Smoked Chicken	2 oz	1	60	15%
Smoked Ham	2 oz	1	60	15%
Smoked Turkey	2 oz	1	60	15%
Turkey Ham	2 oz	2	70	26%
Deli-Thin				
Baked Cooked Ham	2 oz	2	70	26%
Bologna	2 oz	2	60	30%
Cooked Ham	2 oz	1	60	15%
Honey Ham	2 oz	2	70	26%
Honey Roasted Smoked Turkey	2 oz	2	70	26%
Oven Roasted Chicken	2 oz	1	60	15%
Oven Roasted Turkey	2 oz	2	60	30%
Smoked Chicken	2 oz	1	60	15%
Smoked Ham	2 oz	1	60	15%
Smoked Turkey	2 oz	1	60	15%
Turkey Ham	2 oz	2	60	30%
(Hillshire Farm)				
Bologna				
large	1 oz	8	90	80%
ring	1 oz	8	89	81%

Food and Description	Amount	Fat Grams	Total Calories	% Fat Calories
Deli Select				
Corned Beef	1 oz	< 1	31	15%
Honey Ham	1 oz	< 1	31	15%
Oven Roasted Cured Beef	1 oz	< 1	31	15%
Oven Roasted Turkey Breast	1 oz	< 1	31	15%
Pastrami	1 oz	< 1	30	15%
Smoked Chicken Breast	1 oz	< 1	31	15%
Smoked Beef	1 oz	< 1	31	15%
Smoked Ham	1 oz	< 1	31	15%
Smoked Turkey Breast	1 oz	< 1	31	15%
Flavorseal				
Beef & Cheddar	2 oz	15	190	71%
Beef Polska Kielbasa	2 oz	17	190	81%
Beef Smoked Sausage	2 oz	16	180	80%
Country Recipe	2 oz	16	180	80%
Hot Smoked Sausage	2 oz	16	180	80%
Lite Polska Kielbasa	2 oz	13	160	73%
Lite Smoked Sausage	2 oz	13	160	73%
Mild Polska Kielbasa	2 oz	17	190	81%
Polska Kielbasa	2 oz	17	190	81%
Smoked Sausage	2 oz	17	190	81%
Smoked Sausage-Italian	2 oz	18	200	81%
Links				
Beef Hot Links	2 oz	17	190	81%
Bun Size Beef Wieners	2 oz	16	180	80%
Bun Size Beef Smoked Sausage	2 oz	16	180	80%
Bun Size Cheddarwurst	2 oz	18	200	81%
Bun Size Cheese Wieners	2 oz	16	180	80%
Bun Size Kielbasa	2 oz	16	180	80%
Bun Size Smoked Sausage	2 oz	16	180	80%
Bun Size Wieners	2 oz	16	180	80%
Cheddarwurst	2 oz	17	190	81%
Fresh Bratwurst	2 oz	17	190	81%
Fully Cooked Brats	2 oz	16	170	85%
Hot Italian Sausage	2 oz	17	180	85%
Hot Links-Lite	2 oz	15	190	71%
Knockwurst	2 oz	16	180	80%
Mild Italian Sausage	2 oz	17	190	81%
Natural Casing Wieners	2 oz	17	180	85%
Polish Sausage Links	2 oz	17	190	81%
Polska Kielbasa Links	2 oz	17	190	81%
Smoked Bratwurst	2 oz	17	190	81%
Smoked Sausage Links	2 oz	18	190	85%
Spicy Bratwurst	2 oz	17	180	85%

Food and Description	Amount	Fat Grams	Total Calories	% Fat Calories
Lunch'n Munch Light				
Cooked Ham	1 sandwich	2	35	51%
Honey Ham	1 sandwich	2	35	51%
Smoked Chicken	1 sandwich	2	35	51%
Smoked Turkey	1 sandwich	2	35	51%
Semi-Dry Sausage				
Beef Summer Sausage	2 oz	17	190	81%
Summer Sausage	2 oz	16	180	80%
Summer Sausage w/ Cheese	2 oz	18	200	81%
Thuringer	2 oz	15	180	75%
Honey Loaf-Pork/Beef	1 oz	1	36	25%
(Eckrich)	1 oz	1	35	26%
(Hormel)	2 slices	5	90	50%
Honey Roll-Sausage/Beef	1 oz	2.98	52	52%
Iowa Brand Loaf (Hormel)	2 slices	6	90	60%
Italian Sausage				
Pork-cooked	3 oz	21	268	71%
Pork-raw	3 oz	28.5	315	81%
(Kahn's)				
Family Pack				
Beef Bologna	1 slice	6	70	77%
Beef Pickle	1 slice	5	60	75%
Beef Salami	1 slice	5	60	75%
Beef Spice	1 slice	5	60	75%
Cotto Salami	1 slice	3	45	60%
Deluxe Club Bologna	1 slice	6	70	77%
Pickle Loaf	1 slice	6	70	77%
Spice Loaf	1 slice	6	70	77%
Links				
Beef Frank	1	13	140	84%
Beef n'Cheddar Frank	1	16	180	80%
Big Red Smokey	1	14	170	74%
Bratwurst	1	17	190	81%
Bun Size Beef Frank	1	17	190	81%
Bun Size Beef Smokey	1	15	180	75%
Bun Size Frank	1	17	190	81%
Bun Size Polska	1	17	190	81%
Cheese Wiener	1	13	150	78%
Wieners	1	13	140	84%
Sliced Pack Luncheon Meats				
Beef Bologna-8 oz	1 slice	8	90	80%
Beef n'Cheddar Bologna-8 oz	1 slice	8	90	80%
Beef Pounder	1 slice	8	90	80%
Beef Salami-8 oz	1 slice	6	70	77%

Food and Description	Amount	Fat Grams	Total Calories	% Fat Calories
Chopped Ham-8 oz	1 slice	3	50	54%
Cooked Ham-5 oz	1 slice	1	30	30%
Cooked Salami-8 oz	1 slice	4	60	60%
Deluxe Club Bologna-8 oz	1 slice	8	90	80%
Deluxe Club Pounder	1 slice	8	90	80%
Dutch Loaf-8 oz	1 slice	7	80	79%
Garlic Bologna-8 oz	1 slice	8	90	80%
Giant Beef Bologna-12 oz	1 slice	8	90	80%
Giant Deluxe-12 oz	1 slice	8	90	80%
Giant Thick Deluxe-12 oz	1 slice	10	110	82%
Ham & Cheese Loaf	1 slice	6	70	77%
Ham Bologna-12 oz	1 slice	8	90	80%
Honey Loaf-8 oz	1 slice	2	40	45%
Jalapeno Loaf-8 oz	1 slice	6	70	77%
Liver Loaf	1 slice	15	170	79%
Low Salt Ham-5 oz	1 slice	1	30	30%
P & B Loaf-8 oz	1 slice	2	40	45%
Pepper Loaf-8 oz	1 slice	2	40	45%
Pickle Loaf-8 oz	1 slice	7	80	79%
Souse Loaf-8 oz	1 slice	7	90	70%
Spiced Luncheon Loaf-8 oz	1 slice	7	80	79%
Thick Deluxe-8 oz	1 slice	13	140	84%
Thin Sliced Deluxe-8 oz	1 slice	5	60	75%
Kielbasa, Kalbassy Sausage				
Pork or Beef	1 oz	7.7	88	79%
(Hormel) skinless	½ link	14	180	70%
Polska (Eckrich)-Lite	1 oz	6	70	77%
Skinless	1 oz	16	180	80%
Polska (Louis Rich)-turkey	1 oz	3	50	54%
Knackwurst, Knockwurst-Pork, Beef	1 oz	7.87	87	81%
(Best's) Beef Lower Fat	3 oz	16	210	69%
(Hebrew National) Beef Franks	3 oz	25	260	87%
Kolbase Polish Sausage (Hormel)	3 oz	19	220	78%
Lebanon Bologna-Beef	1 oz	4	64	56%
Light & Lean (Hormel) Lunch Meats				
BBQ Ham	2 slices	2	50	36%
Black Peppered Ham	2 slices	2	50	36%
Bologna	2 slices	12	140	77%
Bologna-thin sliced	2 slices	6	70	77%
Breast of Turkey	2 slices	2	60	30%
Canadian Style Bacon	2 slices	1	35	26%
Chopped Ham	2 slices	4	70	51%
Cooked Ham	2 slices	2	50	36%
Cotto Salami	2 slices	6	80	68%

Food and Description	Amount	Fat Grams	Total Calories	% Fat Calories
Glazed Ham	2 slices	2	50	36%
Ham & Cheese Loaf	2 slices	6	90	60%
New England Brand Luncheon Meat	2 slices	6	90	60%
Pickle Loaf	2 slices	6	100	54%
Red Peppered Ham	2 slices	2	50	36%
Smoked Cooked Ham	2 slices	2	50	36%
Spiced Luncheon Meat	2 slices	9	120	68%
Summer Sausage	2 slices	8	100	72%
Liver Cheese-Pork	1 oz	7	86	73%
Liver Loaf (Hormel)	2 slices	13	160	73%
Liver Sausage, Liverwurst/Pork (Oscar Meyer)	1 oz	8	93	77%
sliced	1 oz	9	95	85%
tube	1 oz	9	95	85%
(Louis Rich) Cold Cuts				
Chopped Turkey Ham	1 slice	2	40	45%
Deli-Thin				
Hickory Smoked Chicken Breast	1 slice	< 1	12	38%
Hickory Smoked Turkey Breast				
98% fat free	1 slice	< 1	10	45%
Honey Roasted Turkey Breast	1 slice	< 1	12	38%
Oven Roasted Turkey Breast	1 slice	< 1	12	38%
Oven Roasted Chicken Breast	1 slice	< 1	12	38%
Turkey Ham-smoked				
96% fat free	1 slice	< 1	12	38%
Mild Turkey Bologna	1 slice	5	60	75%
Turkey Bologna	1 slice	5	60	75%
82% fat free	1 slice	4	45	80%
Turkey Cotto Salami				
90% fat free	1 slice	3	40	68%
Turkey Luncheon Loaf	1 slice	3	45	60%
Turkey Pastrami-round	1 slice	1	35	26%
Turkey Pastrami-square	1 slice	.5	25	18%
Turkey Salami	1 slice	4	55	66%
Turkey Summer Sausage	1 slice	4	55	66%
Lumberjack Beef Roll-dry (Hormel)	1 oz	9	101	80%
Luncheon meat, beef-sliced thin smoked beef (97% fat free)	1 oz 2 slices	.9	35	23%
	~.5 oz	1.5	20	68%
spiced (Hormel)				
canned	3 oz	26	280	84%
pkg	2 slices	9	118	69%
Luncheon Loaf-chicken (Hormel)				
canned	2 oz	10	130	69%

Food and Description	Amount	Fat Grams	Total Calories	% Fat Calories
Luxury Loaf	1 oz	1	40	23%
Macaroni-Cheese Loaf (Eckrich)	1 oz/			
	1 slice	6	75	72%
Minced Roll Sausage (Eckrich)	1 oz/			
	1 slice	7	80	79%
Mortadella-Beef/Pork	1 oz	7	88	72%
Mother's Loaf	1 oz	6	80	68%
New England Brand Sausage	1 oz	2	46	39%
Old Fashioned Loaf-Pork and Beef	1 oz	5	68	66%
(Eckrich)	1 oz	6	70	77%
Olive Loaf-Beef & Pork				
(Eckrich)	1 oz	6	80	68%
Pork	1 oz	4.68	67	63%
(Hormel)	2 slices	7	110	57%
(Oscar Meyer) Cold Cuts				
Bar-B-Que Loaf-93% fat free	1 slice	2	50	36%
Beef-smoked-97% fat-free	1 slice	.5	15	30%
Bologna-Beef & Pork	1 oz	8	90	80%
Wisconsin Made Ring Bologna	1 oz	8	85	85%
w/cheese	1 oz	7	75	84%
Chicken Breast-oven roasted-97% fat-free	1 slice	.5	30	15%
Chicken Breast-smoked-97% fat-free	1 slice	.5	25	18%
Chopped Ham w/natural juices	1 slice	4	50	72%
Corned Beef-98% fat-free	1 slice	.5	15	30%
Corned Beef Loaf, jellied-93% fat-free	1 slice	2	40	45%
Cotto Salami	1 slice	4	50	72%
Cotto Salami-beef	1 slice	4	45	80%
Genoa Salami	1 slice	3	35	77%
Ham-baked w/natural juices (97% fat-free)	1 slice	.5	20	23%
Ham-boiled w/natural juices (96% fat-free)	1 slice	.5	25	18%
Ham-chopped, peppered w/ natural juices	1 slice	4	55	66%
Ham-Cracked Black Pepper (96% fat-free)	1 slice	1	25	36%
Ham-Honey w/natural juices (96% fat-free)	1 slice	< 1	25	18%
Ham-Lower Salt-95% fat free (water added)	1 slice	1	25	36%
Ham-Smoked Cooked-96% fat-free	1 slice	< 1	20	18%
Ham & Cheese Loaf	1 slice	5	70	64%
Head Cheese	1 slice	4	55	66%

Food and Description	Amount	Fat Grams	Total Calories	% Fat Calories
Honey Loaf-95% fat-free	1 slice	1	35	26%
Honey Roll Sausage-beef-90% fat-free	1 slice	2	35	51%
Jalapeno Loaf	1 slice	6	70	77%
Liver Cheese, pork fat wrapped	1 slice	10	115	78%
Lunchables				
Deluxe				
Lean Chicken & Lean Roast Beef	1 pkg	25	420	54%
Lean Chicken & Lean Turkey	1 pkg	24	410	53%
Lean Ham & Lean Roast Beef	1 pkg	27	430	57%
Lean Honey Ham & Lean Chicken	1 pkg	22	400	50%
Lean Turkey & Lean Ham	1 pkg	23	390	53%
Original				
Bologna & American	1 pkg	38	480	70%
Chicken & Monterey Jack	1 pkg	22	360	55%
Ham & Cheddar	1 pkg	25	370	61%
Ham & Swiss	1 pkg	21	350	54%
Lean Ham & Cheddar	1 pkg	25	325	61%
Lean Turkey & Cheddar	1 pkg	23	360	58%
Salami & Mozzerella	1 pkg	29	420	62%
Smoked Turkey & Monterey Jack	1 pkg	22	360	55%
W/Dessert				
Lean Chicken & Monterey Jack	1 pkg	23	380	54%
Lean Ham & Swiss	1 pkg	23	380	54%
Lean Honey Ham & American	1 pkg	23	450	46%
Lean Honey Turkey & Cheddar	1 pkg	26	460	51%
Luncheon Meat	1 slice	9	100	90%
Luxury Loaf-95% fat-free	1 slice	1	40	23%
New England Brand Sausage				
(92% fat-free)	1 slice	2	30	60%
Old Fashioned Loaf	1 slice	5	70	64%
Olive Loaf	1 slice	4	60	60%
Pastrami-97% fat free	1 slice	.5	15	30%
Peppered Loaf-93% fat-free	1 slice	2	40	45%
Pickle & Pimento Loaf	1 slice	4	60	60%
Picnic Loaf	1 slice	4	60	60%
Salami for Beer	1 slice	5	55	82%
Salami for Beer-beef	1 slice	6	65	83%
Salami-beef-Machiaeh Brand	1 slice	5	60	75%
Salami-hard	1 slice	3	35	77%
Sausage-Beef Smokies	1 link	11	120	83%
Summer sausage				
(Thuringer) Cervelat	1 slice	6	70	77%
Summer sausage-beef				
(Thuringer) Cervelat	1 slice	6	70	77%

Food and Description	Amount	Fat Grams	Total Calories	% Fat Calories
Thin Sliced meats-96% fat free				
Boiled Ham	1 slice	< 1	12	38%
Honey Ham	1 slice	< 1	14	32%
Roast Beef	1 slice	< 1	14	32%
Roast Chicken	1 slice	< 1	14	32%
Roast Turkey	1 slice	< 1	12	38%
Turkey Breast-oven roasted				
(97% fat-free)	1 slice	.5	20	23%
Turkey Breast-smoked (98% fat free)	1 slice	.5	20	23%
Pastrami				
Beef	1 oz	8	99	73%
Thin sliced (Carl Buddig)	1 oz	2	40	45%
Turkey	2 oz	3.5	80	39%
Pate-Chicken Liver/canned	1 Tbs	1.7	26	59%
	1 oz	3.7	57	58%
Pate-generic/canned	1 oz	7.9	90	79%
Pate-Goose Liver (de fois gras)-canned	1 Tbs	5.7	60	86%
	1 oz	12	131	82%
smoked-canned	1 oz	12	131	82%
Pate-Liver, Sells (Underwood) canned	2¼ oz	16	190	76%
Peppered Loaf/Beef, Pork	1 oz	1.8	42	39%
(Eckrich)	1 slice/1 oz	1	35	26%
Pepperoni/Pork, Beef	~ 9 oz	110	1248	79%
	1 oz	12	135	80%
(Hormel)	2 slices	7	80	79%
Bits	1 Tbs	3	35	77%
dry	1 oz	13	140	84%
chunk-chub	1 oz	12	140	77%
Leoni Brand	1 oz	12	130	83%
Rosa	1 oz	13	140	84%
Rosa Grande	1 oz	13	140	84%
Pickle Loaf				
(Eckrich)	1oz/1 slice	6	80	68%
(Hormel)	2 slices	7	102	62%
Pickle & Pimento Loaf-Pork	1 oz	5.99	74	73%
Picnic Loaf-Pork/Beef	1 oz	4.7	66	64%
Polish Sausage/Pork	1 oz	8	92	78%
10" long-1.5" dia	1 sausage	6.5	74	79%
	1 oz	8	92	78%
frozen (Schwan's)	1 link/2.7 oz	24	260	83%
(Hormel)	2 sausages	14	170	74%
(Oscar Meyer) International	~ 2.5 oz	20	230	78%
Pork/Slender sliced (Eckrich)	1 oz	2	45	40%
Pork Luncheon Meat (Hormel)-canned	3 oz	21	240	79%

Food and Description	Amount	Fat Grams	Total Calories	% Fat Calories
Pork & Beef Luncheon Sausage	~ 1 oz	4.8	60	72%
Potted Meat				
(Armour Star)	1.5 oz	6	80	68%
(Hormel)	1 Tbs	2	30	60%
(Libby's)	1.83 oz	9	110	74%
Salami/cooked-Beef	1 oz	5.9	74	72%
(Hormel)	2 slices	5	50	90%
cooked-Beef and Pork	1 oz	5.7	71	72%
cooked-Turkey	2 oz	7.8	111	63%
hard (Hormel)	2 slices	7	80	79%
dry	1 oz	10	110	82%
(Health Valley)	3.5 oz	35	400	79%
(Hebrew National) beef-original				
deli style	1 oz	7	80	79%
party-dry (Hormel)	1 oz	8	90	80%
Piccolo-dry stick (Hormel)	1 oz	11	120	83%
Salami/Pork-dry or hard	2 slices/			
	~1 oz	7	85	74%
Salt Pork/raw	1 oz	22.8	212	97%
Sandwich Spread/Pork, Beef	1 Tbs	3	35	77%
Sausage				
Beef-smoked (Eckrich)	1 oz	9	100	81%
Beef & Pork-smoked links	1 link/~.5 oz	4.9	54	82%
Brown'N Serve (Hormel)/cooked	2	13	140	84%
uncooked	2	17	180	85%
smoked skinless (Eckrich)	1 oz	16	180	80%
New England Brand (Eckrich)	1 slice/1 oz	1	35	26%
Patties (Hormel)/canned-hot	1 pattie	13	150	78%
mild	1 pattie	13	150	78%
Pork-fresh-cooked	~ 1 oz	8	100	72%
Pork (Hormel)				
Little Sizzlers-cooked	2	9	103	79%
Midget Links	2	13	143	82%
Pork-smoked links	1 link/~.5 oz	5	62	73%
Smoked (Eckrich)/Lite	1 link	13	150	78%
	1 oz	6	70	77%
Smoked (Oscar Meyer)-International	1 oz	7	83	76%
Smoked pork (Hormel)	3 oz	27	290	84%
Smoked turkey (Butterball)	1 oz	3	50	54%
Smoked turkey (Louis Rich)	1 oz	3	50	54%
Smoked turkey (Louis Rich)				
w/cheese	1 oz	4	55	66%
Smokie Cheezers (Hormel)	2 sausages	15	168	80%
Smokie Links (Oscar Meyer)	~ 1.5 oz	11	125	79%

Food and Description	Amount	Fat Grams	Total Calories	% Fat Calories
Smokies-Beef (Oscar Meyer)	~ 1.5 oz	11	125	79%
Smokies-Cheese (Oscar Meyer)	~ 1.5 oz	11	125	79%
Smokies-Little (Oscar Meyer)	9 grams	3	30	90%
Smokies Smoked (Hormel)	2 sausages	14	160	79%
Scrapple	1 oz	4	61	59%
Smok-Y-Links (Eckrich)				
Beef	2 links	14	160	79%
Cheese	2 links	14	160	79%
Ham	2 links	15	160	84%
Hot	2 links	14	150	84%
Lite	2 links	10	120	75%
Maple-flavored	2 links	14	160	79%
Original	2 links	14	160	79%
Souse	1 slice/1 oz	3.8	51	67%
Spam (Hormel)/deviled	1 Tbs	3	35	77%
lite	2 oz	12	140	77%
luncheon	1¾ oz	14	150	84%
	2 oz	15	170	79%
smoke-flavored	2 oz	15	170	79%
w/ cheese chunks	2 oz	15	170	79%
Spreads				
Chicken-canned	1 oz	3	55	49%
Chicken (Hormel)	½ oz	2	30	60%
Chicken (Swanson)-chunky	1 oz	4	60	60%
Chicken (Underwood)-chunky				
Light	2⅛ oz	5	100	45%
Original	2⅛ oz	9	150	54%
Smokey-Flavored	2⅛ oz	8	190	38%
Corned Beef (Hormel)	½ oz	3	35	77%
Liverwurst (Hormel)	½ oz	3	35	77%
(Underwood)	2.25 oz	16	190	76%
Roast Beef				
(Hormel)	½ oz	2	31	58%
(Underwood)				
Light	2⅛ oz	6	90	40%
Mesquite Smoked	2⅛ oz	11	140	71%
Original	2⅛ oz	11	140	71%
The Spreadables (Carnation/Libby's)				
Chicken Salad	1.9 oz	6	90	60%
Ham Salad	1.9 oz	3	70	39%
Tuna Salad	1.9 oz	5	80	56%
Turkey Salad	1.9 oz	6	100	54%
Summer Sausage				
Beef	~ 1 oz	7.6	86	80%

Food and Description	Amount	Fat Grams	Total Calories	% Fat Calories
Beef & Pork (Eckrich)	1 slice/1 oz	7	90	70%
(Hormel)	2 slices	11	140	71%
beefy dry	1 oz	9	100	81%
Tangy dry chub	1 oz	7	90	70%
Thuringer dry	1 oz	9	90	90%
Turkey	1 slice/1 oz	3.5	52	61%
Thuringer				
Cervelat	1 oz	8.5	98	78%
Old Smokehouse				
chub	1 oz	9	100	81%
dry (Hormel)	1 oz	8	90	80%
sliced	1 oz	9	100	81%
Tongue, Lunch (Armour Star)	3 oz	14	200	63%
Turkey Breast Meat	~ 1.5 oz	.67	47	13%
(Butterball)				
honey roasted 97% fat free	¾ oz	1	30	30%
oven roasted	1 slice/1 oz	1	30	30%
smoked	1 slice/1 oz	1	35	26%
smoked 97% fat free	¾ oz	1	25	36%
(Danola)				
smoked/deli sliced	1 oz	<1	30	15%
(Eckrich) Lite-oven roasted	1 oz	1	30	30%
Lite-smoked	1 oz	.5	30	15%
(Hormel)	2 slices	2	60	30%
smoked	2 slices	2	60	30%
(Weaver)	1 slice	<1	20	23%
Turkey Ham	2 oz	2.88	73	36%
(Butterball) chopped	1 slice/1 oz	1	35	26%
cold cuts	1 slice/1 oz	1	35	26%
Deli thin	1 oz	1	35	26%
honey cured	1 slice/1 oz	1	35	26%
(Carl Buddig) Thin sliced	1 oz	2	40	45%
(Weaver)	1 slice	1	23	39%
Turkey Pastrami (Butterball)				
cold cuts	1 slice/1 oz	1	30	30%
Deli	1 oz	1	35	26%
Slice'N Serve	1 oz	1	35	26%
Turkey Roll-Light and Dark Meat	1 oz	1.98	42	42%
Turkey Roll-Light Meat	1 oz	2	42	43%
Turkey Salami				
(Butterball)	1 slice/1 oz	4	50	72%
Deli	1 oz	4	50	72%
Slice'N Serve	1 oz	4	50	72%
variety pak	¾ oz	3	40	90%

Food and Description	Amount	Fat Grams	Total Calories	% Fat Calories
(Carl Buddig) Thin sliced	1 oz	2	40	45%
Turkey-Slender sliced (Eckrich)	1 oz	2	45	40%
Thin sliced (Carl Buddig)	1 oz	2	40	45%
Turkey-Smoked (Butterball)				
variety pak	¾ oz	1	25	36%
Turkey Spread	~ 2 oz	6	100	54%
(Underwood) Chunky-Light	2⅛ oz	2	75	24%
(Tyson) Deli Meats				
Chicken Bologna	1 slice	.5	44	10%
Chicken Roll	1 slice	.5	26	17%
Hickory Smoked Breast	1 slice	1	25	36%
Honey Flavored Chicken Breast	1 slice	1	25	36%
Oven Roasted Breast	1 slice	.5	25	18%
Oven Roasted Mesquite Breast	1 slice	1	25	36%
Turkey Breast	1 slice	< 1	20	18%
Turkey Ham	1 slice	< 1	23	8%
Vienna Sausage/canned				
Beef and pork	1 sausage	4	45	80%
(Hormel) no broth	4 sausages	18	200	81%
(Libby's)				
in Barbeque Sauce	2.5 oz	15	180	75%
in Beef Broth				
5 oz can	3½ links	15	160	84%
9 oz can	3½ links	14	160	79%
Chicken				
(Hormel)	4 sausages	16	180	80%
(Libby's)	2 oz	10	130	69%
Generic	7 sausages	28	315	80%
(Weight Watchers)				
Deli Meats				
Honey Roasted Ham	1 oz	< 1	45	10%
Oven Roasted Beef	1 oz	1	30	90%
Oven Roasted Chicken Breast	1 oz	< 1	25	18%
Oven Roasted Turkey Breast	1 oz	< 1	25	18%
Premium Baked Ham	1 oz	2	35	77%
Premium Bologna	1 oz	3	45	60%
Premium Cooked Ham	1 oz	< 1	30	15%
Smoked Turkey Breast	1 oz	< 1	30	15%
Deli Thin Slices				
Oven Roasted				
Cured Beef	⅓ oz	< 1	10	45%
Ham	⅓ oz	< 1	12	38%
Honey Ham	⅓ oz	< 1	12	38%
Premium Smoked Ham	⅓ oz	< 1	12	38%

Food and Description	Amount			
Roasted & Smoked				
Chicken Breast	⅓ oz	< 1	10	45%
Turkey Breast	⅓ oz	< 1	10	45%
Oven Roasted				
Honey Ham	¾ oz	1	25	36%
Smoked Ham	¾ oz	1	25	36%
Turkey Breast	¾ oz	1	25	36%
Turkey Ham	¾ oz	1	25	36%
Premium				
Bologna	¾ oz	2	35	51%
Cooked Ham	¾ oz	1	25	36%
Roasted & Smoked				
Chicken Breast	¾ oz	1	25	36%
Turkey Breast	¾ oz	1	25	36%
LUPINS				
boiled	½ cup	2	98	18%
raw	½ cup	8	330	22%

M

Food and Description	Amount	Fat Grams	Total Calories	% Fat Calories
MACADAMIA NUT				
dried	1 oz	20.9	199	95%
dry roasted	1 oz	21	193	98%
oil roasted	1 oz	21.7	204	96%
MACARONI (*See* PASTA)				
MACARONI AND CHEESE (*See also* PASTA ENTREE/DINNER)				
Canned	1 cup	9.6	228	38%
(Franco-American) frozen	7 oz	9	220	37%
(Golden Grain) dry	1.81 oz	2	190	10%
prepared	½ cup	15	300	45%
Standard Home Recipe (USDA)	1 cup	22	430	46%
(Swanson's) frozen	10 oz	21	400	47%
MACARONI SALAD				
canned (Joan of Arc)	½ cup	13	200	59%
MACAROON (*See* COOKIE)				

Food and Description	Amount	Fat Grams	Total Calories	% Fat Calories
MACE/ground	1 tsp	.6	8	68%
MACKEREL				
Atlantic				
cooked-dry heat	3 oz	15	223	61%
raw	3 oz	11.8	174	61%
Jack-canned	1 cup	11.97	296	36%
King-raw	3 oz	1.7	89	17%
Spanish				
cooked-dry heat	3 oz	5	134	34%
raw	3 oz	5	118	38%
MALT (See individual FAST FOOD listings; MILK MIXES)				
MAMEY or MAMMEE APPLE				
raw, whole	1 med	4.4	446	9%
MANDARIN ORANGE (See also TANGERINE)				
canned in juice	1 cup	–	92	–
canned in light syrup	1 cup	.5	125	4%
(Del Monte)	5.5 oz	< 1	100	5%
(Dole) light syrup	½ cup	< 1	76	6%
(Nutradiet)	½ cup	–	28	
(S&W)				
natural style	½ cup	–	60	–
sections in heavy syrup	½ cup	< 1	76	6%
MANDARIN TANGERINE JUICE (See TANGERINE JUICE)				
MANGO	1	.57	135	4%
diced/sliced	1 cup	.7	109	6%
MANGO NECTAR				
(Kern's)	6 oz	–	110	–
MANICOTTI (See also FROZEN ENTREE/DINNER; PASTA ENTREE/DINNER)				
Standard Home Recipe (USDA)				
w/meat sauce	~ 5 oz	11	235	42%
w/tomato sauce	5 oz	10	223	45%
MARGARINE/MARGARINE SPREAD				
(Autumn) Spread	1 Tbs	8	80	100%
(Blue Bonnet)				
Reduced Calorie	1 Tbs	6	50	100%
Soft or Stick	1 Tbs	11	100	100%
Spread				
52% fat	1 Tbs	8	80	100%
75% fat	1 Tbs	11	90	100%
Whipped				
Soft	1 Tbs	7	70	100%
Stick	1 Tbs	7	70	100%
(Chiffon)				
Soft stick	1 Tbs	11	100	100%

Food and Description	Amount	Fat Grams	Total Calories	% Fat Calories
Soft tub	1 Tbs	10	90	100%
Whipped	1 Tbs	8	70	100%
(Country Crock)				
Churn style	1 Tbs	9	80	100%
Classic 64% Spread Sticks	1 Tbs	9	80	100%
Corn Oil Spread	1 Tbs	9	80	100%
Original	1 Tbs	9	80	100%
Squeeze	1 Tbs	9	80	100%
Whipped Honey Spread	1 Tbs	9	90	90%
(Dairybrook) Sticks	1 Tbs	5.8	50	100%
(Fleischmann's)				
Light Corn Oil Spread				
Soft or Stick	1 Tbs	8	80	100%
Squeeze	1 Tbs	10	90	100%
Move Over Butter Spread				
Sticks	1 Tbs	10	90	100%
Tub	1 Tbs	10	90	100%
Reduced Calorie	1 Tbs	6	50	100%
Soft or Stick	1 Tbs	11	100	100%
Whipped	1 Tbs	7	70	100%
Generic				
Hard	1 Tbs	11	100	100%
	1 Pat	4	35	100%
	4 oz	91	810	100%
Soft	1 Tbs	11	100	100%
	4 oz	92	813	100%
Spread				
40% fat/soft	1 Tbs	5.7	50	100%
	4 oz	44	393	100%
60% fat				
Hard	1 Pat	3	25	100%
	1 Tbs	9	75	100%
	4 oz	69	610	100%
Soft	1 Tbs	9	75	100%
	4 oz	69	613	100%
Squeeze	1 tsp	3.8	34	100%
Whipped/hard & soft	1 Tbs	7	70	100%
(Gold-N-Sweet) Canola	1 Tbs	11	100	100%
(Gregg's) Gold-n-Soft-Lite Spread	1 Tbs	7	70	100%
(Hain) Safflower-Regular and				
Unsalted	1 Tbs	11	100	100%
(Heart Beat) Heart Smart				
Spread (tub)	1 Tbs	3	25	100%
(Heartlight) Canola	1 Tbs	11	100	100%

Food and Description	Amount	Fat Grams	Total Calories	% Fat Calories
I Can't Believe It's Not Butter	1 Tbs	10	90	100%
Light Spread				
Sticks	1 Tbs	7	60	100%
Tub	1 Tbs	7	60	100%
(Imperial)				
A La Mode	1 Tbs	7.5	70	100%
A La Mode Sticks	1 Tbs	11	100	100%
Light	1 Tbs	6	60	100%
Quarters	1 Tbs	11	100	100%
Savory Squeeze				
Buttery	1 Tbs	10	90	100%
Garlic & Herb	1 Tbs	10	90	100%
Soft	1 Tbs	11	100	100%
Soft Diet	1 Tbs	6	50	100%
Whipped	1 Tbs	5.6	50	100%
(Kraft) Touch of Butter				
40% fat-Tub	1 Tbs	6	50	100%
50% fat-Stick	1 Tbs	7	60	100%
(Land O'Lakes)				
Premium Corn Oil	1 tsp	4	35	100%
Soft or Stick	1 tsp	4	35	100%
Soy oil-regular	1 tsp	4	35	100%
Liquid	1 tsp	3.8	34	100%
Regular-80% fat (hard)	1 Tbs	11	100	100%
	1 Pat	4	35	100%
(soft)	1 Tbs	11	100	100%
Spread-40% fat (soft)	1 Tbs	5.7	50	100%
60% fat (hard)	1 Tbs	9	75	100%
	1 Pat	3	25	100%
(soft)	1 Tbs	9	75	100%
Tub	1 tsp	3	25	100%
(Latta)	1 Tbs	5.6	50	100%
(Mazola)	1 Tbs	11	100	100%
Reduced Calorie				
Light Corn Oil	1 Tbs	6	50	100%
Regular	1 Tbs	6	50	100%
(Miracle Brand)				
Whipped				
Soft	1 Tbs	7	60	100%
Stick	1 Tbs	7	70	100%
(Mrs. Filberts)				
Corn Oil Family Spread	1 Tbs	7	65	100%
Golden Quarters	1 Tbs	11	100	100%
Soft Corn	1 Tbs	11	100	100%

Food and Description	Amount	Fat Grams	Total Calories	% Fat Calories
Soft Gold	1 Tbs	11	100	100%
Vegetable Oil	1 Tbs	7	65	100%
(Nucoa)				
Heart Beat-corn oil	1 Tbs	3	25	100%
No burn	1 Tbs	11	100	100%
Soft	1 Tbs	11	100	100%
(Parkay)				
50% vegetable oil	1 Tbs	7	60	100%
Light Corn Oil	1 Tbs	8	70	100%
Liquid				
Regular	1 Tbs	11	100	100%
Spread	1 Tbs	10	90	100%
Reduced Calorie	1 Tbs	6	50	100%
Soft or Stick	1 Tbs	11	100	100%
Whipped				
Soft or Stick	1 Tbs	7	70	100%
(Promise)	1 Tbs	10	90	100%
Extra Light	1 Tbs	6	50	100%
Sunflower oil	1 Tbs	10	90	100%
Ultra (tub) Spread	1 Tbs	4	35	100%
(Shedd's)				
Churn Style	1 Tbs	7	60	100%
Corn Oil	1 Tbs	7	70	100%
Country Crock	1 Tbs	7	70	100%
Whipped	1 Tbs	11	100	100%
(Touch of Butter) spread/stick	1 Tbs	10	90	100%
(Weight Watchers)				
Country Cottage (tub) Spread	1 Tbs	4	45	100%
Extra Light Spread Tubs				
Regular	1 Tbs	6	50	100%
Sweet Unsalted	1 Tbs	6	50	100%
Light Sticks	1 Tbs	7	60	100%
(Willow Run Print) Sticks	1 Tbs	11	100	100%
MARINADES (See also SEASONINGS)				
Bottle or Jar				
(Golden Dipt)				
Cajun Style Barbecue Sauce	1 oz	8	90	80%
Ginger Teriyaki	1 oz	7	120	53%
Lemon Herb	1 oz	14	130	97%
Mix				
(Durkee)	½ cup	.7	28	23%
(French's)	⅛ pkg	–	10	–
(Kikkoman)	1 oz pkg	–	64	–
MARINARA SAUCE (See SAUCE)				

Food and Description	Amount	Fat Grams	Total Calories	% Fat Calories
MARIONBERRIES				
frozen (Schwan's)				
no sugar	3.5 oz	–	60	–
MARJORAM/dried	1 tsp	–	2	–
MARSHMALLOW				
(Campfire)				
large	2	–	40	–
miniature	10	–	17	–
	24	–	40	–
(Kraft)				
Funmallows	1	–	30	–
miniature	10	–	18	–
Jet Puffed	1	–	25	–
miniature	10	–	18	–
Marshmallow Creme (Kraft)	1 oz	–	90	–
Miniature or large	1 oz	–	94	–
MATZO				
(Goodman's)				
Passover Egg	1 piece	1	132	7%
Passover	1 piece	–	129	–
(Manischewitz)				
American	1 board	1.9	115	15%
Egg n/Onion	1 board	1	112	8%
Miniatures	15-20 crackers	.5	90	5%
Passover	1 board	–	129	–
Passover Egg	10 crackers	2	108	17%
Passover Egg	1 board	2	132	14%
Thin Salted	1 board	–	100	–
Thin Tea				
(Daily)	1 board	–	103	–
Thins, dietic	1 board	1	91	10%
Unsalted				
(Daily)	1 board	–	110	–
Wheat	10 crackers	1	90	10%
Whole Wheat w/bran	1 board	.6	110	5%
MATZO MEAL				
(Goodman's) Passover	1 cup	1	514	2%
(Manischewitz)	1 cup	1	510	2%
MAYONNAISE (See also SALAD DRESSING)				
(Bama) Regular	1 Tbs	11	100	100%
(Bennett's) Real	1 Tbs	12	110	98%
(Best Foods)				
Light	1 Tbs	5	50	90%
Real	1 Tbs	11	100	99%

Food and Description	Amount	Fat Grams	Total Calories	% Fat Calories
(Estee)	1 Tbs	10	100	90%
(Hain)				
Canola				
Light Reduced Calorie	1 Tbs	5	60	75%
Regular	1 Tbs	11	100	100%
Cold-Processed	1 Tbs	12	110	98%
Eggless	1 Tbs	12	110	98%
Light	1 Tbs	6	60	90%
Real	1 Tbs	12	110	98%
Safflower	1 Tbs	12	110	98%
(Heart Beat) corn oil	1 Tbs	4	40	90%
(Hellman's)	1 Tbs	11	100	100%
(Hollywood)				
Canola	1 Tbs	12	110	100%
Safflower	1 Tbs	12	110	98%
(Kraft)				
Cholesterol free	1 Tbs	10	90	100%
Kraft Free	1 Tbs	–	12	–
Light	1 Tbs	5	50	90%
Regular	1 Tbs	12	100	100%
(Life All Natural) egg-free	1 Tbs	8	70	100%
(Miracle Whip) Free	1 Tbs	–	20	–
(Weight Watchers)				
Mayonnaise-Style Dressing				
Fat Free	1 Tbs	–	50	–
Light	1 Tbs	5	50	90%
Low Sodium	1 Tbs	5	50	90%

MEAL REPLACEMENT (See NUTRITIONAL SUPPLEMENTS)
MEAT SEASONINGS (See SEASONINGS)
MEAT SPREAD (See LUNCHEON MEAT)
MEAT SUBSTITUTES (See also VEGETARIAN FOOD)

Food and Description	Amount	Fat Grams	Total Calories	% Fat Calories
Numette	2.5 oz	11	150	66%
Tender Cuts	2.2 oz	1	60	15%
MEAT TENDERIZER/seasoned	1 tsp	–	2	–
MEATLESS LOAF	1 oz	.7	90	7%

MEATLOAF (See FROZEN ENTREE/DINNER)
MELBA TOAST (See also CRISPBREAD)

Food and Description	Amount	Fat Grams	Total Calories	% Fat Calories
(Devonsheer)				
Garlic, Sesame,				
Onion, Rye, Honey Bran	1 slice	–	12	–
White, Plain, & Vegetable Toast	1 slice	–	16	–
(Lance) Melba Toast-Oblong	2 slices	–	30	–
Round-garlic	2 slices	1	20	45%
Round-onion	2 slices	1	20	45%

Food and Description	Amount	Fat Grams	Total Calories	% Fat Calories
Round-plain	2 slices	1	20	45%
Sesame	2 slices	1	25	36%
(Old London) Melba Toast				
Onion	3 slices	< 1	50	9%
Pumpernickle	3 slices	< 1	50	9%
Rye	3 slices	< 1	50	9%
Sesame	3 slices	2	50	36%
Sesame-unsalted	3 slices	2	50	36%
Wheat	3 slices	< 1	50	9%
White	3 slices	< 1	50	9%
White-Unsalted	3 slices	< 1	50	9%
Whole Grain	3 slices	< 1	50	9%
Whole Grain unsalted	3 slices	< 1	50	9%
(Old London) Snacks				
Bacon	5 rounds	1	50	18%
Cheese	5 rounds	< 1	50	9%
Garlic	5 rounds	1	50	18%
Onion	5 rounds	1	50	18%
Rye	5 rounds	1	50	18%
Sesame Rounds	5 rounds	2	56	32%
White	5 rounds	1	50	18%
Whole Grain	5 rounds	1	50	18%
MELON (*See* individual listings, such as CANTALOUPE, HONEYDEW, etc.)				
MELON BALLS/frozen	1 cup	.5	58	8%
sweetened	1 cup	.5	245	2%
MEXICAN FOOD (*See also* FROZEN ENTREE/DINNER)				
■ **ACAPULCO DIP** (Ortega)	1 oz	–	8	–
■ **BEAN DIP**				
Hot (Hain)	4 Tbs	1	70	13%
Jalapeno-Flavored (Wise)	2 Tbs	–	25	–
Mexican (Hain)	4 Tbs	1	60	15%
Onion	4 Tbs	1	70	13%
■ **BURRITO**				
Frozen				
(BR Brand)				
Bean & Cheese	5 oz	6	290	19%
Beef & Bean	5 oz	15	400	34%
Green Chili	5 oz	9	340	24%
Red Chili	5 oz	5	290	16%
(El Charrito)				
Bean & Cheese	5 oz	8	320	23%
Grande	6 oz	8	380	19%
Beef & Bean	5 oz	12	350	31%
Beef Grande	6 oz	16	430	33%
Grande	6 oz	16	430	34%

Food and Description	Amount	Fat Grams	Total Calories	% Fat Calories
Green Chili	5 oz	13	350	33%
Green Chili Grande	6 oz	14	410	31%
Jalapeno Grande	6 oz	15	410	33%
Red Chili	5 oz	13	360	33%
Red Chili Grande	6 oz	15	410	33%
Red Hot Beef & Bean	5 oz	11	330	30%
(Hormel)	1	8	205	35%
Burrito Grande	5.5 oz	16	380	38%
Cheese	1	5	210	21%
Chicken & Rice	1	4	200	18%
Hot Chili Burrito	1	8	240	30%
(Old El Paso)				
Beef & Bean				
Hot	1	11	310	32%
Medium	1	13	330	35%
Mild	1	11	320	31%
Bean & Cheese	1	11	330	30%
(Patio)				
Britos				
Beef & Bean	3 oz	9	210	39%
Nacho Beef	3 oz	11	220	45%
Nacho Cheese	3.63 oz	10	250	36%
Spicy Chicken & Cheese	3 oz	9	210	39%
Burritos				
Hot Beef & Bean Red Chili	5 oz	13	340	34%
Medium Beef & Bean	5 oz	16	370	39%
Mild Beef & Bean Green Chili	5 oz	12	330	33%
Red Hot Beef & Bean	5 oz	15	360	38%
(Schwan's) Beef & Bean	4 oz	7	270	23%
(Weight Watchers)	7.62 oz	12	310	35%
Home Recipe - Beefsteak	6 oz	15	250	54%
■ BURRITO FILLING/MIX				
(Del Monte)	½ cup	1	110	8%
■ CHILI & CHILI BEANS				
Beef Chili w/beans				
canned (Chef Boyardee)	7.5 oz	17	330	46%
Chilee Weenee canned (Van Camp's)	1 cup	16	310	47%
Chili				
canned				
Chicken				
(Armour) Premium				
Lite w/Beans	7.5 oz	11	170	37%
(Cimmaron)	7.5 oz	4	190	19%
(Dennison's)	7.5 oz	15	310	44%
	8 oz	17	340	45%

Food and Description	Amount	Fat Grams	Total Calories	% Fat Calories
Chunky	7.5 oz	14	310	41%
EZO	7 oz	19	330	52%
Hot	7.5 oz	16	310	47%
	8 oz	19	350	49%
(Hain) spicy	7.5 oz	2	130	14%
(Hormel)	7.5 oz	3	200	14%
(Stagg)	7 oz	7	200	32%
Fat-free (Health Valley)	5 oz	–	140	–
Lentil				
(Health Valley)	4 oz	5	110	41%
low sodium	4 oz	6	120	45%
Lite chicken (Dennision's)-w/beans	7.5 oz	5	200	23%
no beans	7.5 oz	5	210	21%
No Beans				
(Armour Star)	7.5 oz	31	390	72%
(Dennison's)	7.5 oz	19	310	55%
	9.5 oz	24	380	57%
(Gebhardt) plain	7.5 oz	32	410	70%
(Hain) Tempeh Spicy	7.5 oz	4	160	23%
(Hormel)	7⅜ oz	28	380	66%
(Libby's)	7.5 oz	30	390	69%
(Stagg) Steak House	7.5 oz	16	280	51%
(Van Camp's)	1 cup	34	410	75%
Vegetarian				
(Hain) Spicy	7.5 oz	1	160	6%
reduced sodium	7.5 oz	1	170	5%
(Health Valley)				
mild	4 oz	6	120	45%
spicy	4 oz	6	120	45%
(Wolf)	1 cup	27	390	62%
Extra Spicy	1 cup	25	360	63%
Turkey				
(Healthy Choice)				
spicey w/beans	7.5 oz	5	210	21%
w/beans	7.5 oz	5	200	23%
W/ Beans				
(Armour Star)				
Hot	7.5 oz	26	390	60%
Regular	7.5 oz	26	390	60%
(Cimmaron) Hot	7.5 oz	9	230	35%
(Dennison's)				
Chunky	7.5 oz	14	310	41%
Cook Off	7.5 oz	19	340	51%
(Estee)	7.5 oz	20	370	49%

Food and Description	Amount	Fat Grams	Total Calories	% Fat Calories
(Featherweight)	7.5 oz	13	270	43%
(Heinz) Hot	7¾ oz	16	330	44%
(Hormel)				
Hot	7⅜ oz	11	250	40%
Regular	7⅜ oz	11	250	40%
(Libby's)	7.5 oz	13	270	43%
	8 oz	14	290	43%
(Stagg)				
Chili Laredo	7.5 oz	15	290	47%
Country Chili	7.5 oz	14	280	45%
(Van Camp's)	1 cup	23	350	59%
(Wolf)	1 cup	22	350	57%
Extra Spicy	1 cup	21	330	57%
Frozen				
(Banquet) Cookin' Bag				
Turkey	4 oz	2	80	23%
(Kraft) w/beef & beans	9.7 oz	22	380	52%
Homemade	1 cup	15	400	34%
Microwave				
No Beans (Hormel)	10.5 oz	22	380	52%
Turkey (Healthy Choice)				
Spicy w/Beans	7.5 oz	5	210	21%
w/Beans	7.5 oz	5	200	23%
Vegetarian (Nile Spice)				
Chili'n Beans Mild	7 oz	1	160	6%
Chili'n Beans Spicy	7 oz	2	170	11%
w/beans (Impromptu)	10 oz	10	330	27%
Mixes				
(Durkee)				
Dry	1 pkt	1.6	148	10%
Prepared	1 cups	25	465	48%
	4 cup	100	1859	48%
(Durkee) Texas Chili Seasoning Mix				
dry	1 pkt	4	151	24%
prepared	2 cups	75	1544	44%
(Hain)	¼ pkg	1	30	30%
(McCormick/Schilling)	¼ pkg	–	5	–
(Kraft) prepared - Good Times				
Chili Fixin's Original w/beans	4 oz	1	80	11%
Chili Fixin's Original w/o beans	4 oz	–	50	–
Chili Fixin's Texas Style w/beans	4 oz	1	90	10%
Chili Fixin's Texas Style w/o beans	4 oz	1	60	15%
Manwich Chili Fixins (Hunt's)				
sauce only	5.3 oz	1	110	8%

Food and Description	Amount	Fat Grams	Total Calories	% Fat Calories
w/regular ground beef	8 oz	14	290	43%
Chili Beans				
canned				
Caliente Style-dry				
(Joan of Arc/Green Giant)	½ cup	1	100	9%
in Chili Gravy				
(Dennison's)	7.5 oz	1	180	5%
(Luck's) Hot-pintos	7.5 oz	2	200	9%
in Sauce (Hormel)	5 oz	3	130	21%
(La Loma)	½ cup	4	120	30%
Mexican Style (Van Camp's)	1 cup	2	210	9%
(S&W)	½ cup	1	130	7%
Chili con Carne				
canned (Heinz)	7¾ oz	21	350	54%
canned w/ beans				
(Chef Boyardee)				
EZO	7 oz	20	340	53%
Hot	7 oz	21	350	54%
frozen w/beans				
(Stouffer's)	8.75 oz	10	260	35%
Microwave				
w/ beans				
(Dennison's)	7.5 oz	13	290	40%
Chunky	7.5 oz	13	280	42%
Hot	7.5 oz	15	310	44%
w/ beans	7⅜ oz	11	250	40%
(Lunch Bucket)				
Regular	8.5 oz	16	330	44%
Hot	8.5 oz	16	330	44%
(Swanson) frozen				
Homestyle Recipe	8.25 oz	10	270	33%
w/o beans				
(Dennison's)	7.5 oz	19	310	55%
(Hormel)	8.25 oz	28	380	66%
Chili Dip (La Victoria)	1 Tbs	–	6	–
Chili Hot Dog Sauce				
(Chef Boyardee)	1 oz	1	30	30%
(Wolf)	⅛ cup	2	40	45%
Chili Mac (*See* PASTA ENTREE/DINNER)				
Chili Makin's				
original (S&W)	½ cup	1	100	9%
Chili Sauce				
(Del Monte)	¼ cup	1	70	13%
(Heinz)	1 Tbs	–	17	–

Food and Description	Amount	Fat Grams	Total Calories	% Fat Calories
Tamalitos in Chili Gravy				
canned (Dennison's)	7.5 oz	16	310	47%
■ CHIMICHANGAS				
Beef				
frozen (Schwan's)	5.8 oz	18	370	44%
homemade w/ cheese	4 oz	15.6	282	50%
■ DINNER MIXES				
(Old El Paso) Mexican Rice	½ cup	2	140	13%
(Pritikin) Mexican Dinner Mix	1 cup	1	170	5%
■ DULCITA				
frozen (Hormel)				
Apple	4 oz	10	290	31%
Cherry	4 oz	9	300	27%
■ ENCHILADA SAUCE				
(Gebhardt)	3 Tbs	1	25	36%
(La Victoria)	1 Tbs	5	80	56%
green chili (Old El Paso)	2 Tbs	–	11	–
hot				
(Del Monte)	¼ cup	–	45	–
(El Molino)	2 Tbs	1	16	56%
(Las Palmas)	½ cup	1	25	36%
(Old El Paso)	¼ cup	1	30	30%
mild				
(Del Monte)	¼ cup	–	45	–
(Old El Paso)	¼ cup	1	25	36%
(Rosarita)	3 oz	< 1	19	24%
mix (Durkee)				
mix only	1 pkg	1.8	89	18%
prepared	4 cups	2.4	229	9%
■ ENCHILADAS				
Beef/Box mix				
(International Lites)				
Enchilada Acapulco-prepared	10 oz	8	250	29%
Beef/frozen				
(Hormel)	1	5	140	32%
(Old El Paso)	2	10	170	53%
(Schwan's)	11.3 oz	17	400	38%
(Van de Kamp's)				
Beef Enchilada	1	12	270	40%
Beef Enchilada Family Pack	¼ pkg	5	150	30%
Beef, Shredded	1	14	360	35%
(Weight Watchers)				
Ranchero	9.12 oz	5	190	24%
Cheese/frozen				
(3) (El Charrito)	11 oz	20	470	38%

Food and Description	Amount	Fat Grams	Total Calories	% Fat Calories
(6) (El Charrito)	16.25 oz	30	780	35%
(Hormel)	1	6	151	36%
(Kraft)	9.8 oz	20	390	46%
(Van de Kamp's)				
Enchilada	1	15	300	45%
Enchilada Dinner	½ pkg	9	220	37%
Enchilada Family Pack	¼ pkg	10	200	45%
Enchilada Ranchero	½ pkg	12	260	42%
(Weight Watchers)				
Ranchero	8.87 oz	10	260	35%
Chicken/frozen				
(Van de Kamp's)				
Chicken Enchilada	½ pkg	11	260	38%
Chicken Enchilada Suiza	½ pkg	10	230	39%
(Weight Watchers)				
Chicken Enchilada Suiza	9 oz	7	230	27%
Chicken Ranchero	7.62 oz	13	310	38%
■ **FAJITAS**				
Frozen				
(Weight Watchers)				
Beef	6.75 oz	7	250	25%
Chicken	6.75 oz	5	270	21%
Mixes				
(McCormick/Schilling)	¼ pkg	< 1	28	16%
■ **FLAUTA**				
frozen (Schwan's)				
apple	2 oz	5	150	30%
cherry	2 oz	3	140	19%
■ **FROZEN ENTREE/DINNER** (See also DINNER MIXES, in this listing)				
(Banquet)				
Chili Gravy & Beef Enchiladas	7 oz	13	270	43%
Extra Helping Dinners				
Mexican Style	19 oz	25	680	33%
Family Entrees				
Chili Sauce w/Beef &				
Beef Enchilada	7 oz	13	270	43%
Healthy Balance				
Chicken Enchiladas	11 oz	4	300	12%
Meals & Platters				
Chimichanga	9.5 oz	9	480	17%
Mexican Style	11 oz	17	410	37%
Mexican Style Combination	11 oz	12	360	30%
(Eagle Crest)				
Beef Enchilada Dinner	13.75 oz	31	620	45%
Beef Enchilada Grande Dinner	21 oz	49	950	46%

Food and Description	Amount	Fat Grams	Total Calories	% Fat Calories
Cheese Enchilada Dinner	13.75 oz	24	570	38%
Chicken Enchilada Dinner	13.75 oz	17	510	30%
Grande Entree				
4 Beef Enchiladas & Beans	16.5 oz	47	890	48%
6 Beef & Cheese Enchiladas	16.25 oz	42	880	43%
6 Beef Enchiladas	16.25 oz	49	880	50%
2 Enchiladas, 2 Tacos, & Beans	16.5 oz	35	800	39%
Mexican Style Dinner	14.25 oz	35	690	46%
Mexican Style Grande Dinner	20 oz	47	850	50%
Queso Beef Dinner	13.50 oz	19	530	32%
Queso Dinner	13.25 oz	16	490	29%
Ranchero Cheese Dinner	13.75 oz	17	480	32%
Santa Fe Beef Enchilada				
Roja Dinner	13.75 oz	23	570	36%
Santa Fe Cheese Enchilada				
Roja Dinner	13.75 oz	18	560	29%
Santa Fe Chicken Enchilada				
Verde Dinner	13.75 oz	13	450	26%
Satillo Dinner	13.50 oz	24	570	38%
Satillo Grande Dinner	20.75 oz	34	820	37%
Suiza Chicken Dinner	13.75 oz	19	510	34%
(El Charrito)				
Beef Enchilada Dinner	13.75 oz	31	620	45%
Burrito Dinner	12 oz	16	517	28%
Cheese Enchilada Dinner	13.25 oz	24	570	38%
Chicken Enchilada Dinner	13.75 oz	17	510	30%
Enchilada Grande Beef Dinner	21 oz	49	950	46%
Grande Satillo Dinner	20.75 oz	34	820	37%
Mexican-Style	14.25 oz	35	690	46%
	20 oz	47	850	50%
Queso Dinner	13.25 oz	16	490	29%
Satillo Dinner	13.25 oz	24	570	38%
(Patio) Dinners				
Beef Enchilada	13.25 oz	24	520	35%
Cheese Enchilada	12 oz	10	370	24%
Combination	12 oz	21	468	40%
Fiesta	12 oz	20	540	33%
Mexican-Style	13.25 oz	25	540	42%
Tamale	13 oz	21	470	45%
(Schwan's)				
Beef Enchilada Dinner	13.45 oz	22	500	40%
Supreme Enchilada Dinner	21 oz	39	870	40%
(Stouffer's)				
Pasta Mexicali	10 oz	31	490	57%

Food and Description	Amount	Fat Grams	Total Calories	% Fat Calories
(Swanson)				
Mexican Hungry Man	20.25 oz	41	820	45%
Mexican-Style Combination	14.25 oz	24	520	42%
(Van de Kamp's)				
Mexican-Style	½ pkg	10	220	41%
■ GAZPACHO (See SOUP)				
■ GREEN CHILI SAUCE				
mild (El Molino)	2 Tbs	–	10	–
■ GREEN CHILIES				
whole	1 chili	–	8	–
(Del Monte)	½ cup	–	20	–
whole, sliced, diced, strips (Ortega)	1 oz	–	10	–
■ HOT PEPPERS				
(Ortega) whole, diced	1 oz	–	8	–
(Vlasic) Mexican tiny hot	1 pepper	–	6	–
■ JALAPENO PEPPERS	2 peppers	1	14	64%
(Del Monte)	½ cup	1	30	30%
(La Victoria)				
Marinated	1 Tbs	–	4	–
Nacho	1 Tbs	–	2	–
(Ortega) whole, diced	1 oz	–	10	–
(Vlasic) Mexican Hot	1 pepper	–	8	–
■ MEXICAN CRISPS				
(Old El Paso)	5 crisps	9	150	54%
■ MEXICALI DOGS				
frozen (Hormel)	5 oz	21	400	47%
■ MEXICAN FIESTA				
box mix-prepared				
(Rice-A-Roni) Savory Calssics	1 serving	4	170	21%
■ MEXICORN				
w/peppers - canned	½ cup	1	80	11%
■ NACHO SAUCE				
(Kaukauna) Cheese	1 oz	6	80	68%
■ NACHOS				
Muy Fresco (Real Fresh)				
frozen-microwave	3.5 oz	9	140	51%
Nachos Pronto! (Old El Paso)				
Microwaveable Kit	3 oz	16	240	60%
■ PICANTE SALSA				
(Old El Paso) Mild, Medium, & Hot	2 Tbs	< 1	10	45%
(Ortega)	1 oz	–	10	–
■ PICANTE SAUCE				
(Old El Paso) Mild, Medium, & Hot	2 Tbs	< 1	8	56%
(Wise)	2 Tbs	–	12	–
■ PICANTE STYLE PINTO BEANS				
dry	½ cup	1	100	9%

Food and Description	Amount	Fat Grams	Total Calories	% Fat Calories
■ **REFRIED BEANS**				
Canned				
(Del Monte)				
plain	½ cup	2	130	14%
(Gebhardt)	4 oz	2	130	14%
(Hain)				
vegetarian	4 oz	1	70	13%
(Little Pancho)				
w/green chili	½ cup	–	80	–
(Old El Paso)	¼ cup	1	50	18%
(Rosarita)				
no fat	4 oz	–	80	–
plain	4 oz	2	130	14%
spicy	4 oz	2	120	15%
vegetarian	4 oz	2	100	18%
w/green chiles	4 oz	2	120	15%
Spicy (Del Monte)	½ cup	2	130	14%
vegetarian (Old El Paso)	½ cup	1	90	10%
w/green chilis (Old El Paso)	½ cup	2	100	18%
w/ sausage (Old El Paso)	½ cup	16	360	40%
■ **SALSA** (*See also* SAUCE)				
(Del Monte)				
Burrito & Rojo mild	¼ cup	–	20	–
Green Chili-mild	¼ cup	–	20	–
Picante				
hot	¼ cup	–	20	–
hot chunky	¼ cup	–	15	–
(Hain)				
hot	¼ cup	–	22	–
mild	¼ cup	–	20	–
(Kaukauna)				
Mexican	1 oz	< 1	14	32%
(La Victoria)				
Brava	1 Tbs	–	6	–
Casera	1 Tbs	–	4	–
Green Chili	1 Tbs	–	3	–
Green Jalapeno	1 Tbs	–	4	–
Omelette	1 Tbs	–	6	–
Picante	1 Tbs	–	4	–
Ranchera	1 Tbs	–	6	–
Red Jalapeno	1 Tbs	–	6	–
Suprema	1 Tbs	–	4	–
Victoria	1 Tbs	–	4	–
(Old El Paso)				
Thick 'n Chunky - Mild, Medium, & Hot	2 Tbs	< 1	6	75%

Food and Description	Amount	Fat Grams	Total Calories	% Fat Calories
(Ortega)				
Green Chili				
mild	½ oz	–	8	–
medium	½ oz	–	6	–
hot	½ oz	–	6	–
(Rosarita)				
hot chunky	3 Tbs	< 1	25	18%
medium chunky	3 Tbs	< 1	25	18%
medium chunky taco	3 Tbs	< 1	25	18%
mild chunky	3 Tbs	< 1	25	18%
mild chunky taco	3 Tbs	< 1	25	18%
(Sonora Valley)				
hot	1 oz	–	10	–
mild	1 oz	–	10	–
■ SANCHOS				
Frozen (Schwan's) beef & bean	5.3 oz	13	300	39%
■ SPANISH RICE (See RICE DISHES)				
■ TACO DIP				
(Hain) & sauce	¼ cup	1	35	26%
(Wise)	2 Tbs	–	12	–
■ TACO SAUCE				
(Del Monte) hot & mild	¼ cup	–	15	–
(El Molino) red mild	2 Tbs	–	10	–
(La Victoria)				
Green	1 Tbs	–	4	–
Red	1 Tbs	–	6	–
(Old El Paso)	2 Tbs	–	10	–
(Ortega) Thick & Smooth				
Hot	1 Tbs	–	8	–
Medium,	1 Tbs	–	8	–
Mild	1 Tbs	–	8	–
■ TACO SEASONING MIX				
(Durkee)				
Mix Only	1 pkg	1	67	13%
Prepared as Directed	2 cups	15	1238	11%
(French's) mix only	⅙ pkg	–	20	–
(Hain)	¹⁄₁₀ pkg	–	10	–
(Old El Paso) Mix Only	¹⁄₁₂ pkg	< 1	8	56%
(Ortega)				
Mix Only	1 oz	1	90	10%
Prepared as Directed	1 oz	4	60	60%
■ TACO SHELLS				
Mini (Old El Paso)	1 shell	3	55	49%
Regular				
(Gebhardt)	1 shell	2	50	36%

Food and Description	Amount	Fat Grams	Total Calories	% Fat Calories
(Old El Paso)	1 shell	3	55	49%
(Ortega)	1 shell	2	50	36%
(Rosarita)	1 shell	2	50	36%
Super				
(Azteca)	1 shell	12	200	54%
(Old El Paso)	1 shell	6	100	54%
■ TACOS				
Beef				
Hamburger Helper (Betty Crocker) Tacobake				
box mix/dry	⅙ pkg	4	170	21%
box mix/prepared	⅙ recipe	15	320	42%
Standard Home Recipe (USDA)	~ 3 oz	7	153	41%
w/cheese	~ 3 oz	9	182	45%
Ham/Border Breakfasts				
(Owens) frozen	2 tacos	6	90	60%
Sausage/Border Breakfasts				
(Owens) frozen	2 tacos	12	190	57%
Taco Barquito				
frozen (Schwan's)	5 oz	21	410	46%
Taco Starter				
(Del Monte)	8 oz	1	140	6%
■ TAMALES				
Beef				
canned				
(Gebhardt)	2	19	270	63%
(Hormel)	2	10	140	64%
(Van Camp's)	8 oz	16	290	50%
(Wolf)	1 cup	24	350	62%
frozen				
(Hormel)	1	7	140	45%
(Old El Paso)	2	12	190	57%
(Schwan's)	1	3	80	34%
homemade	~ 2.5 oz	9.5	183	48%
Beef-Hot 'N Spicy				
canned (Hormel)	2	10	140	64%
■ TAQUITOS				
Beef/frozen shredded				
(Van de Kamp's)	8 oz	25	490	46%
■ TOMATILLO ENTERO				
(La Victoria)	1 Tbs	–	6	–
■ TOMATOES & JALAPENOS				
(Ortega)	1 oz	–	8	–
■ TORTILLA				
Corn				
(Azteca)	1 small	–	45	–

Food and Description	Amount	Fat Grams	Total Calories	% Fat Calories
(El Charrito)	2	1	95	10%
(Old El Paso)	1	1	60	15%
(Tyson) Enchilada Style	1	< 1	54	8%
Flour				
(Azteca)				
small	1	2	80	23%
8"	1	3	130	21%
Salad Bake & Fill	1	12	200	54%
Taco Salad Shell	1	12	200	54%
(El Charrito)	2	4	170	21%
(Old El Paso)	1	3	150	18%
(Tyson)				
Burrito Style Large	1	4	173	21%
Fajita Style	1	2	84	21%
Hand Stretched				
Burrito Style Small	1	2	106	17%
Heat Pressed				
Burrito Style Large	1	4	182	20%
Soft Taco	1	3	121	22%
Whole Wheat Tortilla	1-1.5 oz	1.8	93	17%
Mix (Quaker)				
Corn-Masa Harina De Maiz	1 cup	5	411	11%
	2 tortillas	1	140	6%
Wheat-Masa Trigo	1 cup	12	445	24%
	2 tortillas	4	150	24%
■ TORTILLA CHIPS (See TORTILLA CHIPS)				
■ TOSTACO SHELLS				
Corn (Old El Paso)	1 shell	5	100	45%
■ TOSTADA				
Beef				
frozen Supreme				
(Van de Kamp's)	8.5 oz	30	530	51%
homemade	~ 3 oz	7	153	41%
homemade-w/cheese	~ 3 oz	9	182	45%
■ TOSTADA SHELLS				
Corn				
(Old El Paso)	1 shell	3	55	49%
(Ortega)	1 shell	2	50	36%
(Pancho Villa)	1 shell	3	55	49%
(Rosarita)	1 shell	3	60	45%

MICROWAVEABLE NONFROZEN MEALS (See also BEEF DISHES; CHICKEN EN-TREE/DINNER; PASTA ENTREE/DINNER; RICE DISHES; etc.)

Food and Description	Amount	Fat Grams	Total Calories	% Fat Calories
(Hormel)				
Microcup				
Chili Mac	7.5 oz	10	200	45%

Food and Description	Amount	Fat Grams	Total Calories	% Fat Calories
Chili No Beans	7⅜ oz	28	380	66%
Chili With Beans	7⅜ oz	11	250	40%
Dinty Moore Beef Stew	7.5 oz	9	190	43%
Hot Chili W/Beans	7⅜ oz	11	250	40%
Lasagna	7.5 oz	13	250	47%
Macaroni & Cheese	7.5 oz	6	190	28%
Noodles & Chicken	7.5 oz	8	180	40%
Pork & Beans	7.5 oz	5	250	18%
Ravioli in Tomato Sauce	7.5 oz	11	250	40%
Scalloped Potatoes & Ham	7.5 oz	16	260	55%
Spaghetti & Meatballs	7.4 oz	7	204	31%
Top Shelf				
Boneless Beef Ribs	10 oz	13	340	34%
Breast of Chicken w/Spanish Rice	10 oz	15	400	34%
Chicken Ala King	10 oz	12	340	32%
Chicken Cacciatore	10 oz	1	200	5%
Glazed Breast Chicken	10 oz	2	170	11%
Italian Style Lasagna	10 oz	16	350	41%
Linguini	10 oz	19	350	49%
Salisbury Steak	10 oz	15	320	42%
Spaghettini	10 oz	6	260	21%
Tender Roast Beef	10 oz	7	250	25%
Vegetable Lasagna	10 oz	9	280	26%
(Light Balance) Microwaveable Lunch Buckets				
Pasta & Garden Vegetables	8.25 oz	1	170	5%
(Lunch Bucket)				
Chili Mac	8.5 oz	15	270	50%
Fettucini Marinara	8.25 oz	2	210	9%
Lasagna	8.5 oz	5	260	17%
Light Balance				
Beef Americana	8.25 oz	3	170	16%
Beef & Pasta Bordeaux	8.25 oz	1	180	5%
Chicken Cacciatore	8.25 oz	1	200	5%
Chicken Fiesta	8.25 oz	3	210	13%
Mushroom Stroganoff	8.25 oz	5	180	25%
Pasta & Garden Vegetables	8.25 oz	1	180	5%
Macaroni'N Beef	8.5 oz	5	260	17%
Macaroni'N Cheese	8.5 oz	6	230	23%
Pasta Italiano	8.5 oz	9	280	29%
Pasta'N Chicken	8.5 oz	8	210	34%
Ravioli	8.5 oz	4	280	13%
Spaghetti'N Meat Sauce	8.5 oz	5	260	17%
MILK				
Buffalo	1 cup	17	236	65%

Food and Description	Amount	Fat Grams	Total Calories	% Fat Calories
Buttermilk				
cultured	1 cup	2	99	18%
	1 quart	9	396	20%
(A&P)	1 cup	1	90	10%
(Crowley)	1 cup	4	110	33%
dry	1 Tbs	–	25	–
(SACO)	4 Tbs	< 1	80	5%
low-fat				
1½% (Borden)				
Golden Churn	1 cup	4	120	30%
1½% (Friendship)	1 cup	4	120	30%
2% (Knudsen)	1 cup	5	120	38%
Carob-Chocolate Milk 1%	1 cup	3	160	17%
Chocolate				
low-fat 2%	1 cup	5	179	25%
(Borden) Dutch Brand	1 cup	5	180	25%
(Carnation)	1 cup	4	170	21%
(Hershey)	1 cup	5	180	25%
Chocolate-Flavored				
Box Drink	1 cup	2	150	12%
(La Parisian) Light Bavarian				
Fudge Creme Cooler	1 cup	5	130	35%
low-fat 1%				
Generic	1 cup	2.5	158	14%
(Kemps) Swiss Style	1 cup	3	170	16%
(Land O' Lakes)	1 cup	3	160	17%
low-fat ½% (Pevely)	1 cup	1	97	9%
powder (2 Tbs) + water	6 oz	1	100	9%
powder (2 Tbs) + whole milk	8 oz	9	250	32%
(Quik) Lite	8 oz	5	130	35%
skim				
(Anderson & Erickson)	8 oz	1	130	7%
(Land O'Lakes)	8 oz	–	140	–
whole	1 cup	8.5	208	37%
(Meadow Gold)	1 cup	8	210	34%
(Nestle)	1 cup	9	210	39%
(Pevely)	1 cup	8	210	34%
Cocoa/Hot Chocolate w/ whole milk	8 oz	9	218	37%
Condensed/canned-sweetened	¼ cup	6.6	244	24%
(Carnation)	1 oz	3	123	22%
	3.5 oz	8.7	321	24%
	⅓ cup	9	318	26%
(Dairy Sweet)	⅓ cup	9	320	25%
(Eagle Brand)	⅓ cup	9	320	25%

Food and Description	Amount	Fat Grams	Total Calories	% Fat Calories
Dry				
(Milkman) low-fat mixed w/water	8 oz	–	190	–
	1 quart	5	380	12%
Nonfat				
Nonfat/Skim	¼ cup	–	100	–
prepared w/water	8 oz	–	80	–
(Alba) mixed w/water	8 oz	–	80	–
(SACO) mixed w/water	8 oz	–	80	–
(Sanalac) mixed w/water	8 oz	–	80	–
Skim	¼ cup	–	100	–
prepared w/water	8 oz	–	80	–
Whole	¼ cup	8.5	159	48%
Eggnog (*See* EGGNOG)				
Evaporated				
canned-low-fat	¼ cup	1.5	55	25%
canned-skim	¼ cup	–	50	–
canned whole	¼ cup	4.8	84	51%
(Carnation) low-fat	3.5 oz	1.9	85	20%
	½ cup	3	110	25%
(Carnation) skim	3.5 oz	–	80	–
	½ cup	–	100	–
(Carnation) whole	3.5 oz	7.6	134	51%
	½ cup	10	170	53%
(Milnot) whole	½ cup	8	150	48%
(Pet)				
Light	½ cup	–	100	–
whole	½ cup	10	170	53%
Fresh				
Low-fat 2%	1 cup	5	121	37%
(A&P)	8 oz	5	120	38%
(Borden) Hi-Protein	1 cup	5	140	32%
(Crowley)	8 oz	5	120	38%
(Darigold)	8 oz	5	120	38%
(Knudsen)	8 oz	5	140	32%
(Land O'Lakes)	1 cup	5	120	38%
(Viva) w/extra calcium	1 cup	5	120	38%
w/nonfat milk solids added	1 cup	4.7	125	34%
Low-fat 1%	1 cup	2.6	105	22%
(A&P)	8 oz	3	100	27%
(Borden) w/L. Acidophilus	1 cup	2	100	18%
(Crowley)	8 oz	2	100	18%
(Darigold)	8 oz	2	100	18%
(Knudsen) Nice'n Light	8 oz	3	130	21%
(Land O'Lakes)	1 cup	3	100	27%

Food and Description	Amount	Fat Grams	Total Calories	% Fat Calories
w/nonfat milk solids added	1 cup	2.4	104	21%
Low-fat ½% (Pevely)	1 cup	1	90	10%
Skim	1 cup	.6	100	6%
(Borden)				
Skim-Line				
protein fortified	1 cup	1	100	9%
vitamins A & D	1 cup	.6	90	6%
w/nonfat milk solids added	1 cup	.6	90	6%
Whole				
(Borden)	1 cup	8	150	48%
(Real) Real Fresh milk w/vitamins				
A & D-ready to chill box	1 cup	8	150	48%
Vitamin D	1 cup	8	150	48%
w/added calcium-Hi Calcium	1 cup	8	150	48%
Goat	8 oz	10	168	54%
canned (Meyenberg)				
evaporated	8 oz	8	160	45%
carton				
powder mixed w/water	8 oz	8	150	48%
refrigerated	8 oz	8	150	48%
Human	2 oz	2	42	43%
Reindeer	8 oz	48.6	580	75%
Sheep	8 oz	17	264	58%
Soybean "Milk"	8 oz	4.6	79	52%
Substitutes				
(Dairy Ease)				
lactose reduced				
1%	8 oz	2	100	18%
2%	8 oz	5	120	38%
Nonfat	8 oz	–	90	–
(Lactaid)				
Calcium Fortified	8 oz	< 1	90	5%
Lowfat 1%	8 oz	2	100	18%
Lowfat 2%	8 oz	5	120	38%
Nonfat	8 oz	–	90	–
(Meadow Farms)	8 oz	5	120	38%
MILK MIXES				
Carob Mix				
dry	1 Tbs	< 1	45	10%
w/8 oz whole milk	8 oz	9	195	42%
(Caracoa) Instant Carob Drink				
prepared	8 oz	1	145	6%
(El Molino)				
dry	1 Tbs	< 1	40	11%

Food and Description	Amount	Fat Grams	Total Calories	% Fat Calories
w/8 oz whole milk	8 oz	9	190	43%
Chocolate				
(Choco Milk) dry mix	1 oz	1	110	8%
+ 8 oz whole milk	8 oz	10	264	34%
Chocolate syrup	2 Tbs	.5	82	6%
+ whole milk	8 oz	8.5	232	33%
Chocolate-flavored syrup				
(Estee) syrup	1 Tbs	–	6	–
(Hershey's) syrup	2 Tbs	< 1	110	4%
Cocoa				
(Alba)				
Chocolate Marsh	1 pkt	–	60	–
Milk Chocolate	1 pkt	–	60	–
Mocha	1 pkt	–	60	–
(Baker's)	1 oz	2	120	15%
(Carnation)				
Chocolate Fudge-dry	1 oz	1	110	8%
Diet Hot Cocoa Mix	1 env	< 1	25	18%
Milk Chocolate-Dry	1 oz	1	110	8%
Mocha-Sugar-Free-Dry	1 oz	.5	50	9%
Natural Mint-Dry	1 oz	1	110	8%
Rich Chocolate-Dry	1 oz	1	110	8%
Sugar-Free-Dry	1 oz	.5	50	9%
Rich Chocolate w/Marshmallows-Dry	1 oz	1	110	8%
70 Calorie-Dry	3.5 oz	1	353	3%
	3 tsp	–	70	–
w/ Chocolate Marshmallows	1 pkt	1	110	8%
(Land O Lakes) Cocoa Classics-dry				
Chocolate & Cinnamon	1 pkg	5	160	28%
Chocolate & Mint	1 pkg	5	160	28%
Chocolate Supreme	1 pkg	5	160	28%
(Nestle Quik)				
Chocolate				
Dry	¾ oz/ ~2½ tsp	1	90	10%
+ 8 oz whole milk	8 oz	9	240	34%
+ 8 oz 2% milk	8 oz	6	210	26%
+ 8 oz 1% milk	8 oz	4	190	18%
+ 8 oz skim milk	8 oz	1.6	180	8%
Sugarless/dry	.35 oz	1	40	23%
+ 8 oz 2% milk	8 oz	5	160	28%
(Ovaltine) sugar free-dry	1 pkt	1	40	23%
(Swiss Miss) instant				
Amaretto Creme	1 pkt	3	150	18%

Food and Description	Amount	Fat Grams	Total Calories	% Fat Calories
Bavarian Chocolate	1 pkt	3	110	25%
Chocolate Creme	1 pkt	4	110	33%
Chocolate Mint	1 pkt	3	150	18%
Chocolate Mocha Creme	1 pkt	4	140	26%
Cocoa/diet	1 env	< 1	20	23%
Double Rich	1 pkt	1	110	8%
Lite	1 pkt	< 1	70	6%
Milk Chocolate	1 pkt	1	110	8%
Mini Marshmallow	1 pkt	1	110	8%
Sugar Free	1 pkt	1	60	15%
Sugar Free/Fat Free	1 pkt	–	50	–
Sugar Free-w/Mini Marshmallows	1 pkt	1	50	18%
(Ultra Slim Fast)				
Creamy Hot Cocoa	1 pkg	< 1	190	2%
(Weight Watchers) Chocolate &				
Marshmallow	1 pkt	–	60	–
Malted				
(Carnation)				
chocolate-dry	3.5 oz	3.8	375	9%
	3 Heaping Tbs	.8	79	9%
original-dry	3.5 oz	8.5	411	19%
	3 Heaping Tbs	2	90	20%
Generic/chocolate powder	1 Heaping Tbs	1	85	11%
w/whole milk	8 oz	9	235	35%
(Kraft) Instant				
Chocolate	4 tsp	1	90	10%
Natural	3 tsp	2	90	20%
(Ovaltine)				
Classic-Traditional Chocolate Malt				
Dry	¾ oz	–	80	–
w/2% milk	8 oz	5	210	21%
Rich Chocolate				
Dry	¾ oz	–	80	–
w/2% milk	8 oz	5	210	21%
(PDQ) 3-4 tsp w/whole milk	8 oz	5	180	25%
Strawberry (Nestle Quik)				
Dry	¾ oz/ ~2½ tsp	–	80	–
+ 8 oz whole milk	8 oz	8	230	31%
+ 8 oz 2% milk	8 oz	5	200	23%
+ 8 oz 1% milk	8 oz	3	180	15%

Food and Description	Amount	Fat Grams	Total Calories	% Fat Calories
+ 8 oz skim milk	8 oz	.6	170	3%

MILK SHAKE (*See also* individual FAST FOOD listings)
Canned
(Frostee)

Chocolate-Flavored Drink	1 cup	8	200	36%
Strawberry-Flavored Drink	1 cup	7	180	35%

(Real) Sport Shake

Chocolate	10 oz	10	310	29%
Strawberry	10 oz	10	270	33%

Chilled
(Killer) Shake

Choco Loco	8 oz	6	240	23%
Radically Vanilla	8 oz	5	220	20%
Totally Chocolate	8 oz	5	230	20%

Frozen
(Micro Magic)

Chocolate	11.5 oz	8	340	21%
Strawberry	11.5 oz	9	340	24%
Vanilla	11.5 oz	13	380	31%

Mix
(Alba 77) Fit'N Frosty

Chocolate	1 pkt	–	70	–
Chocolate Marshmallow	1 pkt	–	70	–
Double Fudge	1 pkt	–	70	–
Strawberry	1 pkt	–	70	–
Vanilla	1 pkt	–	70	–

(Weight Watchers)

Chocolate Fudge	1 pkt	< 1	70	6%
Orange Sherbet	1 pkt	< 1	70	6%

Regular

Chocolate	10 oz	10	360	25%
Strawberry	10 oz	9	350	23%
Vanilla	10 oz	9	340	27%

MILK SUBSTITUTES (*See* MILK, SOY MILK)

MILKFISH/raw	3 oz	6	125	43%

MILLET (*See also* CEREAL, FLOUR)

(Arrowhead Mills)	1 oz	1	90	10%

Generic

cooked	4 oz	1	135	7%
	1 cup	2	287	6%
dry	1 oz	1	107	8%
	1 cup	8	756	10%
Whole grain	4 oz	3	371	7%

MINERAL WATER (*See* WATER)

Food and Description	Amount	Fat Grams	Total Calories	% Fat Calories
MINESTRONE SOUP (*See* SOUP)				
MISO PASTE	½ cup	8	285	25%
MOLASSES				
Barbados	1 Tbs	–	54	–
	1 oz	–	111	–
	1 cup	–	889	–
Blackstrap (Plantation)				
3rd extraction	1 Tbs	–	43	–
	1 oz	–	87	–
	1 cup	–	699	–
(Brer Rabbit)				
Dark	1 Tbs	–	60	–
Light	1 Tbs	–	60	–
Light-lst extraction	1 Tbs	–	50	–
	1 oz	–	103	–
	1 cup	–	827	–
Medium-2nd extraction	1 Tbs	–	46	–
	1 oz	–	95	–
	1 cup	–	761	–
(Mott's)				
Grandma's Gold Label	1 Tbs	–	70	–
Grandma's Green Label	1 Tbs	–	70	–
Treacle-Black	1 Tbs	–	53	–
MONKFISH/raw	3 oz	1	64	14%
MOOSE/raw-boneless	3 oz	4.8	152	28%
MOTHBEANS				
boiled	½ cup	–	103	–
raw	½ cup	1.5	335	4%
MOUNTAIN YAM/cooked Hawaiian	1 cup	–	119	–
MOUSSE (*See* PUDDING & MOUSSE)				
MUFFINS (*See also* SNACK CAKES)				
(Betty Crocker) Mix only				
Apple Cinnamon	1	3	100	27%
Bake Shop Muffins				
Blueberry Streusel	1	7	190	33%
Banana Nut	1	4	110	33%
Cinnamon Streusel	1	8	190	39%
Oat Bran	1	7	170	37%
Wild Blueberry	1	3	100	27%
Wild Blueberry Light	1	< 1	70	6%
(Dromedary) Corn mix	1	5	130	35%
(Duncan Hines) mix				
Bakery Style Blueberry	1	6	190	28%

Food and Description	Amount	Fat Grams	Total Calories	% Fat Calories
Bakery Style Bran & Honey Nut	1	7	200	32%
Bakery Style Cinnamon Swirl	1	7	200	32%
Bakery Style Cranberry Orange Nut	1	8	200	36%
Bakery Style Pecan Crunch	1	11	220	45%
Bran & Honey	1	4	120	38%
Oat Bran Blueberry	1	5	110	41%
Wild Blueberry	1	3	110	25%
(Dunkin' Donuts)				
Apple N' Spice	1	8	300	24%
Banana Nut	1	10	310	29%
Blueberry	1	8	280	26%
Corn	1	12	340	32%
Cranberry Nut	1	9	290	25%
Oat-bran				
Apple	1	8	320	23%
Blueberry	1	7	270	23%
Plain	1	11	350	28%
Raisin-Nut	1	11	330	30%
(Earth Grains) English				
Plain	1	1	150	6%
Raisin	1	1	150	6%
Wheatberry	1	1	150	6%
Whole Wheat	1	2	170	11%
(Entenmann's) Blueberry	1	8	200	36%
(Flako) Corn mix	1	4	120	30%
Generic				
Corn Mix	1	6	145	37%
English				
Cracked Wheat	1	1	158	6%
Plain	1	1	140	6%
Sourdough	1	1	130	7%
w/Raisins	1	1	146	6%
Whole Wheat	1	1.6	130	11%
(Hain) mix				
Apple Cinnamon	1	3	140	19%
Banana Nut	1	4	140	26%
Raspberry Spice	1	3	140	19%
(Health Valley) Fat Free fruit	1	< 1	65	7%
Oat Bran Almond-Date	1	6	170	32%
Oat Bran Blueberry	1	4	140	26%
Oat Bran Raisin	1	3	140	19%

Food and Description	Amount	Fat Grams	Total Calories	% Fat Calories
(Healthy Choice) Frozen				
Apple Spice	1	4	190	19%
Banana Nut	1	6	180	30%
Blueberry	1	4	190	19%
(Home Pride) Muffin Loaves				
Apple Cinnamon	1 piece	6	110	49%
Blueberry	1 piece	5	110	41%
Raspberry	1 piece	5	110	41%
Homemade				
Apple	~ 1.5 oz	7	135	47%
Blueberry	~ 1.5 oz	5	135	33%
Bran	~ 1.5 oz	4	104	35%
Corn				
w/degermed cornmeal	~ 1.5 oz	4	128	30%
w/whole-ground cornmeal	~ 1.5 oz	4	115	31%
Orange	~ 1.5 oz	5	135	33%
Plain	~ 1.5 oz	4	118	31%
(Hostess)				
Breakfast Bake Shop				
Mini Banana Walnut	5	16	260	55%
Mini Blueberry	5	13	240	49%
Mini Cinnamon Apple	5	16	260	55%
Oat Bran	1	7	170	39%
Oat Bran Banana Nut	1	5	140	32%
97% fat free				
Apple Streusel	1	1	100	9%
Blueberry	1	1	100	9%
(Krusteaz) mix				
Almond Poppyseed	1	5	180	25%
Apple Cinnamon	1	3	180	15%
Blueberry	1	4	160	23%
Chocolate Chocolate Chip	1	5	200	23%
Cornbread	1	7	220	29%
Honey Bran	1	4	140	26%
Oat Bran	1-2.5 oz	6	210	26%
	1-2 oz	5	190	24%
(Martha White) mix				
Apple Cinnamon, Blackberry, Blueberry, Orangeberry, Raspberry, Strawberry	1	3	140	19%
Bran	1	5	150	30%
Double Blueberry Lite				
Cholesterol Free	1	< 1	80	6%
Mix Only	1	< 1	70	6%

Food and Description	Amount	Fat Grams	Total Calories	% Fat Calories
Standard Recipe	1	< 1	80	6%
(Oroweat) English				
Blueberry	1	1	170	5%
Extra Crisp	1	1	130	7%
Health Nut Raisin	1	4	200	18%
Oat Bran	1	1	150	6%
Oat Nut Raisin	1	2	160	11%
Sourdough	1	1	140	6%
(Pepperidge Farm)				
English				
Cinnamon Apple	1	1	140	6%
Cinnamon Chip	1	3	160	17%
Cinnamon Raisin	1	2	150	12%
Plain	1	1	140	6%
Sourdough	1	1	135	7%
Old Fashioned Frozen				
Blueberry	1	7	180	35%
Corn	1	7	180	35%
Oat Bran w/Apple	1	7	190	33%
Raisin Bran	1	6	170	32%
(Robin Hood/Gold Medal) mix/prepared				
Applesauce	1	5	160	28%
Banana	1	5	150	30%
Blueberry	1	6	170	32%
Corn	1	7	180	35%
Honey Bran	1	5	170	26%
(Roman Meal) English-Plain	1	2	145	12%
(Thomas)				
Honey Wheat	1	1	120	8%
Plain & Sourdough	1	1	120	8%
Raisin	1	1.5	153	4%
(Sara Lee) Frozen				
Corn	1	13	250	47%
Hearty Fruit				
Apple Cinnamon Spice	1	8	220	33%
Banana Nut	1	0	200	35%
Blueberry	1	8	200	36%
Golden Corn	1	13	250	47%
Oat Bran	1	8	220	33%
Oatmeal & Fruit	1	9	230	35%
Raisin Bran	1	7	220	29%
(Winchell Donuts) Muffins				
Apple Spice	1	11	327	30%
Banana Nut	1	12	327	33%

Food and Description	Amount	Fat Grams	Total Calories	% Fat Calories
Blueberry	1	10	263	34%
Bran	1	13	353	33%
Cherry	1	10	317	28%
Corn	1	13	347	34%
(Wolferman's) English				
Apple Strudel	1	2	110	16%
Blueberry	1	< 1	110	4%
Cinnamon & Raisin	1	< 1	110	4%
Cranberry	1	1	120	8%
Original	1	< 1	110	4%
MULBERRY	1 cup	.55	61	8%
MULLET/striped				
cooked-dry heat	3 oz	4	127	28%
raw	3 oz	3	99	27%
MUNG BEANS				
boiled	6 oz	–	107	–
raw	½ cup	1	361	3%
Sprouts				
(Arrowhead Mills)	½ cup	–	25	–
canned	½ cup	–	8	–
cooked	½ cup	–	13	S
raw	4 oz	–	40	–
raw	½ cup	–	16	–
stir-fried	½ cup	–	31	–
MUNGO BEANS/boiled	½ cup	–	95	–
MUSHROOM				
Canned				
(B&B)	2 oz	1	25	36%
(Libby's)	1 oz	–	70	–
Marinated (Cara Mia)	1 oz	1	13	69%
Oriental Straw	2 oz	–	12	–
Pieces & Stems Buttons (Green Giant)	½ cup	–	25	–
Seasoned Whole (Cara Mia)	1 oz	–	7	–
Fresh-Boiled	½ cup	–	21	–
Frozen (Freshlike)	3.5 oz	–	30	–
Raw	1	–	5	–
Raw/Pieces	½ cup	–	9	–
Sauteed or Fried	10 Small	10	100	9%
Shiitake Mushroom/Cooked	4	–	40	–
Canned	4 oz	–	45	–
Dried	1	–	11	–
MUSHROOM DISHES				
Mushroom Stroganoff (Light Balance)				
microwaveable	8.25 oz	5	180	25%

Food and Description	Amount	Fat Grams	Total Calories	% Fat Calories
Mushrooms breaded-frozen (Ore Ida)	2⅔ oz	8	140	51%
Mushrooms w/butter sauce-canned	2 oz	1	30	30%
MUSHROOM SOUP (See SOUP)				
MUSKELLUNGE (North American Pike)				
raw	3 oz	2	93	19%
MUSSEL				
Blue				
cooked-moist heat	3 oz	3.8	147	23%
raw	3 oz	1.9	73	23%
	1 cup	3	129	21%
MUSTARD				
Brown				
(Heinz)	1 tsp	< 1	8	56%
(Nabisco)	1 tsp	–	4	–
Dip'N Spread (French's)	1 Tbs	1	40	23%
Prepared				
(French's)				
Bold & Spicy	1 tsp	< 1	6	75%
Creamy Spread	1 tsp	< 1	8	56%
Dijon	1 tsp	< 1	8	56%
w/Horseradish	1 tsp	< 1	6	75%
w/Sweet Onion	1 tsp	< 1	8	56%
Yellow	1 tsp	< 1	4	90%
Grey Poupon				
(Nabisco)	1 tsp	1	18	50%
	1 Tbs	2	30	60%
(Gulden's)				
Creamy Mild	1 Tbs	–	6	–
Diablo	1 Tbs	–	8	–
Spicy Brown	1 Tbs	< 1	9	50%
(Hain)				
No Salt	1 Tbs	1	14	64%
Stone Ground	1 Tbs	1	14	64%
(Heinz)				
Mild	1 tsp	–	5	–
Pourable	1 tsp	–	5	–
Horseradish	1 Tbs	1	14	64%
(Kraft)				
Pure Prepared	1 Tbs	1	11	82%
MUSTARD, DRIED	1 tsp	< 1	12	38%
MUSTARD GREENS				
fresh-boiled	½ cup	–	11	–
frozen-boiled	½ cup	–	14	–
frozen (Pictsweet)	3.3 oz	–	20	–

Food and Description	Amount	Fat Grams	Total Calories	% Fat Calories
raw	½ cup	–	7	–
MUSTARD SAUCE (*See* SAUCE)				
MUSTARD SEED/yellow	1 tsp	1	15	60%
MUSTARD SPINACH				
fresh-boiled	½ cup	–	14	–
raw	½ cup	–	17	–

N

Food and Description	Amount	Fat Grams	Total Calories	% Fat Calories
NACHOS (*See* MEXICAN FOOD)				
NAPOLEON (*See* CAKE AND CAKE PASTRY)				
NATTO	½ cup	9.7	187	47%
NAVY BEAN				
boiled	½ cup	.5	129	4%
canned	½ cup	.57	148	4%
(Joan of Arc)	½ cup	< 1	100	5%
Old Fashioned (Ranch Style)	7.5 oz	2	160	7%
Seasoned w/Pork (Luck's)	7.5 oz	7	230	27%
raw	½ cup	1.5	345	4%
sprouts raw	½ cup	–	35	–
NAVY BEAN SOUP (*See* SOUP)				
NECTARINE/fresh	1	.7	67	9%
NEWBURG SAUCE (*See* SAUCE)				
NON-DAIRY FROZEN DESSERT (*See* FROZEN NON-DAIRY DESSERT)				
NOODLE (*See* PASTA)				
NOODLE SOUP (*See* SOUP)				
NUTMEG/ground	1 tsp	.8	11	66%
NUTRITIONAL SUPPLEMENTS (*See also* BREAKFAST BAR, BREAKFAST DRINK)				
(Carnation) Slender Canned				
Chocolate	10 oz	4	220	16%
Chocolate Fudge	10 oz	4	220	16%
Chocolate Malt	10 oz	4	220	16%
Milk Chocolate	10 oz	4	220	16%

Food and Description	Amount	Fat Grams	Total Calories	% Fat Calories
Vanilla	10 oz	4	220	16%
(California Slim) Mix-Dry				
Chocolate Shake	1 serving	< 1	100	5%
Citrus Juice	1 serving	< 1	90	5%
Fruit Juice	1 serving	< 1	90	5%
Mocha Shake	1 serving	< 1	100	5%
Vanilla Shake	1 serving	< 1	100	5%
(Dynatrim) Mix-Dry				
Dutch Chocolate	1 serving	1	100	9%
Strawberry Royale	1 serving	1	100	9%
Vanilla Royale	1 serving	1	100	9%
(Joe Weider's)				
Carbo Energizer	6 oz	–	140	–
90 Plus sugar-free	8 oz	1	100	9%
(Meritene)				
Milk Chocolate	4 Tbs	1	120	8%
Vanilla	4 Tbs	1	120	8%
(MLO)				
Milk & Egg	1 Tbs	–	100	–
w/8 oz non-fat milk	8 oz	–	190	–
Mus-L-On Vanilla	5 Tbs	4	330	11%
w/16 oz whole milk	16 oz	22	650	30%
Super High Instant	3 Tbs	–	90	–
w/8 oz non-fat milk	8 oz	< 1	180	3%
Vanilla-dry	2 Tbs	1	110	8%
w/8 oz non-fat milk	1 serving	1	200	5%
(Nutrament) Energy Food				
Chocolate	12 oz	10	360	25%
Vanilla	12 oz	10	360	25%
(Resource)				
Chocolate	1 pkt	8.8	250	32%
Vanilla	1 pkt	8.8	250	32%
(Ross) Ensure				
Black Walnut	8 oz	8.8	250	32%
Chocolate	8 oz	8.8	250	32%
Coffee	8 oz	8.8	250	32%
Eggnog	8 oz	8.8	250	32%
Plus chocolate	8 oz	12.6	355	32%
Plus coffee	8 oz	12.6	355	32%
Plus eggnog	8 oz	12.6	355	32%
Plus strawberry	8 oz	12.6	355	32%
Plus vanilla	8 oz	12.6	355	32%
Strawberry	8 oz	8.8	250	32%
Vanilla	8 oz	8.8	250	32%

Food and Description	Amount	Fat Grams	Total Calories	% Fat Calories
(Sego) Liquid Diet Food				
Lite				
Chocolate	10 oz	3	150	18%
Dutch Chocolate	10 oz	3	150	18%
French Vanilla	10 oz	3	150	18%
Strawberry	10 oz	3	150	18%
Vanilla	10 oz	3	150	18%
Very				
Chocolate	10 oz	1	225	4%
Chocolate Malt	10 oz	1	225	4%
Strawberry	10 oz	5	225	20%
Vanilla	10 oz	5	225	20%
(Sustacal)				
Chocolate	32 oz	22	960	21%
(Ultra Diet Quick) Mix-Dry				
Fruit Juice	1 serving	–	90	–
Dutch Chocolate	1 serving	1	100	9%
Strawberry Delight	1 serving	< 1	100	5%
Vanilla Creme	1 serving	< 1	100	5%
(Ultra Slim Fast) Canned				
Original				
Liquid				
Chocolate Royale	11 oz	3	230	12%
French Vanilla	11 oz	3	210	13%
Powder				
Cafe Mocha	1 scoop	< 1	100	5%
w/8 oz skim milk	8 oz	1	200	5%
Chocolate Fantasy	1 scoop	1	120	8%
w/8 oz skim milk	8 oz	2	250	7%
Chocolate Malt	1 scoop	< 1	100	5%
w/8 oz skim milk	8 oz	1	190	5%
Chocolate Royale	1 scoop	< 1	110	4%
w/8 oz skim milk	8 oz	1	200	5%
French Vanilla	1 scoop	< 1	100	5%
w/8 oz skim milk	8 oz	1	190	5%
Fruit Juice	1 scoop	–	90	–
w/8 oz orange juice	8 oz	< 1	200	2%
Pina Colada	1 scoop	< 1	90	5%
w/8 oz skim milk	8 oz	< 1	180	3%
Rich & Delicious Chocolate	1 scoop	< 1	100	5%
w/8 oz skim milk	8 oz	1	190	5%
Rich & Delicious Strawberry	1 scoop	< 1	100	5%
w/8 oz skim milk	8 oz	1	190	5%
Rich & Delicious Vanilla	1 scoop	< 1	100	5%

Food and Description	Amount	Fat Grams	Total Calories	% Fat Calories
w/8 oz skim milk	8 oz	1	190	5%
Strawberry Jubilee	1 scoop	1	110	8%
w/8 oz skim milk	8 oz	2	240	8%
Strawberry Supreme	1 scoop	< 1	100	5%
w/8 oz skim milk	8 oz	1	190	5%
Vanilla Creme	1 scoop	< 1	110	4%
w/8 oz skim milk	8 oz	1	240	4%
Plus				
Powder				
Chocolate Fantasy	1 scoop	1	120	8%
w/8 oz skim milk	8 oz	2	250	7%
Fruit Juice	1 scoop	< 1	80	6%
w/12 oz orange juice	12 oz	1	250	4%
Vanilla Creme	1 scoop	< 1	110	4%
w/8 oz skim milk	8 oz	1	240	4%
(Ultra Slim Fast) Water-Mixable Shake Mix				
Dutch Chocolate	1 envelope	< 1	220	2%
French Vanilla	1 envelope	< 1	220	2%
(Weight Watchers) Shake Mix				
Chocolate Fudge	1 pkt	1	70	13%
Orange Sherbet	1 pkt	–	70	–
NUTS, FORMULATED				
wheat based				
Macadamia-flavored	1 oz	16	176	82%
other flavors	1 oz	18	184	88%
unflavored	1 oz	16	177	81%
NUTS, MIXED (*See also* Individual Names)				
Mixed Nuts				
(Eagle)	1 oz	16	180	80%
Deluxe	1 oz	17	180	85%
(Planters)				
Dry Roasted	1 oz	14	160	79%
Unsalted	1 oz	15	170	79%
Oil Roasted	1 oz	16	180	80%
Deluxe	1 oz	17	180	85%
Unsalted	1 oz	16	180	80%
Select Mix				
Cashews w/Almonds & Peanuts	1 oz	14	170	74%
Cashews w/Almonds & Pecans	1 oz	16	180	80%
Cashews w/Pecans & Peanuts	1 oz	16	180	80%
Mixed Nuts w/Peanuts				
Dry Roasted	1 oz	14.6	169	78%

Food and Description	Amount	Fat Grams	Total Calories	% Fat Calories
(Guy's)	1 oz	16	180	80%
Oil Roasted	1 oz	16	175	82%
Mixed Nuts w/o Peanuts				
Oil Roasted	1 oz	15.95	175	82%

O

Food and Description	Amount	Fat Grams	Total Calories	% Fat Calories
OAT BRAN (See CEREAL)				
OATS (See also CEREAL)				
(Arrowhead Mills)				
Flakes	2 oz	4	220	16%
Groats	2 oz	4	220	16%
Steel Cut	2 oz	4	220	16%
Whole Grain	1 oz	2	110	16%
	1 cup	10.8	607	16%
OCEAN PERCH, ATLANTIC (See also FROZEN ENTREE/DINNER)				
breaded & fried	3 oz	11	185	54%
cooked-dry heat	3 oz	1.8	103	16%
raw	3 oz	1	80	11%
Mixed				
cooked-dry heat	3 oz	1	77	12%
frozen-raw				
(Gorton's)	5 oz	1	110	8%
OCTOBER BEANS				
canned				
Seasoned w/Pork (Luck's)	7.25 oz	6	220	25%
	7.5 oz	7	230	27%
OCTOPUS/raw	3 oz	.88	70	11%
OILS (See also COOKING SPRAY, FAT, LARD, SHORTENING)				
ALL VEGETABLE OILS	1 Tbs	14	120	100%

[NOTE: You need to watch even your use of "healthier"(less saturated) oils in order to keep your total fat intake within acceptable boundaries. Because it is so important for you to select the least saturated oil to fit your needs, I have listed the most commonly used oils and fats below, showing the % of saturated fat, polyunsaturated fat, and monounsaturated fat in each one. Those that contain less saturated fat are listed first

Food and Description	Amount	Fat Grams	Total Calories	% Fat Calories

for both oils and fats. (Data is based on information from USDA Nutritive Value of American Foods in Common Units, 1988.)]

REMEMBER—NO VEGETABLE OIL CONTAINS CHOLESTEROL!

■ OILS & FATS

VEGETABLE OIL/FAT	% SATURATED	% UNSATURATED	
		% POLY	% MONO
CANOLA	7	35	58
ALMOND	8	19	73
SAFFLOWER	9	78	13
SUNFLOWER	11	69	20
CORN	13	62	25
OLIVE	14	12	74
WALNUT	14	67	19
SESAME	15	43	42
SOYBEAN	15	43	42
MARGARINE			
(Liquid/Tub)	17	37	46
(Stick)	20	33	47
(Whipped)	20	30	50
PEANUT	18	33	49
SOYBEAN/COTTONSEED BLEND	19	50	31
WHEAT GERM	20	50	31
SHORTENING (VEGETABLE)	27	26	47
COTTONSEED	27	55	18
PALM	52	10	38
COCOA BUTTER	62	3	35
BUTTER			
(Stick)	66	4	30
(Whipped)	69	3	28
PALM KERNEL	87	2	11
COCONUT	92	2	6

ANIMAL FAT	% SATURATED	% UNSATURATED
GOOSE	27	73
CHICKEN	30	70
TURKEY	30	70
DUCK	34	66
SALT PORK	36	64
LARD	41	59
BEEF TALLOW	52	48

Food and Description	Amount	Fat Grams	Total Calories	% Fat Calories
OKRA				
canned	½ cup	–	25	–
fresh-boiled	½ cup	–	25	–
frozen-cooked	½ cup	–	34	–
frozen-cut				
(Freshlike)	3.3 oz	–	25	–
(Pictsweet)	3.3 oz	–	25	–
frozen-whole				
(Freshlike)	3.3 oz	–	30	–
(Pictsweet) Express				
Microwave	2.5 oz	–	20	–
raw	½ cup	–	19	–
OKRA DISHES				
Okra breaded				
frozen (Ore Ida)	3 oz	10	170	53%
OLIVE				
Pickled/canned or bottled				
Green	10 Small	3.6	33	98%
	10 Large	4.9	45	98%
	10 Giant	8	76	95%
Pitted Ripe				
(Early California) all sizes	~1 oz	3	30	90%
(Janet Lee)	8 small	3	30	90%
	7 medium	3	30	90%
	6 large	3	30	90%
(S&W)				
jumbo	3.5 oz	18	163	99%
large	3.5 oz	18	163	99%
xtra large	3.5 oz	18	163	99%
Ripe-Ascolano	10 Xtra large	6.5	61	96%
	10 Mammoth	7.7	72	96%
	10 Giant	9.5	89	96%
	10 Jumbo	11	105	94%
sliced	1 cup	18.6	174	94%
Ripe-Manzanillo	10 Small	4	38	95%
	10 Medium	4.7	44	96%
	10 Large	5.5	51	97%
	10 Xtra large	6.5	61	96%
sliced	1 cup	18.6	174	96%
Ripe-Mission	10 Small	5.9	54	98%
	10 Medium	6.9	63	99%
	10 Large	8	73	99%
	10 Xtra large	9.5	87	98%
sliced	1 cup	27	248	98%

Food and Description	Amount	Fat Grams	Total Calories	% Fat Calories
Ripe (S&W)				
large	3.5 oz	18	163	99%
xtra large	3.5 oz	18	163	99%
Ripe-Sevillano	10 Giant	6.5	64	91%
	10 Jumbo	7.8	76	92%
	10 Colossal	9.7	95	92%
	10 SuperCol	11.6	114	92%
sliced	1 cup	12.8	126	91%
Ripe-salt cured/Greek style	10 Medium	6.9	65	96%
	10 Xtra large	9.5	89	96%
OLIVE LOAF (See LUNCHEON MEAT)				
OMELETTE (See EGG MEALS)				
ONION				
canned-French Fried Onions				
(Durkee)	1 oz	15	175	77%
canned (S&W)	½ cup	–	35	–
cooked	1 cup	–	60	–
Dehydrated Flakes	1 Tbs	–	16	–
frozen				
chopped (Ore Ida)	2 oz	–	20	–
diced (Freshlike)	1 oz	–	8	–
small whole (Birds Eye)	½ cup	–	40	–
	¼ cup	–	45	–
whole (Freshlike)	3.3 oz	–	95	–
Green-spring	5 Large	–	10	–
(Heinz) sweet onions	1	–	40	–
raw/chopped	1 Tbs	–	3	–
	½ cup	–	27	–
(Vlasic) Lightly Spiced Cocktail	1 oz	–	4	–
ONION DISHES				
Chopped Onions/frozen (Ore Ida)	2 oz	–	20	–
Onions in cream sauce/frozen				
(Birds Eye)	3 oz	6	110	49%
Onion Ringers/frozen (Ore Ida)	2 oz	7	140	45%
Onion Rings				
Frozen, Breaded				
Generic				
Pan fried heated in oven	7 rings	18.69	285	59%
(Mrs. Paul's) Crispy	2.5 oz	12	190	57%
Small Onions w/cream sauce/frozen				
(Birds Eye)	3 oz	6	110	49%
ONION POWDER	1 tsp	–	7	–
ONION SOUP (See SOUP)				
OPOSSUM/braised or roasted	3 oz	8	190	38%

Food and Description	Amount	Fat Grams	Total Calories	% Fat Calories
ORANGE (*See also* MANDARIN ORANGE)				
Oranges	1	–	62	–
Oranges/Navels	1	–	65	–
Oranges/Valencias	1	–	59	–
ORANGE DRINK				
Bottled, Boxed, or Canned				
(Bama)	8.45 oz	–	120	–
(Betty Crocker) Squeezit	6.75 oz	–	110	–
(Hawaiian Punch)	6 oz	–	100	–
(Juice Works)	6 oz	–	90	–
(Kool-Aid) Kooler	8.45 oz	–	110	–
(Mott's) Blend	10 oz	–	144	–
(Tropicana) single serve	10 oz	–	132	–
From Frozen Concentrate				
w/orange pulp	6 oz	–	91	–
Mix				
(Crystal Light)	8 oz	–	4	–
(Tang) Breakfast Drink				
Fruit Box				
Orange	8.45 oz	–	130	–
Tropical Orange	8.45 oz	–	150	–
Regular	4 oz	–	60	–
	6 oz	–	90	–
Sugar-Free	6 oz	–	6	–
ORANGE JUICE				
Bottled, Boxed, or Canned				
(Campbell's) Juice Bowl	6 oz	–	90	–
(Del Monte) unsweetened	6 oz	–	80	–
Generic				
sweetened	8 oz	–	119	–
unsweetened	8 oz	–	104	–
(Kraft) Pure 100%	6 oz	–	80	–
(Libby's) unsweetened	6 oz	–	80	–
(Mott's) blend	9.5 oz	–	139	–
(S&W) unsweetened	6 oz	–	83	–
(Sippin Pak) from concentrate	8.45 oz	–	110	–
(Sunkist)				
fresh squeezed	6 oz	–	77	–
from concentrate	6 oz	–	84	–
	8 oz	–	112	–
(Tree Top)	6 oz	–	90	–
(Tropicana)				
sweetened	8 oz	–	109	–
unsweetened	6 oz	–	75	–

Food and Description	Amount	Fat Grams	Total Calories	% Fat Calories
Fresh	8 oz	.5	111	4%
Frozen				
(Birds Eye)	6 oz	–	80	–
(Gold-N-Rich)	6 oz	–	80	–
undiluted	6 oz	< 1	340	1%
ORANGE PEEL				
candied	1 oz	–	90	–
fresh	1 Tbs	–	–	–
ORANGE-APRICOT DRINK				
Canned	8 oz	–	128	–
(Tropicana) Twister	8 oz	–	114	–
ORANGE-BANANA JUICE				
(Chiquita)	6 oz	< 1	100	5%
(Smucker's)	8 oz	–	120	–
ORANGE-CRANBERRY DRINK				
(Tropicana) Twister	8 oz	–	114	–
ORANGE-GRAPEFRUIT JUICE				
canned (sweetened)	8 oz	–	107	–
(Kraft) Pure 100%	6 oz	–	80	–
ORANGE-LEMON DRINK	8 oz	–	124	–
ORANGE-PASSION FRUIT DRINK				
(Tropicana) Twister	8 oz	–	90	–
ORANGE-PINEAPPLE JUICE				
(Kraft) Pure 100%	6 oz	–	80	–
(Tropicana)	8 oz	–	111	–
unsweetened	6 oz	–	80	–
ORANGE-STRAWBERRY-BANANA DRINK				
(Tropicana) Twister	8 oz	–	90	–
ORANGE-STRAWBERRY-BANANA JUICE				
(Tropicana)	6 oz	–	106	–
OREGANO/ground	1 tsp	–	5	–
ORIENTAL FOOD (*See also* FROZEN ENTREE/DINNER, PASTA, RICE)				
■ **BEEF MANDARIN**				
Frozen (Van de Kamp's)	11 oz	10	310	29%
■ **BEEF PEPPER ORIENTAL**				
canned	¾ cup	2	80	23%
■ **(BETTY CROCKER) BOX MIX**				
Skillet Chicken Helper - prepared				
Stir-Fried Chicken	⅕ box	11	330	30%
■ **(BOOTH) LIGHT ENTREE**				
Shrimp Oriental/frozen	10 oz	3	190	14%
■ **CHOP SUEY**				
Standard Home Recipe (USDA)				
w/beef w/o noodles	1 cup	17	300	51%
w/beef & pork	1 cup	17	300	51%

Food and Description	Amount	Fat Grams	Total Calories	% Fat Calories
■ **CHOW MEIN-BEEF**				
Canned	¾ cup	1	70	13%
Standard Home Recipe (USDA)	1 cup	17	300	51%
■ **CHOW MEIN-CHICKEN**				
canned	¾ cup	3	80	34%
homemade	¾ cup	10	255	35%
microwave (Kid's Kitchen)				
box mix	7.5 oz	1	90	10%
■ **CHOW MEIN-PORK**				
homemade w/noodles	1 cup	24.7	432	51%
homemade w/o noodles	¾ cup	14	223	57%
■ **CHOW MEIN-SHRIMP**				
homemade w/noodles	¾ cup	3.9	141	25%
■ **(CHUN KING)**				
Divider Pak Entrees/Canned-Prepared				
Beef Chow Mein				
40 oz package	7 oz	2	100	18%
24 oz package	8 oz	2	110	16%
Beef Pepper Oriental	7 oz	4	110	33%
Chicken Chow Mein				
40 oz package	7 oz	4	110	33%
24 oz package	8 oz	4	120	30%
Pork Chow Mein	7 oz	4	120	30%
Shrimp Chow Mein	7 oz	2	100	18%
Egg Rolls & Side Dishes/Frozen				
Chicken Egg Rolls	3.5 oz	7	210	30%
Chinese Pea Pods	1.5 oz	–	16	–
Fried Rice w/Chicken	8 oz	4	254	14%
Fried Rice w/Pork	8 oz	5	263	17%
Meat & Shrimp Egg Rolls	3.5 oz	8	214	34%
Pork Restaurant Style				
Egg Rolls	3 oz	6	172	31%
Shrimp Egg Rolls	3.5 oz	6	189	29%
Entrees/Frozen				
Beef Pepper Oriental	13 oz	3	310	9%
Chicken Chow Mein	13 oz	6	370	10%
Crunchy Walnut Chicken	13 oz	5	310	15%
Imperial Chicken	13 oz	1	300	3%
Sweet & Sour Pork	13 oz	5	400	11%
Stir-Fry Entrees/Canned-Prepared				
Chow Mein w/beef	6 oz	19	290	59%
Chow Mein w/chicken	6 oz	11	220	45%
Egg Foo Young	5 oz	8	140	51%
Pepper Steak	6 oz	17	250	61%
Sukiyaki	6 oz	17	260	59%

Food and Description	Amount	Fat Grams	Total Calories	% Fat Calories
■ **EGG FOO YOUNG**				
homemade	~ 5 oz	10	150	60%
■ **EGG ROLL**				
frozen (Chun King)				
Chicken	3.6 oz	8	220	33%
Meat & Shrimp	3.6 oz	8	220	33%
Shrimp	3.6 oz	6	200	27%
homemade w/o meat	2.25 oz	5.9	102	52%
■ **FRIED RICE** (*See* RICE DISHES)				
■ **(HUNT'S) MINUTE GOURMET**				
Oriental Beef/box mix-prepared	6.4 oz	14	290	43%
Sweet & Sour Chicken/box mix	7.8 oz	4	300	12%
■ **(IMPROMTU LITE)**				
■ microwave box mix				
Sweet & Sour Chicken	9 oz	3	290	9%
■ **(INTERNATIONAL LITES)**				
Microwaveable Box				
Beef Peking	10 oz	3	230	12%
Chicken Peking	10 oz	3	230	12%
■ **(JENO'S)**				
frozen				
Chicken egg rolls	3 oz	9	190	43%
Shrimp & Cheese Egg Rolls	3 oz/			
	~ 6 rolls	8	190	38%
■ **(KIBUN)**				
frozen				
Lemon Ginger Beef	8 oz	4	230	16%
■ **(LA CHOY)**				
Canned				
Bi-Packs/prepared as directed				
Beef Chow Mein	¾ cup	1	70	13%
Beef Pepper Oriental	¾ cup	3	100	27%
Chicken Chow Mein	¾ cup	3	80	34%
Pork Chow Mein	¾ cup	4	80	45%
Shrimp Chow Mein	¾ cup	1	70	13%
Sukiyaki	¾ cup	1	70	13%
Vegetable Chow Mein	¾ cup	2	50	36%
Chow Meins				
Beef	¾ cup	1	60	15%
Chicken	¾ cup	2	70	26%
Meatless	¾ cup	1	35	26%
Shrimp	¾ cup	1	45	20%
Entrees				
Beef Pepper Oriental	¾ cup	2	90	20%
Sweet & Sour Oriental				
w/chicken	¾ cup	2	240	8%

Food and Description	Amount	Fat Grams	Total Calories	% Fat Calories
w/pork	¾ cup	4	250	14%
■ (LEAN CUISINE)				
Chicken Chow Mein	9 oz	5	240	19%
Oriental Beef	8.5 oz	7	250	25%
■ (LEAN POCKETS)				
Chicken Oriental/frozen	1	6	250	22%
■ NOODLES (See PASTA)				
■ (ORIENTAL CLASSICS)				
Box mix				
Sweet & Sour Chicken Dinner	¼ pkg	7	470	13%
Stir Fried Rice Dinner	1 serving	14	430	29%
■ (PRITIKIN)				
Box mix				
Oriental Dinner/prepared	1 cup	1	170	5%
■ (SCHWAN'S)/FROZEN				
Pork Egg Roll	2 oz	7	120	53%
Shrimp Egg Roll	2 oz	4	100	36%
■ SUSHI				
■ homemade w/vegetables	4.5 oz	–	181	–
■ SWEET & SOUR CHICKEN				
canned-prepared	¾ cup	2	120	15%
■ SWEET & SOUR PORK				
frozen (Van de Kamp's)	11 oz	15	430	31%
homemade	¾ cup	7.7	187	37%
■ SZECHWAN CHICKEN				
(International Lites)				
microwaveable - box prepared	10 oz	5	270	17%
■ TERIYAKI CHICKEN				
canned-prepared	¾ cup	2	85	21%
■ TERIYAKI SHRIMP				
homemade	¾ cup	1	174	5%
■ (TYSON)				
Gourmet Selection Entrees				
Chicken Oriental	10.25 oz	7	270	23%
Peking Chicken	10 oz	20	390	46%
Sweet & Sour Chicken	11 oz	16	440	33%
Teriyaki Chicken	11 oz	2	130	14%
Teriyaki Chicken Wings	11 oz	14	220	57%
Stir Fry				
Chicken Stir Fry/frozen	4 oz	6	130	42%
Resolutions/frozen				
Beef Stir Fry	5.6 oz	4	180	20%
■ (WEIGHT WATCHERS)/FROZEN				
Beef Cantonese w/Rice	9 oz	4	200	18%
Chicken Polynesian	9 oz	1	190	5%
Imperial Chicken	8.5 oz	3	200	14%

Food and Description	Amount	Fat Grams	Total Calories	% Fat Calories
Jade Garden Beef	9 oz	3	150	18%
Orange Glazed Chicken	9 oz	2	170	11%
Sesame Chicken w/Lo Mein Noodles	9 oz	4	200	18%
Spring Vegetables w/Teriyaki Chicken	9 oz	3	140	19%
Teriyaki Chicken	7.6 oz	4	150	24%
Vegetable Hunan & Ginger Chicken	9 oz	2	160	11%
■ WON TON SOUP (*See* SOUP)				

ORIENTAL FOOD SEASONINGS

Food and Description	Amount	Fat Grams	Total Calories	% Fat Calories
(Durkee)				
Chop Suey-dry	1 pkg	2	128	14%
prepared	3½ cups	42	1113	34%
Fried Rice				
dry	1 pkg	1	62	15%
prepared	2 cups	1.5	430	9%
Sweet & Sour Sauce				
prepared	1 cup	5.7	230	22%
(Kikkoman)				
Baste & Glaze				
Teriyaki	1 tsp	< 1	9	50%
(La Choy)				
Teriyaki Marinade & Sauce	1 oz	–	30	–
(S&B Sunbird)				
Oriental Seasonings/dry				
Beef & Broccoli	1 pkg	–	97	–
Chinese Barbeque	1 pkg	1	54	17%
Chop Suey	1 pkg	.6	85	6%
Chow Mein	1 pkg	.57	84	6%
Fried Rice	1 pkg	–	57	–
Oriental Chicken	1 pkg	7	140	45%
Stir Fry	1 pkg	.5	75	6%
Sukiyaki	1 pkg	.9	84	10%
Sweet & Sour	1 pkg	–	85	–
Tomato Beef	1 pkg	1	131	7%
Teriyaki Marinade	1 pkg	1	100	9%

OYSTER

Food and Description	Amount	Fat Grams	Total Calories	% Fat Calories
Eastern				
battered & fried	3 oz	10	181	50%
	6 Medium	11	175	57%
breaded & fried	3 oz	10.7	167	58%
	6 Medium	11	173	57%
canned	3 oz	2	58	31%
whole (S&W)	2 oz	3	95	28%
meat only	1 cup	4	160	23%
raw	6 Medium	2	58	31%
steamed	3 oz	4	117	31%

Food and Description	Amount	Fat Grams	Total Calories	% Fat Calories
steamed	3 oz	4	117	31%
	6 Medium/			
	~ 1.5 oz	2	58	31%
Pacific/Western				
canned	6-9 Medium/			
	12 oz	7.5	309	22%
	1 cup	5	218	21%
raw	3 oz	2	69	26%

OYSTER STEW (See SOUP)

P

Food and Description	Amount	Fat Grams	Total Calories	% Fat Calories
PANCAKE				
■ FROZEN				
(Aunt Jemima)				
Blueberry	3	4	200	18%
Buttermilk	3	2	180	10%
Original	3	2	180	10%
(Downyflake)				
Blueberry	3	9	290	28%
Buttermilk	3	9	280	29%
Regular	3	9	280	29%
(Krusteaz)				
Blueberry	3	5	300	15%
Buttermilk	3	5	290	16%
Whole Wheat N Honey	3	4	250	14%
(Morningstar Farms) plain	3.5 oz	5	232	19%
(Swanson) Budget Breakfast	3.5 oz	12	290	37%
■ FROZEN MICROWAVEABLE				
(Aunt Jemima)				
Blueberry	3	4	220	16%
Buttermilk	3	3	210	13%
Buttermilk Lite	3	3	140	19%
Homestyle				
4 Pancakes & 2 Sausages	6 oz	16	420	34%

Food and Description	Amount	Fat Grams	Total Calories	% Fat Calories
4 Lite Pancakes & 2 Lite Links	6 oz	10	310	29%
Lite Pancakes & Lite Syrup	6 oz	3	260	10%
Scrambled Eggs & Sausage w/Pancakes	5.2 oz	14	270	47%
Original	3	4	210	17%
(Krusteaz)				
Blueberry	1	2	100	18%
Buttermilk	1	2	96	19%
Whole Wheat	1	1	83	11%
(Microwave Morning)				
w/Whipped Maple Flavored Topping	4.7 oz	13	380	31%
(Pillsbury Hungry Jack)				
Blueberry	3	4	230	16%
Buttermilk	3	4	260	14%
Harvest Wheat	3	4	230	16%
Oat Bran	3	4	230	16%
Original	3	4	240	15%
(Swanson-Great Starts)				
Pancakes w/Bacon	4.5 oz	20	400	45%
Pancakes & Sausages	6 oz	22	460	43%
Silver Dollar Pancakes & Sausage	3¾ oz	14	310	41%
Whole Wheat Pancakes w/Lite Links	5.5 oz	16	350	41%
(Weight Watchers)				
w/links	4 oz	10	220	41%
■ HOMEMADE				
Standard Home Recipe (USDA)				
Buckwheat (6" dia)	3	9	410	20%
Buttermilk (6" dia)	3	15	490	28%
Plain				
(4" dia)	1	2	62	29%
(6" dia)	1	5	169	27%
PANCAKE BATTER				
Frozen				
(Aunt Jemima)				
Blueberry	3.6 oz	4	204	18%
Buttermilk	3.6 oz	2	180	10%
Original	3.6 oz	2	183	10%
PANCAKE/WAFFLE MIX (*See also* WAFFLE)				
(Arrowhead Mills)				
Blue Corn	½ cup	5	330	14%
Buckwheat	½ cup	2	270	7%
Griddle Lite	½ cup	3	260	10%
Multi-grain	½ cup	2	350	5%
Oat Bran	½ cup	2	200	9%

Food and Description	Amount	Fat Grams	Total Calories	% Fat Calories
(Aunt Jemima)				
Buckwheat	3	1.6	143	10%
Buttermilk Pancake & Waffle	3	< 1	122	5%
Complete Pancake & Waffle/Original	3	4	250	14%
Complete Buttermilk	3	3	230	12%
Lite	3	2	130	14%
Original Pancake & Waffle	3	< 1	116	6%
No cholesterol version	3	4	170	21%
Pancake Express				
Blueberry	3	4	230	16%
Buttermilk	3	3	230	12%
Lite	3	2	130	14%
Original	3	3	240	11%
Whole Wheat	3	1	120	8%
(Betty Crocker)				
Buttermilk	3	10	280	32%
Buttermilk Complete	3	3	210	13%
(Bisquick)				
Shake'N Pour				
Apple Cinnamon	3	3	240	11%
Blueberry	3	3	270	10%
Buttermilk	3	3	250	11%
Original	3	4	250	14%
Blue Corn Pancake & Waffle	⅓ cup	2	200	9%
Buckwheat, Generic, w/Whole Milk	1	2	55	33%
(Classique Fare)				
Apple Complete Dry Mix	.83 oz	.5	83	5%
(Estee)	3	–	100	–
(Feam)				
Buckwheat	½ cup	3	235	12%
Rich Earth	½ cup	2	190	10%
7-Grain Buttermilk	½ cup	2	200	9%
Stone Ground Whole Wheat	½ cup	2	220	8%
Unbleached Wheat & Soya	½ cup	2	235	8%
(Featherweight)	3	2	140	13%
(Hungry Jack)				
Buttermilk				
w/Egg	3	9	210	39%
w/Egg Whites	3	7	200	32%
Buttermilk Complete	3	3	180	15%
Extra Lights				
w/Egg	3	6	190	28%
w/Egg Whites	3	4	170	21%
Extra Lights Complete	3	3	180	15%

Food and Description	Amount	Fat Grams	Total Calories	% Fat Calories
Pre-Measured Packets				
Complete	3	3	180	15%
Wild Blueberry	3	14	320	39%
(Krusteaz)				
Blueberry	3	4	205	18%
Buckwheat	3	3	215	9%
Buttermilk	3	3	200	14%
Complete whole wheat/honey	3	1	215	4%
Complete Oat Bran	3	2	200	9%
Lite	3	1	130	7%
(Martha White) FlapStax	1	1	80	11%
Light Crust Pancake/dry mix	2 oz	3	120	23%
Robin Hood (Gold Medal)				
Pouch mix				
Buttermilk-prepared	⅛ mixture	2	100	18%
PANCAKE/WAFFLE SYRUP (*See also* SYRUP)				
(Aunt Jemima)				
Butter Lite	2 Tbs	–	50	–
Lite	2 Tbs	–	50	–
Regular	2 Tbs	–	110	–
(Cary's)				
Low-cal	1 Tbs	–	6	–
Pure Maple	2 Tbs	–	100	–
(Estee)				
all flavors	1 Tbs	–	4	–
(Featherweight) Lite				
All flavors	1 Tbs	–	16	–
(Golden Griddle)	1 Tbs	–	55	–
(Hungry Jack)				
Lite	2 Tbs	–	50	–
Regular	2 Tbs	–	100	–
(Karo) Pancake	1 Tbs	–	60	–
(Log Cabin)				
Buttered	2 Tbs	–	100	–
Country Kitchen	2 Tbs	–	100	–
Lite	2 Tbs	–	50	–
Maple Honey	2 Tbs	–	100	–
Regular	2 Tbs	–	100	–
(Mrs. Butterworth's) Lite	2 Tbs	–	60	–
(Nabisco) Vermont Maid	1 Tbs	–	50	–
(Nutradiet)				
Blueberry	1 tsp	–	4	–
Maple Flavored	1 tsp	–	4	–
Strawberry	1 tsp	–	4	–

Food and Description	Amount	Fat Grams	Total Calories	% Fat Calories
(Polander)				
Blueberry	2 Tbs	* –	100	–
Raspberry	2 Tbs	–	100	–
Strawberry	2 Tbs	–	100	–
(Smucker's)				
All fruit flavors	1 Tbs	–	50	–
(Weight Watchers)				
Reduced calorie	1 Tbs	–	25	–
PAPAW/fresh	½ lb	2	194	84%
PAPAYA/fresh	1	.5	117	4%
	⅔ cup pulp	–	60	–
PAPAYA JUICE				
Papaya Delight/bottled	6 oz	–	90	–
Papaya Juice/canned	8 oz	–	120	–
PAPAYA NECTAR				
Generic	8 oz	–	142	–
(Kern's)	6 oz	–	110	–
(Knudsen)	8 oz	–	100	–
(Libby's)	6 oz	–	110	–
PAPAYA-PINEAPPLE NECTAR				
(Kern's)	6 oz	–	110	–
PAPAYA PUNCH				
(Tropicana)				
single serve	8 oz	–	110	–
PAPRIKA	1 tsp	–	6	–
PARSLEY	10 sprigs	–	3	–
	½ cup	–	10	–
dried	1 tsp	–	1	–
freeze-dried	any amount	–	–	–
PARSNIP				
fresh-cooked	½ cup	–	63	–
raw	½ cup	–	50	–
PASSION FRUIT				
fresh	1	–	18	–
	½ lb	–	106	–
PASSION FRUIT JUICE				
fresh				
purple	1 cup	–	126	–
yellow	1 cup	–	149	–
Passion Fruit Delight/bottled	6 oz	–	90	–
PASSION FRUIT-ORANGE-GUAVA JUICE				
Blend from frozen concentrate	6 oz	–	80	–
PASSION FRUIT-ORANGE JUICE				
From frozen concentrate	6 oz	–	80	–

Food and Description	Amount	Fat Grams	Total Calories	% Fat Calories
PASSION FRUIT-ORANGE NECTAR				
(Kern's)	6 oz	–	120	–
PASTA				
(American Beauty) Dry				
Coiled Vermicelli	2 oz	1	210	4%
Curly Roni	2 oz	1	210	4%
Elbo Roni	2 oz	1	210	4%
Extra Wide Egg Noodles	2 oz	3	220	12%
Fettuccine	2 oz	3	220	12%
Fine Egg Noodles	2 oz	3	220	12%
Krinkly Egg Noodles	2 oz	3	220	12%
Lasagna	2 oz	1	210	4%
Long Spaghetti	2 oz	1	210	4%
Mostaccioli	2 oz	1	210	4%
Rainbow Shells	2 oz	1	210	4%
Rainbow Twirls	2 oz	1	210	4%
Roni Mac	2 oz	1	210	4%
Rotini	2 oz	1	210	4%
Salad Mac	2 oz	1	210	4%
Shell Roni	2 oz	1	210	4%
Shell Roni-Large	2 oz	1	210	4%
Spaghetti	2 oz	1	210	4%
Thin Spaghetti	2 oz	1	210	4%
Vermicelli	2 oz	1	210	4%
Wide Egg Noodles	2 oz	3	220	12%
(Contadina) Fresh Chilled w/o Sauce				
Agnolotti	3 oz	7	270	23%
Angel's Hair	3 oz	3	260	10%
Chicken Ravioli	3 oz	10	260	35%
Fettuccine	3 oz	3	260	10%
Fettucine (Spinach)	3 oz	4	260	14%
Linguine (Egg)	3 oz	3	260	10%
Ravioli				
w/Beef	3 oz	3	270	10%
w/Cheese	3 oz	11	270	37%
Rigatoni	2.0 oz	3	200	14%
Tortellini				
Sausage	3 oz	7	260	24%
w/Cheese (Egg)	3 oz	6	260	21%
w/Cheese (Spinach)	3 oz	6	260	21%
w/Chicken & Prosciutto	3 oz	6	250	22%
w/Meat	3 oz	6	260	21%
Couscous				
(Casbah) Pilaf-prepared	½ cup	–	100	–

Food and Description	Amount	Fat Grams	Total Calories	% Fat Calories
(Near East)				
dry	1.25 oz	–	120	–
(Nile Spice)				
Salad Mix-Lemon Thyme				
dry	¾ oz	–	58	–
prepared	½ cup	5	103	44%
Whole Wheat Pilaf				
Lentil & Onion				
dry	1.27 oz	–	123	–
prepared	½ cup	4	153	24%
(Creamette) Dry				
Egg Noodles				
Homestyle	2 oz	3	220	12%
Pennsylvania Dutch				
Broad	2 oz	3	220	12%
Egg Noodle Dumpling	2 oz	4	220	16%
Enriched Egg Noodles	2 oz	3	220	12%
Enriched Elbow Macaroni	2 oz	1	210	4%
Enriched Fettuccine	2 oz	1	210	4%
Enriched Lasagna	2 oz	1	210	4%
Enriched Linguini	2 oz	1	210	4%
Enriched Mostaccioli	2 oz	1	210	4%
Enriched Rainbow Rotini	2 oz	1	210	4%
Enriched Rigatoni	2 oz	1	210	4%
Enriched Rotini	2 oz	1	210	4%
Enriched Spaghetti	2 oz	1	210	4%
Enriched Spinach Macaroni				
Ribbons	2 oz	1	210	4%
Enriched Thin Spaghetti	2 oz	1	210	4%
Enriched Vermicelli	2 oz	1	210	4%
Enriched Wide Egg Noodles	2 oz	3	220	12%
No Egg Yolk Ribbons	2 oz	1	210	4%
(De Cecco) Prepared				
Capellini	4 oz	1	210	4%
Fusilli	4 oz	1	210	4%
Lasagna	4 oz	1	210	4%
Linguini	4 oz	1	210	4%
Penne Rigati	4 oz	1	210	4%
Pennete	4 oz	1	210	4%
Spaghetti	4 oz	1	210	4%
Spaghettini	4 oz	1	210	4%
(Deboles) Prepared				
Artichoke				
Elbows	4 oz	1	210	4%

Food and Description	Amount	Fat Grams	Total Calories	% Fat Calories
Linguini	4 oz	1	210	4%
Rigatoni	4 oz	1	210	4%
Spinach Fettuccine	4 oz	1	210	4%
Thin Spaghetti	4 oz	1	210	4%
Ziti	4 oz	1	210	4%
Wheat Free Corn				
Elbows	4 oz	2	200	9%
Shells	4 oz	2	200	9%
Thin Spaghetti	4 oz	2	200	9%
Whole Wheat Spaghetti	4 oz	1	200	5%
(Di Giorno) Fresh Chilled w/o Sauce				
Angel's Hair	3 oz	3	250	11%
Fettuccine	3 oz	3	250	11%
Herb Linguine	3 oz	3	260	10%
Lasagna	1 oz	1	80	11%
Linguine	3 oz	3	250	11%
Spaghetti	3 oz	3	250	11%
Spinach Fettuccine	3 oz	2	260	7%
(Eden) Prepared				
Organic Wheat				
Extra Fine Pasta	4 oz	–	228	–
Paella Ribbons w/Saffron	4 oz	–	228	–
Provencal Ribbons	4 oz	–	228	–
Organic Wheat Vegetable				
Shells	4 oz	1	228	4%
Spirals	4 oz	1	228	4%
Organic Whole Wheat				
Sesame Rice Spirals	4 oz	1	212	4%
Spinach Ribbons	4 oz	–	212	–
Vegetable Spirals	4 oz	1	212	4%
Egg Noodle Substitute (Foulds)				
No Yolks-dry	2 oz	2	210	9%
(Golden Grain) Dry				
Egg noodles	2 oz	2	210	9%
Pasta	2 oz	1	200	5%
(Grandma's)				
Wide Egg Noodles				
Country Style				
frozen	4 oz	2	175	10%
(Health Valley) dry				
Amaranth Pasta	2 oz	1	170	5%
Elbows				
Whole Wheat	2 oz	1	202	5%
Whole Wheat w/4 Vegetables	2 oz	1	202	5%

Food and Description	Amount	Fat Grams	Total Calories	% Fat Calories
Lasagna				
Spinach	2 oz	1	170	5%
Whole Wheat w/Wheat Germ	2 oz	1	170	5%
Spaghetti				
100% Organic	2 oz	1	170	5%
Organic Spinach	2 oz	1	170	5%
Whole Wheat	2 oz	1	170	5%
Whole Wheat Amaranth	2 oz	1	200	5%
Whole Wheat w/Spinach	2 oz	1	170	5%
(Hodgson Mill) Prepared				
Semolina Veggie				
Bows	4 oz	1	210	4%
Egg Noodles	4 oz	3	220	12%
Rotini	4 oz	1	210	4%
Wagon Wheels	4 oz	1	210	4%
Whole Wheat				
Elbows	4 oz	1	200	5%
Fettuccine	4 oz	1	200	5%
Lasagna	4 oz	1	200	5%
Medium Shells	4 oz	1	230	4%
Spaghetti	4 oz	1	200	5%
Spinach Spaghetti	4 oz	1	200	5%
Spirals	4 oz	1	230	4%
Whole Wheat Egg Noodles				
Plain	4 oz	3	220	12%
Spinach	4 oz	3	220	12%
(Light Balance) Microwaveable Lunch Buckets				
Pasta & Garden Vegetables	8.25 oz	1	170	5%
Macaroni				
Dry	8 oz	2.7	838	3%
Enriched/Unenriched				
Cooked-Firm	1 cup	1	190	5%
Tender-Cold	1 cup	< 1	115	4%
Tender-Hot	1 cup	1	155	6%
(Martha Gooch) Prepared				
Big Elbow Macaroni	4 oz	1	210	4%
Egg Noodles				
Dumplings	4 oz	3	220	12%
Extra Wide	4 oz	3	220	12%
Wide	4 oz	3	220	12%
Long Spaghetti	4 oz	1	210	4%
Rotini	4 oz	1	210	4%
Shell Macaroni	4 oz	1	210	4%
Thin Spaghetti	4 oz	1	210	4%

Food and Description	Amount	Fat Grams	Total Calories	% Fat Calories
Matzo Farfel				
(Manischewitz) Prepared	1 cup	.8	180	4%
(Mueller's) Dry				
Egg Noodles	2 oz	3	220	12%
Golden Rich Egg Noodles	2 oz	3	220	12%
Lasagna	2 oz	1	210	4%
Macaroni	2 oz	1	210	4%
Spaghetti	2 oz	1	210	4%
Tri-Color Twists	2 oz	1	210	4%
Noodles				
Chow Mein				
Canned	1 cup	11	220	45%
Dry (La Choy)	½ cup	8	150	48%
Egg				
Cooked	1 cup	2	200	9%
Dry	8 oz	10	881	10%
Flakes				
(Goodman's) dry	2 oz	3	220	12%
Frozen				
(Reames)				
Cooked	4 oz	1	150	6%
Dry	2 oz	2	160	11%
Oriental Noodles				
Chinese (Chun King)				
Canned	1 oz	7	140	45%
Chow Funn				
Wheat-dry	1 oz	< 1	102	4%
Saimin				
Wheat-dry	1 oz	–	95	–
Soba (Eden)				
Buckwheat-dry	1 oz	1	100	9%
Pastini				
Carrot-dry	4 oz	2	420	4%
Egg-dry	1 cup	7	651	10%
Spinach-dry	4 oz	2	415	4%
(Pennsylvania Dutch)				
Egg Noodles-dry				
Broad	1 oz	1	110	8%
Kluski	1 oz	1	110	8%
Medium	1 oz	1	110	8%
Stroganoff	1 oz	1	110	8%
(Pritikin) Dry				
Ribbon Pasta				
whole wheat	2 oz	2	220	8%

Food and Description	Amount	Fat Grams	Total Calories	% Fat Calories
Spaghetti				
whole wheat	2 oz	2	220	8%
(Ronzoni) Dry				
Egg Noodles	2 oz	2	210	9%
Spinach	2 oz	3	220	12%
Macaroni	2 oz	< 1	210	2%
Medium Shells	2 oz	1	210	4%
Spinach Macaroni	2 oz	< 1	210	2%
Tri-color Rotini	2 oz	1	210	4%
(San Giorgio) Dry				
Acine Di-Pepe	1 oz	< 1	110	4%
Capellini	1 oz	< 1	110	4%
Cut Fusilli	1 oz	< 1	110	4%
Cut Ziti	1 oz	< 1	110	4%
Elbow Macaroni	1 oz	< 1	110	4%
Jumbo Shells	1 oz	< 1	110	4%
Large Shells	1 oz	< 1	110	4%
Light & Fluffy				
Dumplings	1 oz	< 1	110	4%
Egg Noodles				
Extra Wide	1 oz	2	110	16%
Medium	1 oz	2	110	16%
Spinach	1 oz	2	110	16%
Wide	1 oz	2	110	16%
Linguine	1 oz	< 1	110	4%
Mafalda	1 oz	< 1	110	4%
Manicotti	1 oz	< 1	110	4%
Orzo	1 oz	< 1	110	4%
Rainbow Medley	1 oz	< 1	110	4%
Rainbow Shells	1 oz	< 1	110	4%
Rainbow Twirls	1 oz	< 1	110	4%
Ridged Mostaccioli	1 oz	< 1	110	4%
Rigatoni	1 oz	< 1	110	4%
Rotini	1 oz	< 1	110	4%
Small Shells	1 oz	< 1	110	4%
Spaghetti	1 oz	< 1	110	4%
Spaghettini	1 oz	< 1	110	4%
Spaghetti				
Cooked				
Firm Stage	1 cup	.7	192	3%
Tender Stage	1 cup	.6	155	4%
(Weight Watchers) Dry				
Elbow Style	2 oz	1	160	6%
Spaghettini	2 oz	1	160	6%

Food and Description	Amount	Fat Grams	Total Calories	% Fat Calories
(Westbrae Natural) Whole Wheat - Dry				
Lasagna	2 oz	2	210	9%
Spaghetti				
Plain	2 oz	2	210	9%
Spinach	2 oz	2	210	9%
PASTA ENTREE/DINNER(See also FROZEN ENTREE/DINNER; MICROWAVE-ABLE NONFROZEN MEALS; and individual listings)				
(NOTE: Data for homemade dishes in this table will vary, pending type of ingredients used, i.e. low-fat milk & cheeses. Mixes are prepared as directed unless otherwise stated.)				
(Amy's) Frozen				
Macaroni and Cheese	1 serving	10.8	226	43%
Macaroni and Soy Sauce	1 serving	8.45	228	33%
Vegetable Lasagna	10 oz	7	310	20%
(Betty Crocker) Mix				
Presto Pasta				
Creamy Alfredo	¼ pkg	18	370	44%
Ground Beef in Tomato Herb				
Sauce-dry	¼ pkg	8	280	26%
Italian Sausage in Tomato Herb				
Sauce-dry	¼ pkg	8	280	26%
Tomato Mushroom-dry	¼ pkg	6	240	26%
Suddenly Salad				
Caesar				
Dry	⅙ pkg	1	110	8%
Prepared	½ cup	8	170	42%
Classic Pasta				
Dry	⅙ pkg	1	120	8%
Prepared	½ cup	6	160	34%
Creamy Macaroni				
Dry	⅙ pkg	< 1	100	5%
Prepared	½ cup	10	200	45%
Prepared-lower fat recipe	½ cup	4	140	26%
Italian Pasta				
Dry	⅙ pkg	1	110	8%
Prepared	½ cup	6	160	34%
Pasta Primavera				
Dry	⅙ pkg	< 1	90	5%
Prepared	½ cup	10	190	47%
Prepared-lower fat recipe	½ cup	5	150	30%
Ranch and Bacon				
Dry	⅙ pkg	1	110	8%
Prepared	½ cup	11	210	47%
Prepared-lower fat recipe	½ cup	5	160	28%

Food and Description	Amount	Fat Grams	Total Calories	% Fat Calories
Tortellini Italiano				
Dry	⅕ pkg	2	120	15%
Prepared	½ cup	7	160	39%
(Chef Boy Ar Dee)				
Canned				
ABC's & 1,2,3's				
w/Mini Meatballs	7.5 oz	9	240	34%
in Sauce	7.5 oz	1	160	6%
Beef-O-Getti	7.5 oz	9	220	37%
Beefaroni	7.5 oz	8	220	33%
	8 oz	9	260	31%
	8.7 oz	8	250	29%
Chili Mac	7.5 oz	11	230	43%
Dinosaurs in Cheese Flavored Sauce	8.6 oz	1	200	5%
Dinosaurs in Spaghetti Sauce				
w/cheese flavor	7.5 oz	1	160	6%
Dinosaurs w/Meatballs	8.6 oz	11	280	35%
Dinosaurs w/Mini Meatballs	7.5 oz	8	230	31%
Lasagna	7.5 oz	8	240	30%
Lasagna	8 oz	10	250	36%
Macaroni Shells in Tomato Sauce	7.5 oz	1	150	6%
Mini Bites	7.5 oz	12	260	42%
Mini Cannelloni	7.5 oz	7	230	27%
Pac Man in Chicken Sauce	7.5 oz	7	170	37%
Pac Man in Tomato Sauce	7.5 oz	1	150	6%
Pac Man w/Meatballs	7.5 oz	9	230	35%
Ravioli Products				
Beef Ravioli in Sauce	8 oz	5	220	21%
	8.7 oz	6	240	23%
Beef Ravioli				
in Tomato & Meat Sauce	7.5 oz	5	220	21%
Cheese Ravioli				
in Beef & Tomato Sauce	7.5 oz	3	200	14%
Cheese Ravioli in Tomato Sauce	7.5 oz	5	200	23%
Chicken Ravioli	7.5 oz	4	180	20%
Mini Ravioli-Beef	7.5 oz	5	210	38%
Mini Ravioli-Beef	8 oz	6	230	24%
Mini Ravioli-Chicken	7.5 oz	8	220	33%
Roller Coasters	7.5 oz	10	230	39%
Smurf Beef Raviioli & Pasta				
in Meat Sauce	7.5 oz	5	230	20%
Smurf Pasta in Spaghetti Sauce				
w/cheese flavor	7.5 oz	1	150	6%
Smurf Pasta w/Meatballs	7.5 oz	9	240	34%

Food and Description	Amount	Fat Grams	Total Calories	% Fat Calories
Spaghetti & Meatballs-25.5 oz	8.5 oz	11	250	40%
Spaghetti & Meatballs w/tomato sauce-15 oz	7.5 oz	9	230	35%
Spaghetti & Meatballs w/tomato sauce-39 oz	7.8 oz	10	240	38%
Spaghetti'n Beef in tomato sauce	7.5 oz	9	240	34%
Tic Tac Toes in Spaghetti Sauce w/cheese flavor	7.5 oz	1	160	6%
Tic Tac Toes w/Mini Meatballs	7.5 oz	9	240	34%
Zooroni w/Meatballs in Sauce	7.5 oz	8	240	30%
Dinner Products				
Lasagna Dinner	5.97 oz	8	280	26%
Spaghetti Dinner w/Condensed Meat Sauce	3.25 oz	6	250	22%
Spaghetti packaged Dinner w/prepared Meat Sauce	4.88 oz	3	240	11%
Spaghetti packaged Dinner w/prepared Mushroom Sauce	4.88 oz	1	210	4%
(EZO)				
ABC's & 123's in Sauce	7 oz	1	160	6%
ABC's & 123's w/Meatballs	7 oz	8	230	31%
ABC's & 123's w/Mini Meatballs	7.5 oz	11	260	38%
Beef Ravioli	7 oz	5	180	25%
	7.5 oz	4	190	19%
Beef Stew	7 oz	13	220	53%
Beefaroni	7.5 oz	7	220	29%
Chili Mac	7 oz	10	230	39%
Dinosaurs in Sauce	7 oz	1	160	6%
w/Meatballs	7 oz	7	220	29%
Lasagna	7.5 oz	9	230	35%
	7 oz	8	220	33%
Mini Cannelloni	7.5 oz	9	240	34%
Roller Coasters	7 oz	9	230	35%
Spaghetti'N Beef in Tomato Sauce	7 oz	8	220	33%
Spaghetti w/Meatballs	7 oz	8	210	34%
	7.5 oz	10	240	38%
Tic Tac Toes w/Meatballs	7.5 oz	11	260	38%
Tic Tac Toes w/Mini Meatballs	7 oz	8	210	34%
Tic Tac Toes in Spaghetti Sauce w/Cheese flavor	7 oz	1	160	6%

Food and Description	Amount	Fat Grams	Total Calories	% Fat Calories
(LIDO Club)				
Beef Ravioli	7.5 oz	4	190	19%
Spaghetti & Meatballs	7.5 oz	9	220	37%
Spaghetti Rings & Little Meat Balls	7.5 oz	10	220	41%
(Estee)				
Ravioli Beef	7.5 oz	6	210	26%
Spaghetti & Meatballs	7.5 oz	15	240	56%
(Franco-American)				
Canned				
Beef Ravioli's in Meat Sauce	7.5 oz	8	250	29%
Hearty Pasta Beef Ravioli in Meat Sauce	7.5 oz	11	280	35%
Hearty Pasta Macaroni w/Beef in Tomato Sauce	7.5 oz	5	200	23%
Hearty Pasta Twists in Pizza Sauce	7.5 oz	7	220	29%
Macaroni & Cheese	7⅜ oz	5	170	27%
Spaghetti w/Meatballs in Tomato Sauce	7⅜ oz	8	220	33%
Spaghetti in Tomato Sauce w/cheese	7⅜ oz	2	190	10%
Spaghettio's in Tomato & Cheese Sauce	7.5 oz	2	170	7%
Spaghettio's w/Meatballs in Tomato Sauce	7⅜ oz	8	210	66%
Spaghettio's w/Sliced Beef Franks in Tomato Sauce	7⅜ oz	9	220	37%
Sporty O's	7⅜ oz	8	210	34%
Teddy O's	7.5 oz	2	170	11%
(Golden Grain)				
Lunch-In-One Microwave				
Fettuccine Alfredo	1 package	13	350	33%
Macaroni & Cheese	1 package	10	340	26%
Pasta Broccoli Au Gratin	1 package	10	330	27%
Pasta & Three Cheeses	1 package	12	340	32%
Shells & Creamy Sauce	1 package	12	340	32%
Noodle Roni Mix				
Angel Hair Pasta				
w/herbs-dry	1 serving	2	120	15%
w/herbs-prepared	1 serving	8	200	36%
w/parmesan cheese-dry	1 serving	3	140	19%
w/parmesan cheese-prepared	1 serving	9	210	39%
Broccoli Au Gratin	½ cup	9	190	43%

Food and Description	Amount	Fat Grams	Total Calories	% Fat Calories
Broccoli & Mushroom	½ cup	14	240	53%
Chicken & Mushroom	½ cup	8	180	40%
Creamy Chicken	½ cup	8	180	40%
Creamy Garlic	½ cup	14	240	53%
Fettuccine	½ cup	15	250	54%
Herb & Butter	½ cup	13	240	49%
Mild Cheddar	½ cup	9	190	43%
Parmesano	½ cup	14	250	50%
Romanoff	½ cup	10	200	45%
Sour Cream & Chives	½ cup	14	240	53%
Stroganoff	½ cup	9	200	41%
Vegetable Alfredo	½ cup	14	240	53%
(Green Giant) Frozen				
Entrees				
Lasagna	12 oz	20	490	37%
Macaroni & Cheese	9 oz	10	290	31%
Garden Gourmet–"Right for Lunch"				
Fettucine Primavera	1 pkg	8	230	31%
Pasta Dijon	1 pkg	17	260	59%
Rotini Cheddar	1 pkg	10	230	39%
Pasta Accents				
Cheddar Cheese Seasoning	½ cup	3	90	30%
Garden Herb Seasoning	½ cup	3	80	34%
Garlic Seasoning	½ cup	4	100	36%
Primavera	½ cup	4	110	33%
(Hain) Mix				
Pasta & Sauce (prepared)				
Creamy Dill Multi Bran	½ cup	6	150	36%
Creamy Parmesan	½ cup	7	160	39%
Creamy Swiss	½ cup	9	180	45%
Fettuccini Alfredo	½ cup	10	190	47%
Italian Herb	½ cup	10	170	53%
Italian Multi Bran	½ cup	7	120	53%
Primavera	½ cup	10	180	50%
Salsa Multi Bran	½ cup	7	130	48%
Tangy Cheddar	½ cup	11	190	52%
(Healthy Choice)				
Canned				
Lasagna w/Meat Sauce	7.5 oz	5	220	20%
Spaghetti w/Meat Sauce	7.5 oz	3	150	18%
Spaghetti Rings	7.5 oz	–	140	–
Microwaveable Cups				
Lasagna w/Meat Sauce	7.5 oz	5	220	20%
Spaghetti w/Meat Sauce	7.5 oz	3	150	18%

Food and Description	Amount	Fat Grams	Total Calories	% Fat Calories
Spaghetti Rings	7.5 oz	–	140	–
(Heinz)				
Chili-Mac	7.5 oz	12	250	43%
Macaroni'N Beef in Tomato Sauce	7.25 oz	8	200	36%
Macaroni & Cheese	7.5 oz	8	190	38%
Noodles & Beef in Sauce	7.5 oz	8	170	42%
Noodles & Chicken	7.5 oz	7	160	39%
Noodles & Tuna	7.5 oz	5	170	27%
Spaghetti in Tomato Sauce				
w/cheese	7.75 oz	2	160	11%
Spaghetti in Tomato Sauce w/meat	7.5 oz	6	170	32%
(Kid's Kitchen)				
Microwave				
Macaroni & Cheese	7.5 oz	5	170	27%
Macaroni & Chicken	7.5 oz	2	120	15%
(Kraft) Mix				
Dinners-Prepared				
Egg Noodles w/Cheese Dinner	¾ cup	17	340	45%
Egg Noodles w/Chicken Dinner	¾ cup	9	240	34%
Macaroni & Cheese	¾ cup	13	290	40%
Deluxe	¾ cup	8	260	28%
Family Size	¾ cup	13	290	40%
Micromac-dry	¼ pkg	2	150	12%
Micromac-prepared	½ cup	7	210	30%
Macaroni & Cheese				
Dinomac	¾ cup	14	310	41%
Spirals	¾ cup	18	340	48%
Teddy Bears	¾ cup	14	310	41%
Wild Wheels	¾ cup	14	310	41%
Spaghetti Dinner				
American Style	1 cup	7	300	21%
Tangy Italian Style	1 cup	8	310	23%
w/Meat Sauce	1 cup	14	360	35%
Spiral Macaroni & Cheese	¾ cup	17	330	46%
Velveeta				
Bits of Bacon Shells	½ cup	10	240	38%
Rotini & Cheese Broccoli-prepared	½ cup	8	210	34%
Touch of Mexico Shells	½ cup	8	210	34%
Pasta & Cheese-prepared				
Cheddar Broccoli	½ cup	8	180	40%
Chicken w/Herbs	½ cup	7	170	37%
Fettuccine Alfredo	½ cup	9	180	45%
Parmesan	½ cup	8	180	40%
3-Cheese & Vegetable	½ cup	8	180	40%

Food and Description	Amount	Fat Grams	Total Calories	% Fat Calories
Pasta Salad-prepared				
Broccoli & Vegetable	½ cup	16	210	69%
Creamy Dill	½ cup	11	200	50%
Garden Primavera	½ cup	7	170	37%
Herb & Garlic	½ cup	12	210	51%
Homestyle	½ cup	16	240	60%
Light Italian	½ cup	3	130	21%
Rancher's Choice				
Light	½ cup	7	170	37%
Regular	½ cup	16	250	58%
(Lipton)				
Hearty Ones Microwave				
Beef Vegetable	11 oz	3	230	12%
Garden Medley	11 oz	4	320	11%
Homestyle Chicken	11 oz	4	230	16%
Italiano	11 oz	2	330	5%
Minestrone	11 oz	3	190	14%
Shells & Cheddar	11 oz	7	370	17%
Noodles & Sauce (as packaged)				
Alfredo	½ cup	3	130	21%
Beef	½ cup	2	120	15%
Butter	½ cup	4	140	26%
Butter & Herb	½ cup	3	140	19%
Carbonara Alfredo	½ cup	3	130	21%
Cheese	½ cup	2	140	13%
Chicken Broccoli	½ cup	2	125	14%
Chicken Flavored	½ cup	2	125	14%
Creamy Chicken	½ cup	2	125	14%
Parmesan	½ cup	4	140	26%
Romanoff	½ cup	3	135	20%
Sour Cream & Chive	½ cup	3	140	13%
Stroganoff	½ cup	2	110	16%
Tomato Alfredo	½ cup	3	130	21%
Pasta & Sauce (as packaged)				
Cheddar Broccoli	½ cup	5	130	35%
Creamy Garlic	½ cup	2	145	12%
Creamy Mushroom	½ cup	3	145	19%
Herb Tomato	½ cup	1	130	7%
Pasta Salad (as packaged)				
Creamy Broccoli	½ cup	1	120	8%
Robust Italian	½ cup	1	125	7%
(Little Chef) Mix				
Entree Pasta Italiano				
dry	¼ pkg	–	110	–

Food and Description	Amount	Fat Grams	Total Calories	% Fat Calories
w/chicken	1 cup	10	290	31%
w/tofu	1 cup	11	250	40%
Looney Tunes (Tyson) Pastas				
Bugs Bunny & Tazmanian Devil	8 oz	8	290	25%
Daffy Duck & Elmer Fudd	8 oz	7	270	23%
Foghorn Leghorn & Henry Hawk	8 oz	4	230	16%
Sylvester & Tweety	8 oz	4	250	14%
(McCormick/Schilling) Mix				
Pasta Prima				
Alfredo				
Dry	1 pkg	–	169	–
Prepared	½ cup	13	253	46%
Creamy Garlic-dry	1 pkg	5.3	107	45%
Creamy Seafood-dry	1 pkg	1.8	135	12%
Herb & Garlic				
Dry	1 pkg	–	65	–
Prepared	½ cup	12	326	33%
Marinara				
Dry	1 pkg	–	74	–
Prepared	½ cup	8	329	22%
Pasta Salad				
Dry	1 pkg	–	78	–
Prepared	½ cup	23	390	53%
Pesto				
Dry	1 pkg	–	37	–
Prepared	½ cup	6	193	28%
(Minute Microwave) Mix				
Prepared w/Butter				
Chicken Flavored Noodles				
Family Size	½ cup	5	160	23%
Single Size	½ cup	4	160	23%
Noodles Alfredo				
Family Size	½ cup	6	170	32%
Single Size	½ cup	5	160	28%
Parmesan Noodles				
Family Size	½ cup	6	170	17%
Single Size	½ cup	5	160	23%
Pasta & Cheddar Cheese				
Family Size	½ cup	7	160	39%
Single Size	½ cup	6	160	34%
(Nile Spice) Meals In A Cup				
Pasta'N Sauce				
Mediterranean	7 oz	4	210	17%
Parmesan	7 oz	4	210	17%

Food and Description	Amount	Fat Grams	Total Calories	% Fat Calories
Primavera	7 oz	3	210	13%
(Ragu)				
Pasta Meals				
Elbows in Sauce w/Ground Beef, Mushrooms,				
& Green Peppers	7.5 oz	4	200	18%
Mini Lasagna in Sauce	7.5 oz	1	160	6%
Shells in Sauce w/Ground Beef	7.5 oz	4	190	19%
Spaghetti in Sauce	7.5 oz	1	170	5%
Spaghetti in Sauce				
w/Ground Beef	7.5 oz	4	210	17%
Twists in Sauce	7.5 oz	1	160	6%
(Ramen) Noodles (*See* SOUP/DEHYDRATED MIX)				
(Rice-A-Roni) Lunch For One				
Broccoli Au Gratin	1 pkg	10	330	27%
Fettuccine Alfredo	1 pkg	13	350	33%
Macaroni & Cheese	1 pkg	10	340	26%
Pasta & Three Cheeses	1 pkg	12	340	32%
Shells & Creamy Sauce	1 pkg	8	290	25%
(Ultra Slim Fast) Microwaveable-Prepared				
Macaroni & Cheese Sauce	1 cup	3	230	12%
Noodles & Alfredo Sauce	8 oz	4	240	15%
Pasta w/Beef Flavored Sauce	8 oz	3	230	12%
Pasta w/Chicken Flavored Sauce	8 oz	3	220	12%
Pasta w/Tomato Herb Sauce	8 oz	3	220	12%
Pasta w/Zesty Cheese Sauce	8 oz	4	230	16%
(Van Camp's)				
Canned Products				
Chili-Mac	1 cup	20	320	56%
Noodlee Weenee	1 cup	8	240	30%
Spaghettee Weenee	1 cup	7	240	26%
(Wolf)				
Chili-Mac-canned	1 cup	20	320	56%
PASTA SAUCE (*See* SAUCE)				
PASTRAMI (*See also* LUNCHEON MEAT)				
	1 oz	8	99	73%
PASTRY (*See* CAKE AND CAKE PASTRY)				
PASTRY SHEET				
Fillo-all purpose dough	1⅓ leaves	–	80	–
(Pepperidge Farm) Puff Pastry Sheets	¼ sheet	17	260	59%
PASTRY SHELL				
(Pepperidge Farm) frozen	1 shell	15	210	64%
PASTRY, TOASTER				
(Kellogg's) Pop Tarts				
Frosted blueberry	1	6	210	26%

Food and Description	Amount	Fat Grams	Total Calories	% Fat Calories
Frosted brown sugar/cinnamon	1	7	210	30%
Frosted cherry	1	5	200	23%
Frosted chocolate fudge	1	5	200	23%
Frosted cinnamon	1	7	210	30%
Frosted dutch apple	1	6	210	26%
Frosted raspberry	1	5	200	23%
Frosted strawberry	1	5	200	23%
Frosted vanilla cream	1	5	200	23%
Unfrosted blueberry	1	6	210	26%
Unfrosted milk chocolate	1	6	210	26%
Unfrosted raspberry	1	6	210	26%
Unfrosted strawberry	1	6	210	26%
(Nabisco) Toastettes Pastry				
Apple	1	5	190	24%
Blueberry	1	5	190	24%
Cherry	1	5	190	24%
Frosted				
Apple	1	5	190	24%
Blueberry	1	5	190	24%
Brown Sugar Cinnamon	1	5	190	24%
Cherry	1	5	190	24%
Fudge	1	5	200	23%
Strawberry	1	5	190	24%
Fruit Punch	1	5	190	24%
Strawberry	1	5	190	24%
(Pepperidge Farm) Toaster Tarts				
Apple cinnamon	1	7	170	37%
Cheese	1	10	190	47%
Strawberry	1	7	190	33%
(Pillsbury)				
Toaster Muffins				
Apple spice	1	5	130	35%
Banana nut	1	6	130	42%
Old fashioned corn	1	5	120	38%
Raisin bran	1	5	120	38%
Wild Maine blueberry	1	3	120	23%
Toaster Strudel Breakfast Pastry				
Apple spice, Blueberry, Cinnamon,				
Raspberry, Strawberry	1	8	190	38%
Cherry	1	9	190	43%
PEA (See also PEA & CARROT, PEA DISHES, PIGEON PEA, SNOW PEA)				
Alaska (Early or June)				
canned				
not drained	½ cup	–	67	–

Food and Description	Amount	Fat Grams	Total Calories	% Fat Calories
drained	½ cup	–	75	–
canned				
(Festal)	½ cup	–	70	–
(Green Giant)	½ cup	–	50	–
(S&W) Petit Pois	½ cup	–	70	–
(Tendersweet)	½ cup	–	70	–
frozen				
(Green Giant)	½ cup	–	50	–
(Harvest Fresh)	½ cup	–	60	–
Edible Podded				
fresh-cooked	½ cup	–	34	–
frozen-boiled	½ cup	–	54	–
frozen (Chun King)	1.5 oz	–	16	–
frozen (La Choy)	1 pkg	–	70	–
Green Peas				
canned	½ cup	–	59	–
fresh-cooked	½ cup	–	67	–
frozen				
(Birds Eye)	3.3 oz	–	80	–
(Health Valley)	5.5 oz	–	126	–
raw	½ cup	–	63	–
Split Peas				
boiled	½ cup	–	115	–
raw	½ cup	1	348	3%
Sweet Peas (wrinkled peas, sugar peas)				
canned				
Garden				
(Freshlike)	½ cup	–	50	–
(Green Giant)				
50% Less Salt	½ cup	–	50	–
Mini (Green Giant)	½ cup	–	60	–
Perfection				
(S&W)	½ cup	–	70	–
Small				
(Del Monte)	½ cup	–	50	–
(Freshlike)	½ cup	–	50	–
canned-drained				
(Del Monte)	½ cup	–	60	–
Generic	½ cup	–	68	–
(Green Giant)	½ cup	–	50	–
(Libby)	½ cup	–	60	–
canned-not drained				
Generic	½ cup	–	71	–
(Nutradiet)	½ cup	–	40	–

Food and Description	Amount	Fat Grams	Total Calories	% Fat Calories
frozen				
(Green Giant)	½ cup	–	50	–
(Harvest Fresh)	½ cup	–	50	–
Tender Tiny Peas				
frozen (Birds Eye)	½ cup	–	60	–
PEA & CARROT				
canned (Nutradiet)	½ cup	–	35	–
Sweet Peas & Sliced Carrots/canned				
(Freshlike)	½ cup	–	50	–
PEA DISHES (*See also* PEA & CARROT)				
Early Peas in Butter Sauce				
frozen microwave (Green Giant)	4.5 oz	2	80	23%
Field Peas w/Snaps seasoned w/pork				
canned (Luck's)	7.5 oz	7	200	32%
Green Peas & Rice w/mushrooms				
frozen (Birds Eye)	2.3 oz	–	110	–
Green peas in cream sauce				
frozen (Birds Eye)	2.6 oz	6	120	45%
Green peas, potatoes in cream sauce				
frozen (Bird's Eye)	2.6 oz	6	130	42%
Mini Peas, Pea Pods & Water Chestnuts				
in Butter Sauce				
frozen (LeSueur)	½ cup	2	80	23%
Peas & potatoes w/cream sauce				
frozen (Birds Eye)	½ cup	6	127	43%
Peas in Cream Sauce				
frozen (Green Giant)	½ cup	4	90	40%
Peas in Butter Sauce				
frozen Micro Quick (Freshlike)	5 oz	2	110	16%
Peas, Onions, & Carrots in butter sauce				
frozen (LeSueur)	½ cup	3	80	34%
Peas, Pearl Onions in cheese sauce				
frozen (Birds Eye)	½ cup	5	140	32%
Peas, Pearl Onions, Mushrooms				
frozen (Pictsweet) Express microwave	2.5 oz	–	45	–
Peas-Seasoned				
canned (Del Monte)	½ cup	–	60	–
Sweet Pea Cauliflower Medley				
frozen				
(Green Giant) Valley Combinations	½ cup	–	30	–
Sweet Peas in Butter Sauce				
frozen (Green Giant)	½ cup	2	80	23%
Sweet Peas & Diced Carrots				
canned (S&W)	½ cup	–	50	–

Food and Description	Amount	Fat Grams	Total Calories	% Fat Calories
Sweet Peas & Onions				
canned (Green Giant)	½ cup	–	50	–
Sweet Peas & Sliced Mushrooms				
in Butter Sauce				
Vegetable Classics (Del Monte)				
microwave	½ cup	2	60	30%
Sweet Peas & Tiny Onions				
canned (Freshlike)	½ cup	–	60	–
Sweet Peas & Tiny Pearl Onions				
canned (S&W)	½ cup	1	60	15%
PEA SOUP (*See* SOUP)				
PEA SPROUT/cooked	½ cup	–	80	–
PEACH				
Canned				
in Heavy Syrup	1 cup	–	190	–
in Juice	1 cup	–	109	–
in Water	1 cup	–	58	–
(Del Monte)				
Freestone Halves or Slices	½ cup	–	90	–
Lite Freestone	½ cup	–	60	–
Lite Yellow Cling	½ cup	–	50	–
Yellow Cling Halves or Slices	½ cup	–	80	–
Dried				
Cooked Halves				
No Sugar	½ cup	< 1	100	5%
w/Sugar	½ cup	< 1	165	3%
Uncooked Halves	10 large	1	380	2%
	10 medium	.9	341	2%
	½ cup	.6	191	2%
(Del Monte)	2 oz	–	140	–
(Mariani)	¼ cup	–	140	–
(Sun Maid)	2 oz	–	140	–
Fresh	1	–	37	–
Slices	1 cup	–	73	–
Frozen				
No Sugar	3.5 oz	< 1	45	10%
Sliced	1 cup	< 1	132	3%
Sweetened				
Sliced	1 cup	< 1	235	2%
Fruit Cup				
(Del Monte)				
Yellow Cling Peaches, Diced	5 oz	–	110	–
(Nutradiet)				
Halves	½ cup	–	30	–

Food and Description	Amount	Fat Grams	Total Calories	% Fat Calories
Sliced	½ cup	–	30	–
(S&W)				
Clingstone				
Halves in Heavy Syrup	½ cup	–	100	–
Freestone				
Halves in Heavy Syrup	½ cup	–	100	–
Slices in Heavy Syrup	½ cup	–	100	–
Natural	½ cup	–	90	–
Yellow Cling				
Sliced in Heavy Syrup	½ cup	–	100	–
Spiced				
Canned in Syrup	1 cup	–	180	–
(Del Monte) w/Pits	3.5 oz	–	80	–
(S&W) Yellow Cling				
Whole in Heavy Syrup	½ cup	–	90	–
PEACH BUTTER				
(Smucker's)	1 tsp	–	15	–
PEACH JUICE				
Bottled or Canned				
(Dole) Pure & Light				
Orchard Peach	6 oz	–	90	–
Peach Delight	6 oz	–	90	–
(Smucker's)	8 oz	–	120	–
PEACH NECTAR				
Generic/canned	8 oz	–	134	–
(Kern's)	6 oz	–	110	–
(Libby's) Ripe Peach	8 oz	–	130	–
PEANUT				
■ ALL TYPES				
Boiled	½ cup	7	102	62%
Dried	1 oz	13.97	161	78%
Dry Roasted	1 oz	13.9	164	76%
Lite	1 oz	9	135	60%
Honey Roasted	1 oz	13	170	69%
Oil Roasted	1 oz	13.8	163	76%
	½ cup	35.5	418	76%
■ BY BRAND NAME				
(Eagle)				
Cinnamon Roasted	1 oz	13	170	69%
Cinnamon Honey Roasted	1 oz	13	170	69%
Dry Honey Roasted	1 oz	13	170	69%
Fancy Virginia	½ oz	8	90	80%
Lightly Salted	1 oz	15	170	79%
Maple Roasted	1 oz	13	170	69%
Maple Honey Roasted	1 oz	13	170	69%

Food and Description	Amount	Fat Grams	Total Calories	% Fat Calories
Oil Honey Roasted	1 oz	13	170	69%
Salted	1 oz	14	170	74%
Roaster's Choice-Salted	1 oz	15	170	79%
(Frito Lay's)	1 oz	15	170	79%
(Guy's)				
Dry Roasted	1 oz	14	170	74%
Spanish-Salted	1 oz	14	170	74%
(Laura Scudder's) Virginia	1 oz	15	182	74%
(Little Debbie)				
Honey Roasted	1.13 oz	13	190	62%
Salted	1.25 oz	18	230	70%
(Planters)				
Dry Roasted				
Salted	1 oz	14	160	79%
Unsalted	1 oz	14	160	79%
Honey Roasted	1 oz	13	170	69%
Honey Dry Roasted	1 oz	13	160	73%
In Shell				
Salted	1 oz	14	160	79%
Unsalted	1 oz	14	160	79%
Oil Roasted Cocktail	1 oz	15	170	79%
Unsalted	1 oz	15	170	79%
Oil Roasted Redskin	1 oz	15	170	79%
Sweet "N Crunchy	1 oz	8	140	51%
Oil Roasted Salted	1 oz	15	170	79%
(Weight Watchers) Honey Roasted	.7 oz	6	100	54%
PEANUT, SPANISH	1 oz	13.7	162	76%
	½ cup	36	425	76%
(Laura Scudder's)	1 oz	15	181	75%
(Planters)				
Dry Roasted	1 oz	14	160	79%
Oil Roasted	1 oz	15	170	79%
Raw	1 oz	12	150	
PEANUT, VALENCIA				
Oil Roasted	1 oz	14	165	76%
	½ cup	37	424	79%
PEANUT, VIRGINIA				
Oil Roasted	1 oz	4.5	161	25%
PEANUT BUTTER				
■ CHUNKY				
(Country Pure)	2 Tbs	16	190	76%
(Erewhon)	2 Tbs	14	190	66%
(Erewhon) No Salt	2 Tbs	14	190	66%
(Estee)	1 Tbs	8	100	72%
(Featherweight)	1 Tbs	7	90	70%

Food and Description	Amount	Fat Grams	Total Calories	% Fat Calories
Generic	2 Tbs	16	188	77%
	½ cup	64	760	76%
	1 cup	131.9	1526	78%
(Health Valley)	2 Tbs	14	170	74%
No Salt	2 Tbs	14	170	74%
(Nu Made)	2 Tbs	16	190	76%
(Peter Pan)	2 Tbs	16	180	80%
Whipped				
Creamy	2⅔ Tbs	16	190	76%
Crunchy	2⅔ Tbs	16	190	76%
(Skippy) Super Chunk	2 Tbs	17	190	81%
	1 cup	137	1540	80%
(Smucker's) Natural	2 Tbs	16	200	72%
■ CREAMY/SMOOTH				
(Arrowhead Mills)	2 Tbs	16	190	76%
(Bama)	2 Tbs	17	200	77%
(Country Pure)	2 Tbs	16	190	76%
(Erewhon)	2 Tbs	14	190	66%
(Featherweight)	2 Tbs	15	180	75%
Generic	2 Tbs	16	188	77%
	½ cup	64	760	76%
	1 cup	131.9	1526	78%
(Health Valley)	2 Tbs	14	170	74%
No Salt	2 Tbs	14	170	74%
(Jif)	2 Tbs	16	190	76%
(Laura Scudder's)				
Roasted				
Honey Nut	2 Tbs	16	200	72%
(Nu Made)	2 Tbs	16	190	76%
(Nutradiet)	1 Tbs	8	93	87%
(Peter Pan)	2 Tbs	16	180	80%
no sugar	2 Tbs	17	180	85%
(President's Choice)				
Too Good To Be True	2 Tbs	18	210	77%
(Skippy)	2 Tbs	17	190	81%
Roasted Honey Nut	2 Tbs	17	190	81%
■ CRUNCHY				
(Arrowhead Mills)	2 Tbs	16	190	76%
(Bama)	2 Tbs	17	200	77%
(Jif)	2 Tbs	17	190	81%
(Laura Scudder's)				
Roasted Honey Nut	2 Tbs	16	200	72%
(Peter Pan)	2 Tbs	16	180	80%
(President's Choice)				
Too Good To Be True	2 Tbs	18	210	77%

Food and Description	Amount	Fat Grams	Total Calories	% Fat Calories
(Skippy)				
Roasted Honey Nut	2 Tbs	17	190	81%
■ MIXED				
w/fudge (Smucker's)				
Goober Fudge	2 Tbs	13	240	49%
w/honey (Smucker's)				
Goober Honey	2 Tbs	10	180	50%
w/jelly				
(Bama)	2 Tbs	7	150	42%
(Smucker's)				
Goober Grape	2 Tbs	10	180	50%
Goober Strawberry	2 Tbs	10	180	50%
■ NO SALT NATURAL				
(Smucker's)	2 Tbs	17	200	77%
■ NUTTY				
(Laura Scudder's)	2 Tbs	16	200	72%
PEANUT BUTTER FLAVORED BAKING CHIPS				
(Reese's)	¼ cup	13	230	51%
PEANUT FLOUR				
Low Fat	1 oz	6	120	45%
	1 cup	13	257	46%
PEAR				
Fresh				
Bartlett	1	1	100	9%
D'Anjou	1	1	120	8%
Slices	1 cup	.66	97	6%
Candied	1 oz	–	86	–
Canned				
in Water	1 cup	< 1	71	6%
in Juice	1 cup	< 1	123	4%
in Light Syrup	1 cup	< 1	130	4%
in Heavy Syrup	1 cup	< 1	188	2%
(Del Monte)				
Halves or Slices	½ cup	–	80	–
Lite Halves or Slices	½ cup	–	50	–
Dried				
Cooked	1 cup	.78	325	0%
Uncooked	1 cup	1	472	2%
(Mariani) dried	¼ cup	–	150	–
(Nutradiet)				
Peeled Halves	½ cup	–	35	–
Peeled Quarters	½ cup	–	35	–
(S&W)				
Bartlett Halves In Heavy Syrup	½ cup	–	100	–
Natural-Sliced	½ cup	–	80	–

Food and Description	Amount	Fat Grams	Total Calories	% Fat Calories
PEAR NECTAR				
Canned	1 cup	–	149	–
Ripe Nectar (Libby's)	8 oz	–	150	–
PEAR-PINEAPPLE NECTAR				
(Kern's)	1 cup	–	112	–
PECAN				
(Azar)				
Chips	1 oz	21	210	90%
Halves	1 oz	21	210	90%
Pieces	1 oz	21	210	90%
Dried	1 oz	19	190	90%
	1 cup/ halves	73	721	91%
Dry Roasted	1 oz	18	187	87%
	10 Xtra large	28.7	277	93%
(Eagle)				
Honey Roasted	1 oz	19	200	86%
In Shell	10 large	24.5	236	93%
Oil Roasted	1 oz	20	195	92%
(Planters)				
Chips	1 oz	20	190	95%
Halves	1 oz	20	190	95%
Pieces	1 oz	20	190	95%
Shelled				
Chopped	1 cup	84	811	93%
	1 Tbs	5	52	87%
Ground	1 cup	67.6	653	93%
Halves	10 large	6	62	87%
	10 jumbo	10	96	94%
	10 mammoth	12.8	124	93%
	1 cup	76.9	742	93%
PECAN FLOUR	1 oz	–	93	–
PEPPER (See also MEXICAN FOOD)				
Greek Pepperoncini Salad (Vlasic)				
Mild	1 oz	–	4	–
Hot	1 oz	–	10	–
(Heinz)	1	–	8	–
Hot Banana				
(Heinz)	1	–	6	–
(Vlasic)	1 oz	–	4	–
Hot Cherry (Vlasic)	1 oz	–	10	–
Hot Chili-Red				
raw	1 pepper	–	18	–

Food and Description	Amount	Fat Grams	Total Calories	% Fat Calories
raw/chopped	½ cup	–	17	–
Hot Chili-Green/raw	½ cup	–	16	–
Hot Pepper Rings/slices (Heinz)	1	–	4	–
Jalapeno				
canned/whole	2 peppers	1	14	64%
chopped	½ cup	1	20	45%
Mexican Hot (Vlasic)	1 oz	–	8	–
Mexican Tiny Hot (Vlasic)	1 oz	–	6	–
Mild	1 oz	–	8	–
(Heinz) sweet	1	–	8	–
(Vlasic) Cherry	1 oz	–	8	–
Sweet (Green & Red)				
raw	1 pepper	–	18	–
raw/chopped	½ cup	–	12	–
freeze-dried	½ cup	–	10	–
	1 Tbs	–	1	–
(Heinz) rings/slices	1	–	4	–
Sweet Pepper Mementos (Heinz)	1	–	6	–
PEPPER DISHES				
Standard Home Recipe (USDA)				
Stuffed green pepper				
w/beef & bread crumbs	1 medium	10.5	325	29%
w/beef & rice	½ medium	13	219	53%
w/rice only	~ 5 oz	11.9	198	54%
PEPPER POT SOUP (See SOUP)				
PEPPER SEASONING				
black	1 tsp	–	9	–
chili	1 tsp	–	9	–
red (cayenne)	1 tsp	–	9	–
white	1 tsp	–	9	–
PEPPERONI (See LUNCHEON MEAT)				
PERCH (See OCEAN PERCH)				
PERSIMMON				
fresh/native	1	–	32	–
Japanese (or Kaki)				
fresh	1	< 1	118	4%
dried	1	< 1	93	5%
PESTO SAUCE (See SAUCE)				
PHEASANT				
breast meat only-raw	~ 6 oz	5.9	243	22%
giblets-raw	3 oz	4	119	30%
leg meat only-raw	~ 4 oz	4.6	143	29%
meat & skin-raw	~ 1 lb	37	723	46%
meat only-raw	~ ¾ lb	12.8	470	25%

Food and Description	Amount	Fat Grams	Total Calories	% Fat Calories
PICANTE SALSA (*See* MEXICAN FOOD, SAUCE)				
PICKLE				
Bread & butter pickles	3 slices	–	16	–
	1 oz	–	25	–
(Claussen) Dill	1 oz	–	6	–
(Del Monte) Dill Halves	1 oz	–	3	–
Deli Style Dill halves	1 oz	–	4	–
Dill pickles	1 medium	–	15	–
(Featherweight) Whole Dill	1 piece	–	4	–
Genuine Dill	1 oz	–	2	–
Gherkin pickles	1 Small	–	22	–
Hamburger Chips	1 oz	–	2	–
Hamburger Dill	1 oz	–	2	–
(Heinz) Baby Kosher Dill	1 oz	–	4	–
Hot Garlic	1 oz	–	6	–
Kosher	2 oz	–	7	–
halves	1 piece	–	9	–
slices	1 oz	–	3	–
whole	1 oz	–	2	–
Kosher Dill	1 oz	–	4	–
Kosher Dill Chips	1 oz	–	4	–
Kosher Dill Spears	1 oz	–	4	–
Old Fashioned Kosher Chips	1 oz	–	4	–
Old Fashioned Kosher Deli Halves	1 oz	–	4	–
Old Fashioned Whole Kosher	1 oz	–	4	–
Picalilli	1 oz	–	30	–
Pickled cucumbers	2 spears	–	13	–
Polish Style Dill	1 oz	–	4	–
Polish Style Dill Spears	1 oz	–	4	–
Polskie Ogorki	1 oz	–	6	–
Processed Dill	1 oz	–	2	–
Sour	1 oz	–	3	–
Sweet Cucumber Slices	1 oz	–	20	–
Sweet Cucumber Stix	1 oz	–	25	–
Sweet Gherkins	1 oz	–	35	–
Sweet Midget Gherkins	1 oz	–	35	–
Sweet Mixed	1 oz	–	40	–
Sweet Pickles	1 oz	–	35	–
Sweet Pickle Slices	1 oz	–	35	–
Sweet Salad Cubes	1 oz	–	30	–
(Vlasic)				
Bread & Butter Chunks	1 oz	–	25	–
Sweet Butter Chips	1 oz	–	30	–

Food and Description	Amount	Fat Grams	Total Calories	% Fat Calories
Sweet Butter Stix	1 oz	–	18	–
Half-The-Salt Pickles				
Hamburger Dill Chips	1 oz	–	2	–
Kosher Crunchy Dills	1 oz	–	4	–
Kosher Dill Spears	1 oz	–	4	–
Sweet Butter Chips	1 oz	–	30	–
Kosher Pickles				
Baby Dills	1 oz	–	4	–
Crunchy Dills	1 oz	–	4	–
Dill Gherkins	1 oz	–	4	–
Dill Spears	1 oz	–	4	–
Snack Chunks	1 oz	–	4	–
No-Garlic Pickles				
Crunchy Dills	1 oz	–	4	–
Dill Spears	1 oz	–	4	–
Original Dills				
Original Dills	1 oz	–	2	–
Polish Snack Chunks	1 oz	–	4	–
Zesty Crunchy Dills	1 oz	–	4	–
Zesty Dill Spears	1 oz	–	4	–
Zesty Dill Snack Chunks	1 oz	–	4	–
Refrigerated Pickles				
Deli Bread & Butter	1 oz	–	25	–
Deli Dill Halves	1 oz	–	4	–

PIE & COBBLER (*See also* PIE CRUST, PIE FILLING, SNACK CAKES)
(NOTE: All homemade pie crusts were made with enriched flour & vegetable shortening.)

Apple				
(Amy's)-frozen	1 pie	14	282	45%
(Banquet)-frozen	3.33 oz	11	250	40%
(Entenmann's)-homestyle	2.1 oz	7	140	45%
homemade (9" dia)	⅙ pie	18	405	40%
(Mrs. Smith's)				
Apple Raisin	⅛ pie	28	560	45%
Dutch Apple Crumb	⅛ pie	13	420	28%
Natural Juice	⅐ pie	22	420	47%
Old Fashioned	⅛ pie	27	530	46%
Ready to Bake	⅛ pie	17	390	39%
Streusel	⅐ pie	16	420	34%
Thaw'N'Serve-Lattice	⅛ pie	11	280	35%
(Pet-Ritz)-frozen	⅙ pie	12	330	33%
(Weight Watchers)-frozen	3.5 oz	4	165	22%
Apple cobbler-frozen				
(Pet-Ritz)	⅙ cobbler	9	290	28%

Food and Description	Amount	Fat Grams	Total Calories	% Fat Calories
(Stilwell)	4 oz	4	200	18%
Apple Crumb-mix (Dromedary)	1 piece	6	237	23%
Apple-Dutch (Little Debbie)	2.17 oz	8	230	31%
Apple-Homestyle (Entenmann's)	2.1 oz	7	140	45%
Apple Streusel-frozen				
(Sara Lee) Free & Light	1 slice	2	170	11%
Banana-frozen				
(Banquet)	2.33 oz	10	180	50%
(Mrs. Smith's) Thaw'N Serve	⅛ pie	12	240	45%
Banana Cream				
homemade (9" dia)	⅙ pie	13	300	39%
(Pet-Ritz)-frozen	⅙ pie	9	170	48%
Banana Custard-homemade (9" dia)	⅙ pie	14	336	38%
Berry-frozen (Mrs. Smith's)				
Ready To Bake	⅛ pie	16	400	36%
Blackberry				
(Banquet)-frozen	3.33 oz	11	270	37%
homemade (9" dia)	⅙ pie	17	384	40%
Blackberry cobbler-frozen				
(Pet-Ritz)	⅙ cobbler	10	250	36%
(Stilwell)	4 oz	8	280	26%
Blueberry				
(Banquet)-frozen	3.33 oz	11	270	37%
homemade (9" dia)	⅙ pie	17	380	40%
(Mrs. Smith's) Old Fashioned				
frozen	⅛ pie	17	460	33%
Ready to Bake	⅛ pie	17	380	40%
Thaw'N Serve-Lattice	⅛ pie	11	290	34%
(Pet Ritz)-frozen	⅙ pie	12	370	29%
Blueberry cobbler-frozen				
(Pet-Ritz)	⅙ cobbler	12	370	29%
Boston Cream-frozen				
(Mrs. Smith's) Thaw'N Serve	⅛ pie	4	240	15%
(Weight Watchers)	3 oz	4	190	19%
Butterscotch-homemade (9" dia)	⅛ pie	12.5	304	37%
Cherry				
(Banquet)-frozen	3.33 oz	11	250	40%
homemade (9" dia)	⅙ pie	18	410	40%
(Mrs. Smith's)-frozen				
Natural Juice	⅐ pie	18	410	40%
Old Fashioned	⅛ pie	19	460	37%
Ready To Bake	⅛ pie	16	400	36%
Thaw'N Serve-Lattice	⅛ pie	10	300	30%
(Pet Ritz)-frozen	⅙ pie	12	300	36%

Food and Description	Amount	Fat Grams	Total Calories	% Fat Calories
Cherry cobbler-frozen				
(Pet-Ritz)	⅙ cobbler	10	280	32%
Cherry Crumb-mix				
(Dromedary)	1 piece	6	231	23%
Cherry Streusel-frozen				
(Sara Lee) Free & Light	1 slice	2	160	11%
Chess-homemade (9" dia)	⅙ pie	24	485	45%
Chocolate				
frozen (Banquet)	2.33 oz	10	185	49%
homemade (9" dia)	⅙ pie	22	433	46%
Chocolate Chiffon-homemade (9" dia)	⅛ pie	12	266	41%
Chocolate Cream-frozen				
(Mrs. Smith's) Thaw'N Serve	⅛ pie	13	270	43%
(Pet-Ritz)	⅙ pie	8	190	38%
Chocolate Meringue-homemade (9" dia)	⅙ pie	18	383	42%
Chocolate Mocha-frozen				
(Weight Watchers)	2.75 oz	4	160	23%
Chocolate Mousse Pie				
box mix				
(Jell-O)	⅛ pie	17	260	59%
(Royal)	⅛ pie	4	130	28%
frozen (Weight Watchers)	2.5 oz	6	170	32%
Chocolate Pecan-frozen				
(Mrs. Smith's) Thaw'N Serve	⅛ pie	20	570	32%
Coconut-frozen (Banquet)	2.33 oz	11	190	52%
Coconut Cream				
box mix				
(Jell-O) No Bake	⅛ pie	17	260	59%
frozen				
(Mrs. Smith's) Thaw'N Serve	⅛ pie	14	270	47%
(Pet-Ritz)	⅙ pie	8	190	38%
Coconut Custard (Entenmann's)	1.8 oz	8	140	51%
Coconut Custard				
frozen				
(Mrs. Smith's) Ready To Bake	⅛ pie	15	330	41%
homemade (9" dia)	⅙ pie	19	357	48%
Cream-homemade (9" dia)	⅙ pie	23	455	46%
Custard-homemade (9" dia)	⅙ pie	17	330	46%
Egg Custard-frozen				
(Mrs. Smith's) Ready To Bake	⅛ pie	9	300	27%
(Pet-Ritz)	⅙ pie	8	200	36%
Flan (*See* CUSTARD)				
Fried				
(Break Cake)	1	19	410	42%

Food and Description	Amount	Fat Grams	Total Calories	% Fat Calories
apple	1	14	255	49%
cherry	1	14	250	50%
homemade	1	19	410	42%
Grasshopper-homemade (9" dia)	⅙ pie	23	460	45%
Key Lime-homemade (9" dia)	⅙ pie	19	460	37%
Lemon-frozen (Banquet)	2.33 oz	11	190	52%
Lemon Chiffon-homemade (9" dia)	⅙ pie	13.6	338	36%
Lemon Cream-frozen				
(Mrs. Smith's) Thaw'N Serve	⅛ pie	12	245	44%
(Pet-Ritz)	⅙ pie	9	190	43%
Lemon Meringue				
frozen				
(Mrs. Smith's) Thaw'N Serve	⅛ pie	6	290	19%
homemade (9" dia)	⅙ pie	14	355	36%
Mix-No Bake (Royal)	⅛ pie	5	210	21%
Mince-frozen				
(Mrs. Smith's) Ready To Bake	⅛ pie	19	470	36%
(Pet-Ritz)	⅙ pie	9	280	29%
Mincemeat				
frozen				
(Banquet)	3.33 oz	11	260	38%
homemade	⅙ pie	18	428	38%
Neopolitan Cream-frozen				
(Pet-Ritz)	⅙ pie	10	180	50%
Peach				
frozen				
(Banquet)	3.33 oz	11	245	40%
(Mrs. Smith's)				
Old Fashioned	⅛ pie	16	365	40%
Thaw'N Serve-Lattice	⅛ pie	12	300	36%
(Pet-Ritz)	⅙ pie	12	320	34%
homemade (9" dia)	⅙ pie	17	405	38%
Peach cobbler-frozen				
(Pet-Ritz)	⅙ cobbler	10	260	35%
(Stilwell)	4 oz	5	270	17%
Pecan				
frozen				
(Mrs. Smith's) Thaw'N Serve	⅛ pie	16	480	30%
homemade (9" dia)	⅙ pie	32	575	50%
Pineapple-homemade (9" dia)	⅙ pie	17	400	38%
Pineapple Chiffon-homemade (9" dia)	⅙ pie	13	311	38%
Pineapple Custard-homemade (9" dia)	⅙ pie	13	334	35%
Praline Pecan Mousse-frozen				
(Weight Watchers)	7 oz	7	190	33%

Food and Description	Amount	Fat Grams	Total Calories	% Fat Calories
Pumpkin				
frozen (Banquet)	3.33 oz	8	200	36%
homemade (9" dia)	⅙ pie	17	320	48%
mix (Jell-O)/No Bake	⅛ pie	11	230	43%
mix-canned (Libby's)	⅙ pie	17	330	46%
Pumpkin Custard-frozen				
(Mrs. Smith's)				
Ready To Serve	⅛ pie	11	310	32%
Thaw'N Serve	⅛ pie	8	300	24%
(Pet-Ritz)	⅙ pie	9	250	32%
Raisin-homemade (9" dia)	⅙ pie	17	427	36%
Raspberry Mousse-frozen				
(Weight Watchers)	2.5 oz	2	150	12%
Red Raspberry-frozen				
(Mrs. Smith's) Ready To Bake	⅛ pie	15	390	35%
Rhubarb-homemade (9" dia)	⅙ pie	17	400	38%
Shoo-fly-homemade (9" dia)	⅛ pie	13	395	30%
Snack-packaged				
(Hostess)				
Apple	1	20	430	42%
Blackberry	1	18	420	39%
Blueberry	1	18	420	39%
Cherry	1	20	460	39%
French Apple	1	20	430	42%
Lemon	1	20	440	41%
Peach	1	19	420	41%
Strawberry	1	19	410	42%
(Hostess) Pudding Pies				
Chocolate	1	19	490	35%
Vanilla	1	17	470	33%
(Little Debbie)				
Marshmallow pies				
Banana	9 oz	12	360	30%
	1.4 oz	6	170	32%
Chocolate	3 oz	13	370	32%
	1.38 oz	6	170	32%
Oatmeal Cream	1.33 oz	6	160	34%
	2.75 oz	14	350	36%
Pecan	3 oz	3	280	10%
	1.83 oz	2	170	11%
Raisin Creme	2.5 oz	10	290	31%
(McMillin's) Individual				
Apple	4 oz	23	430	48%
Berry	4 oz	23	430	48%

Food and Description	Amount	Fat Grams	Total Calories	% Fat Calories
Cherry	4 oz	24	430	50%
Chocolate Pudding	4 oz	21	420	45%
Coconut Pudding	4 oz	26	450	52%
Lemon	4 oz	25	450	50%
Peach	4 oz	24	430	50%
Strawberry	4 oz	20	400	45%
(Sara Lee) frozen				
Country Apple	1	7	230	32%
Fudge Brownie	1	14	280	45%
Southern Pecan	1	13	260	45%
(Tastykake)				
Apple	1 pkg	12	300	36%
Banana Creme	1 pkg	16	380	38%
Blueberry	1 pkg	9	310	26%
Cherry	1 pkg	10	300	30%
Coconut Creme	1 pkg	20	380	47%
French Apple	1 pkg	11	350	28%
Lemon	1 pkg	13	320	37%
Lemon Lime	1 pkg	13	320	37%
Peach	1 pkg	12	300	36%
Pineapple Cheese	1 pkg	13	340	34%
Pumpkin	1 pkg	14	320	39%
Strawberry	1 pkg	11	340	29%
Tasty Klair	1 pkg	20	400	45%
Squash-homemade (9" dia)	⅙ pie	20	360	50%
Strawberries'N Cream-frozen				
(Mrs. Smith's) Thaw'N Serve	⅛ pie	16	330	44%
Strawberry				
(Banquet)-frozen	2.33 oz	9	170	48%
homemade (9" dia)	⅙ pie	10	246	37%
Strawberry cobbler-frozen (Pet-Ritz)	⅙ cobbler	9	290	28%
Strawberry Cream-frozen				
(Pet-Ritz)	⅙ pie	9	170	48%
Strawberry-rhubarb				
homemade (9" dia)	⅛ pie	23	430	48%
(Mrs. Smith's) Ready To Bake-frozen	⅛ pie	17	410	37%
Sweet Potato				
homemade (9" dia)	⅙ pie	17	324	47%
(Pet-Ritz)-frozen	⅙ pie	7	150	42%
PIE CRUST				
(Flako) (9" dia)	⅙ crust	15	250	54%
Frozen				
(Mrs. Smith's)	⅛ of 9⅝ shell	8	130	55%

Food and Description	Amount	Fat Grams	Total Calories	% Fat Calories
(Oronoque)				
Deep Dish (9" dia)	1/6 shell	9	130	62%
Regular (9" dia)	1/6 shell	8	120	60%
(Pepperidge Farm) Patty shells	1 shell	15	210	64%
(Pet-Ritz)				
Deep Dish				
All Vegetable Shortening	1/6 shell	9	140	58%
9" dia	1/6 shell	9	130	62%
Graham Cracker	1/6 shell	6	110	49%
9 5/8" dia	1/6 shell	11	170	58%
Regular				
All Vegetable Shortening	1/6 shell	8	120	60%
9" dia	1/6 shell	8	120	60%
Tart Shells (3")	1 shell	10	150	60%
(Keebler) Ready Crust				
Butter flavored	1/8 crust	5	110	41%
Chocolate	1/8 crust	5	120	38%
Graham Cracker	1/8 crust	6	120	45%
Single Serve	1 tart	5	100	45%
(Krusteaz) baked	~ 1 oz	6	100	54%
(Pillsbury)				
Mix	1/8 crust	13	200	59%
Refrigerated-all ready	1/8 two crust pie	15	240	56%
Standard Home Recipe (USDA) (9" dia)	1 shell	60	900	60%
PIE FILLING				
■ **PIE FILLING-CREAM-CANNED**				
(Comstock)				
Banana	3.5 oz	2	110	16%
Chocolate	3.5 oz	3	130	21%
Coconut	3.5 oz	3	120	23%
Lemon	3.5 oz	1	140	13%
■ **PIE FILLING-FRUIT**				
Box				
(Borden) mincemeat	2.5 oz	2	220	8%
Canned				
(Comstock)				
Apricot	3.5 oz	–	110	–
Blueberry	3.5 oz	–	110	–
Cherry	3.5 oz	–	110	–
Mincemeat	3.5 oz	1	150	6%
Mountain fresh peach	3.5 oz	–	110	–
Pineapple	3.5 oz	–	100	–
Orchard fresh apple	3.5 oz	–	120	–
Pumpkin	3.5 oz	–	100	–

Food and Description	Amount	Fat Grams	Total Calories	% Fat Calories
Raisin	3.5 oz	–	120	–
Strawberry	3.5 oz	–	100	–
(Libby's)				
Baked	⅙ pie	17	330	46%
Pumpkin	1 cup	–	210	–
Pumpkin-Solid pack	1 cup	1	80	11%
Pumpkin pie mix	1 cup	–	282	–
(S&W) Mincemeat-Old Fashioned				
Mellowed w/brandy	3.5 oz	2	206	9%
(Thank You)				
Apple	3.5 oz	–	90	–
Cherry	3.5 oz	–	100	–
Jar (None Such)				
Mincemeat				
plain	⅓ cup	1	200	5%
w/brandy & rum	⅓ cup	2	220	8%
■ PIE FILLING-INSTANT				
Mixes prepared w/whole milk (Jell-O)				
Banana cream	½ cup	4	160	23%
Butter pecan	½ cup	5	170	27%
Butterscotch	½ cup	4	140	26%
Chocolate	½ cup	4	130	28%
Chocolate fudge	½ cup	5	180	25%
Coconut cream	½ cup	6	180	30%
French vanilla	½ cup	4	160	23%
Lemon	½ cup	4	140	26%
Milk chocolate	½ cup	5	180	25%
Pineapple cream	½ cup	4	160	23%
Pistachio	½ cup	4	150	24%
Vanilla	½ cup	4	140	26%
■ PIE FILLING-INSTANT SUGAR-FREE				
Mixes prepared w/2% low-fat milk (Jell-O)				
Banana	½ cup	2	90	20%
Butterscotch	½ cup	2	90	20%
Chocolate	½ cup	3	100	27%
Chocolate fudge	½ cup	3	100	27%
Pistachio	½ cup	3	100	27%
Vanilla	½ cup	2	90	20%
■ PIE FILLING-MICROWAVE				
Prepared as directed (Jell-O)				
Banana cream	½ cup	4	170	21%
Butterscotch	½ cup	4	170	21%
Chocolate	½ cup	5	170	27%
Milk chocolate	½ cup	6	160	34%
Mint chocolate	½ cup	5	160	28%

Food and Description	Amount	Fat Grams	Total Calories	% Fat Calories
Vanilla	½ cup	4	160	23%
■ **PIE FILLING-MIX**				
Prepared w/whole milk				
(Jell-O)				
Banana cream (8" pie)				
excluding crust	⅙ pie	3	100	27%
Butterscotch	½ cup	4	170	21%
Chocolate	½ cup	5	180	25%
Chocolate fudge	½ cup	4	160	23%
Coconut cream (8" pie)				
excluding crust	⅙ pie	2	200	9%
Coconut Cream Pie Dessert				
(no crust)	⅛ pie	7	162	39%
Deluxe chocolate almond				
(no crust)	⅛ pie	7	162	39%
Deluxe chocolate mint				
(no crust)	⅛ pie	7	162	39%
Deluxe double chocolate				
(no crust)	⅛ pie	7	162	39%
French vanilla	½ cup	4	170	21%
Lemon (9" pie)/excluding crust	⅙ pie	2	200	9%
Milk chocolate	½ cup	4	140	26%
Vanilla	½ cup	4	160	23%
(Royal)				
Banana cream	½ cup	4	160	23%
Butterscotch	½ cup	4	160	23%
Chocolate	½ cup	4	180	20%
Custard	½ cup	5	150	30%
Dark'n sweet	½ cup	4	180	20%
Flan w/ caramel sauce	½ cup	5	150	30%
Key lime	½ cup	3	160	17%
Lemon	½ cup	3	160	17%
Vanilla	½ cup	4	160	23%
Vanilla tapioca	½ cup	4	160	23%
■ **PIE FILLING-MIX-SUGAR-FREE**				
Prepared w/2% milk (Jell-O)				
Chocolate	½ cup	3	90	30%
Vanilla	½ cup	2	80	30%
PIGEON PEA				
fresh-cooked	½ cup	1	86	11%
raw	½ cup	1.5	350	4%
PIKE				
Northern				
cooked-dry heat	3 oz	.75	96	7%
raw	3 oz	1	75	12%

Food and Description	Amount	Fat Grams	Total Calories	% Fat Calories
roe-raw	3 oz	1.7	110	14%
Walleye				
raw	3 oz	1	79	11%
PIMIENTO				
canned	1	–	11	–
	4 oz	–	30	–
diced or slices				
(Dromedary)	1 oz	–	10	–
(Dunbar's)	½ oz	–	4	–
PINA COLADA FRUIT DRINK				
Nice & Natural	6 oz	–	80	–
PINE NUTS				
dried				
pignolia	1 oz	14	146	86%
pinyon	1 oz	17	161	95%
PINEAPPLE				
candied	4 oz	.5	357	1%
	1 oz	–	90	–
canned				
(Del Monte)				
chunks, crushed,tidbits, slices				
in juice	½ cup	–	70	–
chunks, crushed, slices				
in syrup	½ cup	–	90	–
spears in juice	2 spears	–	50	–
(Dole)				
all cuts in juice	½ cup	.5	70	6%
all cuts in syrup	½ cup	< 1	95	5%
Generic				
in water	1 slice	–	19	–
	1 cup	< 1	79	6%
in juice	1 slice	–	35	–
	1 cup	.5	150	3%
in heavy syrup	1 slice	–	45	–
(Nutradiet) sliced	½ cup	–	60	–
	1 cup	.9	199	4%
(S&W)				
Hawaiian sliced				
in heavy syrup	2 slices	–	90	–
in pineapple juice	½ cup	–	70	–
fresh	1 slice	–	42	–
	1 cup	.66	77	8%
(Del Monte)	2 slices	–	90	–
	½ cup	–	52	–

Food and Description	Amount	Fat Grams	Total Calories	% Fat Calories
frozen				
sweetened chunks	½ cup	–	104	–
unsweetened	3.5 oz	< 1	50	9%
PINEAPPLE JUICE				
Bottled, Boxed, or Canned				
(Del Monte) unsweetened	6 oz	–	100	–
(Dole) unsweetened	6 oz	–	103	–
Generic	8 oz	–	139	–
(Mott's)	9.5 oz	–	169	–
(S&W) unsweetened	6 oz	–	100	–
(Tree Top)	6 oz	–	100	–
Frozen				
From frozen concentrate	8 oz	–	129	–
Undiluted	6 oz	< 1	385	1%
PINEAPPLE NECTAR				
(Libby's)	6 oz	–	110	–
PINEAPPLE SAUCE				
(Dole)				
Chunky	½ cup	–	90	–
Smooth	½ cup	–	90	–
PINEAPPLE-GRAPE JUICE DRINK	8 oz	–	117	–
PINEAPPLE-GRAPEFRUIT JUICE				
(Del Monte)	6 oz	–	90	–
(Dole)	6 oz	–	90	–
(Tropicana)	6 oz	–	90	–
PINEAPPLE-GRAPEFRUIT JUICE COCKTAIL				
(Ocean Spray)	6 oz	–	110	–
PINEAPPLE-GRAPEFRUIT JUICE DRINK				
(Tropicana) single serve	10 oz	–	159	–
PINEAPPLE-ORANGE JUICE				
(Del Monte)	6 oz	–	90	–
(Dole)	6 oz	–	100	–
PINEAPPLE-ORANGE JUICE DRINK				
Canned	8 oz	–	125	–
Mix (Tropical Sno)	6 oz	–	110	–
PINEAPPLE-ORANGE-BANANA JUICE				
(Dole)	6 oz	< 1	00	5%
PINEAPPLE-ORANGE-GUAVA JUICE				
from frozen concentrate	6 oz	< 1	100	5%
PINEAPPLE-PINK GRAPEFRUIT JUICE				
(Del Monte)	6 oz	–	90	–
(Dole)	6 oz	–	100	–
PINEAPPLE-PINK GRAPEFRUIT JUICE DRINK				
(Dole)	6 oz	–	100	–

Food and Description	Amount	Fat Grams	Total Calories	% Fat Calories
PINK BEANS				
boiled	½ cup	–	125	–
raw	½ cup	1	360	3%
PINTO BEAN				
boiled	½ cup	–	117	–
canned	½ cup	–	93	–
Dry (Joan of Arc/Green Giant)	½ cup	1	90	10%
Dry-picante style				
(Joan of Arc)	½ cup	1	100	9%
(Green Giant)	½ cup	1	100	9%
(Gebhardt)	7.5 oz	1	370	3%
(Hain)	4 oz	1	70	13%
(Progresso)	8 oz	1	165	6%
Seasoned w/pork				
(Luck's)	7.25 oz	6	220	25%
w/Jalapeno (Ranch Style)	7.5 oz	2	180	10%
cooked from dry	½ cup	.5	133	3%
raw	½ cup	1	325	3%
sprouts-raw	½ cup	1	65	14%
PINTO BEAN DISHES				
Canned w/Onions Seasoned w/Pork				
(Luck's)	7.5 oz	6	220	25%
PISTACHIO NUT				
(Dole) shelled dry roasted	1 oz	14	163	77%
Generic				
dried	1 oz	13.7	164	
	1 cup	61.9	739	75%
dry roasted	1 oz	15	172	79%
	1 cup	67.6	776	78%
in shell	1 oz	7	84	75%
shelled	1 oz	15	168	80%
(Planters)				
dry roasted	1 oz	15	170	79%
natural	1 oz	15	170	79%
red	1 oz	15	170	79%
PITANGA/Surinam or Brazilian cherry				
fresh	1 lb	1.6	132	11%
	2 pieces	–	5	–
	1 cup	.7	57	11%
PIZZA & PIZZA SNACK (*See also* FAST FOOD)				
(ACT II)				
Pizza Pockets-Pepperoni	1	20	400	45%
■ (CELENTANO)				
9-slice pizza	2.7 oz	4	150	24%
ThickCrust Pizza	4.3	11	290	34%

Food and Description	Amount	Fat Grams	Total Calories	% Fat Calories
(CELESTE)				
Original				
Cheese	¼ pizza	17	315	49%
Deluxe	¼ pizza	22	380	52%
Pepperoni	¼ pizza	29	370	71%
Sausage	¼ pizza	22	375	53%
Suprema	¼ pizza	24	380	57%
Pizza-For-One				
Cheese	1 pizza	25	500	45%
Deluxe	1 pizza	32	580	50%
Pepperoni	1 pizza	30	545	50%
Sausage	1 pizza	32	570	51%
Suprema	1 pizza	39	680	52%
Vegetable	1 pizza	44	490	81%
■ **(CHEF BOY-AR-DEE)**				
Box Mix				
Cheese Pizza				
Complete (15⅜) oz	3.84 oz	6	230	24%
2 Complete (28⅞) oz	3.61 oz	5	210	21%
Pepperoni Pizza				
Complete (13.5 oz)	3.38 oz	6	230	24%
Complete (16⅝) oz	4.16 oz	9	250	32%
2 complete (30 oz)	3.75 oz	7	210	30%
Plain Pizza Mix (14 oz)	3.5 oz	3	180	15%
Sausage Pizza				
Complete (16⅞ oz)	4.22 oz	10	270	33%
■ **(ELIO'S) HEALTHY SLICE**				
Cheese	2.67 oz	2	160	11%
Mixed Vegetable	3.1 oz	2	150	12%
■ **(FOX) DELUXE PIZZA**				
Golden Topping (6.8 oz)	½ pizza	11	240	41%
Hamburger (7.6 oz)	½ pizza	12	260	42%
Pepperoni (7 oz)	½ pizza	13	250	47%
Sausage (7.2 oz)	½ pizza	13	260	45%
Sausage & Pepperoni Combination				
(7.2 oz)	½ pizza	13	260	45%
■ **(GRAINDANCE)**				
Cheese w/whole wheat crust	¼ pizza	8	190	38%
■ **(HEALTHY CHOICE) FRENCH BREAD PIZZA**				
Cheese	5.6 oz	3	300	9%
Deluxe	6.25 oz	8	330	22%
Italian Turkey Sausage	6.45 oz	7	320	20%
Pepperoni	6.25 oz	8	320	23%
■ **(JACLYN'S)**				
Fat-Free Pizza	⅛ pizza	–	120	–

Food and Description	Amount	Fat Grams	Total Calories	% Fat Calories
■ **(JENO'S)**				
Crisp 'n Tasty Pizza				
Canadian Style Bacon (7.7 oz)	½ pizza	10	240	38%
Cheese(7.4 oz)	½ pizza	10	240	38%
Combination(7.8 oz)	½ pizza	15	280	48%
Hamburger (8.1 oz)	½ pizza	14	280	45%
Pepperoni (7.6 oz)	½ pizza	15	280	48%
Sausage (7.8 oz)	½ pizza	15	280	48%
4-Pack Pizzas				
Cheese	1 pizza	8	160	45%
Combination	1 pizza	9	180	45%
Hamburger	1 pizza	9	180	45%
Pepperoni	1 pizza	9	170	48%
Sausage	1 pizza	9	180	45%
Pizza Pocketjs				
Pepperoni	1	20	370	49%
Sausage	1	19	360	48%
Sausage & Pepper	1	20	360	50%
Supreme	1	19	370	46%
Pizza Rolls				
Cheese	3 oz	5	200	23%
Hamburger	3 oz	8	220	33%
Pepperoni	3 oz	9	220	37%
Sausage	3 oz	7	210	30%
■ **(JOHN'S) PIZZA**				
Cheese 3-pack	1 pizza	12	300	36%
Deluxe Sausage	½ pizza	13	260	45%
Golden Topping	½ pizza	11	240	41%
Sausage	½ pizza	13	260	45%
Sausage 3-pack	1 pizza	12	300	36%
■ **(KID CUISINE)**				
Cheese	6.85 oz	12	380	28%
Hamburger	6.85 oz	10	330	27%
■ **(LEAN CUISINE)**				
French Bread Pizza				
Cheese	5⅛ oz	9	300	27%
Deluxe	6⅛ oz	8	320	23%
Pepperoni	5¼ oz	11	330	30%
Sausage	6 oz	9	330	25%
Three-Cheese	5.5 oz	10	330	27%
■ **(LEAN POCKETS)**				
Pizza Deluxe				
w/pepperoni & sausage	1 pocket	13	280	42%
■ **LOONEY TUNES (TYSON)**				
Foghorn Leghorn Pepperoni Pizza	6.35 oz	13	400	29%

Food and Description	Amount	Fat Grams	Total Calories	% Fat Calories
■ (MICRO MAGIC)				
Deep Dish Combination Pizza	6.5 oz	34	605	51%
Deep Dish Pepperoni Pizza	6.5 oz	32	610	47%
Deep Dish Sausage Pizza	6.5 oz	31	590	47%
■ (MR. P'S PIZZA)				
Combination (7.2 oz)	½ pizza	13	260	45%
Golden Topping (6.8 oz)	½ pizza	11	240	41%
Hamburger (7.6 oz)	½ pizza	12	260	42%
Pepperoni (7 oz)	½ pizza	13	250	47%
Sausage (7.2 oz)	½ pizza	13	260	45%
■ (PAPPALO'S)				
Pan Pizza				
Pepperoni	⅕ pizza	11	350	28%
Sausage	⅕ pizza	11	350	28%
Sausage & Pepperoni	⅕ pizza	12	360	30%
Supreme	⅙ pizza	12	340	32%
Three Cheese	⅕ pizza	8	310	23%
Traditional				
9"				
Pepperoni	½ pizza	14	390	32%
Sausage	½ pizza	13	380	30%
Sausage & Pepperoni	½ pizza	15	390	34%
Supreme	½ pizza	16	400	36%
Three Cheese	½ pizza	11	350	28%
12"				
Pepperoni	½ pizza	11	350	28%
Sausage	½ pizza	12	350	31%
Sausage & Pepperoni	½ pizza	12	360	30%
Supreme	½ pizza	12	350	31%
Three Cheese	½ pizza	7	310	20%
■ (PEPPERIDGE FARM) CROISSANT CRUST PIZZA				
Cheese	1	23	430	48%
Deluxe	1	23	440	47%
Pepperoni	1	22	440	45%
■ (PILLSBURY) OVEN LOVIN'				
Microwave French Bread Pizza				
Cheese	1 pizza	14	350	36%
Combination	1 pizza	21	420	45%
Pepperoni	1 pizza	21	410	46%
Sausage	1 pizza	20	400	45%
Microwave Pizza				
Cheese	½ pizza	12	250	43%
Combination	½ pizza	18	310	52%
Pepperoni	½ pizza	17	300	51%
Sausage	½ pizza	16	290	50%

Food and Description	Amount	Fat Grams	Total Calories	% Fat Calories
Supreme	½ pizza	18	310	52%
■ (RED BARON)				
Deep Dish Single Serve Pizza				
Cheese	5.5 oz	22.5	448.8	45%
Pepperoni	6 oz	26.9	479	51%
Sausage	6 oz	24.8	459.6	49%
Supreme	6 oz	25	466	48%
12 Inch Pizza				
Canadian Bacon	22 oz	75	1446.5	47%
Cheese	21 oz	73.6	1429	46%
Hamburger	22 oz	65.6	1418.7	42%
Pepperoni	22 oz	93	1623.6	52%
Pepperoni Deluxe	22 oz	95	1875.7	46%
Sausage	22 oz	82.6	1525	49%
Sausage & Mushroom	24 oz	82	1541	48%
Sausage & Pepperoni	22.75 oz	94	1656.9	51%
Special Deluxe	23.6 oz	91	1858	44%
Supreme	24.5 oz	86	1581	49%
Microwave Pizza				
Hamburger	3.5 oz	13	290	40%
Pepperoni	3.5 oz	15	320	42%
Sausage	3.5 oz	14	300	42%
Sausage & Pepperoni	3.5 oz	16	310	47%
Supreme	3.5 oz	14	290	43%
■ SNACK TRAY PIZZAS				
Cheese (12)	4 pizzas	7	130	49%
Pepperoni (12)	4 pizzas	8	140	51%
Sausage (12)	4 pizzas	8	140	51%
■ (SCHWAN'S)				
Deep Dish Single Serve Pizza				
Cheese	6 oz	24	520	42%
Mexican Style	5.5 oz	18	430	38%
Pepperoni	6 oz	29	580	45%
Sausage	6 oz	27	560	43%
Supreme	6 oz	29	590	44%
7 ¼" Microwave Pizza				
Pepperoni	3.5 oz	17	310	49%
Supreme	3.5 oz	15	280	48%
Special Recipe Pizza				
Canadian Bacon	3.5 oz	14	280	45%
Cheese	3.5 oz	15	290	47%
Hamburger	3.5 oz	15	280	48%
Pepperoni	3.5 oz	17	310	49%
Sausage	3.5 oz	15	280	48%
Sausage & Pepperoni	3.5 oz	18	290	56%

Food and Description	Amount	Fat Grams	Total Calories	% Fat Calories
Supreme	3.5 oz	16	280	51%
■ (STOUFFER'S)				
French Bread Pizza				
Canadian Style Bacon (11⅝ oz)	½ pizza	15	370	36%
Cheese (10⅜ oz)	½ pizza	14	350	36%
Deluxe (12⅜ oz)	½ pizza	19	420	41%
Double Cheese (11¾ oz)	½ pizza	18	420	39%
Hamburger (12¼ oz)	½ pizza	18	410	40%
Pepperoni (11¼ oz)	½ pizza	19	400	43%
Pepperoni & Mushroom (12¼ oz)	½ pizza	19	410	42%
Sausage (12 oz)	½ pizza	21	430	44%
Sausage & Pepperoni (12.5 oz)	½ pizza	23	460	45%
Vegetable Deluxe (12.75 oz)	½ pizza	20	420	43%
■ (TOMBSTONE)				
Double Top 12"				
Pepperoni w/Double Cheese	4.8 oz	20	360	50%
Sausage w/Double Cheese	4.8 oz	16	330	44%
Sausage & Pepperoni	4.8 oz	18	340	48%
Italian Style Thin Crust				
Cheese & Italian Sausage	3.2 oz	13	220	53%
Cheese & Pepperoni	3.04 oz	14	230	55%
Supreme	3.38 oz	14	230	55%
Three Cheese	3 oz	12	230	47%
Light 8"				
Chicken	4.5 oz	8	240	30%
Italian Sausage	4.1 oz	9	240	30%
Italian Sausage & Pepperoni	4.1 oz	9	250	32/5
Pepperoni	4 oz	10	250	36%
Supreme	4.6 oz	9	250	32%
Vegetable	4.4 oz	8	240	30%
Light 12"				
Chicken Deluxe	4.31 oz	6	240	23%
Pepperoni	3.9 oz	10	260	35%
Sausage	4.05 oz	8	240	30%
Supreme	4.5 oz	9	250	32%
Vegetable	4.3 oz	7	230	27%
Mexican Style Thin Crust				
Ranchero Deluxe	3.4 oz	13	230	51%
Microwave 7"				
Cheese	7.7 oz	24	500	43%
Cheese & Pepperoni	7.5 oz	32	550	52%
Italian Sausage	8 oz	32	550	52%
Sausage & Pepperoni	8 oz	32	570	51%
Supreme	8.5 oz	31	550	51%
Taco	8.4 oz	34	590	52%

Food and Description	Amount	Fat Grams	Total Calories	% Fat Calories
Original 9"				
Cheese	5.6 oz	17	380	40%
Cheese & Hamburger	6.3 oz	21	440	43%
Cheese & Pepperoni	6.3 oz	26	480	49%
Cheese & Sausage	6.3 oz	19	420	41%
Deluxe	7 oz	20	440	41%
Pepperoni & Sausage	6.6 oz	26	490	51%
Original 12"				
Canadian Style Bacon	3.6 oz	10	230	39%
Cheese	3.4 oz	10	230	39%
Cheese & Hamburger	3.7 oz	12	250	43%
Cheese & Pepperoni	3.6 oz	14	260	48%
Cheese & Sausage	3.7 oz	11	240	41%
Cheese, Sausage, & Mushroom	3.8 oz	11	240	41%
Deluxe	3.9 oz	11	240	41%
Sausage & Pepperoni	3.7 oz	13	260	45%
Supreme	3.8 oz	14	270	47%
Special Order				
Four Cheese	4.3 oz	14	300	42%
Four Meat	4.6 oz	15	320	42%
Italian Sausage	4.5 oz	13	300	39%
Pepperoni	4.4 oz	16	320	45%
Supreme	4.4 oz	15	320	42%
Special Order 9"				
Four Meat	3.9 oz	14	280	45%
Pepperoni	3.7 oz	14	280	45%
Supreme	4 oz	14	280	45%
Three Sausage	3.8 oz	12	260	42%
Vegetable	3.9 oz	10	230	39%
Special Order 12"				
Bacon Cheeseburger	4.7 oz	16	330	44%
Veggie	4.6 oz	11	270	37%
■ **(TONY'S)**				
Deli Style				
Pepperoni	3.5 oz	10	250	36%
Sausage	3.5 oz	9	240	34%
Sausage & Pepperoni	3.5 oz	10	240	38%
Supreme	3.5 oz	9	230	35%
French Bread				
Cheese	5.5 oz	8	360	20%
Pepperoni	5.9 oz	15	430	31%
Sausage	6.2 oz	12	410	26%
Supreme	6.3 oz	13	420	28%
Italian Style				
Canadian Bacon	3.5 oz	12	300	36%

Food and Description	Amount	Fat Grams	Total Calories	% Fat Calories
Cheese	3.5 oz	14	290	43%
Hamburger	3.5 oz	16	290	50%
Pepperoni	3.5 oz	14	320	39%
Pepperoni & Mushroom	3.5 oz	14	320	39%
Pepperoni & Sausage	3.5 oz	16	290	50%
Sausage	3.5 oz	16	290	50%
Sausage & Pepperoni	3.5 oz	16	290	50%
Supreme	3.5 oz	15	280	48%
Kidstuff				
Cheeseburger	5 oz	29	560	47%
Extra Cheesy	5 oz	21	460	41%
Pepperoni	5 oz	27	520	47%
Sausage	5 oz	24	500	43%
Taco	5 oz	25	490	46%
Microwave				
Canadian Style Bacon	3.5 oz	15	280	48%
Sausage & Pepperoni	3.5 oz	17	300	51%
Taco	3.5 oz	16	290	50%
Pizza Creations				
Bring Home the Bacon	15.25 oz	33.3	1094	27%
Drag It Through the Garden	16 oz	23.5	903	23%
Give Me the Works	16 oz	46.6	1398	30%
Hold the Tequila	16 oz	51.5	1199	39%
Plain Ol' Pepperoni (You Coward)	14.5 oz	40.9	1073	34%
Udder Delight	14.5 oz	41.1	1350	27%
■ (TOTINO'S)				
Microwave (Small)				
Cheese	1	10	250	36%
Combination	1	13	290	40%
Pepperoni	1	13	270	43%
Sausage	1	13	280	42%
Party Pizza w/Leaner Meats				
Canadian Bacon	½ pizza	13	330	35%
Cheese	½ pizza	10	290	31%
Combination	½ pizza	17	370	41%
Hamburger	½ pizza	17	350	44%
Pepperoni	½ pizza	19	000	46%
Sausage	½ pizza	17	370	41%
Pan Pizza				
Cheese	⅙ pizza	10	290	31%
Pepperoni	⅙ pizza	15	330	41%
Sausage	⅙ pizza	13	320	37%
Sausage & Pepperoni Combination	⅙ pizza	15	330	41%
Party Pizza-Family Size				
Cheese	⅓ pizza	11	320	31%

Food and Description	Amount	Fat Grams	Total Calories	% Fat Calories
Combination	⅓ pizza	18	400	41%
Pepperoni	⅓ pizza	20	410	44%
Sausage	⅓ pizza	18	410	40%
■ (WEIGHT WATCHERS)				
French Bread Pizza				
Deluxe	5.94 oz	7	260	24%
Pizza				
Cheese	6.03 oz	7	300	21%
Deluxe Combination	7.32 oz	9	320	25%
Pepperoni	6.08 oz	8	320	23%
Sausage	6.43 oz	10	340	26%
Pocket Pizza Deluxe Sandwich	4 oz	5	200	23%
■ (ZAP)				
French Bread Pizza				
Cheese French Bread	4.5 oz	10	308	29%
Deluxe French Bread	4.8 oz	13	323	36%
Pepperoni French Bread	4.5 oz	16	347	42%
PIZZA CRUST				
(Chef Boyardee) mix				
Crust only	¼ pizza	2	150	12%
Quick & Easy	¼ mix	2	150	12%
(Gold Medal) mix				
prepared	⅙ crust	1	110	8%
(Jiffy) mix	.81 oz	2	90	20%
(Ragu)				
Crust only-mix	¼ pizza	2	170	11%
Pizza Quick Canned Mix				
Dry	1½ scoops	2	170	11%
Pizza Recipe	¼ pizza	11	300	33%
Ready-to-Use				
Boboli-cheese	4" dia	6.5	301	19%
	8" dia	13	602	19%
	12" dia	26	1205	19%
Refrigerated (Pillsbury)	⅛ crust	1	90	10%
PIZZA SAUCE (See SAUCE)				
PLANTAIN (See BANANA)				
PLUM				
Canned				
in Water	1 cup	–	102	–
in Juice	1 cup	–	146	–
in Heavy Syrup	1 cup	–	230	–
Fresh	1	< 1	36	13%
(Nutradiet)				
Halves Unpeeled	½ cup	–	52	–
Whole Unpeeled	½ cup	–	52	–

Food and Description	Amount	Fat Grams	Total Calories	% Fat Calories
(S&W)				
Halves Unpeeled				
in Heavy Syrup	½ cup	–	135	–
Whole Fancy Unpeeled				
in Extra Heavy Syrup	½ cup	–	135	–
PLUM NECTAR				
(Kern's)	6 oz	–	110	–
POI	4 oz	–	134	–
POKEBERRY				
fresh-cooked	½ cup	–	16	–
raw	½ cup	–	20	–
POLLACK or Pollock (See also SEAFOOD ENTREE/DINNER)				
Atlantic				
raw	3 oz	.83	78	10%
Walleye				
cooked-dry heat	3 oz	.95	96	9%
raw	3 oz	.68	68	9%
POMEGRANATE/fresh	1	.5	104	4%
POMPANO/Florida				
breaded & fried	3 oz	16.8	271	56%
cooked-dry heat	3 oz	10	179	50%
raw	3 oz	8	140	51%
POP TART (See PASTRY, TOASTER)				
POPCORN				
(Act I) Microwave				
Butter	3 cups	8	140	51%
Extra Butter	3 cups	10	160	56%
(Act II)				
Frozen				
Butter Flavored	3 cups	10	190	47%
Real Butter	3 cups	8	140	51%
Microwave				
Butter	3 cups	8	140	51%
Caramel	3 cups	14	280	45%
Lite				
Butter	3 cups	3	100	27%
50% less Salt	3 cups	3	100	27%
Natural	3 cups	3	100	27%
Natural	3 cups	8	140	51%
Sour Cream & Onion	3 cups	8	150	48%
Tangy Ranch	3 cups	8	140	51%
White Cheddar Cheese	3 cups	9	160	51%
Airpopped-no butter added				
Generic	1 cup	–	30	–

Food and Description	Amount	Fat Grams	Total Calories	% Fat Calories
(Betty Crocker) Pop Secret-popped				
Butter Flavor				
Light	3 cups	3	70	39%
Regular	3 cups	6	100	54%
Salt Free	3 cups	6	100	54%
Singles				
Light	6 cups	6	140	39%
Regular	6 cups	12	200	54%
Natural Flavor				
Light	3 cups	6	100	54%
Regular	3 cups	3	70	39%
Singles-Light	6 cups	6	150	36%
Pop Qwiz				
Butter	3 cups	6	100	54%
Natural	3 cups	6	100	54%
(Blue Heaven) Microwaveable				
Blue Corn	2 cups	8	130	55%
(Borden) Cracker Jack				
Butter Toffee	1 oz	5	130	35%
Original	1 oz	3	120	23%
(Cape Cod) Ready To Eat				
White Cheddar	1 oz	10	160	56%
Caramel Coated-Generic				
Plain	1 oz	3	122	22%
w/Peanuts	1.5 oz	5	180	25%
(Deli Express) Lite Pop				
Butter	3.2 cups	3	100	27%
Natural	3.2 cups	3	100	27%
(Eagle) Ready-to-Eat				
Cheese	½ oz	6	80	68%
White Cheddar	½ oz	6	80	68%
(Jiffy Pop) Popped				
Bag				
Butter				
Light	3 cups	3	80	34%
Regular	3 cups	5	100	45%
Microwave				
Butter	4 cups	7	140	45%
Regular	4 cups	7	140	45%
(Jolly Time) Microwave				
Butter	3 cups	5	90	50%
Light	3 cups	2	60	30%
Cheddar Cheese	3 cups	11	180	55%
Natural	3 cups	7	120	53%

Food and Description	Amount	Fat Grams	Total Calories	% Fat Calories
Light	3 cups	2	70	26%
Regular				
White-no butter	4 cups	.6	77	7%
Yellow-no butter	4 cups	.8	77	9%
(Keebler) Ready to Eat				
Pop Deluxe				
Honey Caramel Glazed	1 oz	3	120	23%
White Cheddar	1 oz	10	140	64%
(Michael Season's) Ready-To-Eat				
White Cheddar Cheese	1 oz	10	161	56%
(Newman's Own)				
Butter	3 cups	8	150	48%
Natural	3 cups	8	150	48%
(Old Vienna)				
Butter	1 oz	10	160	56%
Cheese	1 oz	10	160	56%
(Orville Redenbacher's)				
Frozen				
Butter				
As Packaged	3 cups	8	110	65%
Popped	3 cups	6	100	54%
Natural				
As Packaged	3 cups	8	110	65%
Popped	3 cups	6	100	54%
Microwave				
Butter				
As Packaged	3 cups	8	110	65%
Popped	3 cups	6	100	54%
Butter-Salt Free				
As Packaged	3 cups	8	110	65%
Popped	3 cups	6	100	54%
Butter Toffee				
As Packaged	3 cups	15	300	45%
Popped	3 cups	12	210	51%
Caramel				
As Packaged	3 cups	18	310	52%
Popped	3 cups	14	240	53%
Cheddar Cheese				
As Packaged	3 cups	10	150	60%
Popped	3 cups	8	130	55%
Light				
Butter				
As Packaged	3 cups	4	80	45%
Popped	3 cups	3	70	39%

Food and Description	Amount	Fat Grams	Total Calories	% Fat Calories
Natural				
As Packaged	3 cups	4	80	45%
Popped	3 cups	3	70	39%
Natural				
As Packaged	3 cups	8	110	65%
Popped	3 cups	6	100	54%
Natural-Salt Free				
As Packaged	3 cups	8	110	65%
Popped	3 cups	6	100	54%
Smart Pop				
As Packaged	3 cups	2	60	30%
Popped	3 cups	1	40	23%
Sour Cream 'n Onion				
As Packaged	3 cups	13	180	65%
Popped	3 cups	12	160	68%
Original				
Hot Air	3 cups	< 1	40	11%
Popping Corn	3 cups	4	80	45%
White	3 cups	4	80	45%
Ready-to-Eat Light	1 oz	5	100	45%
(Pillsbury) Micro Wave				
Butter Flavor				
Frozen	3 cups	13	210	56%
Grocery Shelf	3 cups	13	210	56%
Original				
Frozen	3 cups	13	210	56%
Grocery Shelf	3 cups	13	210	56%
Salt Free-frozen	3 cups	7	170	37%
(Planter's) Microwave				
Butter	3 cups	8	140	51%
Natural	3 cups	9	140	58%
Popcorn Snack Cakes (*See also* RICE CAKES)				
(Chico-San) Popcorn				
Butter	1 cake	–	40	–
Cheddar	1 cake	2	50	36%
Lightly Salted	1 cake	–	40	–
Plain	1 cake	–	35	–
(Quaker) Popped Corn				
Butter	1 cake	–	35	–
Caramel Corn	1 cake	–	50	–
Popped in oil-no butter added	1 cup	3	55	49%
(Pops-Rite)				
Butter-Light				
As Packaged	3 cups	4	90	40%

Food and Description	Amount	Fat Grams	Total Calories	% Fat Calories
Prepared	3 cups	3	70	39%
(Smartfood)				
Cheddar Cheese	½ oz	5	80	56%
Light Butter	½ oz	3	70	39%
Syrup-Coated-Generic	1 cup	1	135	7%
(Ultra Slim Fast) Ready To Eat	½ oz	2	60	30%
(Vic's) Corn Popper Gourmet				
Caramel	½ cup	3	110	25%
Cheese	⅔ cup	8	90	80%
White				
Lite	1 cup	2	40	45%
Regular	1 cup	4	60	60%
(Weight Watchers)				
Microwave	1 oz pouch	1	90	10%
Ready-to-eat				
Butter	.7 oz	3	90	30%
Caramel	½ oz	2	60	30%
White Cheddar	.7 oz	4	90	40%
(Wise)				
Tender Eating Baby Popcorn	.5 oz	6	70	77%
w/Real White Cheddar Cheese	.5 oz	5	70	64%
POPCORN SNACK CAKE (See POPCORN)				
POPPY SEED	1 tsp	1	13	35%
POPSICLES (See FRUIT ICES)				
PORGY				
breaded & fried	3 oz	13	246	48%
cooked-dry heat	3 oz	8.7	172	46%

PORK (See also BACON, HAM, LUNCHEON MEAT, SAUSAGE)
(NOTE: The information listed below on "Today's Leaner Pork" was provided by the National Pork, Livestock, and Meat Board. Following this is information on "Miscellaneous Cuts," which was provided by the United States Department of Agriculture. Please note that the data listed under "Today's Leaner Pork" apply to meat that has been roasted and trimmed of all separable fat.)

■ **TODAY'S LEANER PORK**

Food and Description	Amount	Fat Grams	Total Calories	% Fat Calories
Blade Steaks	3 oz	10.7	193	50%
Center Loin Chop	3 oz	6.9	165	38%
Center Rib Chop	3 oz	6.5	179	43%
Loin Chops	3 oz	6.9	172	36%
Loin Chops (Boneless)	3 oz	6.6	173	34%
Loin Roast (Boneless)	3 oz	6	165	33%
Rib Chops	3 oz	8.3	186	41%
Rib Roast (Boneless)	3 oz	8.6	182	43%
Ribs (Country Style)	3 oz	12.6	210	54%
Sirloin Chops (Boneless)	3 oz	5.7	164	31%
Sirloin Roast	3 oz	8.7	184	43%

Food and Description	Amount	Fat Grams	Total Calories	% Fat Calories
Tenderloin	3 oz	4	139	26%
Top Loin Chop	3 oz	6.6	165	36%
■ MISCELLANEOUS CUTS				
Brains				
Braised	3 oz	8	117	62%
Canned In Milk Gravy (Armour Star)	2.75 oz	8	110	65%
Chitterlings				
Cooked-Simmered	3 oz	24	258	84%
	1 lb	73	923	71%
Ears				
Cooked-Simmered	1 Ear	11.88	183	58%
Feet				
Cooked-Simmered	2.5 oz	8.8	138	57%
Feet				
Cured, Pickled	1 oz	4.58	58	71%
Simmered	3 oz	10.6	166	57%
Heart				
Braised	1 Heart	6.5	191	31%
Jowl				
Raw	4 oz	78.66	740	96%
	1 oz	19.7	186	95%
Kidney				
Braised	3 oz	4	128	28%
Liver				
Braised	3 oz	3.7	141	24%
Lungs				
Braised	3 oz	2.65	85	28%
Spleen				
Braised	3 oz	2.7	128	19%
Stomach				
Raw	3 oz	8	135	53%
Tail				
Cooked-Simmered	3 oz	30	336	80%
Tongue				
Braised	3 oz	14.8	215	62%
Cured-Canned (Hormel) 8 lb	3 oz	13	190	62%
PORK ENTREE/DINNER (See also FROZEN ENTREE/DINNER)				
Breaded Pork Steaks/frozen (Hormel)	3 oz	15	220	61%
Breakfast Strips (Sizzlean)-Cooked				
Brown Sugar	2 strips	9	110	74%
Plain	2 strips	8	90	80%
Cajun Pork/Hunt's Minute Gourmet box	6.6 oz	23	460	45%
Great Beginnings (Hormel) Box prepared	5 oz	8	140	51%

Food and Description	Amount	Fat Grams	Total Calories	% Fat Calories
Ham & Swiss Cheese Croissant/frozen				
(Sara Lee)	1	18	340	48%
Ham Croquette/homemade	1/~2 oz	9.8	163	54%
Pork Loin-sliced w/gravy/homemade	4 oz	9	162	50%
Scalloped Potatoes & Ham/frozen	9 oz	16	340	42%
(Schwan's) frozen-Center Cut Pork Loin				
Chops	7 oz	14	300	42%
Chopped pork fritter	2.66 oz	9	200	41%
Ham Steak Patties	2 oz	16	180	80%
Pork Dinner Loin	4 oz	4	230	16%

PORK & BEANS (*See* BEAN, BAKED & VARIETY; BEAN MEALS, BAKED)
POT PIE (*See* individual listing under BEEF DISHES, CHICKEN ENTREE/DINNER, or TURKEY ENTREE/DINNER)
POTATO
White

baked-skin only	1 medium	–	115	–
baked w/ skin	~ 7 oz	–	220	–
baked w/o skin	~ 5.5 oz	–	145	–
boiled w/ skin	½ cup	–	68	–
boiled w/o skin	½ cup	–	67	–
	~ 4.75 oz	–	116	–
canned w/o skin	½ cup	–	54	–
small whole new (S&W)	½ cup	–	45	–
whole new potatoes (Del Monte)	½ cup	–	45	–
flakes/dry				
(Arrowhead Mills)	2 oz	–	140	–
(Borden) Country Store	⅓ cup	–	70	–
Generic	1 cup	–	164	–
french fries/from restaurant	10 pieces	8	158	46%
frozen/cottage cut				
cooked in oven	10 pieces	4	109	33%
fried in vegetable oil	10 pieces	8	158	46%
french-fried/heated	10 pieces	4	109	33%
granules/dry	1 cup	1	704	1%
microwaved w/ skin	1 large	–	212	–
microwaved w/o skin	1 large	–	156	–
raw w/ skin	1 medium	–	110	–
raw w/o skin	1 medium	–	88	–

POTATO CHIPS

(Cottage Fries) no salt added	1 oz	11	160	62%
(Deli Style)				
Mesquite Bar-B-Q	1 oz	8	150	48%
Regular	1 oz	8	150	48%
Sour Cream & Onion	1 oz	8	150	48%

Food and Description	Amount	Fat Grams	Total Calories	% Fat Calories
(Eagle)				
Barbeque Flavored	1 oz	8	150	48%
Crispy Cut	1 oz	10	150	60%
Extra Crunchy	1 oz	8	150	48%
Hawaiian	1 oz	8	150	48%
Lattice Cut	1 oz	10	150	60%
Mesquite Barbecue	1 oz	10	150	60%
Onion Ridged	1 oz	10	150	60%
Plain	1 oz	10	150	60%
Ridged-plain	1 oz	10	150	60%
Russet	1 oz	8	150	48%
Sour Cream & Onion	1 oz	10	150	60%
Thins	1 oz	10	150	60%
Barbeque Flavored	1 oz	10	150	60%
(Health Valley)				
Country	1 oz	10	160	56%
Country-no salt	1 oz	10	160	56%
Country Ripples	1 oz	10	160	56%
Dip-no salt	1 oz	10	160	56%
Plain	1 oz	10	160	56%
(Keebler) Ripplin's-all flavors	1 oz	9	150	54%
(Laura Scudder)				
Bar-B-Q	1 oz	9	150	54%
For Dips	1 oz	10	150	60%
Hawaiian	1 oz	9	150	54%
Natural Style	1 oz	10	150	60%
Plain	1 oz	10	150	60%
Sour Cream & Onion	1 oz	9	150	54%
(Lay's)				
Crunch Tators				
Hoppin Jalapeno	1 oz	7	140	45%
Mighty Mesquite	1 oz	7	140	45%
Original	1 oz	8	140	51%
Regular Chips				
Bar B Q	1 oz	9	150	54%
Cheddar Cheese	1 oz	10	150	60%
Flamin' Hot	1 oz	9	150	54%
Italian Cheese	1 oz	9	150	54%
Jalapeno'N Cheddar	1 oz	9	150	54%
Original	1 oz	10	150	60%
Salt & Vinegar	1 oz	10	150	60%
Sour Cream & Onion	1 oz	10	160	56%
Tangy Ranch	1 oz	10	160	56%
Unsalted	1 oz	10	150	60%

Food and Description	Amount	Fat Grams	Total Calories	% Fat Calories
(Michael Season's) Hand-Cooked				
Barbecue	1 oz	10	150	60%
Lightly Salted	1 oz	10	150	60%
Unsalted	1 oz	10	150	60%
Wave-Cut	1 oz	10	150	60%
Yogurt & Green Onion	1 oz	10	150	60%
(New York Deli)	1 oz	11	160	62%
(O'Boises)				
Original	1 oz	9	150	54%
Sour Cream & Onion	1 oz	9	150	54%
(O'Grady's)				
Au Gratin	1 oz	8	150	48%
Hearty Seasoning	1 oz	8	140	51%
Plain	1 oz	9	150	54%
(Old Vienna) Plain	1 oz	9	150	54%
(Poore Brothers)				
Bar-B-Que	1 oz	10	150	60%
Cajun	1 oz	10	150	60%
Chili & Lemon	1 oz	10	150	60%
Dill Pickle	1 oz	10	150	60%
Jalapeno	1 oz	10	150	60%
Regular	1 oz	10	150	60%
no salt	1 oz	10	150	60%
Sour Cream & Onion	1 oz	10	150	60%
(Pringle's)				
BBQ	1 oz	11	160	62%
Cheez-ums	1 oz	11	160	62%
Idaho Rippled				
Cheddar'N Sour Cream	1 oz	11	160	62%
Mesquite BBQ	1 oz	11	160	62%
Original	1 oz	11	160	62%
Light				
BBQ	.9 oz	6	130	42%
Cheddar	.9 oz	6	130	42%
Original	.9 oz	6	130	42%
Ranch	.9 oz	6	130	42%
Original	1 oz	11	160	62%
Sour Cream'N Onion	1 oz	11	160	62%
(Ruffles)				
Cheddar & Sour Cream	1 oz	10	160	56%
Light				
plain	1 oz	6	130	42%
sour cream & onion	1 oz	6	130	42%
Mesquite Grille B-B-Q	1 oz	10	160	56%

Food and Description	Amount	Fat Grams	Total Calories	% Fat Calories
Monterey Jack Cheese Attack	1 oz	10	160	56%
Original	1 oz	10	150	60%
Ranch	1 oz	10	160	56%
Sour Cream & Onions	1 oz	10	160	56%
Tato Skins (*See* POTATO SNACKS)				
(Wise) Natural	1 oz	11	160	62%
Ridges-Barbecue	1 oz	10	150	60%
POTATO DISHES				
Au Gratin				
box mix	1 cup	10	230	39%
frozen (Banquet)	½ cup	2	98	18%
homemade w/butter	½ cup	9	160	51%
microwaveable				
(Green Giant) Pantry Express	½ cup	5	120	38%
Baked-Frozen				
(Brighton's)				
Broccoli & Cheese	10.2 oz	12	337	32%
Classic Combination	9.6 oz	13	326	36%
Cheese Sauce/Bacon	9.5 oz	13	352	33%
Cheese Sauce/Ham	10.2 oz	12	347	31%
(Healthy Choice)				
Broccoli & Cheese Sauce				
w/Baked Potato Wedges	9.5 oz	5	240	23%
(Larry's)				
Cheese	5 oz	9	190	43%
Deluxe	6 oz	9	200	41%
Sour Cream & Chives	5 oz	9	190	43%
(Oh Boy!)				
w/Cheddar Cheese	6 oz	4	142	25%
w/Real Bacon	6 oz	3	116	23%
w/Sour Cream, Onion, & Chives	6 oz	5	129	35%
(Pillsbury)				
w/Cheese Flavored Topping	5 oz	6	200	27%
w/Sour Cream & Chives	5 oz	10	230	39%
(Weight Watchers)				
Broccoli & Cheese	10.5 oz	6	270	20%
Chicken Divan	11.25 oz	7	280	23%
Ham Lorraine	11.5 oz	5	240	19%
Homestyle Turkey	11.25 oz	7	230	27%
Vegetable Primavera	11.15 oz	9	320	25%
(Betty Crocker) box mixes				
Microwave-prepared				
Au Gratin	1 serving	5	140	24%
Cheddar & bacon	1 serving	5	140	24%

Food and Description	Amount	Fat Grams	Total Calories	% Fat Calories
Cheesy Scalloped	1 serving	5	140	32%
Hash browns w/onions	1 serving	6	160	34%
Homestyle Skin-On Potatoes				
American Cheese				
Prepared	⅛ box	5	140	32%
Unprepared	⅛ box	1	90	10%
Cheddar Cheese				
Prepared	⅛ box	5	140	32%
Unprepared	⅛ box	2	100	17%
Julienne	1 serving	5	130	39%
Potato Buds	1 serving	6	130	42%
Scalloped	1 serving	5	140	32%
Scalloped w/Ham	1 serving	6	160	32%
Smokey Cheddar	1 serving	5	140	36%
Sour Cream & Chive	1 serving	5	140	39%
Twice Baked				
Bacon & Cheddar	1 serving	11	210	47%
Herbed Butter	1 serving	13	220	53%
Mild Cheddar w/onion	1 serving	11	190	52%
Sour Cream & Chive	1 serving	11	200	50%
Escalloped Potatoes/Vegetable Classics				
(Del Monte) microwave	4.5 oz	9	140	58%
(French's)				
Box Mixes-prepared				
Cheddar & Bacon Casserole	1 serving	5	130	35%
Creamy Italian Scalloped	1 serving	3	120	23%
Creamy Stroganoff	1 serving	4	130	28%
Crispy Top Scalloped w/Savory Onion	1 serving	5	140	32%
Real Cheese Scalloped	1 serving	5	140	32%
Real Sour Cream & Chives	1 serving	7	150	42%
Tangy Au Gratin	1 serving	5	130	35%
Hash Browns				
frozen-generic				
plain	½ cup	8.97	170	48%
w/butter sauce	3.5 oz	8.9	178	45%
homemade w/vegetable oil	½ cup	10.05	163	60%
refrigerated (Simply Potatoes)	4 oz	< 1	100	5%
(Kraft) Box Mixes-prepared				
Broccoli Au Gratin	½ cup	5	150	30%
Potatoes & Cheese-Two Cheese	½ cup	4	130	28%
Scalloped Potatoes				
Plain	½ cup	5	140	32%
w/Ham	½ cup	5	150	30%

Food and Description	Amount	Fat Grams	Total Calories	% Fat Calories
Mashed				
w/whole milk	½ cup	.6	81	7%
w/whole milk & margarine	½ cup	4	94	38%
from dehydrated flakes				
w/milk & butter added	½ cup	6	165	33%
Instant Mix-Prepared				
(Instamash) Microwave	½ cup	1	80	11%
(French's)	½ cup	6	130	42%
(Hungry Jack)	½ cup	7	140	45%
Potato Buds (Betty Crocker)				
Box Mix-dry	½ cup	–	70	–
Box Mix-prepared	½ cup	6	130	42%
Spuds (French's)	½ cup	7	140	45%
(Micromagic) Frozen				
Crinkle Cut	3 oz	10.5	220	43%
French Fries	3 oz	13	290	40%
Skinny Fries	3.5 oz	15	350	39%
Tater Sticks	4 oz	22	390	51%
Microwave				
(Del Monte) Vegetable Classics				
Potatoes Au Gratin in Tangy				
Chili Sauce	½ cup	11	190	52%
(Ore Ida) frozen				
Cheddar browns	3 oz	2	90	23%
Cottage Fries	3 oz	4	130	38%
Crinkle Cuts, Microwave	3.5 oz	8	190	40%
Crispers!	3 oz	13	220	59%
Crispy Crowns	3 oz	11	190	53%
Crispy Crunchers	3 oz	9	180	45%
Deep Fries-for the oven				
Crinkle Cuts				
Lites	3 oz	2	90	20%
Original	3 oz	7	160	34%
Regular Cuts	3 oz	7	170	39%
French Fries-Golden Crinkles	3 oz	3	120	23%
French Fries-Golden Fries	3 oz	3	120	23%
French Fries-Pixie Crinkles	3 oz	5	140	32%
French Fries-Shoestrings	3 oz	6	150	36%
Fries Country Style Dinner	3 oz	2	110	16%
Golden Patties	2.5 oz	7	130	51%
Golden Twirls	3 oz	6	160	39%
Hash Browns-Microwave	2 oz	7	120	60%
Hash Browns-Shredded	3 oz	–	70	–
Hash Browns-Southern Style	3 oz	–	70	–

Food and Description	Amount	Fat Grams	Total Calories	% Fat Calories
Hash Browns-Toaster	1.75 oz	5	100	54%
Potatoes O'Brien	3 oz	–	60	–
Small Whole Potatoes	3 oz	–	70	–
Tater Tots				
Bacon Flavored	3 oz	7	150	36%
Microwave	2 oz	9	210	41%
Regular	3 oz	8	160	42%
w/Onion	3 oz	7	150	36%
Topped Baked				
Broccoli & Cheese	5⅞ oz	4	160	23%
Vegetable Primavera	6⅛ oz	5	160	28%
Twice Baked				
Butter Flavor	5 oz	8	200	36%
Cheddar Cheese	5 oz	9	210	39%
Sour Cream & Chives	5 oz	8	190	38%
Wedges Home Style	3 oz	2	110	16%
Whole Small	3 oz	–	70	–
Zesties!	3 oz	8	160	45%
Pierogi (dumpling)-frozen				
(Mrs. T's)				
Potato Cheese	1	1	70	13%
Potato Onion	1	–	50	–
(Pillsbury) box mixes/prepared				
Cheddar & Bacon	1 serving	5	130	35%
Creamy Italian Style	1 serving	3	120	23%
Potato Pancake	3 pancakes	2	90	20%
Scalloped w/Cheese	1 serving	5	140	32%
Scalloped w/Creamy White Sauce	1 serving	5	140	32%
Sour Cream & Chives	1 serving	7	150	42%
Tangy Au Gratin	1 serving	5	130	35%
Potato Fillets/frozen				
(Gorton's)	2 fillets	20	310	58%
Potato Pancakes				
(French's)				
Box Mix	3 cakes	2	90	20%
Dinner Pancakes	3-3" pancakes	2	90	20%
Homemade				
w/Butter & Milk	1 pancake	12.6	495	23%
Potato Puffs/frozen	1 puff	.8	16	45%
Potato Salad w/Mayonnaise				
Canned German Style				
(Read)	½ cup	3	120	23%
Canned Home Style				
(Read)	1 cup	22	340	58%

Food and Description	Amount	Fat Grams	Total Calories	% Fat Calories
Homemade	½ cup	10	179	50%
Potato Sticks/Frozen				
(Gorton's)	4 sticks	16	260	55%
Potatoes O'Brien w/Bread Crumbs & Butter				
Homemade	½ cup	1	79	11%
Scalloped				
Homemade				
w/Butter	½ cup	4.5	105	39%
w/Cheese	½ cup	9.5	175	49%
Scalloped Potatoes & Ham				
Frozen				
Generic				
Plain	½ cup	6	123	44%
w/Cheese	½ cup	9.6	177	49%
(Swanson's)	9 oz	13	300	39%
Microwaveable				
(Hormel) Microcup	7.5 oz	16	260	55%
(Lunch Bucket)	8.5 oz	13	260	45%
POTATO SNACKS (See also POTATO CHIPS)				
(Keebler) Tato Skins-all flavors	1 oz	8	150	48%
(Planter's)				
BBQ	1 oz	10	160	56%
Plain	1 oz	10	160	56%
Potato Sticks-Generic	1 cup	12	190	57%
	1 oz	9	148	55%
(Durkee) Shoestring	1 oz	9	160	51%
POTATO SOUP (See SOUP)				
POTATO STARCH (Manischewitz)	½ cup	–	385	–
POULTRY SEASONING	1 tsp	–	5	–
POUT-OCEAN/raw	3 oz	1	70	13%
PRESERVES (See JAM/JELLY/PRESERVES)				
PRETZELS				
(Eagle)				
Beer	1 oz	2	110	16%
Plain	1 oz	2	110	16%
(Estee) unsalted	5 pieces	< 1	25	18%
(Featherweight) unsalted pretzels	1 oz	1	110	8%
(Laura Scudder's) Bavarian	1 oz	1	110	8%
Unsalted	1 oz	1	120	8%
Sticks	1 oz	1	110	8%
Twists	1 oz	1	110	8%
(Michael Season's) Twist				
Lightly Salted	1 oz	1	114	8%
Unsalted	1 oz	1	114	8%

Food and Description	Amount	Fat Grams	Total Calories	% Fat Calories
(Nabisco)				
Mr. Phipps Pretzel Chips				
Fat Free	8 pieces	–	50	–
Lightly Salted	8 pieces	1	60	15%
Original	8 pieces	1	60	15%
Sesame	8 pieces	1	60	15%
Mister Salty				
Butter Flavored	1 oz	1	110	8%
Dutch Pretzels	1 oz	1	110	8%
Fat Free	1 oz	–	100	–
Junior Pretzels	1 oz	2	110	16%
Mini	1 oz	1	110	8%
Pretzel Rings	1 oz	2	110	16%
Pretzel Sticks	1 oz	1	90	10%
Pretzel Twists	1 oz	2	110	16%
Very Thin Pretzel Sticks	1 oz	1	110	8%
(Planter's) Pretzels	1 oz	1	110	8%
(Pocket Pretzels) Peanut Butter-Filled	1 oz	4	126	29%
(Rokeach) Dutch	1 oz	< 1	110	5%
No Salt	1 oz	< 1	110	5%
(Rold Gold)				
Bavarian	1 oz	2	120	15%
Rods	1 oz	2	110	16%
Sticks	1 oz	2	110	16%
Twists	1 oz	1	110	8%
Tiny Twist	1 oz	1	110	8%
(Seyfert's) Butter-rods	1 oz	1	110	8%
(Snyder's) Hard Pretzels				
Old Fashioned	1 oz	–	110	–
Sour Dough	1 oz	–	110	–
(Super Pretzel) frozen-baked soft				
Oat Bran	2.25 oz	–	178	–
Original	2.25 oz	–	190	–
(Ultra Slim Fast)	1 oz	< 1	100	5%
PRICKLY PEAR	1	.5	42	11%
PRUNE				
(Del Monte)				
moist pack	2 oz	–	120	–
uncooked				
w/pits	2 oz	–	120	–
w/o pits	2 oz	–	140	–
Generic				
canned in heavy syrup	5	–	90	–
	1 cup	< 1	240	2%

Food and Description	Amount	Fat Grams	Total Calories	% Fat Calories
cooked-dried				
no sugar	1 cup	< 1	225	2%
w/sugar	1 cup	< 1	294	2%
uncooked	10 Pitted	< 1	201	2%
(Mariani) dried				
large	¼ cup	1	140	6%
pitted	¼ cup	1	140	6%
(Sunsweet) dried				
bite size				
breakfast	2 oz	–	120	–
extra large	2 oz	–	120	–
large	2 oz	–	120	–
medium	2 oz	–	120	–
pitted	2 oz	–	140	–
PRUNE JUICE				
canned	4 oz	–	90	–
(Del Monte)				
unsweetened	6 oz	–	120	–
(Mott's)				
country style	6 oz	–	129	–
unsweetened	6 oz	–	130	–
(S&W) unsweetened	6 oz	–	120	–
(Sunsweet)	6 oz	–	130	–
w/prune pulp	6 oz	–	130	–
PUDDING & MOUSSE (*See also* CUSTARD)				
Apple Brown Betty				
Homemade	1 cup	7.6	325	21%
Bread				
Homemade w/ raisins	1 cup	16	495	29%
Canned				
Banana	½ cup	4	150	24%
Butterscotch	½ cup	4	150	24%
Chocolate	½ cup	4	190	19%
Egg Custard	½ cup	6	140	39%
Fudge	½ cup	4	190	10%
Lemon	½ cup	2	170	11%
Rice	½ cup	3	150	18%
Tapioca	½ cup	4	140	26%
Vanilla	½ cup	4	150	24%
Corn				
Homemade	1 cup	9.8	255	35%
(Del Monte) Pudding Cups				
Banana	5 oz	5	180	25%
Butterscotch	5 oz	5	180	25%

Food and Description	Amount	Fat Grams	Total Calories	% Fat Calories
Chocolate	5 oz	6	190	28%
Chocolate Fudge	5 oz	6	190	28%
Tapioca	5 oz	4	180	20%
Vanilla	5 oz	5	180	25%
(Featherweight) Sweet Pretenders/canned				
Butterscotch	½ cup	1	100	9%
Chocolate	½ cup	1	100	9%
Vanilla	½ cup	2	100	18%
Indian Pudding/homemade-baked	½ cup	4.5	120	34%
Mix				
(D-Zera) Reduced Calorie-prepared w/skim milk				
Butterscotch	½ cup	–	70	–
Chocolate	½ cup	–	60	–
Vanilla	½ cup	–	70	–
(Estee)				
Mousse				
Amaretto	½ cup	3	70	39%
Orange/Chocolate	½ cup	3	70	39%
Pudding				
Chocolate	½ cup	1	70	13%
Vanilla	½ cup	.5	70	6%
(Jell-O) Deluxe Chocolate Collection				
Chocolate Almond & Chocolate Creme Dessert/				
Prepared as Directed	½ cup	8	220	33%
(Jell-O) Instant - Prepared w/Whole Milk				
Banana Cream	½ cup	4	160	23%
Butter Pecan	½ cup	5	170	27%
Butterscotch	½ cup	4	140	26%
Chocolate	½ cup	4	130	28%
Chocolate Fudge	½ cup	5	180	25%
Coconut Cream	½ cup	6	180	30%
French Vanilla	½ cup	4	160	23%
Lemon	½ cup	4	140	26%
Milk Chocolate	½ cup	5	180	25%
Pineapple Cream	½ cup	4	160	23%
Pistachio	½ cup	4	150	24%
Vanilla	½ cup	4	140	26%
(Jell-O) Instant-Sugar Free-Prepared w/2% Low-Fat Milk				
Banana	½ cup	2	90	20%
Butterscotch	½ cup	2	90	20%
Chocolate	½ cup	3	100	27%
Chocolate Fudge	½ cup	3	100	27%
Pistachio	½ cup	3	100	27%
Vanilla	½ cup	2	90	20%

Food and Description	Amount	Fat Grams	Total Calories	% Fat Calories
(Jell-O) Microwave Puddings-Prepared w/Whole Milk				
Banana Cream	½ cup	4	170	21%
Butterscotch	½ cup	4	170	21%
Chocolate	½ cup	5	170	27%
Milk Chocolate	½ cup	6	160	34%
Mint Chocolate	½ cup	5	160	28%
Vanilla	½ cup	4	160	23%
(Jell-O) Regular Puddings-Prepared w/Whole Milk				
Banana Cream	½ cup	3	100	27%
Butterscotch	½ cup	4	170	21%
Chocolate	½ cup	5	180	25%
Chocolate Fudge	½ cup	4	160	23%
Coconut Cream	½ cup	6	170	32%
French Vanilla	½ cup	4	170	21%
Lemon	½ cup	2	200	9%
Milk Chocolate	½ cup	4	160	23%
Vanilla	½ cup	4	140	26%
(Jell-O) Regular Sugar-Free Puddings-Prepared w/2% Milk				
Chocolate	½ cup	3	90	30%
Vanilla	½ cup	2	80	23%
(Jell-O) Mousse-Rich & Luscious-Prepared w/Whole Milk				
Chocolate	½ cup	6	150	36%
Chocolate Fudge	½ cup	6	150	36%
(Jell-O) Rice Pudding				
Americana Prepared w/Whole Milk	½ cup	4	170	21%
(Jell-O) Whip'N Chill Deluxe Dessert Mix				
Chocolate	½ cup	2	70	26%
Lemon	½ cup	2	70	26%
Mint	½ cup	2	70	26%
Strawberry	½ cup	2	70	26%
Vanilla	½ cup	2	70	26%
(My-T-Fine) Dry Mix to Make ½ Cup Serving				
Almond	.9 oz	1	100	9%
Butterscotch	.9 oz	–	90	–
Chocolate	.9 oz	–	100	–
Fudge	.9 oz	–	100	–
Lemon (pudding & pie)	.9 oz	–	90	–
Tapioca	.9 oz	–	80	–
Vanilla	.9 oz	–	90	–
(Royal) Instant Pudding				
Banana Cream-				
Prepared w/Whole Milk	½ cup	5	180	25%
Butterscotch-				
Prepared w/Whole Milk	½ cup	5	180	25%

Food and Description	Amount	Fat Grams	Total Calories	% Fat Calories
Chocolate-				
Prepared w/Whole Milk	½ cup	4	190	19%
Chocolate Almond-				
Prepared w/2% Milk	½ cup	3	180	15%
Chocolate Chocolate Chip-				
Prepared w/Whole Milk	½ cup	4	190	19%
Chocolate Mint-				
Prepared w/Whole Milk	½ cup	4	190	19%
Dark'N Sweet-				
Prepared w/Whole Milk	½ cup	4	190	19%
Lemon-Prepared w/Whole Milk	½ cup	5	180	25%
Pistachio Nut-				
Prepared w/Whole Milk	½ cup	4	170	21%
Toasted Butter Almond-				
Prepared w/Whole Milk	½ cup	4	170	21%
Toasted Coconut				
Prepared w/Whole Milk	½ cup	4	170	21%
Vanilla				
Prepared w/Whole Milk	½ cup	5	180	25%
(Royal) Instant-Sugar-Free/Prepared w/2% Milk				
Butterscotch	½ cup	2	100	18%
Chocolate	½ cup	3	110	25%
Vanilla	½ cup	2	100	18%
(Royal) Regular (Cooked)-Prepared w/Whole Milk				
Banana Cream	½ cup	4	160	23%
Butterscotch	½ cup	4	160	23%
Chocolate	½ cup	4	180	20%
Custard	½ cup	4	150	24%
Dark'N Sweet	½ cup	5	180	25%
Flan w/Caramel Sauce	½ cup	5	150	30%
Vanilla	½ cup	4	160	23%
Vanilla Tapioca	½ cup	4	160	23%
(Weight Watchers) Instant-Prepared w/Skim Milk				
Chocolate	½ cup	–	100	–
Vanilla	½ cup	–	90	–
(Weight Watchers) Mousse-Frozen				
Chocolate	2.5 oz	0	150	18%
Praline Pecan	2.71 oz	4	160	23%
Triple Crown Caramel	2.75 oz	4	170	21%
(Weight Watchers) Mousse-Instant-				
Prepared w/Skim Milk				
Chocolate	½ cup	3	70	39%
White Chocolate Almond	½ cup	3	70	39%
Rice-homemade-w/ raisins	½ cup	6	245	22%

Food and Description	Amount	Fat Grams	Total Calories	% Fat Calories
Snack				
(Hershey's) Chocolate Bar Flavor-in the dairy case				
Chocolate	4 oz	6	180	30%
Chocolate & Almond	4 oz	6	180	30%
Kisses-Chocolate & Vanilla	4 oz	6	180	30%
York Peppermint Pattie	4 oz	6	180	30%
(Hershey's) Chocolate Bar Flavor, Free (fat-free)				
Chocolate Fudge	4 oz	–	100	–
Kisses	4 oz	–	100	–
(Hunt's) Snack Pack				
Banana	4.25 oz	6	145	25%
Butterscotch	4.25 oz	6	170	21%
Chocolate	4.25 oz	6	170	21%
Chocolate Fudge	4.25 oz	6	165	22%
Chocolate Marshmallow	4.25 oz	6	165	22%
Lemon	4.25 oz	4	150	24%
Tapioca	4.25 oz	5	150	30%
Vanilla	4.25 oz	6	170	21%
(Hunt's) Snack Pack-Light				
Chocolate	4 oz	2	100	18%
Tapioca	4 oz	2	100	18%
(Jell-O) Free				
Chocolate	4 oz	–	100	–
Chocolate Vanilla Swirls	4 oz	–	100	–
(Jell-O) in the Dairy Case				
Chocolate	4 oz	6	170	32%
Chocolate Caramel Swirls	4 oz	6	170	32%
Chocolate Vanilla Swirls	4 oz	6	170	32%
Double Chocolate Swirls	4 oz	6	170	32%
Vanilla	4 oz	7	180	35%
Vanilla Chocolate Swirls	4 oz	6	180	32%
(Jell-O) Light-Pudding Snacks				
Chocolate	4 oz	2	100	18%
Chocolate Fudge	4 oz	1	100	9%
Chocolate Vanilla Combo	4 oz	2	100	18%
Vanilla	4 oz	2	100	17%
(Swiss Miss) Light-Pudding Snacks				
Chocolate	4 oz	2	100	18%
Chocolate Fudge	4 oz	1	100	9%
Vanilla	4 oz	1	100	9%
Vanilla/Chocolate Parfait	4 oz	1	100	9%
(Swiss Miss) Original-Pudding Snacks				
Butterscotch	4 oz	6	180	30%
Chocolate	4 oz	6	180	30%

Food and Description	Amount	Fat Grams	Total Calories	% Fat Calories
Chocolate Fudge	4 oz	6	220	16%
Tapioca	4 oz	5	160	28%
Vanilla w/Fudge Topping	4 oz	7	190	33%
(Swiss Miss) Parfait-Pudding Snacks				
Chocolate	4 oz	6	170	32%
Vanilla	4 oz	6	180	30%
(Swiss Miss) Sundae-Pudding Snacks				
Chocolate	4 oz	7	220	29%
Vanilla	4 oz	7	220	29%
(Ultra Slim Fast)				
Butterscotch	4 oz	< 1	100	5%
Chocolate	4 oz	< 1	100	5%
Vanilla	4 oz	< 1	100	5%
(Yoplait) Pudding Snacks				
Double Chocolate	4 oz	4	150	24%
Milk Chocolate	4 oz	4	170	21%
Vanilla	4 oz	4	150	24%
Tapioca				
Canned	5 oz	5	160	28%
Homemade	1 cup	8	221	33%
Apple	1 cup	–	293	–
(Jell-O) Americana Prepared w/Whole Milk				
Chocolate	½ cup	5	170	27%
Vanilla	½ cup	4	160	23%
1-Minute	1 Tbs	–	35	–
PUDDING POPS				
(Jell-O) Pudding Pops				
Chocolate	1	2	80	23%
Chocolate Caramel Swirl	1	2	80	23%
Chocolate-Covered Chocolate	1	7	130	49%
Chocolate-Covered Vanilla	1	7	130	49%
Chocolate Vanilla Swirl	1	2	70	26%
Chocolate w/Chocolate Chips	1	3	80	34%
Vanilla	1	2	70	26%
Vanilla w/Chocolate Chips	1	3	80	34%
PUMMELO/raw	1	–	228	–
	1 cup		71	–
PUMPKIN				
canned				
(Del Monte)	½ cup	–	35	–
(Festal)	½ cup	1	40	23%
solid pack (Libby's)	1 cup	1	80	11%
fresh-boiled-mashed	1 cup	–	48	–
raw-cubed	1 cup	–	30	–

Food and Description	Amount	Fat Grams	Total Calories	% Fat Calories
PUMPKIN BUTTER				
(Smucker's)	1 tsp	–	12	–
PUMPKIN FLOWERS				
cooked	½ cup	< 1	10	45%
raw	½ cup	< 1	5	90%
PUMPKIN LEAVES/cooked	½ cup	< 1	7	64%
PUMPKIN PIE MIX/canned (Libby's)	1 cup	< 1	260	2%
PUMPKIN PIE SPICE	1 tsp	–	6	–
PUMPKIN SEEDS				
dried/hulled	1 oz	13	155	75%
	1 cup	63	747	76%
kernels-roasted	1 oz	11.96	148	73%
	1 cup	95.6	1184	73%
whole-roasted	1 oz	5.5	127	39%
	1 cup	12	285	38%
PUNCH(*See also* FRUIT JUICE PUNCH; FRUIT PUNCH DRINK)				
Dietetic or low-calorie				
(Kool-Aid) Soft Drink Mix				
Sugar-Free	8 oz	–	4	–
Sweetened	8 oz	–	90	–
Tropical Punch	8 oz	–	100	–
PURSLANE				
boiled	½ cup	–	10	–
raw	1 cup	–	7	–

Q

Food and Description	Amount	Fat Grams	Total Calories	% Fat Calories
QUAIL				
breast meat only-raw	~ 2 oz	1.67	69	22%
meat & skin-raw	~ 4 oz	13	210	56%
meat only-raw	~ 3 oz	4	123	29%
QUICHE (*See* EGG MEALS)				
QUINCE	1	–	53	–
QUINOA				
(Eden Foods)	2 oz	4	200	18%

Food and Description	Amount	Fat Grams	Total Calories	% Fat Calories
Generic	1 oz	1.6	106	14%
	1 cup	10	637	14%
QUINOA SEED (Arrowhead Mills)	2 oz	3	200	14%

R

Food and Description	Amount	Fat Grams	Total Calories	% Fat Calories
RABBIT				
Domestic				
breaded & fried/boneless	3 oz	8.8	199	40%
chopped/diced	1 cup	14	302	42%
ground	1 cup	11	238	42%
stewed	4 oz	11.5	245	42%
	1 lb	45.8	980	42%
Wild/raw-boneless	3 oz	8.5	182	42%
RADISH/raw	10 pieces	–	7	–
Chinese	½ cup	–	13	–
Oriental				
raw	½ cup	–	8	–
dried	¼ cup	–	75	–
White Icicle	1 piece	–	14	–
RAISIN				
Golden				
seedless	1 cup	.75	453	2%
(Del Monte)	3 oz	–	260	–
(Dole)	½ cup	–	262	–
(Sun Maid)	½ cup	–	260	–
Muscat (Sun Maid)	⅓ cup	1	270	3%
natural (Del Monte)	3 oz	–	250	–
seedless	1 cup	.68	434	1%
	1 pack/			
	½ oz	–	40	–
cooked w/sugar	1 cup	–	628	–
(Sun Maid)	1 oz	–	96	–
uncooked ground				
packed	1 cup	< 1	780	1%

Food and Description	Amount	Fat Grams	Total Calories	% Fat Calories
unpacked	1 cup	–	578	–
sun-dried				
(Dole)	½ cup	–	250	–
(Sun Maid)	½ cup	–	250	–
with seeds	1 cup	.8	428	2%
RASPBERRY				
Black				
canned in water	1 cup	2	110	16%
fresh	1 cup	2	100	18%
Red				
canned in heavy syrup	1 cup	< 1	234	2%
fresh	1 cup	.66	61	10%
	1 pint	1.7	154	10%
frozen				
Lite Syrup (Birds Eye)	5 oz	< 1	90	5%
sweetened	1 cup	< 1	256	2%
unsweetened	3.5 oz	< 1	50	9%
RASPBERRY JUICE				
Black				
Raspberry/fresh	4 oz	–	49	–
Raspberry,Country				
from frozen conc	6 oz	–	90	–
Raspberry (Dole) Pure & Light	6 oz	–	87	–
Red				
Red Raspberry				
(Smucker's)	8 oz	–	120	–
Red Raspberry Delight/bottled	6 oz	–	90	–
RASPBERRY-CRANBERRY JUICE COCKTAIL				
(Seneca)	6 oz	–	110	–
RAVIOLI (*See also* BEEF DISHES; FROZEN ENTREE/DINNER; PASTA ENTREE/DINNER)				
Canned, Beef				
(Chef Boyardee)	7 oz	5	180	25%
(Estee)	7.5 oz	11	230	43%
(Franco-American)	7.5 oz	4.7	223	19%
Hearty Beef	7.5 oz	11	290	34%
Hearty Pasta	7.5 oz	11	280	35%
Raviolio's-canned	7.5 oz	8	250	29%
w/Meat Sauce	7.5 oz	10.8	284	34%
Homemade				
Cheese				
w/meat sauce	~9 oz	17	360	43%
w/tomato sauce	~9 oz	15	340	40%
w/o sauce	~8.5 oz	17	430	36%

Food and Description	Amount	Fat Grams	Total Calories	% Fat Calories
Meat				
w/tomato sauce	~9 oz	17	385	40%
w/o sauce	~8.5 oz	23	550	38%
RED BEAN				
canned	½ cup	–	100	–
(Van Camp's)	1 cup	1	190	5%
dry				
(Joan of Arc/Green Giant)	½ cup	1	90	10%
RED BEAN SOUP (*See* SOUP)				
REFRIED BEANS (*See* MEXICAN FOOD)				
RELISH				
(Claussen)	1 Tbs	–	14	–
(Heinz)				
Hamburger relish	1 oz	–	30	–
Hot Dog relish	1 oz	–	35	–
India relish	1 oz	–	35	–
Sweet relish	1 oz	–	30	–
Pickle Relish	1 Tbs	–	12	–
(Vlasic)				
Dill relish	1 oz	–	2	–
Green tomato piccalilli	1 oz	–	35	–
Hamburger relish	1 oz	–	40	–
Hot Dog relish	1 oz	<1	40	11%
Hot piccalilli relish	1 oz	–	35	–
India relish	1 oz	–	30	–
Sweet relish	1 oz	–	30	–
RENNIN				
Rennin Products (Coagulates milk used in making cheese)	1 tablet	–	1	–
	1 pkg	–	12	–
RHUBARB				
cooked-sweetened	1 cup	–	280	–
frozen-cooked w/sugar	1 cup	–	278	–
raw-diced	½ cup	–	13	–
RICE				
(A Taste of Thai) Soft Jasmine Rice				
cooked	¼ cup	–	160	–
dry	1.5 oz	–	160	–
(Arrowhead Mills) Brown Rice				
quick	2 oz	1	200	5%
Brown				
cooked				
long grain				
cold	1 cup	.9	173	5%

Food and Description	Amount	Fat Grams	Total Calories	% Fat Calories
hot	1 cup	1	232	4%
raw				
long grain	1 cup	3.5	666	5%
short grain	1 cup	3.8	720	5%
Long grain				
cooked	½ cup	–	90	–
Long Grain & Wild Rices				
Brown & Wild				
dry	½ cup	1	130	7%
prepared w/butter	½ cup	4	150	24%
Chicken Stock Sauce				
dry	½ cup	2	140	13%
prepared w/butter	½ cup	5	160	28%
Original				
dry	½ cup	< 1	100	5%
prepared w/butter	½ cup	2	120	15%
Original Fast Cooking Recipe				
dry	½ cup	< 1	100	5%
prepared w/butter	½ cup	4	130	28%
Rice In An Instant				
dry	⅔ cup	< 1	120	4%
prepared w/butter	⅔ cup	2	130	14%
Whole Grain Brown				
dry	⅔ cup	1	130	7%
prepared w/butter	⅔ cup	3	150	18%
(MJB) brown rice				
Quick/cooked	½ cup	1	110	8%
(Mahatma)				
Brown/dry	1 oz	–	110	–
Instant/dry	1 oz	–	110	–
cooked/no butter	½ cup	–	110	–
White/dry	1 oz	–	100	–
(Minute Rice)				
Boil In Bag				
prepared	½ cup	–	90	–
Brown/instant				
prepared	½ cup	1	120	8%
Premium Long Grain				
prepared	⅔ cup	–	120	–
White/prepared	⅔ cup	< 1	120	4%
(New Frontier)				
Standard				
Brown Rice				
cooked	1 serving	.9	111	7%

Food and Description	Amount	Fat Grams	Total Calories	% Fat Calories
dry	3.5 oz	1.9	354	5%
Wild Rice				
cooked	1 serving	< 1	147	3%
dry	3.5 oz	.7	353	2%
Ultra Roast				
Brown Rice				
cooked	1 serving	.9	111	7%
dry	3.5 oz	3	395	7%
Wild Rice				
cooked	1 serving	.9	147	3%
dry	3.5 oz	1	394	2%
(Success)				
Brown				
Boil In Bag/prepared	½ cup	–	103	–
10 Minute/prepared	½ cup	–	103	–
Natural Long Grain				
pre-cooked/prepared	½ cup	< 1	90	5%
(Texmati)				
Brown	½ cup	–	85	–
Lite Bran	½ cup	–	84	–
White Long Grain	½ cup	–	82	–
(Uncle Ben's)				
Boil In Bag/as packaged	½ cup	< 1	90	5%
Aromatica/prepared	½ cup	–	100	–
Converted				
dry	⅔ cup	< 1	120	4%
prepared w/butter	⅔ cup	2	140	13%
Microwave				
(Vita Fiber)				
Rice Grain	1 oz	6	100	54%
White				
cooked/long grain				
cold	1 cup	< 1	158	3%
hot	1 cup	< 1	223	2%
parboiled/long grain				
cooked-cold	1 cup	–	154	–
cooked-hot	1 cup	–	186	–
dry	1 cup	.6	683	1%
raw				
long grain	1 cup	.7	672	1%
medium grain	1 cup	.8	708	1%
short grain	1 cup	.8	726	1%
Wild Rice/raw	4 oz	< 1	400	1%
RICE BRAN (*See also* CEREAL)	4 oz	18	315	51%

Food and Description	Amount	Fat Grams	Total Calories	% Fat Calories
RICE CAKES				
■ **MINI RICE CAKES**				
(Chico San)				
all flavors	5 pieces	–	50	–
(Hain)				
Apple Cinnamon	5 pieces	< 1	60	8%
Barbeque	5 pieces	3	70	39%
Cheese	5 pieces	2	60	30%
Honey Nut	5 pieces	< 1	60	8%
Nacho	5 pieces	2	70	26%
Popcorn				
Butter Flavored	5 pieces	2	60	30%
Mild Cheddar	5 pieces	2	60	30%
White Cheddar	5 pieces	2	60	30%
Ranch	5 pieces	3	70	39%
Teriyaki	5 pieces	< 1	50	9%
(Hollywood)				
Apple Cinnamon & Plain	~ 5 pieces	< 1	50	9%
Cheese	~ 5 pieces	2	60	30%
Honey Nut	~ 5 pieces	1	60	15%
(Pacific Rice) Mini Crispys)				
Apple Spice	2	–	30	–
Barbecue	2	–	30	–
Honey Sesame	1	–	12	–
Teriyaki	1	–	12	–
■ **STANDARD SIZE RICE CAKES**				
(El Molino) Carob Rice				
Mint	1⅞ oz	6	125	43%
Plain	1⅞ oz	6	125	43%
(Hain)				
5-Grain	1	< 1	40	11%
Plain				
No Salt Added	1	< 1	40	11%
Regular	1	< 1	40	11%
Popcorn				
Butter Flavored	1	1	45	20%
Nacho Cheese	1	1	45	20%
Plain	1	–	35	–
White Cheddar	1	1	45	20%
Sesame				
No Salt	1	< 1	40	11%
Regular	1	< 1	40	11%
(Lundberg)				
Mochi Sweet	1	.5	60	8%
Wild Rice	1	.5	60	8%

Food and Description	Amount	Fat Grams	Total Calories	% Fat Calories
(Pacific Grain)				
Apple Cinnamon	1	–	30	–
Cheddar	1	–	35	–
Toasted Brown	1	–	35	–
(Pritikin)				
Plain	1	–	35	–
Sesame	1	–	35	–
(Quaker)				
Apple Cinnamon	1	–	40	–
Corn				
Butter Popped	1	–	35	–
Caramel	1	–	50	–
Nacho	1	–	40	–
White Cheddar	1	–	40	–
Low Sodium	1	–	35	–
Plain	1	–	35	–
Wheat	1	–	35	–
(Westbrae Natural)				
Double Sesame	1	< 1	30	15%
Sesame Garlic	1	< 1	30	15%
Teriyaki	1	< 1	30	15%
RICE DISHES (See also FROZEN ENTREE/DINNER, MEXICAN FOOD, ORIENTAL FOOD)				
(Birds Eye) International Rice Recipes				
frozen				
French Style	3.3 oz	–	110	–
Italian Style	3.3 oz	1	120	8%
Spanish Style	3.3 oz	–	110	–
(Casbah)				
Pilaf				
dry	2 oz	–	90	–
Pilaf nutted				
prepared	½ cup	2	160	11%
Spanish Pilaf				
dry	1 oz	–	90	–
Tabouly Mix (See TABOULI)				
(Chun King) mix-dry	.25 oz	–	20	–
(Country Inn) as packaged w/o butter				
Broccoli Rice Au Gratin	½ cup	3	130	21%
Chicken Rice Royale	½ cup	1	120	8%
Chicken Stock Rice	½ cup	1	130	7%
Herbed Rice Au Gratin	½ cup	3	140	19%
Rice Alfredo	½ cup	4	140	26%
Rice Florentine	½ cup	3	140	19%

Food and Description	Amount	Fat Grams	Total Calories	% Fat Calories
Vegetable Pilaf	½ cup	1	120	8%
Vegetable Rice Medley	½ cup	1	140	6%
(Country Inn) 10 Minute Recipes as packaged w/o butter				
Asparagus Au Gratin	½ cup	3	130	21%
Broccoli Almondine	½ cup	2	130	14%
Cauliflower Au Gratin	½ cup	3	130	21%
Creamy Chicken & Mushroom	½ cup	3	140	19%
Creamy Mushroom & Wild Rice	½ cup	3	140	19%
Green Bean & Almondine Casserole	½ cup	2	120	15%
Homestyle Chicken & Vegetables	½ cup	3	140	19%
Chicken & Cheese Risotto	½ cup	2	120	15%
(Featherweight)				
Spanish Rice	7.5 oz	–	140	–
(Golden Grain) Rice-A-Roni				
Beef Flavor				
dry	1.13 oz	1	110	8%
prepared	½ cup	4	140	26%
Beef & Mushroom				
dry	1.27 oz	< 1	120	4%
prepared	½ cup	3	150	18%
Chicken Flavor				
dry	1.13 oz	1	110	8%
prepared	½ cup	4	150	24%
Chicken & Broccoli				
dry	1.23 oz	1	120	8%
prepared	½ cup	3	150	18%
Chicken & Mushroom				
dry	1.17 oz	1	130	7%
prepared	½ cup	7	180	35%
Chicken & Vegetables				
dry	1.20 oz	< 1	120	4%
prepared	½ cup	3	140	19%
Fried Rice w/Almonds				
dry	1.04 oz	1	110	8%
prepared	½ cup	5	110	41%
Herb & Butter				
dry	1.04 oz	1	110	8%
prepared	½ cup	4	130	28%
Long Grain & Wild Chicken w/almonds				
dry	1.20 oz	1	120	8%
prepared	½ cup	4	140	26%

Food and Description	Amount	Fat Grams	Total Calories	% Fat Calories
Original				
dry	1.1 oz	–	110	–
prepared	½ cup	3	130	21%
Rice Pilaf				
dry	1.2 oz	–	120	–
prepared	½ cup	4	150	24%
Risotto				
dry	1.5 oz	1	160	6%
prepared	½ cup	6	200	27%
Spanish				
dry	1.07 oz	1	110	8%
prepared	½ cup	4	150	24%
Stroganoff				
dry	1.35 oz	3	150	18%
prepared	½ cup	8	200	36%
Wild Rice Pilaf				
dry	1.06 oz	–	100	–
prepared	½ cup	3	130	21%
Yellow				
dry	1.16 oz	–	110	–
prepared	½ cup	4	140	26%
(Golden Grain) Rice-A-Roni				
Savory Classics				
Almond Chicken & Wild Rice				
dry	1.13 oz	1	110	8%
prepared	½ cup	4	140	26%
Broccoli Au Gratin				
dry	1.12 oz	3	130	21%
prepared	½ cup	9	180	45%
Cauliflower Au Gratin				
dry	1.2 oz	4	140	26%
prepared	½ cup	7	170	37%
Chicken & Broccoli Dijon				
dry	1.2 oz	1	120	8%
prepared	1 serving	5	160	28%
Chicken Florentine				
dry	1.12 oz	1	110	8%
prepared	½ cup	4	130	28%
Creamy Parmesan & Herbs				
dry	1.22 oz	4	140	26%
prepared	½ cup	7	170	37%
Garden Pilaf				
dry	1.12 oz	1	110	8%
prepared	½ cup	4	140	26%

Food and Description	Amount	Fat Grams	Total Calories	% Fat Calories
Green Bean Salad Almondine				
dry	1.25 oz	5	150	30%
prepared	½ cup	11	210	45%
Oriental Stir Fry				
dry	1.08 oz	–	100	–
prepared	½ cup	6	150	34%
Spring Vegetables & Cheese				
dry	1.22 oz	4	140	26%
prepared	½ cup	7	170	37%
Zesty Cheddar				
dry	1.30 oz	4	150	24%
prepared	½ cup	7	180	40%
(Green Giant)				
One Serving Vegetables/frozen				
Rice Medley	4.5 oz	4	130	28%
Rice'n Broccoli in Cheese Sauce	4.5 oz	5	160	28%
Rice Originals/frozen				
Rice Florentine	½ cup	4	140	26%
Rice Medley	½ cup	1	100	9%
Rice'n Broccoli in Flavored Cheese				
Sauce	½ cup	4	120	30%
Rice Pilaf	½ cup	1	110	8%
Rice w/Herb Butter Sauce	½ cup	5	150	30%
White & Wild Rice	½ cup	2	130	14%
(Hain)				
3-Grain Side Dishes				
Chicken Meatless Style	½ cup	4	130	28%
Herb	½ cup	4	120	30%
Rice Almondine	½ cup	4	130	28%
Rice Oriental 3-Grain Goodness	½ cup	5	130	35%
(Heinz)				
Beef Flavored				
dry	1 oz	–	100	–
Chicken Flavored				
dry	1 oz	1	100	9%
Long Grain Wild-prepared	½ cup	1	100	9%
Rice Pilaf-dry	1 oz	–	100	–
Spanish-canned	7.25 oz	5	150	30%
Spanish Pilaf-dry	1 oz	–	100	–
(Kashhi)				
7 Whole Grain & Sesame Pilaf				
dry	2 oz	1	177	5%
(Konriko)				
Wild Pecan Rice	½ cup	1	89	10%

Food and Description	Amount	Fat Grams	Total Calories	% Fat Calories
(Kraft)				
Rice & Cheese-prepared				
Cheddar & Chicken	½ cup	4	150	24%
Cheddar Broccoli	½ cup	5	150	30%
Cheddar Pilaf	½ cup	4	150	24%
3-Cheese & Herbs	½ cup	4	150	24%
(La Choy)				
Chinese Fried Rice				
canned	¾ cup	1	190	5%
(Lipton)				
Golden Saute (as packaged)				
Beef Flavor Fried Rice	½ cup	2	125	14%
Chicken Flavor Fried Rice	½ cup	2	130	14%
Oriental Fried Rice	½ cup	2	130	14%
Rice & Sauce				
Beef	¼ pkg	< 1	120	4%
Broccoli & Cheddar	¼ pkg	2	125	14%
Cajun Beans	¼ pkg	< 1	123	4%
Chicken	¼ pkg	1	125	7%
Chicken Broccoli	¼ pkg	2	130	14%
Creamy Chicken	¼ pkg	2	140	13%
Herb & Butter	¼ pkg	2	125	14%
Long Grain & Wild				
Mushrooms & Herbs	½ pkg	< 1	125	4%
Original	¼ pkg	–	120	–
Mushroom	¼ pkg	< 1	123	4%
Pilaf	¼ pkg	< 1	120	4%
Rice Asparagus w/Hollandaise				
Sauce	¼ pkg	1	123	7%
Skillet Style Spanish	¼ pkg	1	100	9%
Spanish	¼ pkg	< 1	120	4%
(MJB)				
Fried Rice Oriental/cooked	½ cup	1	110	8%
Herb & Butter/cooked	½ cup	1	100	9%
Mexican Style/cooked	½ cup	–	120	–
Rice Pilaf/cooked	½ cup	1	110	8%
Savory Beef/cooked	½ cup	1	100	9%
Savory Chicken/cooked	½ cup	1	100	9%
(Minute Microwave)				
Beef Flavored				
family	½ cup	3	160	17%
single	½ cup	2	150	12%
Cheddar Cheese & Broccoli				
family	½ cup	5	160	28%

Food and Description	Amount	Fat Grams	Total Calories	% Fat Calories
single	½ cup	4	160	23%
Chicken Flavored				
family	½ cup	4	160	23%
single	½ cup	3	150	18%
French Style Pilaf				
family	½ cup	3	130	15%
single	½ cup	2	120	15%
(Minute Rice)				
Drumstick-prepared w/butter	½ cup	4	150	24%
Fried-prepared w/oil	½ cup	5	160	28%
Long Grain & Wild-prepared w/				
butter	½ cup	4	150	24%
Rib Roast-prepared w/butter	½ cup	4	150	24%
(Near East)				
Chicken Flavored Pilaf				
dry	1 oz	–	100	–
prepared	½ cup	4	140	26%
Rice Pilaf Mix				
dry	1 oz	–	100	–
Spanish				
dry	1½ oz	–	110	–
prepared	½ cup	4	160	23%
Taboule (*See* TABOULI)				
(Nile Spice)				
Rozdali				
Spicy Currant				
dry	1.34 oz	–	131	–
prepared	½ cup	4	161	22%
Vegetable Curry				
dry	1.23 oz	–	124	–
prepared	½ cup	4	154	23%
(Pritikin)				
Pilaf Brown	½ cup	< 1	90	5%
Spanish Brown	½ cup	< 1	100	5%
Spanish Rice				
(Van Camp's)				
canned	1 cup	3	150	18%
(Suzi Wan)				
Honey Lemon Chicken mix	1 serving	1	200	5%
w/added ingredients	7.5 oz	11	370	27%
Stir Fry Broccoli mix	1 serving	3	200	14%
w/added ingredients	7.5 oz	15	370	37%
Sweet'n Sour mix	1 serving	1	220	4%
w/added ingredients	7.5 oz	5	340	13%

Food and Description	Amount	Fat Grams	Total Calories	% Fat Calories
Teriyaki mix	1 serving	1	180	5%
w/added ingredients	7.5 oz	12	360	30%
As packaged w/o butter				
Chicken & Broccoli	½ cup	1	120	8%
Chicken & Vegetables	½ cup	1	120	8%
Sweet'n Sour Rice	½ cup	1	130	7%
Teriyaki Rice	½ cup	1	120	8%
Three Flavor Rice	½ cup	1	120	8%
(Ultra Slim Fast) Microwaveable				
Prepared				
Rice w/Chicken Flavored Sauce	8 oz	1	240	4%
Rice w/Oriental Style Sauce	8 oz	1	240	4%
(Weight Watchers)				
Spanish Rice				
dry	½ cup	1	100	9%
prepared	½ cup	3	120	23%
(Wick Fowler's)				
Rice Kits, dry				
Cajun	1 serving	1	120	8%
Jalapeno	1 serving	1	130	7%
Ranchero	1 serving	1	110	8%
RICE DRINK				
(Don Jose) Hor chata				
Non dairy rice drink	6 oz	4	120	30%
RICE NOODLES				
canned	½ cup	5	130	35%
RICE POLISH				
stirred & spooned into cup	1 cup	13	278	42%
RICE PUDDING (See PUDDING & MOUSSE)				
RICE TOPPINGS				
(Mayacamas)				
Mix prepared				
Calcutta	2 oz	1	22	41%
Chicken Herb	2 oz	1	23	39%
Creolo	2 oz	1	23	39%
Garden Pea	2 oz	1	22	41%
Mediterranean	2 oz	1	22	41%
Mexicali	2 oz	1	20	39%
RIGATONI				
homemade w/meat sauce	1 cup	16	347	41%
ROAST BEEF (See BEEF, LUNCHEON MEAT)				
ROAST BEEF HASH				
Canned (Mary Kitchen)	7.5 oz	22	350	57%
ROAST BEEF SPREAD (See LUNCHEON MEAT)				

Food and Description	Amount	Fat Grams	Total Calories	% Fat Calories
ROCKFISH				
Pacific				
cooked	3 oz	1.7	103	15%
raw	3 oz	1	80	11%
ROLLS				
Brown & Serve				
(Country Hearth) Krusty Rolls				
Italian	1	4	170	21%
Plain	1	4	170	21%
(Pepperidge Farm) frozen				
Butter Crescent	1	6	110	49%
Club Enriched	1	1	100	9%
French Enriched-3 per pkg	½	1	120	8%
Hearth Enriched	1	1	50	18%
(Roman Meal)	1	2	77	23%
(Wonder)				
Crusty Italian Rolls du Jour	1	1	80	11%
Gem Style	1	2	80	23%
Petite French Rolls du Jour	1	2	230	8%
W/Buttermilk	1	2	80	23%
Butterflake-refrigerated				
(Pillsbury)	1	5	140	32%
Cloverleaf				
commercial				
brown & serve	1	1.9	84	20%
ready to serve	1	1.6	83	17%
homemade-2½" dia	1	3	119	23%
Colonial Wheat (Rainbo)	1	19	300	57%
Cracked Wheat	1	.8	95	8%
Crescent-refrigerated (Pillsbury)	1	6	100	54%
Dinner				
(Pepperidge Farm)	1	2	60	30%
Country Style Classic	1	1	50	18%
Fancy Rolls				
Butter Crescent Enriched	1	6	110	49%
Golden Twist Enriched	1	5	110	41%
Finger Poppy Seed	1	2	50	36%
Hearty Potato Classic	1	3	90	30%
Old Fashioned Enriched	1	2	50	36%
Parker House Enriched	1	1	60	15%
Party Enriched	1	1	30	30%
Soft Family Enriched	1	2	100	18%
(Roman Meal)	1	1	45	20%
(Wonder)	1	1	80	11%

Food and Description	Amount	Fat Grams	Total Calories	% Fat Calories
French Roll	1	1	130	7%
(Earth Grains)	1	1	100	9%
(Pepperidge Farm)				
Hard				
French Style-9 per pkg	1	1	100	9%
Sourdough-9 per pkg	1	1	100	9%
Garlic Rolls/frozen				
(Cole's)	1	5	100	45%
Health Nut Rolls (Oroweat)	1	3	160	17%
Honey & Wheat Rolls				
(King's Hawaiian)	1	3	90	30%
Hot Roll Mix				
(Pillsbury)	2	2	120	15%
Italian Crispy Dinner				
(Lewis)	1	2	100	18%
Kaiser				
(Brownberry) Hearth	1	2	110	16%
(Purity)	1	2	150	12%
(Earth Grains)	1	2	190	10%
Onion				
(Earth Grains)	1	2	190	10%
Pan				
(Wonder)	1	1	80	11%
Parkerhouse/from frozen dough	1	1	75	12%
Popover				
homemade	1	3.7	90	37%
mix	1	5	170	27%
Potato Roll	1	2	130	14%
Rye	1	–	87	–
Sandwich Quartet (Pepperidge Farm)				
Croissant	1	7	170	37%
Sandwich Rolls				
(Pepperidge Farm)				
Dijon Frankfurter	1	5	160	28%
Frankfurter Enriched				
side sliced	1	3	140	19%
Frankfurter Enriched				
top sliced	1	3	140	19%
Onion Buns w/poppy seeds	1	3	150	18%
Potato Sandwich	1	4	160	23%
Salad Sandwich	1	4	110	33%
Sandwich Buns w/sesame seeds	1	3	140	19%
Sliced Hamburger Enriched	1	2	130	14%
Soft Hoagie	1	5	210	41%

Food and Description	Amount	Fat Grams	Total Calories	% Fat Calories
(Weight Watchers)				
Hamburger Buns	1	< 1	80	6%
Hot Dog	1	< 1	80	6%
Reduced Calorie Wheat Buns	1	< 1	80	6%
(Wonder)				
Hamburger Buns	1	2	120	15%
Light	1	1	80	11%
Hoagie Rolls	1	7	400	16%
Hot Dog Buns-Light	1	1	80	11%
Hot Dog Rolls	1	1	80	11%
Country Grain Hot	1	1	100	9%
Scone				
homemade	1.5 oz	6.5	140	42%
(Krusteaz mix)	1 scone	9	180	45%
Sourdough	1	1	130	7%
Steak Rolls (Circle S)	1/1.6 oz	3	150	18%
Submarine (Earth Grains)	½ roll	1	180	5%
Sub, Hoagie	1/~3.5 oz	7	400	45%
Wheat Dinner Rolls (Home Pride)	1	1	70	13%
White-hard	1	1.6	156	9%
White-soft				
hamburger and/or hotdog	1	2	150	12%
hamburger (Holsum)	1	2	120	15%
hamburger (Roman Meal)	1	2	113	16%
hotdog (Roman Meal)	1	2	104	17%
hotdog (Wonder)	1	1	80	11%
White-soft dinner	1	2	85	21%
frozen homestyle (Rich's)	1	1	75	12%
(Home Pride)	1	2	80	23%
homemade	1/~1 oz	3	120	23%
Whole Wheat	1	1	93	10%
ROMAN BEAN				
(Progresso)	8 oz	1	210	4%
ROSEMARY/dried	1 tsp	–	4	–
ROUGHY				
Orange				
raw	3 oz	5.95	107	49%
RUM (*See* LIQUOR, DISTILLED)				
RUTABAGA				
fresh-boiled	½ cup	–	39	–
raw	½ cup	–	25	–
RYE (*See* LIQUOR, DISTILLED)				

S

Food and Description	Amount	Fat Grams	Total Calories	% Fat Calories
SABLEFISH				
raw	3 oz	13	165	71%
smoked	3 oz	17	220	70%
SAFFRON	1 tsp	–	2	–
SAGE/ground	1 tsp	–	4	–
SALAD DRESSING				
■ MIXES & HOME RECIPE				
(NOTE: Mixes were prepared as directed on package.)				
Bleu Cheese (Estee)	1 Tbs	< 1	8	34%
Bleu Cheese & Herbs				
(Good Seasons)				
Prepared	1 Tbs	8	70	100%
Unprepared	1 packet	–	4	–
Blue Cheese				
Chunky	1 Tbs	8	75	96%
(Hidden Valley)	1 Tbs	6	58	93%
Thick 'n Creamy	1 Tbs	9	100	81%
Buttermilk Farm Style (Good Seasons)				
Prepared	1 Tbs	6	60	90%
Unprepared	1 packet	–	4	–
Cheese Garlic (Good Seasons)				
Prepared	1 Tbs	8	70	100%
Unprepared	1 packet	–	4	–
Cheese Italian (Good Seasons)				
Lite				
Prepared	1 Tbs	3	25	100%
Unprepared	1 packet	–	4	–
Regular				
Prepared	1 Tbs	8	70	100%
Unprepared	1 packet	–	4	–
Classic Herb (Good Seasons)				
Prepared	1 Tbs	8	70	100%
Unprepared	1 packet	–	2	–
Cooked/Standard Home Recipe (USDA)				
w/regular margarine	1 Tbs	2	25	72%

Food and Description	Amount	Fat Grams	Total Calories	% Fat Calories
Creamy Italian-Fat Free (Good Seasons)				
Prepared				
w/regular mayonnaise	1 Tbs	1	16	56%
w/o mayonnaise	1 Tbs	–	8	–
Unprepared	1 Tbs	–	6	–
Creamy Style (Good Seasons)				
Prepared	1 Tbs	5	50	90%
Unprepared	1 packet	–	2	–
French/Standard Home Recipe (USDA)	1 Tbs	9.8	88	100%
French, Creamy (Estee)	1 Tbs	–	16	–
French, Old Fashion	1 Tbs	9	85	95%
French, Thick 'n Creamy	1 Tbs	9	100	81%
Garlic	1 Tbs	9	85	95%
Garlic, Creamy (Estee)	1 Tbs	–	2	–
Garlic & Herbs (Good Seasons)				
Prepared	1 Tbs	8	70	100%
Unprepared	1 packet	–	4	–
(Hain) No Oil				
Bleu Cheese	1 Tbs	1	14	64%
Buttermilk	1 Tbs	< 1	11	11%
Caesar	1 Tbs	< 1	6	75%
French	1 Tbs	–	12	–
Garlic & Cheese	1 Tbs	< 1	6	75%
Herb	1 Tbs	–	2	–
Italian	1 Tbs	–	2	–
1,000 Island	1 Tbs	< 1	12	38%
(Hidden Valley)				
Creamy Herb-prepared	1 Tbs	6	58	93%
Honey Dijon Ranch-dry	1 pkg	–	85	–
Original Buttermilk-prepared				
Reduced calorie	1 Tbs	–	35	–
Regular	1 Tbs	6	60	90%
Ranch Italian-dry	1 pkg	–	85	–
Ranch w/Bacon-prepared				
Reduced Calorie	1 Tbs	3	35	77%
Regular	1 Tbs	6	58	93%
Honey Mustard-Fat Free (Good Seasons)				
Prepared	1 Tbs	1	18	50%
Unprepared	1 Tbs	–	10	–
Italian (Good Seasons)				
Prepared	1 Tbs	8	70	100%
Unprepared	1 packet	–	2	–

Food and Description	Amount	Fat Grams	Total Calories	% Fat Calories
Italian-Fat Free				
(Good Seasons)				
Prepared	1 Tbs	1	14	64%
Unprepared	1 Tbs	–	6	–
Italian-Lite (Good Seasons)				
Prepared	1 Tbs	3	25	100%
Unprepared	1 packet	–	4	–
Italian-Mild (Good Seasons)				
Prepared	1 Tbs	8	70	100%
Unprepared	1 packet	–	4	–
Italian-No Oil (Good Seasons)	1 Tbs	–	6	–
Italian-Style (Weight Watchers)				
Individual packets	1 packet	–	9	–
Italian-Zesty				
(Estee)	1 Tbs	–	4	–
(Good Seasons)				
Lite				
Prepared	1 Tbs	3	25	100%
Unprepared	1 packet	–	4	–
Regular				
Prepared	1 Tbs	8	70	100%
Unprepared	1 packet	–	2	–
Lemon & Herbs (Good Seasons)				
Prepared	1 Tbs	8	70	100%
Unprepared	1 pkt	–	2	–
(Macayamas) dry mix				
Blue Cheese	1 Tbs	1	8	56%
Buttermilk & Herb	1 Tbs	1	8	56%
Cheese Garlic	1 Tbs	1	12	38%
Garlic-Lemon-Dill	1 Tbs	1	8	56%
Honey Herb	1 Tbs	1	8	56%
Italian Supreme	1 Tbs	1	8	56%
Ranch (Good Seasons)				
Lite				
Prepared	1 Tbs	2	30	60%
Unprepared	1 packet	–	4	–
Regular				
Prepared	1 Tbs	6	60	90%
Unprepared	1 packet	–	4	–
Spicy Peanut (A Taste of Thai)				
Unprepared	1 packet	1.5	40	34%
Thousand Island (Estee)	1 Tbs	–	8	–
Vinegar & Oil/Standard Home				
Recipe (USDA)	1 Tbs	8	70	100%

Food and Description	Amount	Fat Grams	Total Calories	% Fat Calories
Zesty Herb-Fat Free (Good Seasons)				
Prepared	1 Tbs	1	12	75%
Unprepared	1 Tbs	–	6	–
■ READY TO USE				
(Arcobasso's)				
Bleu Vinaigrette	1 Tbs	6	57	95%
Creamy Caesar	1 Tbs	9	86	94%
Creamy Italian	1 Tbs	8	77	94%
Poppy Seed	1 Tbs	9	87	93%
Ranch	1 Tbs	6	56	96%
Bacon & Buttermilk	1 Tbs	8	80	90%
Bacon & Tomato				
(Estee)	1 Tbs	< 1	8	56%
(Kraft)				
Reduced calorie	1 Tbs	2	30	60%
Regular	1 Tbs	7	70	90%
Bacon, Creamy				
(Kraft) reduced calorie	1 Tbs	2	30	60%
(Bama)	1 Tbs	4	50	72%
(Barondorf) Lite				
Italian Cheese	1 Tbs	< 1	6	75%
Thousand Island	1 Tbs	–	9	–
Vinaigrette	1 Tbs	< 1	5	90%
(Bernstein)				
Caesar	1 Tbs	5	48	94%
Cheese Fantastico	1 Tbs	5	50	95%
French Vinaigrette	1 Tbs	5	48	94%
Italian				
Low-cal	1 Tbs	< 1	4	100%
Restaurant Recipe	1 Tbs	7	60	100%
w/cheese-low-cal	1 Tbs	3	45	60%
w/cheese & garlic	1 Tbs	5	45	100%
Light Fantastico				
Cheese Fantastico	1 Tbs	1	15	60%
Classico Italian	1 Tbs	–	20	–
Creamy Dijon	1 Tbs	1	25	36%
Parmesan Garlic Ranch	1 Tbs	2	35	51%
Restaurant Ranch	1 Tbs	1	25	36%
Roquefort	1 Tbs	7	65	96%
Thousand Island	1 Tbs	6	62	87%
Vinaigrette-Low-cal	1 Tbs	< 1	2	100%
(Bertolli)				
Creamy Olive Oil	1 Tbs	6	60	90%
Original Olive Oil	1 Tbs	8	80	90%
Zesty Olive Oil	1 Tbs	7	70	90%

Food and Description	Amount	Fat Grams	Total Calories	% Fat Calories
Blue Cheese				
(Estee)	1 Tbs	< 1	8	56%
Generic	1 Tbs	8	75	96%
(Nutradiet)	1 Tbs	2	25	72%
Blue Cheese Chunky				
(Kraft)				
Reduced calorie	1 Tbs	2	30	60%
Regular	1 Tbs	6	60	90%
(Nutradiet)	1 Tbs	2	25	72%
(Wish Bone)				
Lite	1 Tbs	4	40	90%
Regular	1 Tbs	8	70	100%
(Bob Evans)	1 Tbs	7	80	79%
Buttermilk, Creamy				
(Estee)	1 Tbs	–	6	–
(Kraft)				
Reduced calorie	1 Tbs	3	30	90%
Regular	1 Tbs	8	80	90%
Buttermilk & Chives, Creamy	1 Tbs	8	80	90%
Buttermilk Ranch (Nutradiet)	1 Tbs	2	25	100%
Buttermilk Recipe (Seven Seas)				
Light	1 Tbs	1	50	18%
Regular	1 Tbs	8	80	90%
Caesar				
(Weight Watchers)				
Bottled	1 Tbs	–	4	–
Individual packets	1 packet	–	6	–
(Wish Bone)	1 Tbs	8	78	92%
Lite w/ olive oil	1 Tbs	3	30	90%
Caesar Ranch				
(Kraft)	1 Tbs	7	70	90%
Catalina French (Kraft)				
Reduced calorie	1 Tbs	1	18	50%
Regular	1 Tbs	5	60	75%
Coleslaw Dressing (Kraft)	1 Tbs	6	70	77%
(Cook's Classic) Cook's Caesar	1 Tbs	5	50	90%
Cucumber, Creamy				
(Kraft)				
Reduced calorie	1 Tbs	2	25	72%
Regular	1 Tbs	8	70	100%
(Nutradiet)	1 Tbs	2	20	72%
Dijon, Creamy (Estee)	1 Tbs	< 1	8	56%
Dijon Vinaigrette-Classic (Wish Bone)				
Lite	1 Tbs	3	30	90%

Food and Description	Amount	Fat Grams	Total Calories	% Fat Calories
Regular	1 Tbs	6	60	90%
(Dorothy Lynch) Homestyle				
Reduced calorie	1 Tbs	< 1	30	15%
(El Molino) Herbal Secrets No-Oil				
Bleu Cheese	1 Tbs	< 1	12	38%
Creamy Italian	1 Tbs	< 1	7	64%
French	1 Tbs	< 1	10	45%
Herb & Spice	1 Tbs	< 1	6	75%
Italian	1 Tbs	< 1	5	90%
Vinaigrette	1 Tbs	< 1	5	90%
(Featherweight)				
Caesar	1 Tbs	1	14	64%
Creamy Cucumber	1 Tbs	–	4	–
French	1 Tbs	–	14	–
Healthy Recipes				
Creamy Dijon	1 Tbs	2	20	90%
Garden Herb	1 Tbs	2	25	72%
Italian Cheese	1 Tbs	2	20	90%
Herb	1 Tbs	–	6	–
Italian	1 Tbs	–	4	–
New Bleu	1 Tbs	–	4	–
Red Wine Vinegar	1 Tbs	–	6	–
Russian	1 Tbs	–	6	–
Thousand Island	1 Tbs	–	18	–
Zesty Tomato	1 Tbs	–	2	–
French				
(Kraft) Miracle				
Reduced calorie	1 Tbs	1	20	45%
Regular	1 Tbs	6	60	90%
(Nutradiet)	1 Tbs	–	18	–
(Pritikin)	1 Tbs	–	10	–
(Weight Watchers)	1 Tbs	–	10	–
(Wish Bone) Lite	1 Tbs	< 1	20	23%
French, Deluxe (Wish Bone)	1 Tbs	5.5	60	83%
French, Garlic (Wish Bone)				
Lite	1 Tbs	2.5	30	75%
Regular	1 Tbs	5	55	82%
French, Red (Wish Bone)				
Lite	1 Tbs	< 1	18	25%
Original	1 Tbs	6	65	83%
French, Sweet 'N Spicy (Wish Bone)				
Lite	1 Tbs	< 1	18	25%
Regular	1 Tbs	5	60	75%

Food and Description	Amount	Fat Grams	Total Calories	% Fat Calories
(Garard's)				
Cabernet	1 Tbs	7	68	93%
Caesar				
Light	1 Tbs	3	37	73%
Regular	1 Tbs	7	69	91%
Champagne				
Light	1 Tbs	5	47	96%
Regular	1 Tbs	7	71	89%
Chardonnay	1 Tbs	5	52	87%
Chenin Blanc	1 Tbs	6	57	95%
Cilantro	1 Tbs	6	59	92%
Olde San Francisco French	1 Tbs	6	59	92%
Olde Venice Italian	1 Tbs	6	57	95%
Original French				
Light	1 Tbs	4	38	95%
Regular	1 Tbs	6	58	93%
Parisian French	1 Tbs	8	79	91%
Rancho California	1 Tbs	8	75	96%
Romano Cheese Italian	1 Tbs	6	57	95%
Garlic, Creamy				
(Estee)	1 Tbs	–	2	–
(Kraft)	1 Tbs	5	50	90%
(Wish Bone)	1 Tbs	8	74	97%
Golden Caesar (Kraft)	1 Tbs	7	70	90%
(Hain)				
Canola Oil Dressings				
Garden Tomato Vinaigrette	1 Tbs	6	60	90%
Italian	1 Tbs	5	50	90%
Spicy French Mustard	1 Tbs	5	50	90%
Tangy Citrus	1 Tbs	5	50	90%
Creamy Caesar	1 Tbs	6	60	90%
Low salt	1 Tbs	6	60	90%
Creamy French	1 Tbs	6	60	90%
Creamy Italian	1 Tbs	8	80	90%
No salt	1 Tbs	8	80	90%
Cucumber Dill	1 Tbs	8	80	90%
Dijon Vinaigrette	1 Tbs	5	50	90%
Garlic & Sour Cream	1 Tbs	7	70	00%
Old Fashioned Buttermilk	1 Tbs	7	70	90%
Poppyseed Ranchers	1 Tbs	7	60	100%
Savory Herb	1 Tbs	10	90	100%
Swiss Cheese Vinaigrette	1 Tbs	7	60	100%
Thousand Island	1 Tbs	5	50	90%
Traditional Italian	1 Tbs	8	80	90%

Food and Description	Amount	Fat Grams	Total Calories	% Fat Calories
No salt	1 Tbs	6	60	90%
(Henri's)				
Chef's Ranch House	1 Tbs	7	70	90%
Hearty French	1 Tbs	6	70	77%
Light				
Chef's Recipe Ranch	1 Tbs	2	40	45%
Cucumber & Onion	1 Tbs	2	35	51%
Original French	1 Tbs	2	40	45%
Parmesan Ranch	1 Tbs	2	35	51%
Private Blend Tas-tee	1 Tbs	2	30	60%
Thousand Island	1 Tbs	2	30	60%
Original French	1 Tbs	6	60	90%
Sweet & Saucy French	1 Tbs	6	70	77%
Tas-Tee Dressing	1 Tbs	4	50	72%
(Herb Magic)				
Creamy Cucumber	1 Tbs	–	8	–
Italian	1 Tbs	–	4	–
Sweet & Sour	1 Tbs	–	18	–
Vinaigrette	1 Tbs	–	6	–
Zesty Tomato	1 Tbs	–	14	–
Herb Vinaigrette (Pritikin) Fat Free	1 Tbs	–	8	–
(Hidden Valley)				
Cole Slaw Dressing	2 Tbs	16	160	90%
Original-reduced calorie	1 Tbs	4	40	90%
Original Creamy	1 Tbs	6	80	90%
Original Ranch-reduced calorie	1 Tbs	4	40	90%
Original w/bacon	1 Tbs	8	80	90%
Ranch Italian-reduced calorie	1 Tbs	3	30	90%
South Western Ranch	1 Tbs	7	66	95%
Take Heart-Nonfat				
Blue Cheese	1 Tbs	–	10	–
French	1 Tbs	–	20	–
Honey Dijon Ranch	1 Tbs	1	20	45%
Italian	1 Tbs	–	14	–
Italian Parmesan	1 Tbs	–	16	–
Original	1 Tbs	1	20	45%
Ranch	1 Tbs	1	20	45%
Thousand Island	1 Tbs	–	25	–
Italian				
Generic				
Low cal	1 Tbs	1.5	16	84%
Regular	1 Tbs	7	69	91%

Food and Description	Amount	Fat Grams	Total Calories	% Fat Calories
(Kraft)				
House				
Original	1 Tbs	6	60	90%
Reduced calorie	1 Tbs	2	30	60%
Oil-free	1 Tbs	–	4	–
Presto	1 Tbs	7	70	90%
Regular	1 Tbs	6	60	90%
w/Olive Oil	1 Tbs	6	60	90%
(Nutradiet) no oil	1 Tbs	–	2	–
(Pritikin) Fat Free	1 Tbs	–	8	–
(Weight Watchers)				
Bottled	1 Tbs	–	6	–
Individual packets	1 packet	–	9	–
(Wish Bone)				
Lite	1 Tbs	< 1	6	45%
Regular	1 Tbs	4	45	80%
w/Olive Oil	1 Tbs	3	35	77%
Italian, Blended (Wish Bone)	1 Tbs	4	40	90%
Italian, Creamy				
(Estee)	1 Tbs	–	4	–
(Kraft)				
Reduced calorie	1 Tbs	2	25	72%
w/real sour cream	1 Tbs	5	50	90%
Lite	1 Tbs	2	25	72%
(Nutradiet)	1 Tbs	1	10	90%
(Wish Bone)				
Lite	1 Tbs	2	25	70%
Regular	1 Tbs	5	55	82%
Italian, Dijon (Nutradiet)	1 Tbs	1	8	100%
Italian French (Estee)	1 Tbs	–	4	–
Italian, Herbal (Wish Bone)	1 Tbs	7	70	90%
Italian Light-Reduced Calorie				
(Newman's Own)	1 Tbs	4	40	90%
Italian Robusto (Wish Bone)	1 Tbs	5	50	90%
Italian, Zesty (Kraft)				
Reduced calorie	1 Tbs	2	20	90%
Regular	1 Tbs	5	50	90%
Italian w/Cheese (Wish Bone)	1 Tbs	9	85	95%
Italian w/olive oil				
(Seven Seas) Light	1 Tbs	3	30	90%
(Wishbone)	1 Tbs	3	33	83%
(Ken's) Steak House Lite				
Buttermilk Ranch	1 Tbs	6	60	90%
Caesar	1 Tbs	3	30	90%

Food and Description	Amount	Fat Grams	Total Calories	% Fat Calories
Country French	1 Tbs	3	45	60%
Creamy Parmesan	1 Tbs	5	55	82%
Honey Mustard Vinaigrette	1 Tbs	5	50	90%
Red Wine Vinegar & Olive Oil	1 Tbs	2	25	72%
(Kraft)				
Deliciously Light-Reduced Calorie				
Catalina	1 Tbs	2	35	51%
Creamy Italian	1 Tbs	2	25	72%
Cucumber Ranch	1 Tbs	2	25	72%
Italian	1 Tbs	3	35	51%
Ranch	1 Tbs	6	60	90%
Thousand Island	1 Tbs	2	30	60%
Free-Nonfat				
Blue Cheese	1 Tbs	–	16	–
Catalina	1 Tbs	–	16	–
French	1 Tbs	–	20	–
Italian	1 Tbs	–	6	–
Ranch	1 Tbs	–	16	–
Thousand Island	1 Tbs	–	20	–
House Italian w/Olive Oil	1 Tbs	6	60	90%
(Life All Natural)				
Avocado w/tofu	1 Tbs	7	70	90%
Creamy salad egg free	1 Tbs	4	39	92%
Garlic w/tofu	1 Tbs	7	70	90%
Tofu	1 Tbs	7	75	84%
(Maple Grove Farms) Lite				
Dijon Maple Vinaigrette	1 Tbs	2	35	51%
Vermont Caesar	1 Tbs	2	35	51%
(Marie's)				
Chunky Blue Cheese	1 Tbs	10	100	90%
Creamy Italian	1 Tbs	10	100	90%
Creamy Ranch				
Lite & Luscious	1 Tbs	3	45	60%
Original	1 Tbs	10	100	90%
Fat-free				
Herb Vinaigrette	1 Tbs	–	16	–
Red Wine Vinaigrette	1 Tbs	–	20	–
Thousand Island	1 Tbs	8	80	90%
(Marzetti)				
Bacon Ranch	1 Tbs	10	93	97%
Buttermilk Blue Cheese	1 Tbs	10	90	100%
Buttermilk Ranch	1 Tbs	10	93	97%
Caesar	1 Tbs	8	75	96%
Celery Seed	1 Tbs	6	72	88%

Food and Description	Amount	Fat Grams	Total Calories	% Fat Calories
Chunky Blue Cheese	1 Tbs	8	78	92%
Fat-Free				
California French	1 Tbs	–	16	–
Italian	1 Tbs	–	5	–
Ranch	1 Tbs	–	12	–
Sweet & Sour	1 Tbs	–	20	–
Garlic Italian	1 Tbs	9	81	89%
Greek	1 Tbs	10	90	100%
Gusto Italian	1 Tbs	6	58	93%
Honey Dijon	1 Tbs	6	67	81%
Honey French	1 Tbs	6	74	85%
Honey Mustard	1 Tbs	6	68	93%
Lite				
Chunky Blue Cheese	1 Tbs	5	45	100%
Honey French	1 Tbs	3	45	60%
Ranch	1 Tbs	5	45	100%
Parmesan	1 Tbs	9	86	94%
Peppercorn	1 Tbs	7	63	100%
Peppercorn Ranch	1 Tbs	9	90	100%
Poppyseed	1 Tbs	5	65	83%
Potato	1 Tbs	7	80	79%
Romano Italian	1 Tbs	8	75	96%
Slaw	1 Tbs	8	80	90%
Southern Slaw	1 Tbs	5	66	68%
Spinach	1 Tbs	10	90	100%
Sweet & Sour	1 Tbs	6	72	88%
Thousand Island	1 Tbs	5	82	55%
Vegetable	1 Tbs	10	90	100%
Miracle French (Kraft)	1 Tbs	6	70	77%
(Miracle Whip)				
Cholesterol-free	1 Tbs	7	70	90%
Coleslaw Dressing	1 Tbs	6	70	77%
Free	1 Tbs	–	20	–
Light	1 Tbs	4	45	80%
Reduced Calorie	1 Tbs	4	45	80%
Regular	1 Tbs	7	70	90%
(Naturally Fresh) Refrigerated				
Bleu Cheese	1 Tbs	8	90	80%
Honey Mustard	1 Tbs	6	80	68%
Italian Herb Vinaigrette	1 Tbs	6	60	90%
Poppy Seed	1 Tbs	4	80	45%
Ranch-Lite	1 Tbs	3	30	90%
Slaw Dressing	1 Tbs	5	70	64%
Thousand Island	1 Tbs	5	50	90%

Food and Description	Amount	Fat Grams	Total Calories	% Fat Calories
Oil & Vinegar (Kraft)	1 Tbs	8	70	100%
(Old Dutch) Oil/Fat Free				
Sweet-Sour	1 Tbs	–	25	–
Olive Oil Vinaigrette				
(Wish Bone)				
Lite	1 Tbs	2	20	90%
Original	1 Tbs	3	30	90%
Onion & Chive				
(Wish Bone) Lite	1 Tbs	3	35	77%
Onion & Chives, Creamy (Kraft)	1 Tbs	7	70	90%
(Oriental Chef)				
Honey Orange	1 Tbs	3	40	68%
Original French	1 Tbs	3	40	68%
Snappy Ginger	1 Tbs	4	40	90%
Tangy Soy	1 Tbs	4	35	100%
(Ott's)				
Buttermilk Ranch	1 Tbs	7	70	90%
Italian	1 Tbs	9	80	100%
Original	1 Tbs	3	40	90%
Reduced calorie	1 Tbs	1	25	36%
(Peggy Jane's)				
Garden Herb	1 Tbs	4	45	80%
Honey Mustard	1 Tbs	6	60	90%
Honey Sesame	1 Tbs	5	60	75%
Pepper Cream	1 Tbs	8	80	90%
Poppy Seed	1 Tbs	4	60	60%
Peppercorn (Kraft)	1 Tbs	9	90	90%
(Pfeiffer)				
Bacon Ranch	1 Tbs	10	93	97%
Buttermilk Blue Cheese	1 Tbs	10	90	100%
Buttermilk Ranch	1 Tbs	10	93	97%
Caesar	1 Tbs	8	75	96%
Celery Seed	1 Tbs	6	72	88%
Chunky Blue Cheese	1 Tbs	8	78	92%
Fat-Free				
California French	1 Tbs	–	16	–
Italian	1 Tbs	–	5	–
Ranch	1 Tbs	–	12	–
Sweet & Sour	1 Tbs	–	20	–
Garlic Italian	1 Tbs	9	81	89%
Greek	1 Tbs	10	90	100%
Gusto Italian	1 Tbs	6	58	93%
Honey Dijon	1 Tbs	6	67	81%
Honey French	1 Tbs	6	74	85%

Food and Description	Amount	Fat Grams	Total Calories	% Fat Calories
Honey Mustard	1 Tbs	6	68	93%
Lite				
Chunky Blue Cheese	1 Tbs	5	45	100%
Honey French	1 Tbs	3	45	60%
Ranch	1 Tbs	5	45	100%
Parmesan	1 Tbs	9	86	94%
Peppercorn	1 Tbs	7	63	100%
Peppercorn Ranch	1 Tbs	9	90	100%
Poppyseed	1 Tbs	5	65	83%
Potato	1 Tbs	7	80	79%
Romano Italian	1 Tbs	8	75	96%
Slaw	1 Tbs	8	80	90%
Southern Slaw	1 Tbs	5	66	68%
Spinach	1 Tbs	10	90	100%
Sweet & Sour	1 Tbs	6	72	88%
Thousand Island	1 Tbs	5	82	55%
Vegetable	1 Tbs	10	90	100%
Ranch				
(Pritikin) Fat Free	1 Tbs	–	16	–
(Weight Watchers) creamy				
Bottled	1 Tbs	–	25	–
Individual packets	1 packet	–	35	–
(Wish Bone)				
Lite	1 Tbs	4	45	80%
Original	1 Tbs	8	80	90%
Rancher's Choice, creamy (Kraft)				
Reduced calorie	1 Tbs	3	30	90%
Regular	1 Tbs	10	90	100%
Red Wine Olive Oil Vinaigrette				
(Wish Bone)	1 Tbs	3	35	77%
Red Wine Vinegar (Estee)	1 Tbs	–	2	–
Red Wine, Vinegar and Oil (Kraft)	1 Tbs	4	60	60%
(Richard Simmons) Salad Spray				
Dijon Vinaigrette	1 spray	–	1	–
	18 sprays	1	14	64%
French	1 spray	–	1	–
	18 sprays	1	14	64%
Italian	1 spray	–	1	–
	18 sprays	1	14	64%
Roma Cheese	1 spray	–	1	–
	18 sprays	1	14	64%
Roka Blue Cheese (Kraft)				
Reduced calorie	1 Tbs	1	16	56%
Regular	1 Tbs	6	60	90%

Food and Description	Amount	Fat Grams	Total Calories	% Fat Calories
Roquefort	1 Tbs	8	77	94%
Russian				
(Kraft)				
Reduced calorie	1 Tbs	1	30	30%
Regular	1 Tbs	5	60	75%
(Nutradiet)	1 Tbs	1	25	36%
(Wish Bone)				
Lite	1 Tbs	< 1	20	23%
Regular	1 Tbs	3	50	54%
Russian, Creamy (Kraft)	1 Tbs	5	60	75%
Sesame Seed-generic	1 Tbs	6.9	68	91%
(Seven Seas)				
Buttermilk Recipe Ranch				
Light	1 Tbs	5	50	90%
Regular	1 Tbs	8	80	90%
Free				
Ranch	1 Tbs	–	6	–
Red Wine Vinegar	1 Tbs	–	16	–
French, Creamy	1 Tbs	6	60	90%
French-Light	1 Tbs	3	35	77%
Italian w/Olive Oil	1 Tbs	3	30	90%
Ranch Light Buttermilk Recipe	1 Tbs	5	50	90%
Thousand Island-Light	1 Tbs	2	30	60%
Thousand Island-Creamy	1 Tbs	5	50	90%
Viva				
Herbs & Spices				
Light	1 Tbs	3	30	90%
Regular	1 Tbs	6	60	90%
Italian				
Creamy				
Light	1 Tbs	4	45	80%
Regular	1 Tbs	7	70	90%
Free-Fat Free	1 Tbs	–	4	–
Light-Reduced Calorie	1 Tbs	3	30	90%
Regular	1 Tbs	5	50	90%
Ranch				
Light	1 Tbs	5	50	90%
Regular	1 Tbs	8	80	90%
Red Wine Vinegar & Oil				
Light	1 Tbs	4	45	80%
Regular	1 Tbs	7	70	90%
Sweet & Spicy (Pritikin) Fat Free	1 Tbs	–	18	–
Thousand Island				
(Bob's) Famous Thousand Island	1 Tbs	6	66	82%

Food and Description	Amount	Fat Grams	Total Calories	% Fat Calories
(Estee)	1 Tbs	–	8	–
(Kraft)				
Reduced calorie	1 Tbs	1	30	30%
Regular	1 Tbs	5	60	75%
(Nutradiet)	1 Tbs	2	25	72%
(Wish Bone)				
Lite	1 Tbs	< 1	20	23%
Regular	1 Tbs	6	60	90%
Thousand Island & Bacon				
(Kraft)	1 Tbs	6	60	90%
Thousand Island Lite				
Less Oil	1 Tbs	3	40	68%
Tomato Vinaigrette				
(Weight Watchers)	1 Tbs	–	8	–
Tomato Zesty				
(Pritikin) Fat Free	1 Tbs	–	18	–
(Ultra Slim Fast)				
French	1 Tbs	< 1	20	23%
Italian	1 Tbs	< 1	6	45%
Thousand Island	1 Tbs	< 1	18	25%
Vinaigrette (Pritikin) Fat Free	1 Tbs	–	10	–
(Walden Farms)				
Bleu Cheese	1 Tbs	1.9	27	63%
Creamy Italian	1 Tbs	2.5	35	64%
French	1 Tbs	2.4	33	65%
Italian				
No Sugar Added	1 Tbs	–	6	–
Original	1 Tbs	–	9	–
Sodium Free	1 Tbs	–	9	–
Ranch	1 Tbs	2	35	51%
Thousand Island	1 Tbs	1.7	24	64%
(Weight Watchers)				
Caesar Salad	1 Tbs	–	4	–
Creamy Cucumber	1 Tbs	–	18	–
Creamy Italian	1 Tbs	–	12	–
Creamy Peppercorn	1 Tbs	–	8	–
Western (Richelieu)				
Reduced calorie	1 Tbs	1	35	26%
Regular	1 Tbs	5	70	64%
(Western) 98% Fat Free				
French	1 Tbs	1	35	26%
(Wish Bone)				
Fat Free				
French	1 Tbs	< 1	20	23%

Food and Description	Amount	Fat Grams	Total Calories	% Fat Calories
Food Service				
Blue Cheese	1 Tbs	8	73	99%
Blue Cheese-Lite	1 Tbs	< 1	20	23%
Creamy Italian	1 Tbs	2	26	69%
Deluxe French	1 Tbs	6	60	90%
French-Lite	1 Tbs	< 1	22	20%
Italian	1 Tbs	4.5	45	90%
Italian-Lite	1 Tbs	< 1	6	75%
Ranch	1 Tbs	8	75	96%
Russian	1 Tbs	3	45	60%
Healthy Sensations				
Blue Cheese	1 Tbs	< 1	20	23%
French	1 Tbs	< 1	20	23%
Honey Dijon	1 Tbs	< 1	25	18%
Italian	1 Tbs	< 1	6	75%
Ranch	1 Tbs	< 1	15	30%
Thousand Island	1 Tbs	< 1	20	23%
SALAD TOPPINGS				
(McCormick/Schilling)				
Bac'n Pieces				
Bits	1 Tbs	< 1	25	18%
Chips	1 Tbs	< 1	26	17%
Cheese	1 Tbs	.7	31	20%
Garden Vegetable	1 Tbs	.7	34	19%
Regular	1 Tbs	.8	32	23%
SALAMI (*See also* LUNCHEON MEAT)				
Beerwurst/Beer Salami				
4" dia-⅛" thick	1 slice	6.76	75	81%
Salami/cooked	1 oz	5.9	7	42%
SALMON (*See also* SEAFOOD ENTREE/DINNER)				
Atlantic				
canned	3 oz	2.8	173	15%
canned solids & liquid	8 oz	6	268	20%
	15 oz	11.9	502	21%
cooked-dry heat	3 oz	6	155	35%
raw	3 oz	5	121	37%
Blueback-fancy				
(Nutradiet)	½ cup	11	188	53%
Chinook				
raw	3 oz	8.88	153	52%
smoked	3 oz	3.67	99	33%
Chum				
canned	3 oz	4.68	120	35%
raw	3 oz	3	102	27%

Food and Description	Amount	Fat Grams	Total Calories	% Fat Calories
Coho				
cooked-moist heat	3 oz	6	157	34%
raw	3 oz	5	124	36%
Pink				
canned	3 oz	5	118	38%
(Bumble Bee)	3.5 oz	8	160	45%
(Chicken Of The Sea) spring water	3.5 oz	2	97	19%
(Del Monte)	½ cup	7	160	39%
(Featherweight)	2 oz	3	70	39%
(Libby's)	7¾ oz	13	310	38%
raw	3 oz	2.9	99	26%
Red				
canned	3 oz	8	154	47%
(Bumble Bee)	3.5 oz	10	180	50%
(Del Monte)	½ cup	9	180	45%
(Nutradiet)	½ cup	11	188	53%
(S&W) Fancy	½ cup	10	190	47%
cooked-dry heat	3 oz	5	140	32%
Smoked	3 oz	8	150	48%
Sockeye				
canned				
(Libby's)	7¾ oz	21	380	50%
cooked dry heat	3 oz	9	183	44%
raw	3 oz	7	143	44%
SALSIFY/cooked/sliced	½ cup	–	46	–
SALT	Any amount	–	–	–
SALT SUBSTITUTE				
Generic				
Seasoned	1 tsp	–	2	–
Seasoned No-Salt	1 tsp	–	4	–
Unseasoned	1 tsp	–	–	–
(Health Valley) Instead of Salt	1 tsp	–	–	–
SANDWICH SPREAD (*See also* LUNCHEON MEAT)				
(Best Foods)	1 Tbs	5	50	90%
(Hellman's)	1 Tbs	5	50	90%
(Kraft)	1 Tbs	5	50	90%
SAPODILLO				
Tropical American	1	1.9	140	12%
	1 cup	2	178	10%
SARDINES				
Atlantic				
canned in Olive Oil				
(Crown Prince) Brisling				
includes oil	3.75 oz	42	460	82%

Food and Description	Amount	Fat Grams	Total Calories	% Fat Calories
(S&W) Norwegian Brisling drained	2 oz	10	130	69%
(Underwood) drained	3.75 oz	20	260	69%
canned in sardine oil (Crown Prince)				
includes oil	3.75 oz	42	460	82%
canned in soya oil				
Generic	2 pieces	2.75	50	50%
(Underwood)	3.75 oz	18	230	70%
canned in tobasco sauce (Underwood)				
drained	1 can/ ~ 3 oz	18	220	74%
canned in tomato sauce (Crown Prince)				
incudes sauce	3.75 oz	18	240	68%
(Del Monte)	½ cup	12	360	30%
Pacific				
canned in mustard sauce (Underwood)				
includes sauce	3.75 oz	16	220	66%
canned in tomato sauce	1	4.5	68	60%
(includes bone)	1 can/ ~ 13 oz	44	658	60%
(Underwood)				
includes sauce	3.75 oz	16	220	66%

SAUCE (*See also* GRAVY, MARINADES, MEXICAN FOOD, PASTA ENTREE/DINNER, SEASONINGS, SOUP)

■ **DEHYDRATED MIXES**

(NOTE: Prepared servings are made according to package directions.)

Food and Description	Amount	Fat Grams	Total Calories	% Fat Calories
A la King (Durkee) Prepared	1 cup	8	133	54%
Alfredo (Knorr)				
Prepared	2 oz	6	100	54%
Unprepared	1 serving	2	45	40%
(Mayacamas) Dry mix for one serving	1 Tbs	< 1	8	56%
Bearnaise				
Generic prepared w/milk and butter	1 cup	68	701	87%
(Great Impressions)				
Prepared	2 Tbs	21	192	98%
	½ cup	34	351	87%
Unprepared	9 oz pkg	2	90	20%
(Knorr)				
Prepared w/4 oz margarine and 1 cup whole milk	2 oz	17	180	85%

Food and Description	Amount	Fat Grams	Total Calories	% Fat Calories
Prepared w/2 oz margarine and ½ cup whole milk	2 oz	10	120	75%
Unprepared	1 serving	< 1	15	30%
(Mayacamas)				
Prepared	1 Tbs	3	32	84%
Unprepared	1 Tbs	< 1	35	13%
(McCormick/Schilling)				
Prepared	¼ cup	11	129	77%
Unprepared	1 pkg	< 1	88	5%
Bouillabaisse				
(Knorr)				
Prepared	⅙ pkg	1	140	6%
Unprepared	1 serving	1	25	36%
Cheddar Cheese (Mayacamas)				
Prepared	1 Tbs	3	31	87%
Unprepared	1 Tbs	< 1	8	56%
Cheese				
(Durkee)				
Prepared	1 cup	16.9	316	48%
Unprepared	1 pkg	8	157	46%
(French's)				
Prepared	⅓ cup	5	110	41%
Unprepared	¼ pkg	2	50	36%
Generic (1.2 oz)				
Prepared w/milk	1 cup	17	307	50%
Unprepared	1 pkg	9	158	51%
(McCormick/Schilling) Dry				
Nacho	¼ pkg	1.5	42	32%
Original	¼ pkg	1.5	35	39%
Curry				
Generic (1 oz)				
Prepared w/milk	1 cup	14.7	270	49%
Unprepared	1 pkg	6.5	121	48%
(Knorr) Prepared	2 oz	2	35	51%
(Mayacamas)				
Prepared	1 Tbs	3	32	84%
Unprepared	1 Tbs	< 1	35	13%
Demi-Glace				
(Knorr)				
Prepared	2 oz	1	30	30%
Unprepared	1 serving	1	30	30%
(Mayacamas) Dry mix for one serving	1 Tbs	–	< 1	–
Dill Sauce, Creamy for Fish				
(Durkee) Roastin' Bag	1 pkg	14	153	82%

Food and Description	Amount	Fat Grams	Total Calories	% Fat Calories
Green Pepper (Knorr)				
Prepared	2 oz	1	20	45%
Green Peppercorn (McCormick/Schilling)				
Prepared	¼ cup	4	86	42%
Unprepared	1 pkg	3	117	23%
Hollandaise				
(Durkee) Prepared	¾ cup	14	173	73%
(French's) Prepared	¼ pkg	1	30	30%
Generic				
Prepared w/butter & water	1 cup	19.74	237	75%
Prepared w/vegetable oil, milk & butter	1 cup	68	703	87%
(Knorr) Prepared	2 oz	1	18	20%
(Macayamas)				
Prepared	1 Tbs	3	32	84%
Unprepared	1 Tbs	< 1	35	13%
(McCormick/Schilling)				
Prepared	¼ cup	13	137	85%
Unprepared	1 pkg	6	141	38%
Honey Mustard (Mayacamas)				
Prepared	1 Tbs	3	32	84%
Unprepared	1 Tbs	< 1	35	13%
Hunter				
(Knorr)				
Prepared	2 oz	< 1	25	18%
Unprepared	1 serving	< 1	25	18%
(McCormick/Schilling)				
Prepared	¼ cup	9	104	69%
Unprepared	1 pkg	< 1	114	4%
Lemon Dill (Knorr) Prepared	2 oz	1	30	30%
Mushroom				
Generic				
Prepared w/milk	1 cup	10	228	40%
Unprepared	1 oz pkg	3	99	27%
(Knorr)				
Prepared w/milk	2 oz	3	60	45%
Unprepared	1 serving	1	20	45%
Mustard Herb (Knorr)				
Prepared w/milk	2 oz	4	90	40%
Unprepared	1 serving	1	40	23%
Napoli (Knorr)				
Prepared w/tomato puree & oil	2 oz	3	100	27%
Unprepared	1 serving	< 1	20	23%
Newberg (Knorr) Prepared	2 oz	1	20	45%

Food and Description	Amount	Fat Grams	Total Calories	% Fat Calories
Parma Rosa (Knorr)				
Prepared w/milk & margarine	2 oz	6	90	60%
Unprepared	1 serving	1	35	26%
Peanut Sauce				
Generic-Unprepared	2 Tbs	.5	25	18%
Pepper (Knorr)				
Prepared w/water	2 oz	1	20	45%
Unprepared	1 serving	1	20	45%
Pesto				
(Knorr) Prepared	2 oz	1	18	50%
(Mayacamas) Dry mix for one serving				
Creamy	1 Tbs	< 1	8	56%
Tomato	1 Tbs	< 1	8	56%
Sour Cream				
Generic (1.2 oz)				
Prepared w/milk	1 cup	30	509	53%
Unprepared	1 pkg	11	180	55%
Spaghetti				
(Durkee)				
Mushroom				
Prepared	2⅔ cups	.8	208	4%
Unprepared	1 pkg	–	69	–
Regular				
Prepared	2½ cups	1	224	4%
Unprepared	1 pkg	< 1	85	5%
Thick & Rich				
Prepared	2¼ cups	1	212	4%
Unprepared	1 pkg	< 1	72	9%
(French's)				
Regular				
Prepared	½ cup	4	90	40%
Unprepared	⅕ pkg	< 1	20	23%
Mushroom				
Prepared	½ cup	4	100	36%
Unprepared	⅕ pkg	< 1	30	15%
Thick				
Prepared	⅞ cup	7	170	37%
Unprepared	¼ pkg	1	150	0%
(Knorr) Prepared	2 oz	1	12	75%
(Mayacamas) Dry mix for one serving				
Alfredo	1 Tbs	< 1	8	56%
Butter Basil	1 Tbs	< 1	8	56%
Clam Sauce	1 Tbs	< 1	6	75%
Creamy Italian	1 Tbs	< 1	8	56%

Food and Description	Amount	Fat Grams	Total Calories	% Fat Calories
Marinara	1 Tbs	< 1	6	75%
Mushroom	1 Tbs	< 1	6	75%
(McCormick/Schilling) Unprepared				
Plain	¼ pkg	–	6	–
Thick & Zesty	¼ pkg	–	34	–
Spare Rib (Durkee) Roastin' Bag	1 pkg	2	162	11%
Stroganoff				
(Durkee)				
Prepared	4 cups	285	3280	78%
	1 cup	71	820	78%
Unprepared	1 pkg	< 1	90	7%
Generic				
Prepared w/milk & water	1 cup	10.7	271	36%
Unprepared	1.6 oz pkg	4	161	22%
Sweet & Sour				
(A Taste of Thai) Tangy Hot	2 Tbs	–	30	–
(Chun King) Glaze Entree Mix	3.8 oz pkg	–	370	–
Generic-Prepared	1 cup	–	294	–
(Kikkoman) Prepared	2⅛ oz pkg	–	228	–
Taco (Old El Paso)	1 pkg	1	100	9%
Teriyaki Sauce-Generic				
Prepared	1 Tbs	–	8	–
	1 cup	1	131	7%
Unprepared	1 pkg	1	30	30%
White				
(Durkee)				
Prepared	1 cup	19.7	317	56%
Unprepared	1 pkg	11	155	64%
(French's)				
Prepared	⅓ cup	5	110	41%
Unprepared	¼ pkg	2	50	36%
(Knorr)				
Unprepared	1 serving	2	30	60%
Prepared w/milk & water	2 oz	4	70	51%
(Mayacamas) Dry mix for				
one serving	1 Tbs	–	< 1	–
(McCormick/Schilling)				
Prepared	¼ cup	3	59	46%
Unprepared	1 pkg	3	127	21%
■ READY-TO-USE & HOMEMADE				
Barbecue				
(Bull's Eye)	2 Tbs	–	50	–
(Chris' & Pitt's)	1 Tbs	–	15	–
(Estee)	1 Tbs	–	18	–
(Featherweight)	1 Tbs	–	14	–

Food and Description	Amount	Fat Grams	Total Calories	% Fat Calories
(French's)				
Cattleman's mild	1 Tbs	–	25	–
Cattleman's smoky	1 Tbs	–	25	–
(Hain)				
Honey	1 Tbs	1	14	64%
(Heinz) Thick & Rich				
Cajun	1 oz	–	35	–
Chunky	1 oz	–	30	–
Hawaiian	1 oz	–	40	–
Hickory Smoke	1 oz	–	35	–
Hot	1 oz	–	30	–
Mesquite	1 oz	–	30	–
Mushroom	1 oz	–	30	–
Old Fashioned	1 oz	–	35	–
Onion	1 oz	–	30	–
Original	1 oz	–	35	–
(Hunt's)				
Country Style	1 Tbs	< 1	20	23%
Hickory	1 Tbs	< 1	20	23%
Homestyle	1 Tbs	< 1	20	23%
Kansas City Style	1 Tbs	< 1	20	23%
Light Hickory Flavor	1 Tbs	< 1	16	28%
Light Original	1 Tbs	–	16	–
New Orleans Style	1 Tbs	< 1	20	23%
Original	1 Tbs	< 1	20	23%
Southern Style	1 Tbs	< 1	20	23%
Texas Style	1 Tbs	< 1	20	23%
Western Style	1 Tbs	< 1	20	23%
(Kingsford)				
Masterpiece Mesquite	1 Tbs	–	30	–
Masterpiece Original	1 Tbs	–	30	–
(Kraft)				
Garlic	2 Tbs	1	40	23%
Hickory Smoke	2 Tbs	1	45	20%
Hickory Smoke Onion Bits	2 Tbs	1	50	18%
Hot	2 Tbs	1	45	20%
Hot Hickory Smoke	2 Tbs	1	45	20%
Italian Seasonings	2 Tbs	1	50	18%
Kansas City Style	2 Tbs	1	50	18%
Mesquite Smoke	2 Tbs	1	40	23%
Onion Bits	2 Tbs	1	50	18%
Original	2 Tbs	1	45	20%
Thick'n Spicy	2 Tbs	1	50	18%
Thick'n Spicy Chunky	2 Tbs	1	60	15%

Food and Description	Amount	Fat Grams	Total Calories	% Fat Calories
Thick'n Spicy Hickory Smoke	2 Tbs	1	50	18%
Thick'n Spicy Kansas City Style	2 Tbs	1	60	15%
Thick'n Spicy Mesquite Smoke	2 Tbs	1	50	18%
Thick'n Spicy Original	2 Tbs	1	50	18%
Thick'n Spicy w/Honey	2 Tbs	1	60	15%
(Maull's)	3.5 oz	2	123	15%
Beer Flavor	1 Tbs	< 1	20	23%
Genuine	1 Tbs	< 1	20	23%
Kansas City Style	1 Tbs	< 1	30	15%
Lite	1 Tbs	< 1	12	38%
Onion	1 Tbs	< 1	20	23%
Smoky	1 Tbs	< 1	20	23%
Sweet/mild	1 Tbs	< 1	30	15%
Sweet/smoky	1 Tbs	< 1	30	15%
(Mowrar's) Gourmet Diet	1 oz	< 1	11	41%
(Open Pit)				
Hickory Smoke	1 Tbs	–	25	–
Hickory thick'n tangy	1 Tbs	–	25	–
Hot'n Tangy	1 Tbs	–	25	–
Mesquite'n Tangy	1 Tbs	–	25	–
Original	1 Tbs	–	25	–
Original w/onions	1 Tbs	–	25	–
Sweet'n Tangy	1 Tbs	–	25	–
Chicken Tonight (Ragu)				
Simmer Sauce				
Country French Chicken	4 oz	12	140	77%
Creamy Chicken Primavera	4 oz	6	90	60%
Creamy Chicken w/ Mushrooms	4 oz	10	110	82%
Herbed Chicken w/ Wine	4 oz	4	100	36%
Oriental Chicken	4 oz	1	70	13%
Salsa	4 oz	–	35	–
Spanish	4 oz	2	70	26%
Chili	1 Tbs	–	17	
(A Taste of Thai)				
Garlic Chili Pepper Sauce	1 Tbs	–	10	–
(Del Monte)	¼ cup	–	70	–
(Featherweight)	1 Tbs	–	8	–
(Heinz)	1 Tbs	–	17	–
Chili Hot Dog Sauce	1.25 oz	2	44	41%
(Chef Boyardee) w/beef	1 oz	1	30	30%
(Gebhardt)	2 Tbs	1	20	45%
(Wolf)	⅙ cup	2	40	45%

Food and Description	Amount	Fat Grams	Total Calories	% Fat Calories
Clam Sauce				
generic				
red	2 oz	1.6	41	35%
white	2 oz	4.8	61	71%
homemade	½ cup	22	275	72%
Cocktail Sauce				
(Del Monte) Seafood	¼ cup	–	70	–
(Estee)	1 Tbs	–	10	–
(Golden Dipt) Seafood Cocktail				
Extra Hot	1 Tbs	–	20	–
Original	1 Tbs	–	20	–
(Heinz) Seafood	1 Tbs	–	20	–
(Sauceworks)	1 Tbs	–	14	–
Creole				
(Golden Dipt)	1 oz	1	20	45%
Dijonaisse				
(Golden Dipt)	1 oz	4	52	69%
(Durkee) Famous Sauce	1 Tbs	6	70	77%
Enchilada (See also MEXICAN FOOD)				
(Del Monte)				
hot	½ cup	–	45	–
mild	½ cup	–	45	–
(La Victoria)	1 cup	5	80	56%
(Old El Paso)				
Green Chili	¼ cup	1	30	30%
Hot	¼ cup	1	25	36%
Plain	¼ cup	–	18	–
(Escoffier)				
Diable Sauce	1 Tbs	–	20	–
Robert Sauce	1 Tbs	–	20	–
French White Sauce				
(Golden Dipt)	1 oz	4	55	65%
Heinz 57	1 Tbs	–	15	–
Horseradish				
(Heinz)	1 Tbs	7	75	84%
(Kraft)				
Creamy Style & Prepared	1 Tbs	1	12	75%
Mustard	1 Tbs	1	14	64%
(Sauceworks)	1 Tbs	5	50	90%
Lemon Butter Dill (Golden Dipt)	1 oz	9	100	81%
Manwich (Hunt's)				
Sauce only	2.5 oz	1	35	26%
w/Ground Beef on Hamburger				
Roll	5.8 oz	13	310	38%

Food and Description	Amount	Fat Grams	Total Calories	% Fat Calories
Sauce only				
Extra Thick & Chunky	2.5 oz	.5	60	8%
Marinara (tomato)	4 oz	4	86	42%
Mustard Sauce-Hot (Sauceworks)	1 Tbs	2	35	51%
Newberg Sauce w/sherry (Snow's)	⅓ cup	8	120	60%
Picante Salsa (*See also* MEXICAN FOOD)				
(Del Monte)				
Hot	¼ cup	–	20	–
Hot & Chunky	¼ cup	–	15	–
(Old El Paso)	2 Tbs	–	10	–
Picante Sauce (*See also* MEXICAN FOOD)				
(Azteca)				
Medium	1 Tbs	–	4	–
Mild	1 Tbs	–	4	–
(Del Monte)				
Burrito	¼ cup	–	20	–
Green Chili Mild	¼ cup	–	20	–
Rojo Mild	¼ cup	–	20	–
(Estee)	2 Tbs	–	8	–
(Old El Paso)	2 Tbs	–	8	–
Pizza				
canned				
(Chef Boyardee) w/cheese	2.5 oz	2	50	36%
	3.88 oz	6	90	60%
(Contadina)				
Quick & Easy	¼ cup	1	30	30%
w/Italian Cheese	¼ cup	1	30	30%
w/Pepperoni	¼ cup	2	40	45%
w/Tomato Chunks	¼ cup	1	25	36%
(Ragu) Extra Tomatoes	3 Tbs	1	25	36%
Pizza Quick Sauce				
(Ragu)				
chunky style	3 Tbs	2	45	40%
garlic & basil	3 Tbs	2	40	45%
pepperoni	½ cup	2	35	51%
traditional	3 Tbs	2	35	51%
w/ cheese	3 Tbs	2	40	45%
Recipe Sauce (Betty Crocker)				
Chicken Cacciatore	3.8 oz	< 1	40	11%
Pepper Steak	3.8 oz	1	45	20%
Stroganoff	4 oz	4	60	60%
Rib Sauce (Gold's)	1 oz	–	60	–
Salsa				
Thick 'N Chunky (Old El Paso)	2 Tbs	–	6	–

Food and Description	Amount	Fat Grams	Total Calories	% Fat Calories
Seafood (*See* Cocktail Sauce, in this listing)				
Sloppy Joe Barbecue Sauce (Libby's)				
w/beef	⅓ cup	7	110	57%
w/pork	⅓ cup	8	120	60%
Soy	1 Tbs	–	11	–
	1 oz	–	23	–
	¼ cup	–	30	–
(Chun King)	1 tsp	–	6	–
(Kikkoman)				
Lite	1 Tbs	–	12	–
Milder	1 Tbs	–	12	–
Regular	1 Tbs	–	18	–
(La Choy)	1 Tbs	< 1	8	56%
Spaghetti Sauce-Canned				
(Campbell's) Healthy Request				
Extra Garlic & Onion	4 oz	< 1	50	2%
Fresh Mushrooms	4 oz	< 1	50	2%
Homestyle	4 oz	–	40	–
Traditional	4 oz	–	50	–
(Chef Boyardee)				
Original w/meat	3.75 oz	3	80	34%
Original w/mushrooms	3.75 oz	3	80	34%
w/ meat	3.75 oz	2	80	23%
w/ mushrooms	3.75 oz	1	60	15%
Generic	1 cup	11.9	272	39%
(Healthy Choice)				
Flavored w/Meat	4 oz	< 1	50	9%
w/Green Pepper	4 oz	< 1	40	11%
(Hunt's)				
Chunky Style	4 oz	< 1	50	9%
Homestyle	4 oz	2	60	30%
w/ meat	4 oz	2	60	30%
w/ mushroom	4 oz	1	50	18%
Light				
Flavored w/Meat	4 oz	< 1	45	10%
Garlic & Onion	4 oz	< 1	40	11%
Traditional	4 oz	< 1	40	11%
w/Mushrooms	4 oz	< 1	40	11%
Meat	4 oz	2	60	30%
Mushroom	4 oz	2	70	26%
Traditional	4 oz	2	70	26%
(Progresso)				
Clam				
Red	½ cup	3	70	39%

Food and Description	Amount	Fat Grams	Total Calories	% Fat Calories
White	½ cup	8	110	65%
Marinara	½ cup	5	90	50%
Meat Flavor	½ cup	5	110	42%
Mushroom	½ cup	5	110	42%
Original	½ cup	5	110	42%
Spaghetti Sauce-Fresh Chilled				
(Contadina)				
Alfredo	4 oz	34	350	87%
Bolognese	5 oz	7	130	48%
Four Cheese	4 oz	27	300	81%
Garden Vegetable	5 oz	3	80	34%
Italian Sausage	5 oz	6	110	49%
Marinara	5 oz	4	80	45%
Pesto	2⅓ oz	34	350	87%
Plum Tomato	5 oz	4	80	45%
(Di Giorno)				
Alfredo	1 oz	10	100	90%
Bolognese	1 oz	2	30	60%
Four Cheese	4 oz	32	350	82%
Marinara	5 oz	6	110	49%
Pesto	1 oz	13	140	84%
Rigoletto	5 oz	8	120	60%
(Fresh Chef)				
Bolognese	4 oz	7	130	49%
Clam				
Red	4 oz	4	90	40%
White	4 oz	10	130	69%
Pesto	4 oz	60	630	86%
Spaghetti Sauce-From Jars				
(Chef Boyardee)				
Meatless	4 oz	1	60	15%
w/ ground beef	4 oz	3	90	30%
	4.14 oz	3	100	27%
w/ mushrooms	4 oz	2	70	26%
(Classico)				
Di Abruzzi	4 oz	4	70	51%
Di Bologna	4 oz	4	70	51%
Di Napoli	4 oz	4	70	51%
Di Roma Arrabiata	4 oz	3	60	45%
Di Sicilia	4 oz	2	50	36%
Di Veneto	4 oz	3	60	45%
(Conca Dioro)				
Marinara	8 oz	6	130	42%
Puttanesca	8 oz	6.8	111	55%

Food and Description	Amount	Fat Grams	Total Calories	% Fat Calories
Napoletana	8 oz	6.6	110	54%
Sicilian	8 oz	4.9	111	40%
(Enrico's) All Natural				
no salt	4 oz	1	60	15%
plain	4 oz	1	60	15%
(Estee)	4 oz	2	60	30%
(Featherweight) Healthy Recipes	4 oz	1	60	15%
(Hain)				
Marinara	4 oz	1	40	23%
Mushroom	4 oz	1	40	23%
(Prego)				
Extra Chunky				
Garden Combination	4 oz	2	80	23%
Mushroom & Green Pepper	4 oz	4	100	36%
Mushroom & Onion	4 oz	4	100	36%
Mushroom & Tomato	4 oz	5	110	41%
Mushroom w/Extra Spice	4 oz	3	100	27%
Sausage & Green Pepper	4 oz	8	160	45%
Tomato & Onion	4 oz	5	110	41%
Marinara	4 oz	6	100	54%
Meat Flavored	4 oz	6	140	39%
Mushroom	4 oz	5	130	35%
No Salt Added	4 oz	6	110	49%
Onion & Garlic	4 oz	4	110	33%
Regular	4 oz	5	130	35%
Three Cheese	4 oz	2	100	18%
Tomato & Basil	4 oz	2	100	18%
(Pritikin)				
Chunky Garden Style	4 oz	–	50	–
plain	4 oz	–	50	–
(Ragu)				
Chunky Garden Style				
Chunky Green & Red Peppers	4 oz	5	110	41%
Green Peppers & Mushrooms	4 oz	2	80	23%
Italian Garden Combination	4 oz	2	80	23%
Mushrooms and Onions	4 oz	2	80	23%
Sweet Green & Red Bell Peppers	4 oz	2	80	23%
Xtra tomatoes, garlic & onions	4 oz	2	80	23%
Extra Thick & Zesty				
flavored w/meat	4 oz	4	100	36%
plain	4 oz	4	100	36%
w/ mushrooms	4 oz	5	110	41%
Fresh Italian				
Garden Medley	4 oz	3	80	34%

Food and Description	Amount	Fat Grams	Total Calories	% Fat Calories
Garlic & Basil	4 oz	3	80	34%
Hot & Spicy	4 oz	3	70	39%
Parmesan	4 oz	4	90	40%
Sliced Mushrooms	4 oz	3	70	39%
Tomatoes & Herbs	4 oz	3	80	34%
Homestyle				
flavored w/meat	4 oz	2	70	26%
plain	4 oz	2	70	26%
w/ mushrooms	4 oz	2	70	26%
Old World Style				
marinara sauce	4 oz	4	90	40%
plain	4 oz	3	80	34%
w/ meat	4 oz	2	80	23%
w/ mushrooms	4 oz	4	80	45%
w/ extra cheese	4 oz	3	80	34%
w/ extra garlic	4 oz	3	80	34%
Slow Cooked Homestyle				
tomato & herbs	4 oz	5	110	33%
w/meat	4 oz	4	110	33%
w/mushrooms & meat	4 oz	5	110	33%
Thick & Hearty				
flavored w/meat	4 oz	4	120	30%
plain	4 oz	4	110	33%
w/ leaner ground beef	4 oz	4	120	30%
w/ mushrooms	4 oz	4	110	33%
Today's Recipe Pasta Sauce				
Garden Harvest	4 oz	1	50	18%
Tomato Herb	4 oz	1	50	18%
(Weight Watchers)				
Flavored With Meat	⅓ cup	1	45	20%
w/ Mushrooms	⅓ cup	–	35	–
Steak Sauce				
(A-1)	1 Tbs	–	14	–
(Estee)	½ oz	–	15	–
(French's)	1 Tbs	–	16	–
(Maull's)				
Mild	1 Tbs	–	20	–
Regular	1 Tbs	–	20	–
Stir Fry				
(Kikkoman)	1 Tbs	–	18	–
Sweet'n Sour Sauce				
(Chun King)	1.8 oz	–	60	–
(Contadina)	4 oz	3	150	18%
(Kikkoman)	1 Tbs	–	16	–

Food and Description	Amount	Fat Grams	Total Calories	% Fat Calories
(LaChoy)	1 Tbs	–	25	–
(Sauceworks)	1 Tbs	–	25	–
(Tabasco)	½ tsp	–	2	–
Taco (*See also* MEXICAN FOOD)				
(Del Monte)				
Hot	¼ cup	–	15	–
Mild	¼ cup	–	15	–
(Estee)	2 Tbs	–	14	–
(Heinz)				
Medium	1 Tbs	–	6	–
Mild	1 Tbs	–	6	–
(Old El Paso)	2 Tbs	–	10	–
Tartar				
(Golden Dipt)				
Lite	1 Tbs	4	50	72%
Original	1 Tbs	7	70	90%
(Kraft)				
Free	1 Tbs	–	16	–
Original	1 Tbs	5	50	90%
(Sauceworks)				
Natural Lemon & Herb	1 Tbs	8	70	100%
Original	1 Tbs	5	50	90%
(Weight Watchers)	1 Tbs	3	35	77%
Teriyaki	1 Tbs	–	15	–
	1 oz	–	30	–
(Kikkoman)	1 Tbs	–	18	–
Teriyaki Baste and Glaze				
(Kikkoman)	1 Tbs	–	27	–
Tomato-Canned				
(Del Monte)				
Plain	1 cup	1	70	13%
w/Onions	1 cup	1	100	9%
Generic				
Plain	4 oz	–	37	–
w/ Herbs & Cheese	4 oz	2	72	25%
w/ Onions, Green Peppers, & Celery	4 oz	.9	50	6%
w/ Tomato Tidbits	4 oz	.5	39	12%
(Hidden Valley)	7.5 oz	.5	58	8%
(Hunt's)				
Herb	4 oz	4	80	45%
Italian	4 oz	2	60	30%
Special	4 oz	–	35	–
w/ Bits	4 oz	–	30	–
w/ Cheese	4 oz	1	45	20%

Food and Description	Amount	Fat Grams	Total Calories	% Fat Calories
w/ Mushrooms	4 oz	–	25	–
w/Onions	4 oz	–	40	–
Welsh Rarebit Cheese Sauce				
(Snow's)	½ cup	11	170	58%
White Cream Sauce				
canned	4 oz	9	118	69%
homemade				
thin	1 cup	21.8	303	65%
medium	1 cup	31	405	69%
thick	1 cup	39	495	71%
White Lobster Sauce (Progresso)	½ cup	8	120	60%
Worcestershire				
(French's)				
Hickory	1 Tbs	–	8	–
regular	1 Tbs	–	8	–
(Heinz)	1 Tbs	–	10	–
(Lea & Perrin)	1 oz	–	30	–
SAUERKRAUT				
Canned				
(Del Monte) canned	½ cup	–	25	–
Generic	½ cup	–	22	–
Jar				
(Vlasic) Old Fashioned	1 oz	–	4	–
SAUERKRAUT DISHES				
Pierogi (dumpling) frozen (Mrs. T's)	1	–	60	–
SAUERKRAUT JUICE				
Canned				
Generic	10 oz	–	28	–
(S&W)	5 oz	–	14	–
SAUSAGE (*See also* LUNCHEON MEAT)				
Beef Breakfast Strips (Sizzlean)	2 strips	5	70	64%
Cooked-smoked	1 oz	7.6	89	77%
(Eckrich) Brown 'N Serve-beef	1 link	12	120	90%
Pork Sausage				
brown & serve	1 link/			
	~ 1 oz	5	50	90%
country style-raw	1 patty/			
	2 oz	22.97	238	87%
	1 link/			
	1 oz	11	118	84%
cooked	1 patty/			
	1 oz	8	100	72%
	1 link/			
	.5 oz	8	96	75%

Food and Description	Amount	Fat Grams	Total Calories	% Fat Calories
fresh-link-cooked	1 oz	11	118	84%
fresh-patty-cooked	1 oz	8	100	72%
(Jimmy Dean) 16 oz pkg-all flavors	1 patty	13	140	84%
Light-turkey & pork	1 oz	6	80	68%
Skinless links	2 links	17	180	85%
Square patties	1 patty	13	140	84%
Links/frozen (Schwan's)	1 oz	10	110	82%
Little Sizzlers (Hormel) cooked	2 sausages	9	103	79%
Midget Links (Hormel) cooked	2 sausages	7	143	44%
Patties/frozen (Schwan's)	2 oz	23	240	86%
(Swift)				
Premium brown'n serve smoke-flavored	1 link	11	120	83%
Premium brown'n serve microwave links	1 link	12	120	90%
Lite	1 link	6	90	60%
Premium brown'n serve country recipe links	1 link	12	130	83%
Lite	2 links	11	120	83%
Premium brown'n serve country recipe patties	1 pattie	12	130	83%
Premium brown'n serve links w/bacon	1 link	11	120	83%
Premium brown'n serve links w/ham	1 link	13	130	90%
Premium brown'n serve maple-flavored links	1 link	12	120	90%
Lite	1 link	5	60	75%
Premium brown'n serve original Lite Links	1 link	5	60	75%
Premium brown'n serve original patties	1 pattie	12	120	90%
Smoked Link-4" long-1⅛" dia	1 link	21.59	265	73%
2" long-¾" dia	1 link	5	62	73%
Whole Hog (Tyson Country Pork)	3.5 oz	29	320	82%
SAVORY/ground	1 tsp	–	4	–
SCALLION	5-5" pieces	–	45	–
SCALLOP (See also SEAFOOD ENTREE/DINNER)				
Mixed				
breaded & fried	2 large/ ~ 1 oz	3	67	40%
imitation	3 oz	< 1	85	5%
raw	3 oz	.6	75	7%
SCONE (See ROLLS)				

Food and Description	Amount	Fat Grams	Total Calories	% Fat Calories
SCOTCH (*See* LIQUOR, DISTILLED)				
SCOTCH BROTH (*See* SOUP)				
SCROD (*See* SEAFOOD ENTREE/DINNER)				
SCUP/raw	3 oz	2	90	20%
SEA BASS				
breaded & fried	3 oz	7	176	36%
cooked-dry heat	3 oz	2	105	17%
raw	3 oz	1.7	82	19%
SEA SALT	1 tsp	–	–	–
SEA TROUT/raw	3 oz	3	88	31%
SEAFOOD CHOWDER (*See* SOUP)				

SEAFOOOD ENTREE/DINNER (*See also* FROZEN ENTREE/DINNER)
(NOTE: Serving sizes for box dishes are for prepared portions. The homemade dishes included here are not made with low-fat substitutes.The data listed can vary, pending the type and amount of certain ingredients used.These data are to be used as a viable guide for the same dish you might make in your home. The same goes for the commercial box mixes—the data may vary slightly, pending on the fat and calorie content of the seafood used in preparation.)

Food and Description	Amount	Fat Grams	Total Calories	% Fat Calories
(Booth) frozen				
Block				
Atlantic Flounder	4 oz	1	90	10%
Atlantic Sole	4 oz	1	90	10%
Cod	4 oz	1	89	10%
Ocean Catfish	4 oz	3	115	24%
Ocean Perch	4 oz	1	100	9%
Whiting	4 oz	1	100	9%
Fishburgers	3 oz	9	170	48%
(Fisherboy)				
fish nuggets	2 oz	10	160	56%
fish portions	2 oz	7	130	49%
fish sticks	2.4 oz	11	190	52%
Individually Wrapped Fillets				
Cod	4 oz	1	90	10%
Flounder	4 oz	–	90	–
Haddock	4 oz	–	90	
Perch	4 oz	1	100	9%
Whiting	4 oz	1	80	11%
Clam Fritter				
homemade	1/~1.5 oz	6	124	44%
Clams				
Frozen-breaded & fried				
(Mrs. Paul's)	2.5 oz	13	240	49%
Clams, Crunchy Strips-frozen				
(Gorton's)	3.5 oz	22	330	60%

Food and Description	Amount	Fat Grams	Total Calories	% Fat Calories
Cod				
Baked Scrod				
Microwave w/ toasted bread crumbs				
frozen (Gorton's)	6 oz	18	320	51%
Fillet of/ Frozen				
(Booth Light Entree)				
Au Gratin	9.5 oz	11	280	35%
Mushroom	9.5 oz	11	280	35%
Fillets				
Microwave/crunchy-frozen	1 fillet	22	330	60%
Crab				
cakes				
fried in margarine-homemade	1/~4 oz	10.8	203	48%
Deviled				
canned	4.5 oz	13	252	46%
homemade	½ cup	12	185	58%
Stuffed				
homemade	½ cup	4	86	42%
Fillet Almondine				
frozen (Gorton's)	5.5 oz	25	350	64%
Fish Cakes				
frozen	1 reg size or 5 bite size	10.7	162	59%
homemade-fried	1 reg size or 5 bite size	4.8	103	42%
Fish Fillets in Buttery Herb Sauce				
frozen-microwave (Gorton's)	6.25 oz	8	190	38%
Fish Loaf-homemade	~ 5 oz	5.6	186	27%
Fish'N Chips-frozen (Swanson)	6.5 oz	18	370	44%
Fish'N Fries-frozen (Swanson)	6.5 oz	17	350	44%
Fish Nuggets-frozen (Swanson)	9.5 oz	19	410	42%
Fish Sticks-frozen (4"x2"x½")	1 stick	3	76	36%
(Frionor) frozen - uncooked unless otherwise noted				
Batter Fried Deep Fry				
2 oz Cod Wedge	4 oz	10	210	43%
fried	4 oz	13	250	47%
Batter Fried Oven Ready				
2 oz Cod Wedge	4 oz	11	220	45%
3 oz Cod Wedge	3 oz	8	160	45%
4 oz Cod Long	4 oz	10	210	43%
4 oz Cod Rectangle	4 oz	10	210	43%
3 oz Pollock Wedge	3 oz	8	170	42%
4 oz Pollock Wedge	4 oz	11	220	45%
2 oz Whiting Wedge	4 oz	11	230	43%

Food and Description	Amount	Fat Grams	Total Calories	% Fat Calories
3 oz Whiting Wedge	3 oz	8	170	42%
4 oz Whiting Rectangle	4 oz	7	160	39%
Breaded Precooked				
1 oz Cod Stick, Grade A	4 oz	9	210	39%
3 oz Cod Rectangle, Grade A	3 oz	7	150	42%
3 oz Cod Rectangle	3 oz	8	180	40%
3.2 oz Cod Rectangle, Grade A	3.2 oz	6	140	39%
3.6 oz Cod Rectangle, Grade A	3.6 oz	7	160	39%
4 oz Cod Rectangle, Grade A	4 oz	9	200	41%
1 oz Minced Cod Stick	4 oz	9	210	39%
3 oz Minced Cod Rectangle	3 oz	7	160	39%
1 oz Haddock Stick, Grade A	4 oz	9	210	39%
3 oz Haddock Rectangle, Grade A	3 oz	8	180	40%
3 oz Haddock Rectangle	3 oz	7	130	49%
3 oz Pollock Rectangle	3 oz	8	180	40%
4 oz Pollock Rectangle, Grade A	4 oz	10	230	39%
3 oz Whiting Rectangle, Grade A	3 oz	7	160	39%
3.6 oz Whiting Rectangle, Grade A	3.6 oz	7	160	39%
3 oz Great Silver Smelt Rectangle	3 oz	6	150	36%
Fancy Stuffed Flounder				
9 oz stuffed w/broccoli, cheese, & lobster	9 oz	13	270	43%
9 oz stuffed w/crabmeat	9 oz	16	330	44%
Fishfries				
1.25 oz Country Style Alaska Pollock	3.75 oz	–	120	–
1.25 oz Country Style Cod	3.75 oz	–	130	–
1.25 oz Santa Fe Style Alaska Pollock	3.75 oz	–	120	–
1.25 oz Santa Fe Style Cod	3.75 oz	–	120	–
1.25 oz Southern Cornmeal Style Alaska Pollock	3.75 oz	–	120	–
Fishfries, Golden Broil				
5 oz Cod Fillet Shape	5 oz	8	170	42%
3 oz Cod Tail-r-Cut	3 oz	5	110	41%
4.5 oz Cod Tail-r-Cut	4.5 oz	7	160	39%
Fishfries, Gourmet Raw Breaded				
3 oz Cod Fillet Shape	3 oz	–	110	–
fried	3 oz	9	190	43%
Fishfries, Honey Granola Crunch				
1 oz Alaska Pollock Nugget	4 oz	20	340	53%
3 oz Alaska Pollock Rectangle	3 oz	11	200	50%
1 oz Cod Nugget	4 oz	21	340	56%
3 oz Cod Rectangle	3 oz	16	260	55%

Food and Description	Amount	Fat Grams	Total Calories	% Fat Calories
1 oz Whiting Nugget	4 oz	20	340	53%
3 oz Whiting Rectangle	3 oz	14	240	53%
Fishfries, Microwaveable fully cooked				
Fish Sandwich w/cheese	5 oz	17	330	46%
2.5 oz	2.5 oz	5	130	35%
3 oz	3 oz	6	150	36%
Fishfries, Norwegian Fish Fillets				
Cod Fillets	4 oz	–	70	–
Salmon Sides	4 oz	10	180	50%
Fishfries, Oven Crispy				
1 oz Cod Triangle Nugget	4 oz	11	220	45%
2 oz Cod Wedge	4 oz	9	210	39%
3 oz Cod Wedge	3 oz	7	160	39%
3 oz Great Silver Smelt Wedge	3 oz	7	160	39%
2 oz Whiting Wedge	4 oz	9	210	39%
3 oz Whiting Wedge	3 oz	7	170	37%
3.6 oz Whiting Wedge	3.6 oz	9	190	43%
3.6 oz Whiting Rectangle	3.6 oz	9	190	43%
Fishfries, Oven Crispy Crunchy				
.5 oz Bunch O'Crunch minced Cod Nugget	2.5 oz	13	200	59%
.67 oz Bunch O'Crunch minced Cod Stick	2.7 oz	15	230	59%
1 oz Cod Nugget	4 oz	11	240	41%
1 oz Cod Select Nugget	4 oz	13	240	49%
1 oz Great Silver Smelt Nugget	4 oz	11	220	45%
1 oz Whiting Nugget	4 oz	11	210	47%
1 oz Whiting Select Nugget	4 oz	14	250	50%
Fishfries, Oven Crispy Fish & Cheese				
3.6 oz Cod'N Cheese Rectangle	3.6 oz	15	250	54%
Fishfries, Raw Breaded				
3 oz Cod Rectangle, Grade A	3 oz	–	120	–
fried	3 oz	11	200	50%
4 oz Cod Tail-r-Cut	4 oz	–	160	–
fried	4 oz	12	240	45%
5⅓ Cod Tail-r-Cut	5⅓ oz	–	210	–
fried	5⅓ oz	18	350	46%
Fishfries, Raw Unbreaded				
4 oz Cod English Cut, Glazed, Grade A	4 oz	–	70	–
4 oz Cod Rectangle	4 oz	–	70	–
12.66 Cod Nordic Cut	4 oz	–	70	–
25.6 oz Cod Shim	4 oz	–	70	–

Food and Description	Amount	Fat Grams	Total Calories	% Fat Calories
4 oz Haddock English Cut, Glazed	4 oz	–	70	–
12.66 oz Haddock Nordic Cut	4 oz	–	70	–
Fishfries, Shellfish				
Norwegian Shrimp	4 oz	1	100	9%
Fishfries, Tender Crisp				
3 oz Cod Fillet Shape	3 oz	–	110	–
fried	3 oz	12	200	54%
(Gorton's)				
Frozen				
Crispy Batter Sticks	4 sticks	14	210	60%
Crispy Batter Fillets	2 fillets	20	300	60%
Crunchy Fish Sticks	4 sticks	15	220	61%
Crunchy Fish Fillets	2 fillets	20	320	56%
Fishmarket Fresh				
cod	5 oz	1	110	8%
flounder	5 oz	1	110	8%
haddock	5 oz	1	110	8%
ocean perch	5 oz	3	140	19%
sole	5 oz	1	110	8%
Light Recipe				
Lightly Breaded Fillets	1 fillet	7	170	37%
Tempura Fish Fillets	1 fillet	12	190	57%
Microwave				
Crunch Whole Shrimp	5 oz	20	380	47%
Fillets-2 larger cut	1 fillet	22	330	60%
Fish Sticks	6 sticks	22	340	58%
Fish Fillets	2 fillets	26	350	67%
Haddock in Lemon Butter	1 pkg	19	320	53%
Shrimp Scampi	1 pkg	24	350	62%
Stuffed Flounder	1 pkg	15	300	45%
Sole in Lemon Butter	1 pkg	19	320	53%
Value Pack				
Fish Portion	1 fillet	11	180	55%
Fish Sticks	4 sticks	11	210	47%
(Healthy Choice) breaded				
Frozen				
2 Fillets	3.5 oz	5	160	34%
4 Fillets	3 oz	4	140	26%
8 Fillets	2.5 oz	4	120	30%
8 Sticks	2.4 oz	4	120	30%
16 Sticks	2.4 oz	4	120	30%
24 Sticks	2.4 oz	4	120	30%
Jambalaya				
homemade	1 cup	6.7	250	24%

Food and Description	Amount	Fat Grams	Total Calories	% Fat Calories
(Kibun & Kibun Gold) frozen				
Dill Sauce & Fish	10 oz	5	280	16%
Mediterranean Fish	10 oz	1	230	4%
Piccata	10 oz	25	470	48%
Primavera	10 oz	19	360	48%
Sea Pasta Pacific Fish & Shrimp				
w/ dressing	½ pkg	9	210	39%
w/o dressing	½ pkg.	1	140	6%
Sea Stix	4 oz	< 1	110	4%
Sea Tails	4 oz	< 1	110	4%
Seafood Fettucini Alfredo	10 oz	11	330	30%
Seafood Linguini	10 oz	6	260	21%
Seafood Marinara	11 oz	2	240	8%
Seafood Newburg	10 oz	7	300	21%
Seafood Piccata	1 serving	21	450	42%
Seafood Primivera	1 serving	7	300	21%
(Lean Cuisine) frozen entrees				
Filet of Fish Divan	10⅜ oz	5	210	21%
Tuna Lasagna	9.75 oz	7	240	26%
Lobster Newburg-homemade	~ 6.5 oz	35	455	69%
(Mrs. Paul's) frozen				
Au Natural				
Cod Fillets	5 oz	2	110	16%
Flounder Fillets	5 oz	2	110	16%
Haddock Fillets	5 oz	2	110	16%
Perch Fillets	5 oz	2	110	16%
Sole Fillets	5 oz	2	110	16%
Healthy Treasures				
Breaded Fillets	4 oz	3	170	16%
Light Fillets				
Cod	1 fillet	11	240	41%
Flounder	1 fillet	10	240	38%
Haddock	1 fillet	9	220	25%
Sole	1 fillet	10	240	38%
Light Seafood Entrees				
Fish Dijon	8¾ oz	5	200	23%
Fish Florentine	8 oz	8	220	33%
Fish Mornay	9 oz	10	230	39%
Seafood Lasagna	9.5 oz	8	290	25%
Seafood Rotini	9 oz	6	240	26%
Shrimp & Clams w/Linguini	10 oz	5	240	19%
Prepared Seafoods				
Batter Dipped Fish Fillets	2 fillets	17	330	37%
Battered Fish Portions	2 portions	19	300	57%

Food and Description	Amount	Fat Grams	Total Calories	% Fat Calories
Battered Fish Sticks	4 sticks	12	210	51%
Combination Seafood Platter	9 oz	31	590	47%
Crispy Crunchy Breaded Fish Portions	2 portions	15	230	59%
Crispy Crunchy Breaded Fish Sticks	4 sticks	6	140	39%
Crispy Crunchy Fish Fillets	2 fillets	9	220	51%
Crispy Crunchy Fish Sticks	4 sticks	8	190	45%
Crunch Batter				
Fish Fillets	2 fillets	14	280	45%
Flounder Fillets	2 fillets	9	220	37%
Haddock Fillets	2 fillets	5	190	24%
Deviled Crabs	1 cake	9	180	37%
Deviled Crab Miniatures	3½ oz	12	240	43%
Fish Cakes	2 cakes	7	190	40%
Fried Clams	2.5 oz	9	200	41%
Fried Scallops	3 oz	7	160	35%
Light Fillets in Butter Sauce	1 fillet	6	140	39%
Oyster Stew homemade	1 cup	15	233	58%
Oysters Rockefeller-homemade	4 oysters	2.7	90	27%
Paella homemade-including saffron rice, seafood, & vegetables	~ 8 oz	11	350	28%
Pollack (Mrs. Paul's) Frozen				
Alaskan Batter Dipped Fillets	2 fillets	13	320	37%
Crispy Crunchy Breaded	2 fillets	18	290	56%
Crunchy Batter	3 oz	17	310	49%
Salmon Cake homemade	3.5 oz	15	248	54%
Salmon Casserole homemade	1 cup	35	555	57%
Salmon Patty homemade	3.5 oz	12	239	45%
Salmon Rice Loaf homemade	6 oz	8	212	34%
(Schwan's) frozen				
Batter Crisp-Breaded Cod	2 oz	8	150	48%
Blue Hake Loins	3.5 oz	1	90	10%
Breaded Clam Strips	3.5 oz	11	220	45%
Breaded Fantail Shrimp	3.5 oz	2	210	9%
Breaded Halibut Fillets	4 oz	9	220	37%

Food and Description	Amount	Fat Grams	Total Calories	% Fat Calories
Breaded Round Shrimp	3.5 oz	2	210	9%
Breaded Shrimp Pieces	3.5 oz	2	210	9%
Butterfly Trout Fillets	3.5 oz	7	150	42%
Cajun Style Catfish	3.5 oz	12	180	60%
Catfish Fingers	3.5 oz	13	230	51%
Cod Fillets	3.5 oz	1	70	13%
Cod Fish Nuggets-Breaded	3.5 oz/ 7 nuggets	10	200	45%
Fish 'N Batter-Breaded Haddock	2 oz	8	140	51%
Fancy Seafood Legs	3.5 oz	.5	100	5%
Flounder Fillets	3.5 oz	1	90	10%
Haddock Fillets	3.5 oz	1	90	10%
Haddock Squares-Breaded	4 oz	8	200	36%
Haddock Sticks-Breaded	1 oz	2	60	30%
Halibut Steaks	3.5 oz	2	110	16%
Lobster Tails	3.5 oz	2	110	16%
New England Style Scrod	5 oz	17	280	55%
Ocean Perch	3.5 oz	2	90	20%
Orange Roughy	3.5 oz	7	120	53%
Oven-ready Breaded Shrimp	3.5 oz	1	210	4%
Peeled & De-veined Shrimp	3.5 oz	2	100	18%
Pollock Fillets	3.5 oz	1	90	10%
Red Snapper Steaks	3.5 oz	1	100	9%
Salmon Fillets	5 oz	8	210	34%
Scallops, North Atlantic	3.5 oz	1	90	10%
Shell On Shrimp	3.5 oz	1	90	10%
Slipper Lobster	3.5 oz	1	90	10%
Stuffed Scrod-New England Style	5 oz	15	250	54%
Stuffed Shrimp	2 oz/1 piece	7	150	42%
Stuffed Sole Monterey	6 oz	8	200	36%
Unbreaded Shrimp	3.5 oz	2	100	18%
Walleye Fillets	3.5 oz	2	90	20%
Seafood Creole w/rice frozen (Swanson)	9 oz	6	240	23%
(Seafood Elites) Cole Fillet Frozen				
w/ Broccoli & Mozzarella	1	7	150	42%
w/ Lemon & Wild Rice	1	7	150	42%
w/ Spinach & Cheddar	1	6	130	42%
Seafood Gumbo homemade	5 oz	1	48	19%

Food and Description	Amount	Fat Grams	Total Calories	% Fat Calories
Seafood Linguini				
frozen (Weight Watchers)	9 oz	7	220	29%
Seafood Salad	3½ oz	10	160	56%
Shrimp				
frozen				
(Booth Light Entree)				
Fettucine Alfredo	10 oz	8	260	28%
New Orleans	10 oz	5	230	20%
(Brilliant)				
cooked	2 oz	–	30	–
Shrimp Creole				
homemade w/rice	1 cup	8.7	301	26%
Shrimp Curried				
homemade	¾ cup	11.5	232	45%
Sole				
frozen				
w/ Wine Sauce				
(Gorton's)	6.5 oz	7	180	35%
Sole, Fillet of				
frozen				
(Le Menu)	10 oz	14	360	35%
Tuna Fillets				
(Gorton's Natural Cut)				
25% less fat				
breaded 6 crunchy fillets	2 fillets	14	260	48%
Tuna Helper (Betty Crocker) Prepared				
Buttery Rice 'n Tuna	1 serving	11	280	35%
Creamy Mushroom	1 serving	6	220	25%
Cheesy Noodles'n Tuna	1 serving	8	240	30%
Creamy Noodles 'n Tuna	1 serving	14	300	42%
Fettucini Alfredo	1 serving	13	300	41%
Romanoff	1 serving	8	290	25%
Tuna Au Gratin	1 serving	11	280	35%
Tuna Pot Pie	1 serving	27	420	58%
Tuna Salad	1 serving	27	420	58%
Tuna Tetrazzini	1 serving	8	240	30%
Tuna Loaf, Smoked				
(Neptune) Tunables	1 oz	1.8	40	41%
Tuna Meat Pie, frozen				
(Banquet)	7 oz	33	540	55%
Tuna Noodle Casserole, frozen				
(Swanson's)	9 oz	11	250	40%
Tuna Pattie				
homemade	3 oz	3	80	34%

Food and Description	Amount	Fat Grams	Total Calories	% Fat Calories
(Van de Kamp's) Frozen				
Battered				
Fish Fillets	1 fillet	10	170	53%
Fish Nuggets	4 pieces	9	130	62%
Fish Sticks	4 sticks	9	160	51%
Haddock Fillets	2 fillets	15	250	54%
Halibut Fillets	2 fillets	6	150	36%
Perch Fillets	2 fillets	21	310	61%
Breaded				
Fish Fillets	2 fillets	18	280	58%
Fish Fillets (Snack Pack)	2 fillets	10	220	41%
Fish Sticks	4 sticks	12	200	54%
Fish Sticks (Value Pack)	4 sticks	10	170	53%
Haddock Fillets-oven	2 fillets	16	270	53%
Crisp & Healthy (Baked)				
Breaded Fish Fillets	2 fillets	3	150	18%
Breaded Fish Sticks	4 sticks	2	120	15%
Crispy Microwave				
Fish Fillets	2 fillets	9	140	58%
Fish Sticks	3 sticks	7	130	48%
Large Fillets	1 fillet	17	290	53%
Light Fillets				
Cod	1 fillet	11	250	40%
Flounder	1 fillet	12	260	42%
Haddock	1 fillet	11	240	41%
Ocean Perch	1 fillet	14	280	45%
Sole	1 fillet	12	250	43%
Natural Fillets				
Cod	4 oz	1	90	10%
Flounder	4 oz	2	100	18%
Haddock	4 oz	1	90	10%
Ocean Perch	4 oz	5	130	35%
Sole	4 oz	2	100	18%
SEASONINGS (*See also* individual listings such as PAPRIKA, SAGE, etc.; BAKE & FRY MIX; GRAVY; MEXICAN FOOD; ORIENTAL FOOD SEASONINGS; SAUCE)				
(A Taste of Thai)				
Panang Curry Base Mix				
Dry	1 Tbs	2	25	72%
Red Curry Base Mix				
Dry	1 Tbs	1.5	20	68%
Seasoning Sauce	1 Tbs	–	15	–
Spicy Chicken & Rice				
Seasoning Mix				
Dry	3.5 oz	< 1	236	2%

Food and Description	Amount	Fat Grams	Total Calories	% Fat Calories
(Durkee)				
Beefstew Seasoning				
Mix Only	1 pkg	.5	99	5%
Prepared	8 cups	134	3032	40%
Ground Beef				
Mix Only	1 pkg	.9	91	9%
Prepared	2 cups	97	1037	84%
Ground Beef w/Onions				
Mix Only	1 pkg	.5	102	4%
Prepared	2 cups	96	1318	66%
Hamburger Seasoning				
Mix Only	1 pkg	5	110	41%
Prepared	2 cups	101	1326	69%
Italian Meatball Seasoning				
Mix Only	1 pkg	.7	22	29%
Prepared	2 cups	97	1238	71%
Lemon Roastin' Bag	1 pkg	.7	75	8%
Meat Marinade Sauce Mix				
Prepared	½ cup	.7	47	13%
Meatloaf Roastin' Bag	1 pkg	1	129	8%
Sloppy Joe Seasoning				
Italian				
Mix Only	1 pkg	5	99	45%
Prepared	2.5 cups	102	1492	62%
Original				
Mix Only	1 pkg	< 1	118	4%
Prepared	2.5 cups	97	1453	60%
(French's) Mix				
Beef Stew	⅙ pkg	–	25	–
Chili-O w/Onion Seasoning	⅙ pkg	–	35	–
Fajita Seasoning	⅕ pkg	1	82	11%
Ground Beef w/Onions	¼ pkg	–	25	–
Hamburger	¼ pkg	–	25	–
Meat Marinade	⅛ pkg	–	10	–
Meatball	¼ pkg	–	35	–
Meatloaf	⅛ pkg	–	20	–
Microwave Mixes				
BBQ Chicken	¼ pkg	1	50	18%
Garlic Butter	¼ pkg	2	50	36%
Italian Parmesan	¼ pkg	2	45	40%
Lemon Dill	¼ pkg	1	45	20%
Roastin' Bag				
Au Jus	⅛ pkg	< 1	10	45%
Chicken	⅕ pkg	< 1	25	18%

Food and Description	Amount	Fat Grams	Total Calories	% Fat Calories
Lemon Butter Fish	¼ pkg	< 1	25	18%
Meatloaf	⅙ pkg	< 1	25	18%
Onion Pot Roast	⅛ pkg	< 1	18	25%
Pork	⅙ pkg	< 1	25	18%
Pot Roast	⅛ pkg	< 1	18	25%
Swiss Steak	⅙ pkg	< 1	20	23%
Sloppy Joe Seasoning	⅛ pkg	–	16	–
(Golden Dipt)				
All Purpose Seafood	¼ tsp	–	2	–
Blackened Redfish	¼ tsp	–	2	–
Broiled Fish	¼ tsp	–	2	–
Cajun Style Shrimp & Crab	¼ tsp	–	2	–
Lemon Pepper Seafood	¼ tsp	–	8	–
(Lipton) Microeasy Mix				
Barbeque Style Chicken	¼ pkg	.5	108	4%
Country Style Chicken	¼ pkg	.6	78	7%
Hearty Beef Stew	¼ pkg	.5	70	6%
Homestyle Meatloaf	¼ pkg	1.5	87	16%
(Manwich) Sloppy Joe Mix	⅙ pkg	< 1	20	23%
(McCormick/Schilling) Mix				
Bag'n Season				
Beef Stew	1 pkg	1	87	10%
Chicken	1 pkg	2	122	15%
Country Chicken	1 pkg	5	134	34%
Italian Herb Fish	1 pkg	< 1	94	5%
Lemon & Dill Fish	1 pkg	11	161	61%
Meat Loaf	1 pkg	< 1	111	4%
Oriental Style	1 pkg	8	152	45%
Pork Chops	1 pkg	< 1	102	4%
Pot Roast	1 pkg	< 1	55	8%
Roast Turkey	1 pkg	5	146	31%
Spare Ribs	1 pkg	1.5	185	7%
Swiss Steak	1 pkg	< 1	81	6%
Chicken Blends				
Cacciatore				
Dry	1 pkg	5	132	34%
Prepared	1 serving	35	575	55%
Creamy Curry				
Dry	1 pkg	6	152	36%
Prepared	1 serving	8	237	30%
Creole				
Dry	1 pkg	5	104	43%
Prepared	1 serving	5	229	20%

Food and Description	Amount	Fat Grams	Total Calories	% Fat Calories
Dijon				
Dry	1 pkg	6	151	36%
Prepared	1 serving	8	238	30%
Italian Marinade				
Dry	1 pkg	1	120	8%
Prepared	1 serving	12	324	33%
Mesquite				
Dry	1 pkg	3	132	20%
Prepared	1 serving	41	545	68%
Parmesan				
Dry	1 pkg	7	244	26%
Prepared	1 serving	20	366	49%
Southwest Style				
Dry	1 pkg	1	106	8%
Prepared	1 serving	20	359	50%
Stir Fry				
Dry	1 pkg	–	124	–
Prepared	1 serving	8	237	30%
Sweet & Sour				
Dry	1 pkg	1	204	4%
Prepared	1 serving	5	208	22%
Teriyaki				
Dry	1 pkg	4	172	26%
Prepared	1 serving	6	202	27%
Old Bay Seasoning	~ 3.5 oz	10	182	49%
Seasoning/Sauce Mixes				
Beef Stew	¼ pkg	< 1	33	14%
Beef Stroganoff	¼ pkg	< 1	32	14%
Cheese Sauce	¼ pkg	1.5	35	39%
Chili Seasoning	¼ pkg	< 1	27	17%
Hamburger	¼ pkg	–	33	–
Hollandaise Sauce	¼ pkg	3.8	51	67%
Meat Loaf	¼ pkg	–	38	–
Meat Marinade	¼ pkg	–	28	–
Nacho Cheese	¼ pkg	1.5	42	32%
Sloppy Joe Seasoning	¼ pkg	< 1	26	17%
Sour Cream	¼ pkg	2.75	44	56%
Spaghetti Sauce	¼ pkg	< 1	32	14%
Swedish Meatballs	¼ pkg	1	57	16%
Taco Seasoning	¼ pkg	< 1	31	29%
Spice Blends				
Barbecue Seasoning	¼ tsp	–	< 1	–
Broiled Steak Seasoning	¼ tsp	–	< 1	–
Butter Salt	¼ tsp	–	.5	–

Food and Description	Amount	Fat Grams	Total Calories	% Fat Calories
Chesapeake Bay Seafood Seasoning	¼ tsp	–	2	–
Fried Chicken Seasoning				
Lite	¼ tsp	–	–	–
Original	¼ tsp	–	1	–
Garlic Bread Sprinkle	¼ tsp	< 1	5	90%
Italian Seasoning	¼ tsp	–	1	–
Lemon & Herb	¼ tsp	–	1.5	–
Lemon & Pepper				
Light	¼ tsp	–	–	–
Original	¼ tsp	–	2	–
Mexican Seasoning	¼ tsp	–	–	–
Onion Salt Light	¼ tsp	–	–	–
Salad Supreme	¼ tsp	4	3	–
Salt'n Spice	¼ tsp	–	1	–
Season All				
Garlic	¼ tsp	–	1.5	–
Light	¼ tsp	–	–	–
Original	¼ tsp	–	1	–
Spicy	¼ tsp	–	2	–
Seasoned All Pepper	¼ tsp	–	1.5	–
Seasoning Salt	¼ tsp	–	1	–
(Molly McButter)				
Cheese-flavor sprinkles	½ tsp	–	4	–
Sour Cream-flavor sprinkles	½ tsp	–	4	–
(Shake & Bake)				
Oven Fry Seasoned Coating Mix				
Chicken				
Extra Crispy	¼ pouch	2	190	15%
Homestyle	¼ pouch	2	90	20%
Pork-Extra Crispy	¼ pouch	3	120	23%
Seasoning Mixture				
Country Mild Recipe	¼ pouch	4	80	45%
For Chicken				
Italian Herb Recipe	¼ pouch	1	80	11%
Original Barbecue Recipe	¼ pouch	2	90	20%
Original Recipe	¼ pouch	2	80	23%
For Fish	¼ pouch	1	70	13%
For Pork				
Original Barbecue Recipe	¼ pouch	2	80	23%
Original Recipe	¼ pouch	2	80	23%
Italian Herb	¼ pouch	1	80	11%
SEAWEED				
Agar				
dried	3 oz	< 1	260	2%

Food and Description	Amount	Fat Grams	Total Calories	% Fat Calories
raw	3 oz	< 1	23	20%
Kelp/raw	3 oz	.6	37	15%
Laver	3 oz	< 1	31	15%
Spirulina				
dried	3 oz	6.6	249	24%
raw	3 oz	< 1	22	21%
Wakame/raw	3 oz	< 1	40	11%
SELTZER WATER (See WATER)				
SESAME BUTTER	1 oz	15	169	80%
Tahini	2 Tbs	16	180	80%
Toasted	2 Tbs	20	200	90%
SESAME FLOUR				
high fat	4 oz	42	595	64%
low fat	4 oz	2	380	5%
partially defatted	4 oz	14	440	29%
SESAME NUT MIX				
(Planters)				
dry roasted	1 oz	12	160	68%
oil roasted	1 oz	13	160	73%
SESAME SEEDS				
dried				
ground	1 tsp	–	5	–
kernels	1 Tbs	4	47	77%
whole	1 Tbs	4.5	52	78%
kernels-toasted	1 oz	13.6	161	76%
	1 cup	80	873	83%
whole roasted & toasted	1 oz	13.6	161	76%
SHAD/American				
cooked-dry heat	3 oz	9.6	171	51%
raw	3 oz	11.7	167	63%
roe-raw	3 oz	1.7	111	14%
SHALLOT/raw	1 Tbs	–	7	–
SHARK				
batter dipped & fried	3 oz	11.75	194	55%
raw	3 oz	3.8	111	31%
SHEEPSHEAD				
cooked-dry heat	3 oz	1	107	8%
raw	3 oz	2	92	20%
SHELLIE BEAN/canned	½ cup	–	37	–
Sprouts (La Choy)	⅔ cup	–	8	–
SHERBET	1 cup	4	270	13%
(Borden) orange	½ cup	1	110	8%
(Dreyer's) all flavors-data averaged	½ cup	1	110	8%
(Pet) orange	½ cup	1	130	7%

Food and Description	Amount	Fat Grams	Total Calories	% Fat Calories
(Sealtest)				
Orange	½ cup	1	130	7%
Rainbow	½ cup	1	130	7%
Strawberry	½ cup	1	130	7%
(Thrifty)				
Apricot Mango	½ cup	1	130	7%
Rainbow	½ cup	1	120	8%
SHORTENING/vegetable (*See also* FAT, LARD, OIL)				
(Crisco) Regular & Butter	1 Tbs	12	113	100%
	1 cup	205	1810	100%
Generic-Soybean/Cottonseed	1 Tbs	13	113	100%
	1 cup	205	1812	100%
(Snowdrift)	1 Tbs	12	110	100%
(Wesson)	1 Tbs	12	100	100%
SHRIMP (*See also* SEAFOOD ENTREE/DINNER)				
breaded & fried	3 oz	10	206	44%
	4 large/			
	~ 1 oz	3.68	73	45%
canned	4 large	1.67	102	15%
	1 cup	3	155	17%
canned-deveined-medium/whole (S&W)	2 oz	–	65	–
cooked-moist heat	3 oz	.9	84	10%
	4 large/			
	~ 1 oz	–	22	–
dried	1 oz	.8	82	9%
imitation (from surimi)	3 oz	1	86	10%
paste	3 oz	8	155	47%
raw	3 oz	1	90	10%
SHRIMP SALAD/homemade	¾ cup	11.9	210	51%
SHRIMP SOUP, CREAM OF (*See* SOUP)				
SLOPPY JOE SAUCE (*See* SAUCE; SEASONINGS)				
SMELT				
Rainbow				
breaded & fried	3 oz	10.6	214	45%
cooked-dry heat	3 oz	2.6	106	22%
raw		3 oz	2	83
SMOKED SALMON (*See* SALMON, SMOKED)				
SNACK BARS (*See* GRANOLA/GRANOLA-TYPE BARS)				
SNACK CAKES (*See also* CAKE AND CAKE PASTRY; RICE CAKES)				
(Angela Marie's)				
Marshmallow Munchies Squares	1 square	1.6	70	21%
(Aunt Fanny's)				
Cakes				
Applesauce	2.5 oz	7	234	27%

Food and Description	Amount	Fat Grams	Total Calories	% Fat Calories
Chocolate Fudge	2.5 oz	6	222	24%
Pound	2.5 oz	9	260	31%
Cupcakes-Orange	3 oz	12	334	32%
Fingers				
Devil's Food	3 oz	9	288	28%
Raspberry	3 oz	9	303	27%
Spice	3 oz	9	290	28%
Vanilla	3 oz	9	250	32%
Twirls				
Cinnamon	1 oz	4	110	33%
Pecan (2 twirls)	2 oz	8	210	34%
(Break Cake)				
Angle Food Cake	1 cake	–	70	–
Apple Sandwich Cakes	1-1.83 oz	3	90	30%
Apple Sweet Rolls	2 rolls	5	380	12%
(Multi-Pak)	1-1.43 oz	2	120	15%
Banana Creme	1-2 oz	9	240	34%
Carrot Cake	2 cakes	12	370	29%
(Multi-Pak)	1-1.08 oz	4	120	30%
Cherry Sweet Rolls	2 rolls	6	400	14%
(Multi-Pak)	1-1.43 oz	2	130	14%
Chocolate Cup Cakes				
(Multi-Pak)	1-1.33 oz	4	130	28%
Chocolate Rounds	2 rounds	16	390	37%
(Multi-Pak)	1-1.33 oz	7	160	39%
Cinnamon Nut Rolls	2 rolls	11	330	30%
Cinnamon Sweet Rolls	2 rolls	10	420	21%
(Multi-Pak)	1-1.33 oz	3	120	23%
Dessert Sets	1 cup	1	100	9%
Filled Twins	2 twins	10	310	29%
(Multi-Pak)	1-1.5 oz	5	150	30%
Fried Pies	2 pies	19	410	42%
Honey Buns	1 bun	28	420	60%
(Multi-Pak)	1-2.75 oz	25	380	59%
Oatmeal Creme	1-1.13 oz	5	140	32%
Pecan Sweet Rolls				
(Multi-Pak)	1-1.31 oz	3	120	23%
Raisin Cinnamon Sweet				
Rolls (Multi-Pak)	1-1.25 oz	3	120	23%
100's				
Chocolate cup cakes	1	2	100	18%
Cinnamon Streusel	1	2	100	18%
Peanut Butter Creme	1-2 oz	9	240	34%
Raisin Creme	1-2 oz	9	240	34%

Food and Description	Amount	Fat Grams	Total Calories	% Fat Calories
Raspberry Sandwich Cakes	1-1.83 oz	3	100	27%
Cupcakes				
chocolate				
(Break Cake)	2 cakes	9	350	13%
homemade-plain	1	5	103	44%
homemade-chocolate frosting	1	8	175	41%
white				
homemade-plain	1	5	114	35%
homemade-chocolate frosting	1	8	186	39%
homemade-white frosting	1	6	165	33%
yellow				
homemade-plain	1	5	125	36%
homemade-chocolate frosting	1	8	195	37%
Devil's food w/creme filling	1 cake	4	105	34%
(Dolly Madison)				
Blue Ribbon Creme Filled	1 cake	3	90	30%
Creme Zinger	1 cake	3	90	30%
Pecan Roller	1 roll	5	120	38%
Raspberry Zinger	1 cake	5	130	35%
White Zinger	1 cake	4	140	26%
Yellow Zinger	1 cake	4	140	26%
(Drake's)				
All Butter Pound Cake	1 pkg	12	270	40%
Chocolate Chip Cookies	1 pkg	12	280	39%
Coconut Cookies	1 pkg	10	260	35%
Coconut Macaroons	1 pkg	7	135	47%
Coffee Cake (small)	1 pkg	9	250	32%
Devil Dogs	1 pkg	16	360	40%
Fig Bars	1 pkg	18	380	43%
Fudge Brownies	1 pkg	15	380	36%
Funny Bones	1 pkg	16	300	48%
Oatmeal Cookies	1 pkg	8	240	30%
Oatmeal Creme Cookies	1 pkg	9	240	34%
Old Fashioned Brownie Bars	1 pkg	6	320	17%
Peanut Butter Wafers	1 pkg	16	325	44%
Pies				
Apple	1 pkg	20	420	43%
Blueberry	1 pkg	20	420	43%
Cherry	1 pkg	20	440	41%
Lemon	1 pkg	22	420	47%
Ring Ding	1 pkg	20	360	50%
Sunny Doodle	1 pkg	9	300	27%
Yankee Doodle	1 pkg	12	300	36%
Yodel	1 pkg	18	300	54%

Food and Description	Amount	Fat Grams	Total Calories	% Fat Calories
(Hostess)				
Big Wheels	1 cake	10	173	52%
Brownie Bites				
Plain	5 pieces	15	260	52%
Walnut	5 pieces	15	260	52%
Choco Bliss	1 cake	9	200	41%
Choco Diles	1 cake	11	240	41%
Chocolate Cupcakes	1 cake	8	170	42%
Cookie Cakes, Chocolate Chipe	5 cakes	13	250	47%
Crumb Cake	1 cake	4	160	23%
Crumb Coffee Cakes				
Cinnamon, 97% Fat Free	1 cake	1	80	11%
Original	1 cake	5	120	38%
Cupcakes				
Chocolate	1 cake	6	180	30%
Chocolate, Lights w/cream filling	1 cake	2	130	14%
Devil's Food	1 cake	4	136	27%
Orange	1 cake	5	160	28%
Dessert Cups	1 cake	2	90	20%
Ding Dongs	1 cake	9	170	48%
Fruit Loaf	1	9	400	20%
Grizzly Chomps				
Chocolate, 97% Fat Free	1 cake	1	110	8%
Vanilla, 97% Fat Free	1 cake	1	110	8%
Ho Ho's	1 cake	6	130	42%
Hostess O's	1 cake	8	220	33%
Lights				
Apple Spice	1.5 oz	1	130	7%
Chocolate				
w/chocolatey frosting	1.25 oz	1	110	8%
	1.5 oz	1	130	7%
w/vanilla pudding	1.25 oz	1	110	8%
	1.5 oz	1	140	6%
Raspberry Filled	1.5 oz	1	130	7%
Lil' Angels	1 cake	2	90	20%
Pudding Cakes	1 cake	4	170	21%
Snoball	1 cake	4	150	24%
Suzy Q's	1 cake	10	250	36%
Banana	1 cake	9	240	34%
Chocolate	1 cake	8	250	29%
Tiger Tails	1 cake	8	140	30%
Twinkies				
Banana	1 cake	5	150	30%

Food and Description	Amount	Fat Grams	Total Calories	% Fat Calories
Fruit N Creme, Strawberry	1 cake	3	140	19%
Lights	1 cake	2	110	16%
Original	1 cake	5	150	30%
(Little Debbie)				
Apple Coffee Cakes	1 piece	3	110	25%
Apple Delights	1 piece	8	160	45%
Apple Spice Snack	1 piece	9	150	54%
Appleroos	1 package/ 2 squares	4	160	23%
Baked Apple Pies	3 oz	9	310	23%
Banana Twins	1 piece	6	140	39%
Cake Mates	1 piece	8	170	42%
Choc-O-Jel	1 piece	10	170	53%
Chocolate Chip Snack	1 piece	16	320	45%
Chocolate Twins	1 piece	6	130	42%
Christmas Treecakes	1 piece	11	220	45%
Coconut Cakes	1 piece	18	310	52%
Coconut Rounds	1 piece	10	170	53%
Coffee Cake	1 piece	3	110	25%
Debbie Doodle Dandies	1 piece	16	320	45%
Devil Cremes	1 pkg/1.4 oz	8	170	42%
Devil Squares	1 piece	9	150	54%
Dutch Crisp	1 piece	6	100	54%
Fancy Cakes	1 piece	8	160	45%
Figaroos	1 piece	4	160	23%
Fudge Crispy	1 piece	11	180	55%
Fudge Rounds	1 piece/ 1.19 oz	5	150	36%
	1 piece/ 3.0 oz	13	370	32%
Lemon Stix	1 piece	6	110	49%
Marshmallow Supremes	1 piece	4	130	28%
Mint Sprints	1 piece	8	120	60%
Nutty Bar	1 piece	10	160	56%
Oatmeal II	1 piece	4	150	24%
Oatmeal Creme Pies	1.35 oz	8	170	42%
	3 oz	18	390	42%
Peanut Butter & Jelly Sandwich	1 piece	7	150	42%
Peanut Butter Bars	1 piece	9	150	54%
Peanut Cluster	1 piece	10	200	45%
Raisin Creme Pie	1 piece	9	160	51%
Snack Cakes-chocolate	1 piece	10	170	53%
Snack Cakes-chocolate chip	1 piece	8	160	39%
Snack Cakes-vanilla	1 piece	11	180	55%

Food and Description	Amount	Fat Grams	Total Calories	% Fat Calories
Star Crunch	1 piece	7	150	42%
Swiss Cake Rolls	1 piece	6	130	42%
Teddy Berries	1 piece	5	140	32%
Vanilla Cremes	1 piece	8	170	42%
(Sara Lee)				
All Butter Pound	1 cake	11	200	50%
Chocolate Fudge	1 cake	10	190	47%
Classic Cheesecake	1 cake	14	200	63%
Deluxe Carrot Cake	1 cake	7	180	35%
(Tastykake)				
Banana Treats	1	4	147	25%
Brownie	1 piece	14	340	37%
Chocolate Chip Bar	1 piece	8	190	38%
Creamie				
Banana	1 piece	7	170	37%
Chocolate	1 piece	8	170	42%
Vanilla	1 piece	9	180	45%
Cupcakes				
Butter Cream	1 piece	4	120	30%
Chocolate				
Cream Filled	1 piece	4	120	30%
Plain	1 piece	3	100	27%
Vanilla	1 piece	3	116	23%
Fudge Bar	1 piece	7	200	32%
Honey Bun				
Glazed	1 piece	20	360	50%
Iced	1 piece	15	350	39%
Honey Lemon Bar	1 piece	7	190	33%
Junior				
Chocolate	1 piece	12	340	32%
Coconut	1 piece	6	300	18%
Koffee Kake	1 piece	8	260	28%
Lemon	1 piece	7	310	20%
Orange	1 piece	9	340	24%
Kandy Kake				
Chocolate	1 piece	3	80	34%
Coconut	1 piece	4	80	45%
Peanut Butter	1 piece	4	90	40%
Koffee Kakes-Cream Filled	1 piece	4	110	33%
Kreme Kup	1 piece	3	90	30%
Krimpet				
Butterscotch	1 piece	3	100	27%
Chocolate Cream Filled	1 piece	4	142	25%
Jelly	1 piece	1	90	10%

Food and Description	Amount	Fat Grams	Total Calories	% Fat Calories
Strawberry	1 piece	2	100	18%
Vanilla Cream Filled	1 piece	4	139	26%
Muffins				
Banana Nut, Mini	1 piece	3	60	45%
Blueberry, Mini	1 piece	3	50	54%
Carrot/Raisin/Nut, Mini	1 piece	3	60	45%
English				
Cinnamon Raisin	1 piece	1	150	6%
Sourdough	1 piece	1	130	7%
Traditional	1 piece	1	130	7%
Oatmeal Raisin Bar	1 piece	8	210	34%
Pastry Pockets				
Apple	1 piece	18	320	51%
Cheese	1 piece	19	330	52%
Cherry	1 piece	17	330	46%
Pecan Twirls	1 piece	5	110	41%
Royal Chocolate Cupcake	1 piece	7	170	37%
Soft'n Chewy				
Chocolate Chip	1 piece	7	170	37%
Chocolate, Chocolate Chip	1 piece	7	170	37%
Oatmeal Raisin	1 piece	5	160	28%
Tasty Twist	1 piece	1	18	20%
Tastylite				
Chocolate Creme Filled	1 piece	1	100	9%
Vanilla Creme Filled	1 piece	1	100	9%
Vanilla Sugar Wafer	1 piece	2	35	51%
SNACK CRACKERS (*See* CRACKERS)				
SNACK MIX				
(Lawry's) Flavor Tree-Party Mix	¼ cup	11	163	61%
no salt	¼ cup	10.8	163	60%
(Pepperidge Farm)				
Classic	1 oz	8	140	51%
Lightly Smoked	1 oz	9	150	54%
Spicy	1 oz	8	140	51%
(Ralston) Chex Mix Brand				
Golden Cheddar	1 oz	5	130	35%
Snackn' Bag				
Barbeque	1 oz	5	130	35%
Golden Cheddar Cheese	1 oz	5	130	35%
Sour Cream & Onion	1 oz	5	130	35%
Sour Cream & Onion	1 oz	5	130	35%
Traditional	1 oz	5	120	38%
(Sunshine)				
Cheez-it Party Mix	1 oz	5	130	30%

Food and Description	Amount	Fat Grams	Total Calories	% Fat Calories
SNACKS (*See also* CRACKERS, FRUIT SNACKS, MEXICAN FOOD, POPCORN, POTATO CHIPS, POTATO SNACKS, PRETZELS, RICE CAKES, TORTILLA CHIPS)				
(Borden) Fox Z Doodle O's				
Cheese Corn Puffs	1 oz	10	160	56%
(Bugles)				
Nacho Cheese	1 oz	9	160	51%
Plain	1 oz	8	150	48%
Ranch	1 oz	9	150	54%
Carrot Chips (Hain)				
Barbecue	1 oz	8	140	51%
Plain	1 oz	9	150	54%
No salt added	1 oz	9	150	54%
(Cheetos)				
Cheddar Valley	1 oz	9	160	51%
Crunchy	1 oz	9	150	54%
Curls	1 oz	9	150	54%
Flamin' Hot	1 oz	9	150	54%
Light Cheese Flavored-Crunchy	1 oz	6	140	39%
Paws	1 oz	10	160	56%
Puffed Balls	1 oz	10	160	56%
Puffs	1 oz	9	160	51%
(Combos) Cracker Cheddar Cheese	1 oz	8	150	48%
Nacho Cheese	1 oz	6	130	42%
Peanut Butter	1 oz	9	150	54%
Pizza-Cheese	1 oz	5	130	35%
Extra Cheese	1 oz	7	140	45%
Pepperoni	1 oz	7	140	45%
Pretzel	1 oz	6	130	42%
Corn cake (*See* POPCORN SNACK CAKE)				
(Cornnuts)				
Barbecue	1 oz	4	110	33%
Cheddar Cheese	1 oz	4	110	33%
Original	1 oz	4	120	30%
(Crunch'N Munch)				
Candied	1.25 oz	7	170	37%
Caramel	1.25 oz	5	160	28%
Maple Walnut	1.25 oz	6	160	34%
Toffee	1.25 oz	5	160	28%
(Eagle)				
Cheese Crunch	1 oz	10	160	56%
Mexican Snack Mix	1 oz	9	160	51%
(Featherweight)				
Cheese Curls	1 oz	9	150	54%
(Funyuns) Onion-Flavored Rings	1 oz	7	140	45%

Food and Description	Amount	Fat Grams	Total Calories	% Fat Calories
(Guy's) Tasty Mix	1 oz	7	130	49%
(Health Valley)				
Puffs				
Carrot Lites	½ oz	4	75	48%
Cheddar Lites	¼ oz	2	40	45%
Cheddar Lites w/Green Onion	¼ oz	2	40	45%
Fat-Free				
Caramel Corn Puffs				
Apple Cinnamon	1 oz	< 1	100	5%
Original	1 oz	< 1	100	5%
Peanut Flavor	1 oz	< 1	100	5%
Green Onion Cheese Flavor	1 oz	< 1	100	5%
Original Cheese Flavor	1 oz	< 1	100	5%
Zesty Chili Cheese Flavor	1 oz	< 1	100	5%
(Keebler) Pizza Chips Pizzarias				
Cheese	1 oz	6	140	39%
Zesty Pepperoni	1 oz	6	140	39%
(Laura Scudder)				
Crunchy Cheese-Flavored				
Snacks	1 oz	10	160	56%
Puffed Cheese-Flavored				
Snacks	1 oz	9	150	54%
(Lawry's) Flavor Tree				
Cajun Hot Sticks	¼ cup	9	133	61%
Cheddar Sticks	¼ cup	8	129	56%
Honey Roasted	¼ cup	9	138	59%
Jalapeno & Cheddar	¼ cup	8	129	56%
Oat Bran	¼ cup	7.5	124	54%
Sesame Sticks	¼ cup	9	133	61%
Sesame Sticks-no salt	¼ cup	8	131	55%
Sour Cream & Onion	¼ cup	8	127	57%
(Lawry's) Sesame Chips	¼ cup	9	163	50%
(Lite Munchies)				
Bar B Que	.5 oz	2	60	30%
Nacho Cheese	.5 oz	2	60	30%
Toasted Onion	.5 oz	2	60	30%
(Michael Season's) Puffs				
Oat Bran	1 oz	10	150	60%
White Cheddar	1 oz	11	160	62%
(Nabisco)				
Doo Dads				
Original	1 oz	6	140	39%
Zesty Cheese	1 oz	6	140	39%
Twigs-Sesame & Cheese Sticks	.5 oz	4	70	51%

Food and Description	Amount	Fat Grams	Total Calories	% Fat Calories
(Pepperidge Farm) Snack Sticks				
Pretzel	8 pieces	3	120	23%
Pumpernickel	8 pieces	6	140	39%
Sesame	8 pieces	5	140	32%
Three Cheese	8 pieces	5	130	35%
(Planter's)				
Cheez Balls				
Nacho Cheez	1 oz	10	160	56%
Plain	1 oz	10	160	56%
Cheez Curls				
Nacho Cheez	1 oz	10	160	56%
Plain	1 oz	10	160	56%
Pork skins (Baken-ets)				
Hot'N Spicy	1 oz	9	150	54%
Original	1 oz	10	160	56%
Skinny Munchies (Skinny Haven)				
Chocolate Fudge	.5 oz	2	66	27%
Nacho Cheese	.5 oz	2	59	31%
Smokey Bar B Q	.5 oz	2	59	31%
Toasted Onion	.5 oz	2	59	31%
Snack Mix (Snyder's)	1 oz	5	130	35%
(Spicer's) Crunchy Diet Snacks				
Barbecue	1 oz	5	100	45%
Cheddar	1 oz	5	100	45%
Chocolate	1 oz	4	100	36%
Natural	1 oz	4	100	36%
Sour Cream & Onion	1 oz	5	100	45%
(Ultra Slim Fast) Cheese Curls	1 oz	3	110	25%
(Upper Crust) Croissant Snack Stix				
Garlic	1 piece	2	30	60%
Original	1 piece	2	30	60%
Sesame	1 piece	2	30	60%
(Weight Watchers) Snackers				
Bar-Be-Que	.5 oz	3	70	39%
Cheddar Cheese	.5 oz	3	70	39%
Cheese Curls	.5 oz	2	70	26%
Sour Cream & Onion	.5 oz	3	70	39%
(Wise)				
Cheez Doodles				
Crunchy	1 oz	10	160	56%
Puffed	1 oz	9	150	54%
Cheez Waffles	1 oz	8	140	51%
SNAIL (Escargot)				
cooked-moist heat	3 oz	1	230	4%

Food and Description	Amount	Fat Grams	Total Calories	% Fat Calories
raw	3 oz	< 1	117	4%
SNAPPER				
cooked-dry heat	3 oz	1	109	8%
raw	3 oz	1	85	11%
SNOW PEA	1 cup	–	30	–
frozen (La Choy)	½ pkg	< 1	35	13%
SOCKEYE				
canned (Libby's)	7¾ oz	21	380	50%
cooked-dry heat	3 oz	9	183	44%
raw	3 oz	7	143	44%
SOFT DRINKS (*See also* PUNCH)				
Apple				
(Crush)	12 fl oz	–	180	–
Diet	12 fl oz	–	20	–
(Slice)	12 fl oz	–	196	–
Diet	12 fl oz	–	20	–
(Welch's)	12 fl oz	–	180	–
(Big Red)	12 fl oz	–	163	–
Birch Beer				
(Canada Dry)	12 fl oz	–	166	–
(Shasta) Diet	12 fl oz	–	4	–
Bitter Lemon				
(Canada Dry)	12 fl oz	–	150	–
(Schweppes)	12 fl oz	–	160	–
Black Cherry				
(Cragmont)	12 fl oz	–	180	–
(Diet-Rite)	12 fl oz	–	4	–
(Shasta)	12 fl oz	–	162	–
(Bubble Up)	12 fl oz	–	145	–
Diet	12 fl oz	–	2	–
Sugar Free	12 fl oz	–	2	–
Cactus Cooler (Canada Dry)	12 fl oz	–	180	–
Cherry (Crush)	12 fl oz	–	150	–
Cherry Cola				
(Cragmont)	12 fl oz	–	158	–
(RC)	12 fl oz	–	171	–
Diet	12 fl oz	–	–	–
(Shasta)	12 fl oz	–	140	–
Cherry-Lime (Spree)	12 fl oz	–	158	–
Chocolate-flavored	12 fl oz	–	155	–
Diet	12 fl oz	–	7	–
(Barons)	9.5 oz	–	142	–
(Canfield's) fudge-diet	6 oz	–	2	–
(Yoo Hoo)	9 oz	< 1	150	5%

Food and Description	Amount	Fat Grams	Total Calories	% Fat Calories
Citrus Mist				
(Shasta)	12 oz	–	170	–
Club Soda	12 oz	–	–	–
(Canada Dry)	12 oz	–	–	–
(Schweppes)	12 oz	–	–	–
(Shasta)	12 oz	–	–	–
(Coca Cola)	6 oz	–	77	–
Caffeine Free	6 oz	–	77	–
Cherry	12 oz	–	154	–
	6 oz	–	76	–
Diet	12 oz	–	2	–
Classic	6 oz	–	72	–
Caffeine-Free	6 oz	–	72	–
Diet	6 oz	–	1	–
Caffeine-Free	6 oz	–	1	–
Cola				
(Canada Dry)	12 oz	–	–	–
(Diet Rite)	6 oz	–	–	–
(Jolt)	12 oz	–	170	–
(Like)	12 oz	–	162	–
Sugar Free	12 oz	–	1	–
(RC)	6 oz	–	86	–
100 Caffeine-Free	6 oz	–	87	–
Diet	6 oz	–	–	–
(Shasta)	12 oz	–	147	–
Diet	12 oz	–	–	–
Collins (Shasta)	12 oz	–	118	–
Cream Soda	12 oz	–	191	–
(A&W) Diet	12 oz	–	–	–
(Barqs) Red Creme	12 oz	–	175	–
(Cragmont)	12 oz	–	168	–
Diet	12 oz	–	–	–
(Crush) Vanilla Cream	12 oz	–	180	–
(Dad's) Diet	12 oz	–	2	–
(Shasta)	12 oz	–	154	–
Dr Diablo (Shasta)	12 oz	–	140	–
(Dr Pepper)	12 oz	–	156	–
Diet	12 oz	–	1	–
Pepper-Free	12 oz	–	156	–
Sugar-free Pepper-Free	12 oz	–	1	–
(Fresca)	12 oz	–	8	–
Fruit Punch	12 oz	–	200	–
(Nehi)	12 oz	–	200	–
(Shasta)	12 oz	–	173	–

Food and Description	Amount	Fat Grams	Total Calories	% Fat Calories
Ginger Beer (Schweppes)	6 oz	–	70	–
Gingsing Ginger	12 oz	–	137	–
Gingerale	12 oz	–	124	–
Low-cal	12 oz	–	7	–
(Canada Dry)	12 oz	–	140	–
Diet	6 oz	–	2	–
Golden	12 oz	–	150	–
(Cragmont)	6 oz	–	63	–
(Fanta)	6 oz	–	63	–
(Health Valley)	12 oz	1	153	6%
(Nehi)	12 oz	–	152	–
(Schweppes)	6 oz	–	70	–
Diet	6 oz	–	2	–
Grape	6 oz	–	100	–
Raspberry	6 oz	–	80	–
Diet	6 oz	–	2	–
(Shasta)	8 oz	–	120	–
Diet	8 oz	–	–	–
Grape	12 oz	–	161	–
Low-cal	12 oz	–	3	–
(Canada Dry)	12 oz	–	195	–
(Cragmont)	12oz	–	192	–
(Crush)	12 oz	–	200	–
(Fanta)	6 oz	–	86	–
(Nehi)	12 oz	–	192	–
diet	12 oz	–	3	–
(Schweppes)	6 oz	–	92	–
(Shasta)	12 oz	–	177	–
(Welch's) Sparkling	12 oz	–	180	–
Grapefruit				
(Cragmont)	12 oz	–	168	–
(Schweppes)	6 oz	–	77	–
(Wink)	12 oz	–	180	–
Half & Half (Canada Dry)	8 oz	–	110	–
(Kool-Aid) Kool Busters				
Cherry	6.75 oz	–	130	–
Grape	6.75 oz	–	130	–
Orange	6.75 oz	–	130	–
Tropical Punch	6.75 oz	–	130	–
Rock-A-Dile Red	6.75 oz	–	130	–
Lemon-Lime	12 oz	–	149	–
(Cragmont)	12 oz	–	148	–
Diet	12 oz	–	–	–
(Minute Maid)	6 oz	–	71	–

Food and Description	Amount	Fat Grams	Total Calories	% Fat Calories
Diet	6 oz	–	10	–
(Nehi) Diet	12 oz	–	5	–
(Schweppes)	12 oz	–	142	–
(7-Up)	12 oz	–	144	–
Diet	12 oz	–	4	–
Gold	12 oz	–	155	–
Diet	12 oz	–	4	–
(Shasta)	12 oz	–	146	–
Diet	12 oz	–	–	–
(Slice) Diet	12 oz	–	16	–
(Sprite)	12 oz	–	142	–
Diet	12 oz	–	4	–
Lemon-Lime-Cherry				
(Cragmont)	12 oz	–	164	–
Diet	12 oz	–	–	–
(7-Up)	12 oz	–	155	–
Diet	12 oz	–	4	–
Lemon Sour (Schweppes)	12 oz	–	149	–
Lemon-Tangerine (Spree)	12 oz	–	165	–
Mandarin Lime (Spree)	12 oz	–	154	–
Mandarin Orange (Slice)	12 oz	–	193	–
Low-cal	12 oz	–	12	–
(Mello Yello)	12 oz	–	174	–
Diet	12 oz	–	6	–
(Mountain Dew)	12 oz	–	171	–
Diet	12 oz	–	4	–
(Mr. Pibb)	6 oz	–	71	–
Orange	12 oz	–	177	–
Low-cal	12 oz	–	2	–
(Canada Dry) Diet	12 oz	–	3	–
Sunripe	12 oz	–	195	–
(Cragmont)	12 oz	–	178	–
(Crush)	12 oz	–	200	–
Sugar free	12 oz	–	24	–
(Fanta)	6 oz	–	88	–
(Minute Maid)	12 oz	–	174	–
Diet	12 oz	–	6	–
(Nehi)	12 oz	–	209	–
Diet	12 oz	–	2	–
(Schweppes) Sparkling	12 oz	–	172	–
(Shasta)	12 oz	–	177	–
(Slice) Mandarin	12 oz	–	193	–
(Welch's) Sparkling	12 oz	–	180	–
Peach	12 oz	–	203	–

Food and Description	Amount	Fat Grams	Total Calories	% Fat Calories
(Pepsi) Cola	12 oz	–	160	–
Diet	6 oz	–	–	–
Diet Caffeine Free	6 oz	–	–	–
(Pepsi) Free	12 oz	–	160	–
Diet	12 oz	–	2	–
(Pepsi) Light	12 oz	–	1	–
(Pepsi) Wild Cherry	12 oz	–	163	–
(Pepsi) Wild Cherry-diet	12 oz	–	1	–
Pineapple (Canada Dry)	12 oz	–	166	–
(Crush)	12 oz	–	200	–
Pink Grapefruit (Diet-Rite)	12 oz	–	4	–
Purple Passiion (Canada Dry)	12 oz	–	180	–
Punch (Cragmont)-sparkling	12 oz	–	198	–
Red Berry (Shasta)	12 oz	–	158	–
Red Raspberry (Diet-Rite)	12 oz	–	4	–
Red Pop (Shasta)	12 oz	–	158	–
Root beer	12 oz	–	152	–
(A & W)	12 oz	–	175	–
Low-cal	12 oz	–	–	–
(Canada Dry) Barrelhead	12 oz	–	166	–
Diet	12 oz	–	3	–
(Cragmont)	12 oz	–	168	–
Diet	12 oz	–	–	–
(Dad's) Diet	12 oz	–	2	–
(Fanta)	12 oz	–	156	–
(Health Valley)				
Old Fashioned	12 oz	1	120	8%
Sarsaparilla	12 oz	1	153	6%
(Hires)	12 oz	–	180	–
Sugar Free	12 oz	–	4	–
(IBC) Diet	12 oz	–	2	–
(New Century) Mug Old Fashioned	12 oz	–	168	–
(Ramblin')	12 oz	–	176	–
Diet	12 oz	–	2	–
(Schweppes)	12 oz	–	150	–
(Shasta)	12 oz	–	154	–
(Oproo)	12 oz	–	154	–
Strawberry	6 oz	–	192	–
Low-cal	6 oz	–	3	–
(Canada Dry)	6 oz	–	180	–
(Cragmont)	6 oz	–	176	–
(Crush)	6 oz	–	180	–
(Nehi)	6 oz	–	192	–
Diet	6 oz	–	3	–

Food and Description	Amount	Fat Grams	Total Calories	% Fat Calories
(Shasta)	6 oz	–	147	–
(Welch's) Sparkling	6 oz	–	180	–
(Tab)	6 oz	–	–	–
Caffeine-Free	6 oz	–	–	–
Tangerine (Diet-Rite)	6 oz	–	4	–
Vanilla Cream (Canada Dry)	12 oz	–	195	–
Wild Berry (Health Valley)	12 oz	1	142	6%
Wild Cherry (Canada Dry)	12 oz	–	195	–
SOFT-DRINK MIX (*See also* individual listings)				
(Kool-Aid)				
Sugar Free-all flavors	8 oz	–	4	–
Sugar-Sweetened-all flavors	8 oz	–	70	–
Unsweetened-all flavors				
dry	1 pkg	–	2	–
prepared w/sugar	8 oz	–	100	–
(Twist)				
Fruit Punch	8 oz	–	60	–
Grapeade	8 oz	–	50	–
Lemonade	8 oz	–	60	–
Orangeade	8 oz	–	60	–
Pink Lemonade	8 oz	–	60	–
SOLE (*See also* SEAFOOD ENTREE/DINNER)				
baked w/butter	3 oz	6	120	45%
cooked-dry heat	3 oz	1	80	11%
raw	3 oz	< 1	58	8%
SORBET (*See* FRUIT ICES)				
SORGHUM	1 Tbs	–	53	–
	1 cup	–	848	–
Cane and Maple	1 Tbs	–	50	–
	1 cup	–	794	–
Table blend	1 Tbs	–	59	–
	1 cup	–	951	–
SORGHUM GRAIN	4 oz	4	380	9%

SOUP

(NOTE: Condensed soups were prepared as directed on packaging w/water, unless otherwise stated. When prepared with milk, whole milk was used. If you use low-fat or skim milk, refer to the Quick Reference-Milk on nexjt page to adjust your fat and calorie data. Ready-To-Serve (RTS) soups were heated as directed w/no added liquid.)

(Andersen's)				
Cream of Asparagus	7.5 oz	7	150	42%
Cream of Broccoli	7.5 oz	7	150	42%
Cream of Potato	7.5 oz	11	220	45%
Split Pea	7.5 oz	–	140	–

Food and Description	Amount	Fat Grams	Total Calories	% Fat Calories
Split Pea w/ham	7.5 oz	1	150	6%
Tomato	7.5 oz	4	140	26%
Asparagus				
(Campbell's) Creamy Natural	1 cup	5	100	45%
prepared w/milk	1 cup	9	170	48%
Cream of				
prepared w/milk	1 cup	8	161	45%
prepared w/water	1 cup	4	87	41%
Bacon, Lettuce, & Tomato				
(Pepperidge Farm)	5.3 oz	12	170	64%
5-Bean Vegetable/chunky				
(Health Valley) No Salt	7.5 oz	2	110	16%
Bean, Black	1 cup	1.5	116	12%
(Campbell's)	1 cup	2	110	16%
(Health Valley) Natural-No Salt	7.5 oz	3	150	18%
Bean, Black Turtle	1 cup	–	218	–
Bean, Black w/Sherry				
(Pepperidge Farm)	5.3 oz	1.7	109	14%
Bean, Navy				
(Pritikin)	7⅜ oz	< 1	130	3%
Bean w/Bacon	1 pkg/1 oz	2	105	17%
	1 cup	2	105	17%
(Campbell's)				
Special Request	1 cup	4	140	26%
Bean w/Franks	1 cup	6.98	187	34%
condensed not prepared	11.25 oz	17	454	34%
Bean w/Ham				
(Campbell's)				
Old Fashioned Soup For One	11 oz	7	220	29%

QUICK REFERENCE: MILK	Amount	Fat Grams	Total Calories	% Fat Calories
Whole	½ cup	4	75	48%
	¼ cup	2	38	47%
2% lowfat	½ cup	2.5	61	37%
	¼ cup	1	31	29%
1% lowfat	½ cup	1	55	16%
	¼ cup	.5	26	17%
Skim	½ cup	–	45	–
	¼ cup	–	23	–

Food and Description	Amount	Fat Grams	Total Calories	% Fat Calories
Bean w/Ham Chunky Old Fashioned				
(Campbell's) RTS	11 oz	9	290	28%
	9⅝ oz	8	250	29%
Beans, Red & Rice w/sausage				
Chunky Creole Style				
(Campbell's) ready-to-serve	9.5 oz	13	300	39%
Beef				
(Campbell's)	1 cup	2	80	23%
(Progresso) ready-to-serve	9.5 oz	5	160	28%
(Right Time)	6 oz	–	8	–
Beef, Hearty				
(Campbell's) Home Cookin' RTS	10¾ oz	3	140	19%
	9.5 oz	3	130	21%
(Progresso)	9.5 oz	4	160	23%
Beef Barley				
(Progresso) ready-to-serve	9.5 oz	4	140	26%
Beef Broth				
(College Inn)	1 cup	–	18	–
(Health Valley)	7.5 oz	–	8	–
(Pritikin)	7.25 oz	–	20	–
ready-to-serve	14 oz	1	27	33%
(Swanson)	7¼ oz	1	18	50%
Beef Broth or Bouillon/ready-to-serve	1 cup	.5	16	28%
Beef Broth & Barley (Campbell's)	1 cup	1	59	15%
Beef Cabbage (Manischewitz)	1 cup	–	62	–
Beef Chunky				
(Campbell's) ready-to serve	10¾ oz	5	190	24%
	9.5 oz	4	170	21%
Beef Minestrone				
(Progresso) ready-to-serve	9.5 oz	5	170	26%
Beef Mushroom	1 cup	3	73	37%
Beef Noodle				
(Campbell's)	1 cup	3	70	39%
(Campbell's) Home Cookin' RTS	10.76 oz	3.8	144	24%
(Lunch Bucket) microwave	8.25 oz	2	120	15%
(Weight Watchers) RTS	10.5 oz	2	90	20%
Beef Noodle-homestyle				
(Campbell's)	1 cup	3	80	34%
Beef Ravioli Romano				
(Campbell's) ready-to-serve	9.49 oz	8	231	31%
Beef Stroganoff Style				
(Campbell's) Chunky RTS	10¾ oz	16	320	45%
Beef Vegetable				
(Progresso) Ready-to-Serve	9.5 oz	3	150	18%

Food and Description	Amount	Fat Grams	Total Calories	% Fat Calories
Beefy Mushroom				
(Campbell's)	1 cup	3	60	45%
Borscht				
(Gold's)	1 cup	–	100	–
(Manischewitz)				
Low Cal	1 cup	–	20	–
w/Beets	1 cup	–	80	–
(Mother's) Old Fashioned	1 cup	–	96	–
(Pepperidge Farm)	5.3 oz	–	89	–
Borscht Beverage (Mother's)				
low cal	8 oz	–	25	–
Broccoli				
(Campbell's) Creamy Natural	1 cup	3	70	39%
prepared w/milk	1 cup	7	140	45%
(Pepperidge Farm) Cream of	5.3 oz	6	100	54%
(Campbell's)				
Healthy Request				
Condensed-Prepared				
Bean w/Bacon	8 oz	4	140	26%
Chicken Noodle	8 oz	2	60	30%
Chicken w/Rice	8 oz	2	60	30%
Cream of Mushroom	8 oz	2	60	30%
Tomato	8 oz	2	90	20%
prepared w/skim milk	8 oz	2	130	14%
Vegetable	8 oz	2	90	20%
Vegetable Beef	8 oz	2	70	26%
Ready-to-Serve				
Hearty Chicken Noodle	8 oz	2	80	23%
Hearty Minestrone	8 oz	3	90	30%
Hearty Vegetable	8 oz	3	110	25%
Home Cookin RTS				
Chicken Noodle	9.5 oz	3	110	25%
Country Vegetable	9.5 oz	2	130	14%
New England Clam Chowder	9.5 oz	16	230	63%
Cauliflower				
(Campbell's) Creamy Natural	1 cup	9	130	62%
prepared w/milk	1 cup	13	200	59%
Cauliflower, Creamy	1 cup	5.9	97	55%
Celery, Cream of				
(Campbell's) prepared w/water	1 cup	7	100	63%
Generic				
condensed not prepared	10.75 oz	14	219	58%
prepared w/milk	1 cup	9.68	165	53%
prepared w/water	1 cup	5.59	90	56%

Food and Description	Amount	Fat Grams	Total Calories	% Fat Calories
Cheddar Cheese				
(Campbell's)	1 cup	8	130	55%
Cheese				
condensed not prepared	11 oz	25	377	60%
prepared w/milk	1 cup	14.56	230	57%
prepared w/water	1 cup	10.5	155	61%
Chickarina				
(Progresso) Ready-to-Serve	9.5 oz	5	130	35%
Chickarina w/Tiny Meatballs				
(Progresso) Ready-to-Serve	9.5 oz	6	90	60%
Chicken				
(Manischewitz) Clear	1 cup	–	46	–
Chicken & Dumplings	1 cup	5.5	97	51%
(Campbell's)	1 cup	3	80	34%
Chicken & Stars (Campbell's)	1 cup	2	60	30%
Chicken Alphabet (Campbell's)	1 cup	2	70	26%
Chicken Barley				
(Campbell's)	1 cup	1.8	70	23%
(Progresso)	9.25 oz	2	100	18%
Chicken Broth	1 cup	1	39	23%
(Campbell's)				
Low Sodium RTS	10.5 oz	2	40	45%
Original	1 cup	2	35	51%
(College Inn) condensed				
Prepared	1 cup	1	39	23%
Unprepared	10.75 oz	3	94	29%
(Health Valley) Natural				
No Salt	7.5 oz	1.6	35	41%
(Manischewitz)	1 cup	–	83	–
(Pritikin)	6⅞ oz	< 1	18	55%
(Swanson) RTS	7¼ oz	2	30	60%
Chicken Broth & Noodles (Campbell's)	1 cup	2	60	30%
Chicken Broth & Rice (Campbell's)	1 cup	1	50	18%
Chicken/Chunky Old Fashioned				
(Campbell's) RTS	10¾ oz	5	180	56%
	9.5 oz	4	150	24%
Chicken Corn Chowder/Chunky				
(Campbell's) Ready-to-Serve	10¾ oz	21	340	56%
Chicken Curry (Pepperidge Farm)	5.3 oz	8	170	42%
Chicken Gumbo				
(Campbell's)	1 cup	2	60	30%
(Pritikin)	7⅜ oz	1	80	11%
Chicken, Cream of				
(Campbell's)	1 cup	7	110	57%

Food and Description	Amount	Fat Grams	Total Calories	% Fat Calories
Prepared w/Milk	1 cup	14.97	191	71%
Ready-to-Serve	7.27 oz	5.5	85	58%
Special Request	1 cup	7	110	57%
Chicken, Cream of w/mushrooms				
(Progresso) Ready-to-Serve	9.5 oz	11	190	52%
Chicken, Creamy Mushroom (Campbell's)	1 cup	7	111	57%
Chicken, Golden & Noodles (Campbell's)				
Soup For One	11 oz	4	120	30%
Chicken, Hearty				
(Lunch Bucket) Microwave	8.25 oz	3	110	25%
(Progresso) Ready-to-Serve	9.5 oz	4	130	28%
Chicken Homestyle				
(Progresso) Ready-to-Serve	9.5 oz	3	110	25%
Chicken Minestrone				
(Progresso) Ready-to-Serve	9.5 oz	3	130	21%
Chicken Mushroom	1 cup	9	132	61%
Chicken Mushroom-creamy				
(Campbell's)	1 cup	8	120	60%
Chunky RTS	9.38 oz	21.5	272	71%
Chicken-Curly Noodle (Campbell's)	1 cup	3	80	34%
Chicken Noodle				
(Campbell's)				
Chunky RTS	10¾ oz	7	200	32%
	9.5 oz	6	180	30%
Homestyle	1 cup	3	70	39%
Ready-to-Serve	7.27 oz	2	60	30%
Special Request	1 cup	2	60	30%
(Lipton) Hearty Ones Microwave				
Homestyle	11 oz	4	230	16%
(Lunch Bucket) Microwave	8.25 oz	4	110	33%
(Progresso) Ready-to-Serve	9.5 oz	4	120	30%
(Weight Watchers) Ready-to-Serve	10.5 oz	1	80	11%
	7.5 oz	1	90	10%
Chicken Noodle w/Meatballs				
ready-to-serve	1 cup	3.57	99	33%
	20 oz	8	227	32%
Chicken Noodle-O's (Campbell's)	1 cup	2	70	26%
Chicken Nuggets w/Vegetables & Noodles				
Chunky (Campbell's) RTS	10¾ oz	9	210	39%
	9.5 oz	8	190	38%
Chicken Rice				
(Manischewitz)	1 cup	–	47	–
Ready-to-serve				
(Campbell's)	7.27 oz	2	52	35%

Food and Description	Amount	Fat Grams	Total Calories	% Fat Calories
Chunky	9.5 oz	4	140	26%
(Progresso)	9.5 oz	3	130	21%
Chicken Rice w/Vegetables				
ready-to-serve	9.5 oz	3	140	19%
Chicken w/Noodles				
(Campbell's)				
Home Cookin' RTS	10¾ oz	4	140	26%
	9.5 oz	3	120	23%
Low Sodium RTS	10¾ oz	5	160	28%
Chicken w/Noodles & Mushrooms				
(Campbell's) Ready-to-Serve	10.76 oz	6.6	195	31%
Chicken w/Ribbon Pasta				
(Pritikin)	7.25 oz	1	80	11%
Chicken w/Rice				
(Campbell's)	1 cup	2	60	30%
Special Request	1 cup	3	60	45%
Chicken w/Wild Rice				
(Pepperidge Farm)	5.3 oz	3	85	32%
Chicken Vegetable				
(Campbell's)	1 cup	3	70	39%
(Estee)	7.25 oz	7	130	49%
Generic				
Ready-to-Serve	9.5 oz	4.8	167	26%
(Manischewitz)	1 cup	–	55	–
(Pritikin)	7.25 oz	1	70	13%
(Progresso) Ready-to-Serve	9.5 oz	4	140	26%
Chicken Vegetable, Chunky				
(Campbell's)				
Low Sodium RTS	10¾ oz	11	240	41%
RTS	9.5 oz	6	170	32%
Chicken Vegetable w/Wild Rice				
(Campbell's) Golden Classic	1 cup	3	80	34%
Chicken Vegetable-w/rice				
(Campbell's) Ready-to-Serve	10.76 oz	2.7	131	19%
Chili (See (Lipton) Kettle Ready in this listing, MEXICAN FOODS)				
Chili Beef				
(Campbell's)	1 cup	5	140	32%
Chunky Ready-to-Serve	9.75 oz	6	260	21%
	11 oz	7	290	22%
Generic	1 cup	6.6	169	35%
condensed unprepared	11.25 oz	16	411	35%
Clam Chowder-Manhattan				
(Campbell's)	1 cup	2	70	26%
(Health Valley) Natural-No Salt	7.5 oz	2	100	18%

Food and Description	Amount	Fat Grams	Total Calories	% Fat Calories
(Pepperidge Farm)	5.3 oz	2	80	23%
(Pritikin)	7⅜ oz	–	70	–
Ready-to-Serve				
(Campbell's)	7.27 oz	1.8	67	24%
(Progresso)	9.5 oz	2	120	15%
(Snow's)	7.5 oz	2	70	26%
Chunky/ready-to-serve	1 cup	3	133	21%
Chunky (Campbell's) RTS	10¾ oz	4	160	23%
	9.5 oz	4	150	24%
Clam Chowder-New England				
(Campbell's)	1 cup	3	80	34%
Soup For One	11 oz	4	130	28%
prepared w/milk	11 oz	7	190	33%
(Pepperidge Farm)	5.3 oz	6	133	41%
(Pritikin)	7⅜ oz	–	118	–
(Progresso) Ready-to-Serve	9.25 oz	11	190	52%
(Snow's) prepared w/milk	7.5 oz	6	140	39%
(Stouffer's) frozen	8 oz	9	180	45%
Clam Chowder-New England, Chunky				
Ready-to-Serve				
(Campbell's)	10¾ oz	17	290	53%
	9.5 oz	15	260	52%
(Gorton's)	¼ can	5	140	32%
Consomme (Beef) w/Gelatin				
condensed-not prepared	10.5 oz	–	71	–
(Campbell's)	1 cup	–	25	–
Consomme, Madrilene				
(Pepperidge Farm)	5.4 oz	–	60	–
Corn Chowder				
(Pepperidge Farm)	5.3 oz	12	170	64%
Corn Chowder-New England				
(Snow's)				
prepared w/milk	7.5 oz	6	150	36%
Corn, Golden (Campbell's) RTS	8 oz	3	110	25%
Crab				
(Pepperidge Farm)	5.3 oz	1.7	80	19%
Ready-to-Serve	1 cup	1.5	76	18%
Creole-style (See Beans, Red & Rice in this listing)				
Double Noodle in Chicken Broth				
(Campbell's) prepared	8 oz	2	90	20%
Escarole				
Ready-to-Serve	1 cup	2	27	67%
(Progresso)	9.25 oz	1	30	30%
	19.5 oz	4	61	59%

Food and Description	Amount	Fat Grams	Total Calories	% Fat Calories
Fat-free				
(Hain)				
Black Bean & Vegetable	7.5 oz	< 1	70	6%
Chicken Broth	7.5 oz	< 1	100	5%
Country Corn & Vegetables	7.5 oz	< 1	70	6%
5-Bean Vegetable	7.5 oz	< 1	100	5%
14-Garden Vegetable	7.5 oz	< 1	50	9%
Lentils & Carrots	7.5 oz	< 1	70	6%
Real Italian Minestrone	7.5 oz	< 1	80	6%
Split Pea & Carrots	7.5 oz	< 1	80	6%
Tomato Vegetable	7.5 oz	< 1	50	9%
Vegetable Barley	7.5 oz	< 1	60	8%
(Health Valley)				
Beef Broth-No salt	6.9 oz	< 1	10	45%
Black Bean & Vegetable	7.5 oz	< 1	70	6%
Chicken Broth	6.9 oz	< 1	20	23%
Country Corn & Vegetable	7.5 oz	< 1	70	6%
5-Bean Vegetable	7.5 oz	< 1	100	5%
14-Garden Vegetable	7.5 oz	< 1	50	9%
Lentils & Carrots	7.5 oz	< 1	70	6%
Real Italian Minestrone	7.5 oz	< 1	80	6%
Split Pea & Carrots	7.5 oz	< 1	50	9%
Tomato Vegetable	7.5 oz	< 1	50	9%
Vegetable Barley	7.5 oz	< 1	60	8%
Fish Chowder-New England				
(Snow's) prepared w/milk	7.5 oz	6	130	42%
Fisherman's Chowder/Chunky				
(Pepperidge Farm)	5.3 oz	6	150	36%
French Onion				
(Campbell's)	1 cup	2	60	30%
Ready-to-Serve	9.5 oz	8	120	60%
(Pepperidge Farm)	5.3 oz	4.7	71	60%
Gazpacho				
(Campbell's)	1 cup	–	41	–
(Pepperidge Farm)	5.3 oz	2	68	27%
ready-to-serve	1 cup	2	57	32%
	13 oz	3	87	31%
Greek-homemade	1 cup	2.5	85	27%
(Hain)				
Black Bean 99% Fat-free	9.5 oz	1	120	8%
	10.5 oz	1	140	6%
Chicken Broth				
No Salt Added	9 oz	3	45	60%
Original	9 oz	3	30	90%

Food and Description	Amount	Fat Grams	Total Calories	% Fat Calories
Chicken Noodle Soup				
No Salt Added	8 oz	4	100	36%
Original	8 oz	4	110	33%
Chicken Vegetable				
No Salt Added	8 oz	3	100	27%
Original	8 oz	3	110	25%
Minestrone				
No Salt Added	9.5 oz	4	160	23%
Original	9.5 oz	3	160	17%
Mushroom Barley				
99% Fat-free	9.5 oz	2	100	18%
	10.5 oz	2	90	30%
Original	9.5 oz	2	80	23%
Turkey Rice				
No Salt Added	8 oz	3	100	27%
Original	8 oz	3	80	34%
Vegetable Broth				
Low-Sodium	9.5 oz	–	40	–
Original	9.75 oz	–	45	–
Vegetarian Lentil-99% Fat-free				
No Salt Added	9.5 oz	1	140	6%
	10.5 oz	2	150	12%
Regular	9.5 oz	1	150	6%
	10.5 oz	2	160	11%
Vegetarian Split Pea-99% Fat-free				
No Salt Added	9.5 oz	1	150	6%
	10.5 oz	1	170	5%
Regular	9.5 oz	1	160	6%
	10.5 oz	1	180	5%
Vegetarian Vegetable				
No Salt Added	9.5 oz	5	150	30%
Original	9.5 oz	4	150	24%
Vegetarian Veggie Broth 99% Fat-free				
No Salt Added	9.25 oz	–	40	–
	10.5 oz	–	50	–
Regular	9.25 oz	–	40	–
	10.5	–	45	–
Wild Rice-99% Fat-free	9.5 oz	2	80	23%
	10.5 oz	2	90	20%
Ham & Bean				
(Progresso) Ready-to-Serve	9.5 oz	2	140	13%
Ham & Butter Beans/Chunky				
(Campbell's) Ready-to-Serve	10¾ oz	10	280	32%

Food and Description	Amount	Fat Grams	Total Calories	% Fat Calories
(Healthy Choice)				
Bean & Ham	7.5 oz	4	220	16%
Beef Vegetable, Chunky				
Canned	7.5 oz	1	110	8%
Microwaveable Cup	7.5 oz	1	110	8%
Chicken Noodle & Vegetable, Chunky				
Canned	7.5 oz	4	160	23%
Microwaveable Cup	7.5 oz	4	160	23%
Chicken w/Rice	7.5 oz	4	140	26%
Country Vegetable	7.5 oz	1	120	8%
Hearty Beef	7.5 oz	1	120	8%
Hearty Chicken	7.5 oz	5	150	30%
Minestrone	7.5 oz	2	160	11%
Old Fashioned Chicken Noodle	7.5 oz	3	90	30%
Split Pea & Ham	7.5 oz	3	170	16%
Tomato Garden	7.5 oz	3	130	21%
Vegetable Beef	7.5 oz	1	130	7%
Hunter's				
(Pepperidge Farm)	5.3 oz	4	105	34%
Italian Pasta, Classic				
(Lipton) Hearty Ones Microwave	11 oz	3	190	14%
Italian Tomato (Campbell's)				
prepared	8 oz	–	90	–
Lentil				
(Health Valley) Natural-No Salt	7.5 oz	2	170	11%
(Pritikin)	7⅜ oz	–	100	–
(Progresso) Ready-to-Serve	9.5 oz	4	140	26%
Lentil, Hearty				
(Campbell's) Home Cookin' RTS	10¾ oz	2	170	11%
	9.5 oz	1	150	6%
Lentil w/Ham				
Ready-to-Serve	1 cup	2.78	140	18%
	13 oz	6	320	17%
Lentil w/Sausage				
(Progresso) Ready-to-Serve	9.5 oz	8	170	42%
(Lipton) Kettle Ready-frozen				
Black Bean w/Ham	6 oz	6	154	35%
Boston Clam Chowder	6 oz	7	130	48%
Chicken Gumbo	6 oz	3.5	94	34%
Chicken Noodle	6 oz	2.9	94	28%
Chili-Jalapeno	6 oz	7.8	173	41%
Traditional	6 oz	6.5	161	36%
Corn & Broccoli Chowder	6 oz	5	102	44%
Cream of Asparagus	6 oz	4	62	58%

Food and Description	Amount	Fat Grams	Total Calories	% Fat Calories
Cream of Cauliflower	6 oz	6.9	93	67%
Cream of Broccoli	6 oz	7	94	67%
Cream of Cheddar Broccoli	6 oz	11	137	72%
Cream of Chicken	6 oz	6	98	55%
Cream of Mushroom	6 oz	6	85	64%
Cream of Potato	6 oz	5	120	30%
Creamy Cheddar Cheese	6 oz	12.5	158	71%
French Onion	6 oz	2	42	43%
Garden Vegetable	6 oz	2.8	85	30%
Hearty Beef Vegetable	6 oz	2.8	85	30%
Hearty Minestrone	6 oz	4	104	35%
Manhattan Clam Chowder	6 oz	2.6	69	34%
New England Clam Chowder	6 oz	6.5	116	50%
Savory Bean w/Ham	6 oz	3.6	113	29%
Split Pea w/Ham	6 oz	4	155	23%
Tomato Florentine	6 oz	4	106	34%
Tortellini in Tomato	6 oz	5	122	37%
Lobster Bisque (Pepperidge Farm)	5.3 oz	10.9	158	62%
Macaroni & Bean				
(Progresso) Ready-to-Serve	9.5 oz	5	140	32%
Minestrone				
(Campbell's)	1 cup	2	80	23%
Ready-to-Serve	7.27 oz	2	70	26%
(Health Valley) Natural-No Salt	7.5 oz	3	130	21%
(Pepperidge Farm)	5.3 oz	4	110	33%
(Pritikin)	7⅜ oz	< 1	80	6%
(Progresso) Ready-to-Serve	9.5 oz	4	130	28%
Minestrone/Chunky-ready-to-serve	1 cup	2.8	127	20%
(Campbell's) RTS	9.5 oz	5	170	27%
(Estee)	7.5 oz	8	165	44%
Minestrone, Extra Zesty				
(Progresso) Ready-to-Serve	9.5 oz	8	150	48%
Minestrone, Old World				
(Campbell's) Home Cookin' RTS	10¾ oz	4	150	24%
	9.5 oz	3	130	21%
Minestrone w/Italian Sausage				
ready-to-serve	9.49 oz	8	169	43%
Mushroom (Pritikin)	7⅜ oz	–	60	–
Mushroom Barley	1 cup	2	73	25%
(Health Valley) Natural-No Salt	7.5 oz	2	100	18%
(Manischewitz)	1 cup	–	72	–
Mushroom, Cream of				
condensed unprepared	10.75 oz	23	313	66%
prepared w/milk	1 cup	13.59	203	60%

Food and Description	Amount	Fat Grams	Total Calories	% Fat Calories
prepared w/water	1 cup	8.97	129	63%
(Campbell's)	1 cup	7	100	63%
Low Sodium RTS	10.5 oz	13	190	62%
Special Request	1 cup	7	100	63%
ready-to-serve				
(Progresso)	9.25 oz	8	140	51%
(Weight Watchers)	10.5 oz	2	90	20%
Mushroom, Creamy Chicken/Chunky				
(Campbell's) RTS	10.5 oz	19	270	63%
	9⅜ oz	17	240	64%
Mushroom, Golden				
(Campbell's)	1 cup	3	70	39%
Mushroom, Savory Cream of				
(Campbell's)				
Soup For One	11 oz	13	180	65%
Mushroom w/Beef stock	1 cup	4	85	42%
Nacho Cheese				
(Campbell's)	1 cup	8	110	66%
Prepared w/Milk	1 cup	12	180	60%
Noodles & Ground Beef				
(Campbell's)	1 cup	3.5	90	35%
Onion	1 cup	1.7	57	27%
condensed unprepared	10.5 oz	4	138	26%
Onion, Cream of				
(Campbell's)	1 cup	5	100	45%
Prepared w/Milk	1 cup	7	140	45%
Oyster Stew				
(Campbell's)	1 cup	5	70	64%
Prepared w/Milk	1 cup	9	140	58%
Generic-Prepared w/Milk	10.5 oz	19	325	53%
(Pepperidge Farm)	5.3 oz	6	110	49%
Pea, Green				
prepared w/milk	1 cup	7	239	26%
prepared w/water	1 cup	2.9	164	16%
(Campell's)	1 cup	3	160	17%
Ready-to-Serve)	7.5 oz	2.6	136	17%
(Pepperidge Farm)	5.3 oz	7	210	30%
Pea, Green Split				
(Health Valley) Natural-No Salt	7.5 oz	1	90	10%
(Progresso) Ready-to-Serve	9.5 oz	3	180	15%
Pea, Split				
(Campbell's) Low Sodium RTS	10¾ oz	5	240	19%
(Manischewitz)	1 cup	–	133	–
(Pritikin)	7.5 oz	< 1	140	3%

Food and Description	Amount	Fat Grams	Total Calories	% Fat Calories
Pea, Split w/Ham				
(Campbell's)				
Chunky/Ready-to-Serve	1 cup	3.98	184	20%
	10¾ oz	6	240	23%
	9.5 oz	5	210	21%
Home Cookin' RTS	10¾ oz	6	230	23%
	9.5 oz	4	190	19%
(Lunch Bucket) Microwave	8.25 oz	3	130	21%
(Progresso) Ready-to-Serve	9.5 oz	5	150	30%
Pea, Split w/Ham & Bacon				
(Campbell's)	1 cup	4	160	23%
Pepperpot				
(Campbell's)	1 cup	4	90	40%
Condensed not prepared	10.5 oz	11	251	39%
Pepper Steak/Chunky				
(Campbell's) RTS	10¾ oz	3	180	15%
	9.5 oz	3	160	17%
Potato				
(Campbell's) Creamy Natural	1 cup	7	120	53%
Prepared w/Milk	1 cup	11	190	52%
(Health Valley) RTS	4 oz	1	70	13%
Homemade	1 cup	12	201	54%
Potato, Cream of				
(Campbell's)	1 cup	3	80	34%
Prepared w/2 oz milk & 2 oz water	1 cup	4	120	30%
Potato Leek (Health Valley) Natural				
No Salt	7.5 oz	2	130	14%
Schav (Manischewitz)	1 cup	–	12	–
Scotch Broth (Campbell's)	1 cup	3	80	34%
Condensed not prepared	10.5 oz	6	195	28%
Seafood Chowder-New England (Snow's)				
Prepared w/Milk	7.5 oz	6	130	28%
Shiitake Mushroom (Pepperidge Farm)	5.3 oz	2.7	73	33%
Shrimp, Cream of				
(Campbell's)	1 cup	6	90	40%
Prepared w/Milk	1 cup	10	160	56%
Condensed not prepared	10.75 oz	13	219	53%
Sirloin Beef				
(Campbell's) Golden Classic	1 cup	3	70	39%
Sirloin Burger/Chunky-Ready-to-Serve				
(Campbell's)	9.5 oz	8	200	36%
	10¾ oz	9	220	37%
Spinach				
(Campbell's) Creamy Natural	1 cup	6	90	60%

Food and Description	Amount	Fat Grams	Total Calories	% Fat Calories
Prepared w/Milk	1 cup	10	160	56%
Spinach, Cream of (Stouffer's)-frozen	8 oz	15	210	64%
Split Pea (*See* Pea, Split, in this listing)				
Steak & Potato-Chunky				
ready-to-serve (Campbell's)	1 cup	3.8	169	20%
	10¾ oz	5	200	23%
	9.5 oz	4	170	21%
Stockpot	1 cup	3.9	100	35%
condensed-not prepared	11 oz	9	242	34%
(Tabatchnick) frozen				
Barley/Bean	7.5 oz	2	130	14%
Cabbage	7.5 oz	2	110	16%
Chicken Noodle	7.5 oz	2	65	28%
Cream of Broccoli	7.5 oz	4	90	40%
Cream of Mushroom	6 oz	2	75	24%
Cream of Spinach	7.5 oz	2	85	21%
Cream of Zucchini	6 oz	2	80	23%
Lentil	7.5 oz	2	170	11%
Minestrone	7.5 oz	2	145	12%
Mushroom Barley				
No Salt	7.5 oz	1	97	9%
Regular	7.5 oz	2	100	18%
New England Chowder	7.5 oz	2	98	18%
Northern Bean	7.5 oz	2	164	11%
Pea				
No Salt	7.5 oz	1	175	5%
Regular	7.5 oz	1	175	5%
Potato	7.5 oz	1	95	10%
Tomato Rice	6 oz	1	73	12%
Vegetable	7.5 oz	1	97	9%
No Salt	7.5 oz	2	92	20%
Regular	7.5 oz	1	97	9%
Tomato				
(Campbell's)	1 cup	2	90	20%
Prepared w/Milk	1 cup	4	150	24%
Special Request	1 cup	2	90	20%
(Health Valley) Natural-No Salt	7.5 oz	3	130	21%
(Manischewitz)	1 cup	–	60	–
Ready-to-Serve	7.27 oz	1.7	106	14%
Tomato w/Tomato Pieces				
(Campbell's) Low Sodium RTS	10.5 oz	5	180	25%
(Pritikin)	7.5 oz	< 1	70	6%
Tomato w/Vegetables				
(Progresso)	9.25 oz	5	140	32%

Food and Description	Amount	Fat Grams	Total Calories	% Fat Calories
Ready-to-Serve	9.5 oz	2	110	16%
Tomato Beef				
w/Noodles				
prepared w/water	1 cup	4	140	26%
w/Rotini				
(Progresso) Ready-to-Serve	9.5 oz	6	170	32%
Tomato Bisque				
(Campbell's)	1 cup	3	120	23%
Prepared w/Milk	1 cup	6.6	198	30%
Tomato, Cream of				
(Campbell's) Homestyle	1 cup	3	110	25%
Prepared w/Milk	1 cup	7	180	35%
Tomato Garden				
(Campbell's) Home Cookin' RTS	10¾ oz	3	150	18%
	9.5 oz	3	130	21%
Tomato Garden-Crispy				
(Campbell's)	1 cup	–	78	–
Tomato Rice				
(Campbell's) Old Fashioned	1 cup	2	110	16%
Tomato Royale				
(Campbell's) Soup For One	11 oz	3	180	15%
Tomato, Zesty (Campbell's)	1 cup	1	90	10%
Tortellini				
(Progresso)				
Ready-to-Serve	9.5 oz	3	90	30%
Creamy Regular	9.25 oz	16	240	60%
Tomato	9.25 oz	5	130	35%
Tortellini & Vegetable				
(Campbell's) Golden Classic	1 cup	2	79	23%
Tortilla/Chunky				
(Campbell's) Ready-to-Serve	10.76 oz	9.6	293	30%
Turkey				
(Weight Watchers) RTS	10.5 oz	2	70	26%
Turkey/Chunky				
ready-to-serve	1 cup	4	136	27%
Turkey Noodle (Campbell's)	1 cup	3	70	39%
Turkey Rice				
(Hain) RTS	9.5 oz	3	100	27%
Turkey Vegetable				
(Campbell's)	1 cup	3	70	39%
Chunky RTS	9⅜ oz	6	150	36%
(Weight Watchers) RTS	10.5 oz	2	70	26%
Turkey Vegetable w/Ribbon Pasta				
(Pritikin)	7⅜ oz	.5	50	9%

Food and Description	Amount	Fat Grams	Total Calories	% Fat Calories
Vegetable				
(Campbell's)	1 cup	2	80	23%
Ready-to-Serve	1 cup	3.7	122	27%
	10¾ oz	5	160	28%
	9.5 oz	4	140	26%
Special Request	1 cup	2	90	20%
(Health Valley)				
Chunky	7.5 oz	7	120	52%
Natural-No Salt	7.5 oz	1	110	8%
Homemade	1 cup	–	70	–
(Manischewitz)	1 cup	–	63	–
(Pritikin)	7⅜ oz	1	90	10%
(Progresso) Ready-to-Serve	9.5 oz	2	90	20%
(Weight Watchers)	7.5 oz	1	90	10%
Vegetable Beef				
(Campbell's)	1 cup	2	70	26%
Special Request	1 cup	2	70	26%
Chunky (Estee)	7.5 oz	7	140	45%
homemade	1 cup	25	320	70%
microwave (Lunch Bucket)	8.25 oz	5	140	32%
Vegetable Beef, Old Fashioned				
(Campbell's)				
Chunky RTS	9.5 oz	5	160	28%
	10¾ oz	5	180	25%
Home Cookin' RTS	10¾ oz	3	140	19%
	9.5 oz	3	140	19%
Vegetable Chicken/chunky				
(Health Valley) Natural-No Salt	7½ oz	7	125	50%
Vegetable, Country				
(Campbell's)				
Home Cookin-RTS	10¾ oz	2	120	15%
	9.5 oz	2	110	16%
(Lunch Bucket) Microwave	8.25 oz	1	90	10%
Vegetable, Garden (Campbell's)	1 cup	1.8	63	26%
Vegetable, Homestyle (Campbell's)	1 cup	2	60	30%
Vegetable, Mediterranean/Chunky				
(Campbell's) RTS	9.5 oz	5	160	28%
Vegetable, Old Fashioned (Campbell's)	1 cup	2	60	30%
Vegetable, Old World				
(Campbell's) Soup for One	11 oz	4	130	28%
Vegetable, Vegetarian (Campbell's)	1 cup	2	80	23%
Vichyssoise	1 cup	6	148	37%
(Pepperidge Farm)	5.3 oz	6.9	114	55%
Watercress (Pepperidge Farm)	5.3 oz	3	90	30%

Food and Description	Amount	Fat Grams	Total Calories	% Fat Calories
(Weight Watchers)				
Chunky Beef Stew	7.5 oz	2	120	15
New England Clam Chowder	7.5 oz	–	90	–
Won Ton				
(Campbell's)	1 cup	1	40	23%
Homemade	1 cup	3	205	13%
■ SOUP(DEHYDRATED)/MIX				
(NOTE: Prepared as directed with water, unless otherwise stated. Pkg or cube servings are unprepared.)				
(A Taste of Thai)				
Hot & Sour Chili Pepper	1 cup	2	40	45%
Tangy Coconut Ginger	1 cup	1.5	25	54%
Asparagus, Cream of	1 pkg/2.2 oz	7	234	27%
(Aunt Patsy's Pantry)/Prepared				
Barley	8 oz	–	101	–
Black Bean	8 oz	1	127	7%
C. Thyme	8 oz	–	77	–
Lentil	8 oz	1	128	7%
Many Bean	8 oz	–	98	–
Navy	8 oz	–	123	–
Pea	8 oz	–	129	–
Red Lentil	8 oz	–	82	–
Beef Broth or Bouilon	1 cup	.7	19	33%
Beef Broth (Cubed)	1 cube	–	8	–
w/ water	1 cup	–	8	–
Beef Noodle	1 cup	.79	41	17%
Broth				
(G. Washington's)				
Brown Seasoning	1 pkg	–	48	–
	1 serving	–	6	–
Brown Seasoning				
Kosher for Passover	1 pkg	–	48	–
	1 serving	–	6	–
Golden Seasoning				
Brown Seasoning	1 pkg	–	48	–
	1 serving	–	6	–
Kosher for Passover	1 serving	–	6	–
Onion Seasoning	1 pkg	–	96	–
	1 serving	–	12	–
Vegetable Seasoning	1 pkg	–	96	–
	1 serving	–	12	–
Romanoff (M B T)				
Beef	1 pkt	.5	12	38%
Chicken	1 pkt	.5	14	32%
Onion	1 pkt	.5	16	28%

Food and Description	Amount	Fat Grams	Total Calories	% Fat Calories
Vegetable	1 pkt	.5	12	38%
Caldo Pronto				
(Sanwa)				
Albondigas Meatball w/noodles	1 cup	17	333	46%
Sabor A Camaron Shrimp	1 cup	14	310	41%
Sabor A Pollo Chicken	1 cup	13	310	38%
Sabor A Res Beef	1 cup	12	310	35%
(Campbell's)				
Block Ramen Noodles/prepared				
Low Fat				
Beef	8 oz	1	160	6%
Chicken	8 oz	1	160	6%
Oriental	8 oz	1	150	6%
Pork	8 oz	1	150	6%
Cup-A-Ramen/prepared				
Low Fat				
Beef flavor w/Vegetables	8 oz	2	220	8%
Chicken flavor w/Vegetables	8 oz	2	220	8%
Oriental flavor w/Vegetables	8 oz	2	220	8%
Shrimp flavor w/Vegetables	8 oz	2	230	8%
Regular				
Beef flavor w/Vegetables	8 oz	10	270	33%
Chicken flavor w/Vegetables	8 oz	10	270	33%
Oriental flavor w/Vegetables	8 oz	10	270	33%
Shrimp flavor w/Vegetables	8 oz	10	280	32%
Cup 2 Minute Soup Mix/prepared				
Chicken Vegetable	6 oz	2	90	20%
Creamy Chicken w/white meat	6 oz	4	90	40%
Noodle w/Chicken broth	6 oz	2	90	20%
Microwaveable				
Bean w/Bacon & Ham	8 oz	5	230	20%
Chicken Noodle	7.75 oz	4	100	36%
Chicken w/Rice	7.75 oz	4	100	36%
Chili Beef	7 oz	4	190	19%
Vegetable Beef	7.75 oz	2	100	18%
Microwaveable Cup (as packaged)				
Beef Flavored Noodle	1.35 oz	2	130	14%
Chicken Flavored Noodle	1.35 oz	3	140	19%
Hearty Noodle w/Vegetables	1.7 oz	2	180	10%
Noodle Soup w/Chicken Broth	1.35 oz	2	130	14%
Quality Soup & Recipe Mix/prepared				
Chicken Noodle	8 oz	2	100	18%
Hearty Noodle	8 oz	1	90	10%
Noodle	8 oz	2	110	16%

Food and Description	Amount	Fat Grams	Total Calories	% Fat Calories
Onion	8 oz	–	30	–
Vegetable	8 oz	–	40	–
Ramen Noodles/prepared				
Beef	8 oz	8	190	38%
Chicken	8 oz	8	190	38%
Oriental	8 oz	8	190	38%
Pork	8 oz	8	200	36%
Cauliflower	1 pkg/.7 oz	1.7	68	23%
	1 cup	1.7	68	23%
Celery, Cream of	1 cup	1.6	63	23%
Chicken (Right Time)	6 oz	–	14	–
Chicken Broth, Bouillon, Consomme	1 Pkg.	.8	16	45%
w/water	1 cup	1	21	43%
Chicken Broth (Cubed)	1 cube	–	8	–
w/water	1 cup	–	8	–
Chicken, Cream of	1 pkg/.6 oz	4	80	45%
	1 cup	5	107	42%
Chicken Noodle	1 cup	1	53	17%
(Campbell's)	1 cup	2	100	18%
Chicken Rice	1 cup	1	60	15%
Chicken Rice w/white meat				
(Campbell's)	1 cup	2	90	20%
Chicken Vegetable	1 cup	.79	49	15%
Clam Chowder-Manhattan	1 cup	1.55	65	22%
Clam Chowder-New England	1 cup	3.67	95	35%
Consomme w/Gelatin	1 pkg/2 oz	–	77	–
	1 cup	–	17	–
(Estee)				
Beef Noodle	6 oz	.5	20	23%
Chicken Noodle	6 oz	.5	25	18%
Mushroom	6 oz	2	40	45%
Onion	6 oz	.5	25	18%
Tomato	6 oz	.5	40	11%
(Golden Dipt)				
Clam Chowder				
Manhattan	¼ pkg	2	80	23%
New England	¼ pkg	2	84	21%
Lobster Bisque	¼ pkg	1	30	30%
Seafood Chowder	¼ pkg	2	70	20%
Shrimp Bisque	¼ pkg	1	30	30%
Golden Mushroom	6 oz	1	60	15%
(Hain)				
Savory Soup				
Lentil	¾ cup	2	130	8%

Food and Description	Amount	Fat Grams	Total Calories	% Fat Calories
Minestrone	¾ cup	1	110	8%
Potato Leek	¾ cup	18	260	62%
Split Pea	¾ cup	10	310	29%
Vegetable	¾ cup	1	80	11%
no salt	¾ cup	1	80	11%
Savory Soup & Recipe				
Cheese & Broccoli	¾ cup	22	310	64%
Mushroom	¾ cup	15	210	64%
no salt added	¾ cup	20	250	72%
Tomato	¾ cup	14	220	57%
Savory Soup & Sauce				
Cheese	⅓ pkt	2	90	20%
	¾ cup	16	250	58%
Savory Soup, Dip, & Recipe				
Onion	¾ cup	2	50	36%
no salt added	¾ cup	1	50	18%
(Herb-Ox)				
Bouillon Cubes				
Beef	1 cube	< 1	10	45%
Chicken	1 cube	< 1	10	45%
Instant Bouillon, Low Sodium				
Beef	1 pkg	< 1	12	38%
Chicken	1 pkg	< 1	12	38%
Vegetable	1 pkg	< 1	12	38%
Instant Bouillon, Regular				
Beef	1 tsp	< 1	10	45%
Chicken	1 tsp	< 1	12	38%
Instant Broth/Seasoning				
Beef	1 pkg	< 1	10	45%
Chicken	1 pkg	< 1	12	38%
(Hormel) Micro Cup Hearty Soup				
Bean & Ham	7.5 oz	3	190	14%
Beef Vegetable	7.5 oz	1	80	11%
Chicken Noodle	7.5 oz	3	110	25%
Chicken w/Rice	7.5 oz	2	110	16%
Country Vegetable	7.5 oz	2	90	20%
Minestrone	7.5 oz	2	110	16%
New England Clam Chowder	7.5 oz	5	120	38%
(Knorr) Soup mix				
Asparagus	⅓ pkg	2	60	30%
Prepared w/water & milk	8 oz	3	80	34%
Broccoli	⅓ pkg	4	90	40%
Prepared w/water & milk	8 oz	8	160	45%
Cauliflower	⅓ pkg	2	80	23%

Food and Description	Amount	Fat Grams	Total Calories	% Fat Calories
Prepared w/water & milk	8 oz	3	100	27%
Chicken Flavored Noodle	⅓ pkg	2	100	18%
Prepared	8 oz	2	100	18%
Chick'N Pasta	⅓ pkg	2	90	20%
Prepared	8 oz	2	90	20%
Country Barley	½ pkg	2	120	15%
Prepared	10 oz	2	120	15%
Fine Herb	⅓ pkg	5	110	41%
Prepared w/water & milk	8 oz	6	130	42%
French Onion	⅓ pkg	1	50	18%
Prepared	8 oz	1	50	18%
Hearty Minestrone	½ pkg	2	130	14%
Prepared	10 oz	2	130	14%
Leek	⅓ pkg	2	70	26%
Prepared w/water & milk	8 oz	4	110	33%
Mushroom	⅓ pkg	3	80	34%
Prepared w/water & milk	8 oz	4	100	36%
Oriental Hot & Sour	⅓ pkg	1	50	18%
Prepared w/water & egg	8 oz	3	80	34%
Oxtail Hearty Beef	⅓ pkg	2	70	26%
Prepared	8 oz	2	70	26%
Spinach	⅓ pkg	2	70	26%
Prepared	8 oz	2	70	26%
Spring Vegetable w/Herbs	⅓ pkg	< 1	30	15%
Prepared	8 oz	< 1	30	15%
Tomato Basil	⅓ pkg	3	90	30%
Prepared	8 oz	3	90	30%
Vegetable	¼ pkg	1	35	26%
Prepared	8 oz	1	35	26%
(Lipton)				
Cup-A-Soup				
Chicken & Noodles	6 oz	7	70	13%
Chicken-Flavored Broth	6 oz	.6	20	27%
Chicken'N Rice	6 oz	.7	45	14%
Chicken Noodle				
w/chicken meat	6 oz	1	50	18%
Chicken Vegetable	6 oz	.6	47	11%
Country Style Chicken				
flavor Supreme	6 oz	5.9	107	50%
Country Style Harvest Vegetable	6 oz	1	90	10%
Country Style Hearty Chicken	6 oz	1	70	13%
Cream of Chicken	6 oz	4	80	45%
Cream of Mushroom	6 oz	3	70	39%
Creamy Broccoli	6 oz	2	60	30%

Food and Description	Amount	Fat Grams	Total Calories	% Fat Calories
Creamy Broccoli & Cheese	6 oz	4	70	51%
Creamy Chicken w/vegetables	6 oz	3	93	29%
Green Pea	6 oz	4	113	32%
Lite				
Chicken Dijon	6 oz	1	50	18%
Chicken Florentine	6 oz	.5	42	11%
Creamy Broccoli	6 oz	1	40	23%
Creamy Tomato & Herb	6 oz	< 1	65	7%
Golden Broccoli	6 oz	1	42	21%
Lemon Chicken	6 oz	< 1	47	10%
Oriental	6 oz	1.7	45	34%
Tomato & Herb	6 oz	1	60	15%
Onion	6 oz	.5	27	17%
Ring Noodle	6 oz	1	60	15%
Spring Vegetable	6 oz	.8	40	18%
Tomato	6 oz	.9	103	8%
Lots-A-Noodles				
Hearty Beef	7 oz	1	110	8%
Hearty Garden Vegetable	7 oz	1.5	125	11%
Hearty Chicken	7 oz	1.6	110	13%
Hearty Chicken Noodle	7 oz	2	110	16%
Hearty Creamy Chicken	7 oz	8	180	40%
Recipe Secrets				
Beefy Onion	8 oz	< 1	30	15%
Golden Onion	8 oz	1	60	15%
Onion	8 oz	< 1	20	27%
Savory Herb w/Garlic	8 oz	< 1	35	13%
Soup Mix				
Chicken Noodle	8 oz	2	80	23%
Country Vegetable	8 oz	.7	80	8%
Giggle Noodle w/real chicken broth	8 oz	2	70	26%
Hearty Beef Noodle	8 oz	.9	85	10%
Hearty Chicken Noodle	8 oz	1	82	11%
Hearty Noodle w/vegetables	8 oz	1.6	75	19%
Noodle w/real chicken broth	8 oz	2	70	26%
Ring-O-Noodle w/real chicken broth	8 oz	1.5	67	20%
Soup Mix/Instant				
Beef Flavor Oriental	8 oz	1	180	5%
Chicken Flavor Oriental	8 oz	2	180	10%
Garden Vegetable Oriental	8 oz	1	200	5%
Oriental Noodle	8 oz	1	200	5%

Food and Description	Amount	Fat Grams	Total Calories	% Fat Calories
(Lite-Line) Bouillon				
Low Sodium				
Beef	1 tsp	–	12	–
Chicken	1 tsp	–	12	–
(Lunch Bucket)/Microwaveable				
Beef Noodle	8.25 oz	1	120	8%
Chicken Noodle	8.25 oz	3	110	25%
Country Vegetable	8.25 oz	1	90	10%
Hearty Chicken	8.25 oz	3	120	23%
Split Pea'n Ham	8.25 oz	3	130	21%
Vegetable Beef	8.25 oz	2	110	16%
(Mayacamas) Soup Mix				
Avgholemono	6 oz	< 1	60	8%
Black Bean	6 oz	< 1	65	7%
Broccoli, Creamy	6 oz	< 1	65	7%
Cheddar Cheese	6 oz	5	85	53%
Chicken Style	6 oz	< 1	55	8%
Cockie Leekie	6 oz	5	95	47%
Creamy Mushroom	6 oz	< 1	55	8%
Creamy Tomato	6 oz	< 1	55	8%
Cream Soup	6 oz	< 1	55	8%
French Onion	6 oz	< 1	50	9%
Garden Pea	6 oz	< 1	65	7%
Lentil	6 oz	< 1	65	7%
Minestrone	6 oz	< 1	70	6%
Mulligatawny	6 oz	< 1	55	8%
New England Clam	6 oz	1	65	14%
Potato Leek	6 oz	1	60	15%
Senegalese	6 oz	< 1	55	8%
Vegetable	6 oz	< 1	65	7%
Minestrone				
(Manischewitz)	8 oz	1	70	6%
Mushroom	8 oz	4.86	96	46%
(Nile Spice)				
Lentil Curry	10.5 oz	–	200	–
Tomato Minestrone	10.5 oz	–	190	–
Vegetable Chicken	10.5 oz	–	190	–
Vegetable Parmesan	10.5 oz	1	200	5%
(Nissin)				
Couscous Soups/prepared				
Lentil Curry	10 oz	< 1	220	2%
Tomato Minestrone	10 oz	–	200	–
Vegetable				
Chicken	10 oz	5	220	20%

Food and Description	Amount	Fat Grams	Total Calories	% Fat Calories
Parmesan	10 oz	3	200	14%
Cup O'Noodles				
Single Serving				
Beef	2.25 oz	14	290	43%
Beef Onion	2.25 oz	12	280	39%
Chicken	2.25 oz	14	300	42%
Chicken Mushroom	2.25 oz	12	280	39%
Chicken, Spicy	2.25 oz	12	290	37%
Crab	2.25 oz	13	270	43%
Garden Vegetable	2.25 oz	12	280	39%
Lobster	2.25 oz	13	290	40%
Pork	2.25 oz	12	280	39%
Shrimp	2.25 oz	13	290	40%
Twin Pack				
Beef	1.2 oz	7	150	42%
Chicken	1.2 oz	6	150	36%
Chicken, Spicy	1.2 oz	6	150	36%
Shrimp	1.2 oz	6	150	36%
Hearty Cup O'Noodles				
Beef Vegetable	2.25 oz	13	290	40%
Country Chicken	2.25 oz	14	300	42%
Chicken Oriental	2.25 oz	14	300	42%
Old Fashioned Vegetable	2.25 oz	15	290	47%
Seafood Chowder	2.25 oz	15	300	45%
Shrimp Chow Mein	2.25 oz	14	300	42%
Oodles of Noodles/Top Ramen				
w/Seasoning Packet				
Beef	3 oz	18	390	42%
Chicken	3 oz	18	400	41%
All Other Flavors	3 oz	18	400	41%
w/o Seasoning Packet				
All Flavors	3 oz	16	360	40%
Potato Soups/prepared				
Potato Leek	10 oz	6	160	34%
Potato Romano	10 oz	6	150	36%
Potato Tomato	10 oz	6	160	34%
Noodle-Hearty				
(Campbell's)	8 oz	2	110	16%
Onion	1 pkg	.5	35	13%
(Campbell's)	1 cup	–	50	–
(Lipton)	1 cup	1	35	26%
Onion Mushroom	8 oz	.5	80	6%
(Campbell's)	8 oz	1	50	18%
Oxtail	1 cup	2.55	71	32%

Food and Description	Amount	Fat Grams	Total Calories	% Fat Calories
Pea, Green or Split	1 cup	1.58	133	11%
(Manischewitz)	6 oz	.5	45	10%
(Soup Break) Instant				
Black Bean	6 oz	1	95	10%
Broccoli	6 oz	1	80	11%
Chicken Leek	6 oz	2	85	21%
Garden Pea	6 oz	1	85	11%
New England Clam	6 oz	2	105	17%
Potato Leek	6 oz	1	85	11%
Tomato	1 pkg/.7 oz	2	77	23%
	1 cup	2	102	18%
Tomato Vegetable	1 pkg/1.4 oz	2	125	14%
	1 cup	.87	55	14%
(Ultra Slim Fast) Prepared				
Creamy Chicken Leek	6 oz	< 1	50	9%
Creamy Potato Leek	6 oz	< 1	80	6%
Creamy Tomato	6 oz	< 1	60	8%
Hearty Onion	6 oz	< 1	45	10%
(Union Foods) Smack Ramen Dry				
Oriental Noodles	3 oz	15	370	36%
Vegetable				
(Campbell's)	1 cup	1	60	15%
(Manischewitz) w/Mushrooms	8 oz	1	70	6%
Vegetable Beef	1 cup	1	53	17%
Vegetable, Cream of	1 cup	5.69	105	49%
(Weight Watchers) Instant				
Beef Broth	1 pkg	–	8	–
Chicken Broth	1 pkg	–	8	–
(Wyler's) Bouillon				
Beef	1 tsp	–	6	–
	1 cube	–	6	–
Chicken	1 tsp	–	8	–
	1 cube	–	8	–
Onion	1 tsp	–	10	–
Vegetable	1 tsp	–	6	–
SOUP GREENS				
(Durkee)-Jar	2.5 oz	3	216	13%
SOUR CREAM				
(Kemps)	1 cup	42	450	84%
Cultured	1 oz	5	60	75%
Lite				
Sour Cream	1 oz	2	30	6%
Tator Topper	1 oz	2	30	6%
w/Chives	1 oz	5	60	75%

Food and Description	Amount	Fat Grams	Total Calories	% Fat Calories
(Knudsen)				
Hamshire	4 Tbs	13	130	90%
Nice N'Light	4 Tbs	6	90	60%
(Land O'Lakes)				
Lite				
Plain	1 Tbs	2	40	45%
w/Chives	1 Tbs	2	40	45%
Regular	1 Tbs	3	30	90%
Sour Half & Half	1 Tbs	2	25	72%
(Marzetti)				
Light	1 Tbs	< 1	30	15%
Sour Dress	1 Tbs	2	25	72%
(Nice N Light) Low-Fat-Light Sour Cream	4 Tbs	6	90	60%
Regular (cultured)	1 Tbs	2.5	26	87%
	1 cup	48	493	87%
(Weight Watchers) Light	2 Tbs	2	35	51%
SOUR CREAM SUBSTITUTES				
Sour Cream-flavored sprinkle products				
Best of Butter	½ tsp	< 1	4	100%
Molly McButter	½ tsp	< 1	4	100%
Sour Cream/substitute				
non-butterfat	1 oz	4	42	86%
	1 cup	39	417	84%
non-dairy	1 oz	6	59	92%
(Chivo)	1 Tbs	3	30	90%
(Dean's) Sour Delite	1 oz	5	50	90%
(IMO)	1 Tbs	3	30	90%
(Land O'Lakes)				
Light Dairy Blend	1 Tbs	1	20	45%
(Slender Choice)	1 Tbs	2	26	69%
SOURSOP/pureed	1 cup	.7	146	4%
SOY MEAL/defatted	½ cup	1	206	4%
SOY MILK				
Dry				
(La Loma)/canned				
Soyagen/prepared				
All-Purpose	1 cup	6	130	42%
Carob	¼ cup	6	140	39%
No Sucrose	1 cup	6	130	42%
(Worthington)				
Soyamel	1 oz	7	130	49%
Liquid	1 cup	4.58	79	52%
(Edensoy)				
Carob	1 cup	4.5	160	25%

Food and Description	Amount	Fat Grams	Total Calories	% Fat Calories
Original	1 cup	4	140	26%
Boxed	8.45 oz	4	140	26%
Vanilla	1 cup	2	150	12%
Boxed	8.45 oz	3	150	18%
(Health Valley) Soy Moo	8.5 oz	6	120	45%
(Isomil) infant formula w/iron	5 oz	5	100	45%
(Isoyalac) infant formula	5 oz	5.5	100	50%
(Soyalac) infant formula	5 oz	5.5	100	50%
(Vitasoy)				
Creamy Original	6 oz	< 1	105	9%
Vanilla Delite	6 oz	4	150	24%
(Westsoy)				
Lite 1%				
Plain	8 oz	2	100	18%
Vanilla	8 oz	2	110	16%
Original	1 cup	7	170	37%
SOY PRODUCT				
(Stir Fruity) Non-Dairy Treat				
Chilled				
Black Cherry	6 oz	2	140	13%
Blueberry	6 oz	1	140	6%
Lemon Chiffon	6 oz	3	150	18%
Mandarin Orange	6 oz	2	140	13%
Mixed Berry	6 oz	2	150	12%
Raspberry	6 oz	2	150	12%
Strawberry	6 oz	2	140	13%
SOY PROTEIN CONCENTRATE	1 oz	–	92	–
SOY SAUCE (*See also* SAUCE)				
(Shoyu)	1 Tbs	–	9	–
	¼ cup	–	30	–
(Tamari)	1 Tbs	–	11	–
	¼ cup	–	35	–
SOYA GRANULES (Feam)	¼ cup	–	140	–
SOYBEAN (*See also* individual products of, such as MISO PASTE, TOFU, etc.)				
Green				
boiled	½ cup	5.8	127	41%
(La Loma) canned w/liquid	~ 4 oz	7	120	53%
raw	½ cup	10	387	44%
roasted	½ cup	21.8	405	48%
SOYBEAN NUTS				
roasted-dry	½ cup	18.6	387	43%
roasted-salted or unsalted	1 oz	6.8	129	47%
	½ cup	21.8	405	48%
roasted & toasted	1 oz	6.8	129	47%

Food and Description	Amount	Fat Grams	Total Calories	% Fat Calories
SOYBEAN SPROUTS				
cooked	½ cup	2	38	47%
raw	10 sprouts	.6	12	45%
stir-fried	4 oz	8	143	50%
SPAGHETTI (*See* PASTA)				
SPAGHETTI DINNER (*See also* FROZEN ENTREE/DINNER, PASTA ENTREE/DINNER)				
Spaghetti w/meat sauce				
Box (Kraft)	1 cup	14	360	35%
Canned (Franco-American)	7.5 oz	8	211	34%
Spaghetti w/meatballs & meat sauce				
Canned	1 cup	10	260	35%
(Chef Boyardee)	7.5 oz	9	230	31%
(Estee)	7.5 oz	14	240	53%
(Franco-American)	7⅜ oz	8	220	33%
Standard Home Recipe (USDA)	1 cup	12	330	33%
Spaghetti w/meatballs & tomato sauce				
canned	1 cup	10.8	258	38%
homemade	1 cup	11.7	332	32%
Spaghetti w/red clam sauce (homemade)	1 cup	7	226	28%
Spaghetti w/tomato sauce & cheese				
canned	1 cup	1.5	190	7%
homemade	1 cup	8.8	280	28%
Spaghetti w/white clam sauce (homemade)	1 cup	19	346	49%
SPAGHETTI SAUCE (*See* SAUCE)				
SPAGHETTIO'S				
Canned (Franco-American)				
w/Meat balls	7⅜ oz	8	210	34%
w/Sliced beef franks	7⅜ oz	9	220	33%
SPICE BLENDS (*See also* SEASONINGS)				
(Lawry's)				
Bacon Onion	1 tsp	–	10	–
Garlic Pepper	¼ tsp	–	2	–
Garlic Powder w/parsley	1 tsp	–	12	–
Garlic Salt	1 tsp	–	4	–
Hot'N Spicy Seasoned Salt	1 tsp	–	3	–
Lemon Pepper	1 tsp	–	6	–
Minced Onion	1 tsp	–	7	–
Pinch of Herbs	1 tsp	.5	9	50%
Salt Free 17	1 tsp	–	10	–
Seasoned Pepper	1 tsp	–	9	–
Seasoned Salt	1 tsp	–	4	–
Seasoned Salt Free	1 tsp	–	3	–

Food and Description	Amount	Fat Grams	Total Calories	% Fat Calories
Seasoned Lite Salt	1 tsp	–	8	–
(McCormick/Schilling)				
All-Purpose	1 tsp	–	3	–
Garlic-saltless	1 tsp	–	11	–
It's a Dilly	1 tsp	–	11	–
Lemon Pepper	1 tsp	–	15	–
Popcorn Blend	1 tsp	–	10	–
Sesame All-Purpose	1 tsp	1	15	60%
(Mrs. Dash)				
Extra Spicy	1 tsp	–	12	–
Lemon & Herb	1 tsp	–	12	–
Low Pepper	1 tsp	–	12	–
No Garlic	1 tsp	–	12	–
Original	1 tsp	–	12	–
Table Blend	1 tsp	–	9	–
(Nile Spice)				
Cleopatra's Secret	⅛ tsp	–	–	–
Desert Spice	⅛ tsp	–	–	–
Ginger Curry	⅛ tsp	–	–	–
Maya Maize Popcorn	½ tsp	–	–	–
Nile Spice	⅛ tsp	–	–	–
Seasoning of Garlic	⅛ tsp	–	–	–
Spicy Lemon Pepper	⅛ tsp	–	–	–
SPICES (See SEASONINGS; SPICE BLENDS; individual listings)				
SPINACH				
Spinach				
canned	½ cup	< 1	25	18%
canned-chopped or whole leaf				
(Del Monte)	½ cup	–	25	–
canned-Premium Northwest (S&W)	½ cup	–	25	–
fresh-boiled	½ cup	–	21	–
frozen (Green Giant)	½ cup	–	25	–
(Harvest Fresh)	½ cup	–	25	–
(Pictsweet) Leaf	3.3 oz	–	20	–
Express-Microwave	2.4 oz	–	18	–
frozen-boiled	½ cup	–	27	–
raw/chopped	½ cup	–	6	–
Spinach-New Zealand				
boiled	½ cup	–	12	–
raw	1 lb	1	86	11%
SPINACH DISHES				
Creamed Spinach/frozen (Green Giant)	½ cup	3	70	39%
Spinach, creamed/frozen (Birds Eye)	½ cup	4	60	60%
Spinach Quiche/homemade	~ 5 oz	26	337	69%

Food and Description	Amount	Fat Grams	Total Calories	% Fat Calories
Spinach Souffle w/whole milk, butter, & cheese/homemade	1 cup	18	218	74%
SPOONBREAD (See BREAD)				
SPORTS DRINK				
(Gatorade)				
Fruit Punch	8 oz	–	50	–
Lemon Lime	8 oz	–	50	–
Orange	8 oz	–	50	–
(La Boost)				
Lemon Lime	8 oz	–	35	–
Orange	8 oz	–	35	–
(10-K)				
Fruit Punch	8 oz	–	60	–
Lemon-Lime	8 oz	–	60	–
Orange	8 oz	–	60	–
SPOT FISH				
cooked-dry heat	3 oz	18.6	252	66%
raw	3 oz	13.5	188	65%
SQUAB (Pigeon)				
breast meat only-raw	~ 4 oz	4.57	135	30%
giblets-raw	3 oz	6	132	41%
meat & skin-raw	~ 7 oz	47	584	72%
meat only-raw	~ 6 oz	12.6	239	47%
SQUASH				
Summer/fresh-boiled	½ cup	–	18	–
Crookneck/fresh-boiled	½ cup	–	18	–
frozen	½ cup	–	24	–
Scallop/fresh-boiled	½ cup	–	14	–
mashed	½ cup	–	19	–
Zucchini & Cocozelle/raw	½ cup	–	9	–
canned (S&W) Italian Style	½ cup	–	45	–
fresh				
boiled	½ cup	–	14	–
mashed	½ cup	–	15	–
frozen	½ cup	–	19	–
Winter				
Acorn/fresh-baked	½ cup	–	57	–
fresh-boiled-mashed	½ cup	–	41	–
All Varieties				
fresh-baked	½ cup	.6	39	14%
fresh-boiled-mashed	½ cup	–	47	–
(Birds Eye) frozen-cooked	½ cup	–	45	–
Butternut/fresh-baked	½ cup	–	41	–
fresh-boiled-mashed	½ cup	–	50	–

Food and Description	Amount	Fat Grams	Total Calories	% Fat Calories
frozen	½ cup	–	47	–
Hubbard/fresh-baked	½ cup	.6	51	11%
fresh-boiled-mashed	½ cup	–	37	–
Spaghetti/boiled or baked	½ cup	–	23	–
SQUASH DISHES				
Zucchini, Breaded/frozen				
(Ore Ida)	2.7 oz	8	150	48%
(Stilwell)	3.3 oz	10	200	45%
Zucchini, Italian style/canned	½ cup	–	33	–
SQUASH SEEDS				
dried/hulled	1 oz	13	155	75%
	1 cup	63	747	76%
kernels-roasted	1 oz	11.96	148	73%
	1 cup	95.6	1184	73%
whole-roasted	1 oz	5.5	127	39%
	1 cup	12	285	38%
SQUID				
breaded & fried	3 oz	6	149	36%
dried	3 oz	4.6	260	16%
pickled	1 oz	–	23	–
raw	3 oz	1	78	12%
SQUIRREL/raw-boneless	3 oz	8.5	182	42%
STEAK SAUCE				
(French's)	1 Tbs	–	16	–
STRAWBERRY				
Fresh	1 cup	.56	45	11%
	1 pint	1	97	9%
Frozen				
(Birds Eys)				
Lite Syrup (Birds Eye)	5 oz	< 1	90	5%
Syrup-Halved (Birds Eye)	5 oz	< 1	120	4%
Generic-frozen				
Sweetened				
Sliced	1 cup	< 1	245	2%
Whole	1 cup	< 1	200	2%
Unsweetened				
Thawed	3.5 oz	< 1	50	9%
Unthawed	1 cup	< 1	52	9%
STRAWBERRY DRINK	8 oz	–	125	–
w/ Vitamin C	8 oz	–	89	–
(Juice Works)	6 oz	–	94	–
STRAWBERRY JUICE				
(Smucker's)	8 oz	–	130	–
Strawberry Delight	6 oz	–	80	–

Food and Description	Amount	Fat Grams	Total Calories	% Fat Calories
STRAWBERRY JUICE DRINK				
(Tang) Fruit Box	8.45 oz	–	120	–
STRAWBERRY NECTAR				
(Kern's) bottled	6 oz	–	110	–
(Libby's) Ripe	8 oz	–	150	–
STRAWBERRY-BANANA NECTAR				
Bottled	6 oz	–	100	–
STUFFING				
(Betty Crocker)-mix				
Chicken				
dry	¼ pkg	1	110	8%
prepared	¼ pkg	9	180	45%
Corn Bread				
dry	¼ pkg	1	110	8%
prepared	¼ pkg	9	180	45%
Pork				
dry	¼ pkg	.5	110	4%
prepared	¼ pkg	9	190	43%
Traditional Herb				
dry	¼ pkg	.5	110	4%
prepared	¼ pkg	8	180	40%
(Golden Grains) mix				
prepared as directed				
All Flavors	½ cup	9	180	45%
(Oven Stuffin') mix				
Chicken/dry	1 oz	1	120	8%
Chicken/prepared	½ cup	9	190	43%
Cornbread Flavor/dry	~ 1 oz	1	120	8%
Cornbread Flavor				
prepared	½ cup	9	190	43%
(Pepperidge Farms) dry-pkg				
Corn Bread,Cubed, Herb				
Seasoned	1 oz	1	110	8%
Country Style	1 oz	1	100	9%
Cube	1 oz	1	110	8%
Distinctive Stuffing				
Apples & Raisin	1 oz	1	110	8%
Classic Chicken	1 oz	1	110	8%
Country Garden Herb	1 oz	4	120	30%
Harvest Vegetable & Almond	1 oz	3	110	25%
Wild Rice & Mushroom	1 oz	5	130	35%
Herb Sejasoned	1 oz	1	110	8%
(Pillsbury) Stuffing Originals				
Chicken	½ cup	7	170	37%

Food and Description	Amount	Fat Grams	Total Calories	% Fat Calories
Cornbread	½ cup	6	170	32%
Mushroom	½ cup	7	150	42%
Wild Rice	½ cup	7	160	39%
(Stove Top Stuffing) Microwave				
Broccoli & Cheese/mix	1 serving	5	140	32%
prepared	1 serving	8	170	42%
Homestyle Cornbread/mix	1 serving	3	120	23%
prepared	1 serving	7	160	39%
Mushroom & Onion/mix	1 serving	3	130	21%
prepared	1 serving	7	170	37%
Regular				
prepared w/butter	½ cup	7	160	39%
prepared w/o butter	½ cup	4	130	28%
(Stove Top Stuffing) Mix				
prepared w/butter				
Americana New England	½ cup	9	180	45%
Americana San Francisco	½ cup	9	170	48%
Beef	½ cup	9	180	45%
Chicken Flavor	½ cup	9	180	45%
Chicken Flavor (Flexible Serving)	½ cup	9	170	48%
Cornbread	½ cup	9	170	48%
Cornbread (Flexible Serving)	½ cup	8	170	48%
Homestyle Herb (Flexible Serving)	½ cup	9	170	48%
Long Grain & Wild Rice	½ cup	9	180	45%
Pork	½ cup	9	170	48%
Savory Herbs	½ cup	9	180	45%
Turkey	½ cup	9	170	48%
W/ Rice	½ cup	9	180	45%
prepared w/o butter				
Chicken Flavor	½ cup	1	110	8%
regular	½ cup	1	110	8%
(Stove Top Stuffing) 15 minute Mix				
Long Grain & Wild Rice mix	1 serving	1	110	8%
prepared	1 serving	9	180	45%
Mushroom & Onion mix	1 serving	1	110	8%
prepared	1 serving	9	180	45%
STURGEON				
cooked-dry heat	0 oz	4	115	31%
raw	3 oz	3	90	30%
smoked	3 oz	3.7	147	23%
steamed	3 oz	4.8	135	32%
SUCCOTASH (*See also* VEGETABLES, MIXED)				
Country Style-canned				
(Libby)	½ cup	1	80	11%

Food and Description	Amount	Fat Grams	Total Calories	% Fat Calories
(S & W)	½ cup	1	80	11%
Homemade	½ cup	–	110	–
SUCKER/raw				
White	3 oz	1.97	79	22%
SUET/raw	1 Tbs	13	121	100%
SUGAR				
Brown	1 cup	–	541	–
Firmly packed	1 cup	–	821	–
	1 Tbs	–	52	–
	1 tsp	–	18	–
Maple	1 piece/			
	1 oz	–	99	–
	1 Tbs	–	52	–
Powdered	1 cup	–	462	–
	1 Tbs	–	31	–
	1 tsp	–	10	–
Turbinado (Hain)	1 Tbs	–	50	–
White-granulated	1 cube	–	25	–
	1 tsp	–	15	–
	1 Tbs	–	46	–
	1 cup	–	770	–
SUGAR APPLE/raw				
(Sweetsop)	1 cup	.8	235	3%
SUGAR SUBSTITUTE				
(Equal)	1 pkt	–	4	–
	1 tablet	–	.5	–
Fructose	1 tsp	–	12	–
(Superose)	1 pkt	–	12	–
(Nutradiet) Sweetener	any amount	–	–	–
(Nutrasweet)	1 pkt	–	4	–
Spoonful	1 tsp	–	2	–
Sprinkle Sweet	1 tsp	–	–	–
Sucaryl	1 tsp	–	–	–
Sugar Twin	1 tsp	–	1	–
	1 pkt	–	< 4	–
Brown Sugar	1 tsp	–	1.5	–
Sweet * 10	⅛ tsp	–	–	–
SweetMate	1 pkt	–	3	–
Sweet'N Low	1 tsp	–	12	–
	1 packet	–	4	–
	1 tablet	–	–	–
Brown Sugar	1/10 tsp	–	2	–
Sweet'N Low-liquid	10 drops	–	–	–
Sweet'N Low 2	1 packet	–	4	–

Food and Description	Amount	Fat Grams	Total Calories	% Fat Calories
Sweet'ner (Weight Watchers)	1 pkt	–	3.5	–
	1 measuring spoon	–	4	–
Swiss Sweet (Estee)	1 tablet	–	–	–
	1 packet	–	4	–
SUNFISH/raw	3 oz	.6	76	7%
SUNFLOWER BUTTER	1 Tbs	8	92	78%
(Hain)	2 Tbs	15	180	75%
SUNFLOWER NUTS				
(Planters)				
dry roasted	1 oz	14	160	79%
unsalted	1 oz	15	170	79%
oil roasted	1 oz	15	170	79%
SUNFLOWER SEED				
(Frito Lay's)	1 oz	16	170	85%
Kernels	1 oz	17	180	85%
kernels-dried	1 oz	14	162	78%
	1 cup	71	821	78%
(Planters)	1 oz	14	160	79%
kernels-dry roasted	1 oz	14	165	76%
	1 cup	63.7	745	77%
kernels-oil roasted	1 oz	16	175	82%
	1 cup	77.56	830	84%
kernels-toasted	1 oz	16	176	82%
	1 cup	76	829	83%
(Laura Scudder's)				
dry roasted	1 oz	8.5	144	53%
oil roasted	1 oz	17	190	81%
roasted in shell	1 oz	7	86	73%
SUNFLOWER SEED BUTTER	1 oz	13.6	165	74%
	1 Tbs	7.6	93	74%
SUNFLOWER SEED FLOUR				
(partially defatted)	1 cup	1	261	3%
SURIMI	3 oz	.8	84	9%
SUSHI (*See* ORIENTAL FOOD)				
SWAMP CABBAGE/fresh-boiled	½ cup	–	10	–
SWEET 'N SOUR SAUCE (*See* SAUCE)				
SWEET POTATO				
boiled-no skin-mashed	½ cup	.5	172	3%
canned-mashed	1 cup	.5	258	2%
pieces	1 cup	< 1	183	3%
w/syrup	1 cup	< 1	212	2%
dehydrated flakes/dry	½ cup	< 1	228	2%
prepared w/water	1 cup	< 1	242	2%

Food and Description	Amount	Fat Grams	Total Calories	% Fat Calories
fresh-baked-mashed	½ cup	< 1	103	4%
frozen-baked	½ cup	< 1	88	5%
raw whole potato	½ cup	1	118	5%
SWEET POTATO DISHES				
(Birds Eye) Specialty Classics				
Candied Sweet Potatoes	5 oz	9	220	37%
Homemade				
Candied w/butter & brown sugar	~ 3.5 oz	3	144	19%
(Mrs. Paul's) frozen				
Candied Sweets'N Apples	4 oz	–	160	–
Candied Sweet Potatoes	4 oz	–	170	–
SWEET POTATO LEAVES				
cooked	1 cup	< 1	22	21%
raw-chopped	1 cup	< 1	12	38%
SWEET ROLL (See CAKE AND CAKE PASTRY)				
SWEETENER, ARTIFICIAL (See SUGAR SUBSTITUTE)				
SWORDFISH				
breaded & fried	3 oz	11.9	207	52%
cooked-dry heat	3 oz	4	132	27%
raw	3 oz	3	103	26%
SYRUP (See also PANCAKE/WAFFLE SYRUP)				
Cane	1 Tbs	–	53	–
Corn	1 Tbs	–	59	–
(Karo)				
Dark	1 Tbs	–	60	–
	½ cup	–	480	–
Light	1 Tbs	–	60	–
	½ cup	–	480	–
Maple	1 Tbs	–	50	–

T

Food and Description	Amount	Fat Grams	Total Calories	% Fat Calories
TABASCO SAUCE (See SAUCE)				
TABOULI (TABOULE, TABOULY)				
(Casbah) mix-prepared	1 serving	1	148	6%

Food and Description	Amount	Fat Grams	Total Calories	% Fat Calories
(Near East) wheat salad mix	⅞ oz	–	80	–
TACO SAUCE (*See* SAUCE)				
TAMARIND/fresh	1	–	5	–
TANGELO/fresh	1	–	39	–
TANGELO JUICE/fresh	8 oz	–	101	–
TANGERINE				
fresh	1	–	37	–
canned				
in juice	½ cup	–	46	–
in syrup	½ cup	–	76	–
TANGERINE JUICE				
Mandarin Tangerine Juice				
(Dole) Pure & Light	6 oz	–	100	–
Tangerine Juice				
canned	8 oz	–	107	–
canned (sweetened)	1 cup	–	125	–
fresh	8 oz	–	108	–
from frozen concentrate	8 oz	–	114	–
undiluted	6 oz	< 1	345	1%
TAPIOCA (*See also* PUDDING)				
(Minute)	1 Tbs	–	30	–
	3.5 oz	–	352	–
TARO				
chips	10	5.86	110	48%
fresh-cooked-slices	½ cup	–	94	–
leaves-raw	½ cup	–	12	–
steamed	½ cup	< 1	17	27%
raw	½ cup	–	56	–
shoots	~ 3 oz	< 1	9	50%
Tahitian				
cooked-sliced	½ cup	< 1	30	15%
raw-sliced	½ cup	1	25	36%
TARRAGON/ground	1 tsp	–	5	–
TARTAR SAUCE (*See also* SAUCE)				
Generic	1 Tbs	8	75	96%
TAVERN NUTS				
(Planters)	1 oz	15	170	79%
TEA				
Bottled				
(Iguana Bay)				
Tropical Iced Tea/diet lemon	6 oz	–	2	–
Brewed	6 oz	–	2	–
(Bigelow) Regular/all flavors	6 oz	–	1	–
(Celestial Seasonings)				

Food and Description	Amount	Fat Grams	Total Calories	% Fat Calories
all flavors	1 cup	–	1–7	–
Kafree (Worthington)				
caffeine free	1 bag	–	1	–
(Lipton) Herbal tea bags				
all flavors	1 bag	–	4	–
(Nestea) tea bags	1 bag	–	2	–
Russian tea	8 oz	–	111	–
Canned (Nestea)				
Diet Lemon-Flavored	12 oz	–	2	–
w/Sugar	12 oz	–	146	–
Instant-mixes				
(Country Time)	8 oz	–	70	–
(Crystal Light)				
Iced				
decaffeinated	8 oz	–	4	–
regular	8 oz	–	4	–
(Lipton)	6 oz	–	–	–
decaffeinated	6 oz	–	–	–
sugar-free	8 oz	–	1	–
decaffeinated	8 oz	–	1	–
w/ Nutrasweet	8 oz	–	5	–
decaffeinated	8 oz	–	5	–
lemon flavored-sweetened	6 oz	–	55	–
lemon flavored-unsweetened	8 oz	–	3	–
(Maxwell House) concentrate				
sweetened	8 oz	–	80	–
unsweetened	8 oz	–	2	–
(Maxwell House) instant	6 oz	–	2	–
(Nestea)				
decaffeinated	6 oz	–	–	–
decaffeinated ice tea mix				
sugar-free	8 oz	–	6	–
Iced tea mix-sugar-free	8 oz	–	6	–
Iced tea mix w/sugar &				
lemon	8 oz	–	70	–
Purepak iced tea-sugar-free				
w/lemon	8 oz	–	2	–
Purepak iced tea w/sugar &				
lemon	8 oz	–	70	–
(Nestea) Ice Teasers				
Citrus	8 oz	–	6	–
Lemon	8 oz	–	6	–
Orange	8 oz	–	6	–
Tropical	8 oz	–	6	–

Food and Description	Amount	Fat Grams	Total Calories	% Fat Calories
Wild Cherry	8 oz	–	6	–
sugar-free/all flavors	8 oz	–	4	–
sugar sweetened w/lemon	12 oz	–	120	–
(Wyler's) fruit tea punch				
bottle	6 oz	–	118	–
canned	6 oz	–	118	–
TEMPEH	½ cup	6	165	33%
TEMPURA BATTER MIX				
(Krusteaz)	1 oz	–	102	–
(S&B Sunbird)	1 pkg	.5	112	4%
TEQUILA (See LIQUOR, DISTILLED)				
TERIYAKI SAUCE (See SAUCE)				
TERRAPIN/baked	¾ cup	4	161	22%
THIRST QUENCHER (See SPORTS DRINK)				
THYME/ground	1 tsp	–	4	–
TILEFISH				
cooked-dry heat	3 oz	3	117	23%
raw	3 oz	2	80	23%
TOASTER PASTRY (See PASTRY, TOASTER)				
TOFU				
dried-frozen	~ ½ oz	5	82	55%
fried	~ ½ oz	2.6	35	67%
Okara	½ cup	1	47	19%
raw-firm	¼ block	7	118	53%
	½ cup	10.98	183	54%
(Hinoichi) Chinese	4 oz	3	70	39%
raw-regular	¼ block	5.55	88	57%
	½ cup	5.9	94	57%
(Hinoichi) Japanese	4 oz	2	60	30%
salted & fermented-fuyu	1 block	1	13	69%
soft (Hinoichi)-Kinugoshi	4 oz	2	50	36%
TOFU FROZEN DESSERT PRODUCTS				
(Dreamy Tofu)	½ cup	4.8	135	32%
(Tofruzen) (non-dairy)				
strawberry	4 oz	8	160	5%
praline pecan	4 oz	8	180	40%
vanilla almond	4 oz	8	180	40%
(Le Tofu)				
chocolate	3.5 oz	7.7	155	45%
strawberry	3.5 oz	8.5	163	47%
vanilla	3.5 oz	7.8	155	45%
(Tofulite)	4 oz	7	150	42%
(Tofutti)				
Chocolate Supreme	4 oz	13	230	51%

Food and Description	Amount	Fat Grams	Total Calories	% Fat Calories
Lite-Lite				
Chocolate	4 oz	< 1	90	5%
Chocolate-Vanilla Twirl	4 oz	< 1	90	5%
Vanilla	4 oz	< 1	90	5%
Vanilla, Chocolate,				
Strawberry	4 oz	< 1	90	5%
Love Drops				
Cappuccino	4 oz	12	230	47%
Chocolate	4 oz	13	230	51%
Vanilla	4 oz	12	220	49%
Tofutti O's/Chocolate				
Dipped	1 piece	2	40	45%
Vanilla	4 oz	11	200	50%
Vanilla Almond Bark	4 oz	14	230	55%
Wild Berry	4 oz	12	210	51%
TOMATO				
Green	1	–	30	–
Red	1	–	24	–
Canned				
(Contadina)				
California Sliced	½ cup	–	40	–
Italian Style-Pear	½ cup	–	25	–
Italian Style-Stewed	½ cup	–	35	–
Stewed	½ cup	–	35	–
Whole-Peeled	½ cup	–	25	–
(Del Monte)				
Stewed	½ cup	–	35	–
Wedges	½ cup	–	30	–
Whole-Peeled	½ cup	–	25	–
(Hunt's)				
Crushed	½ cup	< 1	25	18%
Stewed	½ cup	–	35	–
Whole	½ cup	–	20	–
(Nutradiet) Whole	½ cup	–	25	–
(S&W)				
Italian Style-Pear	½ cup	–	25	–
Italian Style Stewed	½ cup	–	35	–
Ready Cut-Peeled	½ cup	–	25	–
Stewed	½ cup	–	35	–
Stewed-50% less salt	½ cup	–	35	–
Stewed-Mexican Style	½ cup	–	40	–
Whole-Peeled	½ cup	–	25	–
TOMATO ASPIC/canned				
Supreme (S&W)	½ cup	–	60	–

Food and Description	Amount	Fat Grams	Total Calories	% Fat Calories
TOMATO DISHES				
Stewed Tomatoes				
homemade	1 cup	2	60	30%
TOMATO JUICE				
canned				
(Campbell's)	6 oz	–	35	–
generic	6 oz	–	32	–
(Hunt's) no salt added	6 oz	–	30	–
(Nutradiet)	6 oz	–	35	–
(S&W) California	6 oz	–	35	–
Tomato w/beef broth				
canned	5.5 oz	–	61	–
Tomato & Chile Cocktail				
(Del Monte) Snap-E-Tom	6 oz	–	40	–
Tomato & Clam/canned	5.5 oz	–	77	–
TOMATO MARINARA SAUCE/canned	1 cup	8	171	42%
TOMATO PASTE/canned	½ cup	1	110	8%
(Contadina)	2 oz	–	50	–
canned Italian style	2 oz	1	65	14%
(Del Monte)	¾ cup	1	150	6%
(Hunt's)	2 oz	–	45	–
Italian Style	2 oz	–	50	–
(S&W)	6 oz	–	150	–
TOMATO POWDER	4 oz	< 1	342	1%
TOMATO PUREE/canned	1 cup	–	102	–
canned (Contadina)	½ cup	–	40	–
w/crushed tomatoes	½ cup	–	30	–
(Hunt's)	4 oz	–	45	–
(S&W)	4 oz	–	60	–
w/diced tomatoes	4 oz	–	35	–
TOMATO SAUCE (*See also* SAUCE)				
Canned				
(Contadina)				
Italian	½ cup	–	30	–
Original	½ cup	–	30	–
Thick & Zesty	½ cup	–	40	–
(Del Monte)				
Original	1 cup	1	70	13%
w/Onions	1 cup	1	100	9%
(S&W)	½ cup	–	40	–
TOMATO SOUP (*See* SOUP)				
TONIC WATER (*See* WATER)				
TORTELLINI SOUP (*See* SOUP)				
TORTILLA (*See* MEXICAN FOOD)				

Food and Description	Amount	Fat Grams	Total Calories	% Fat Calories
TORTILLA CHIPS				
(Arizona) Traditional Rounds	1 oz	6	137	39%
(Arizona Sonoran) Rounds	1 oz	8	139	52%
(Azteca) Buenitos	1 oz	7	140	45%
(Chi-Chi's)	1 oz	8	142	51%
(Doritos)				
Cool Ranch	1 oz	7	140	45%
Jumpin' Jack	1 oz	7	140	45%
Lights				
all flavors	1 oz	4	110	33%
cool ranch	1 oz	4	120	30%
Nacho Cheese	1 oz	7	140	45%
Salsa Rio	1 oz	7	140	45%
Taco Flavor	1 oz	7	140	45%
Traditional	1 oz	6	140	39%
(Eagle)				
Cantina Tortilla				
Nacho	1 oz	8	150	48%
Regular	1 oz	8	150	48%
Restaurant Style Tortilla Strips	1 oz	6	150	42%
(Fritos)				
Bar-B-Q	1 oz	9	150	54%
Chili Cheese Flavored	1 oz	10	160	56%
Crisp'N Thin	1 oz	10	160	56%
Dip Size	1 oz	10	150	60%
Non-Stop Nacho Cheese	1 oz	9	150	'54%
Original	1 oz	10	150	60%
Rowdy Rustlers	1 oz	9	150	54%
Wild'N Mild	1 oz	9	160	51%
(Hain)				
Sesame	1 oz	7	140	45%
no salt	1 oz	7	140	45%
Sesame Cheese	1 oz	8	160	45%
Taco Style-no salt	1 oz	11	160	62%
(Health Valley)				
Cheese	1 oz	10	160	56%
No Salt	1 oz	11	160	62%
Plain	1 oz	11	160	62%
(Keebler)				
Hooplas				
Nacho	1 oz	8	140	51%
Original	1 oz	8	140	51%
(La Famous) Tortilla Chips	1 oz	7	140	45%
no salt	1 oz	7	140	45%

Food and Description	Amount	Fat Grams	Total Calories	% Fat Calories
(Laura Scudder's)				
Corn Chips				
all flavors	1 oz	10	160	56%
Tortilla Chips	1 oz	7	140	45%
Strips	1 oz	7	140	45%
(Mi Ranchito)				
Traditional & Supreme Lights	1 oz	6	140	39%
(Michael Season's) Organic				
Lightly Salted	1 oz	5	140	32%
Nacho	1 oz	5	140	32%
Ranch	1 oz	5	140	32%
Salsa	1 oz	5	140	32%
Tostados Chips Bite Size	1 oz	5	135	34%
Unsalted	1 oz	5	140	32%
White Corn				
Lightly Salted	1 oz	5	135	34%
Unsalted	1 oz	5	135	34%
(Old Vienna)				
Plain	1 oz	6	140	39%
(Planters)				
Nacho	1 oz	8	150	48%
Plain	1 oz	10	160	56%
(Pringles)				
Fresh Roasted	1 oz	7	140	45%
Mild Nacho Cheese	1 oz	7	140	45%
(Santitas) Restaurant Style				
Cantina Style	1 oz	6	140	39%
Chips	1 oz	7	140	45%
Fajita-Flavored	1 oz	7	140	45%
Strips	1 oz	7	140	45%
(Suncheros) Keebler				
all flavors	1 oz	9	150	54%
(Tostitos)				
Bite Size	1 oz	8	150	48%
Lime'N Chile	1 oz	7	150	42%
Traditional	1 oz	8	140	51%
White Corn Rejstaurant	1 oz	6	130	42%
(Tyson)				
Nacho Cheese	1 oz	7	140	45%
Ranch Flavor	1 oz	7	140	45%
Traditional	1 oz	7	140	45%
Unsalted	1 oz	7	140	45%
(Weight Watchers)				
Corn Snackers	.5 oz	2	60	30%

Food and Description	Amount	Fat Grams	Total Calories	% Fat Calories
Nacho Cheese Flavor (Wise)	.5 oz	2	60	30%
Bravos-Nacho Cheese Flavor	1 oz	8	150	48%
Corn Chips/Corn Crunchies	1 oz	10	160	56%
Corn Spirals-Crispy Corn Twists Nacho Cheese	1 oz	11	160	62%
Toasted Corn Spirals-Crispy Corn Twists	1 oz	11	160	62%
TRAIL MIX (See CEREAL, FRUIT SNACKS, SNACK MIX)				
TREACLE (See MOLASSES)				
TROUT				
Mixed				
raw	3 oz	5.6	126	40%
Rainbow				
broiled w/ butter	3 oz	9	175	46%
cooked-dry heat	3 oz	3.66	129	26%
raw	3 oz	2.85	100	26%
smoked	3 oz	3	153	18%
TUMERIC/ground	1 tsp	–	8	–
TUNA (See also SEAFOOD ENTREE/DINNER)				
Bluefin				
cooked-dry heat	3 oz	5	157	29%
fresh-raw	3 oz	4	122	30%
Light				
canned in oil	3 oz	6.98	169	37%
canned in water	3 oz	< 1	111	4%
Light Chunk				
canned in oil				
(Bumble Bee)	2 oz	12	160	68%
(Carnation)	2 oz	8	125	58%
(Chicken of the Sea)	2 oz	13	170	69%
(S&W) Fancy	2 oz	10	140	64%
(Star Kist)	2 oz	13	150	78%
Light Chunk				
canned in water				
(Carnation)	2 oz	2	70	26%
(Chicken of the Sea)	2 oz	1	60	5%
(Chicken of the Sea)	3.5 oz	1	105	9%
(Featherweight)	2 oz	1	60	15%
(S&W) Fancy	2 oz	1	60	15%
(Star Kist)	2 oz	.5	60	8%
(Weight Watchers)	2 oz	< 1	60	8%
canned in distilled water				
(Star Kist)	2 oz	.5	65	7%

Food and Description	Amount	Fat Grams	Total Calories	% Fat Calories
Skipjack				
fresh-raw	3 oz	1	88	10%
White				
canned in oil	2 oz	6.87	158	39%
canned in water	2 oz	2	116	16%
White-chunk				
canned in water				
(Bumble Bee)	2 oz	2	70	26%
White-solid				
canned in oil				
(Star Kist) Prime Catch-Light	2 oz	13	150	78%
canned in water				
(Bumble Bee)	2 oz	2	70	26%
(Star Kist)	2 oz	< 1	60	8%
(Weight Watchers)	2 oz	1	70	13%
White-solid Albacore				
canned Fancy				
in oil (S&W)	2 oz	12	160	68%
canned in water				
(Chicken of the Sea)	3.5 oz	2	120	15%
(Star Kist)	2 oz	.5	70	6%
Yellowfin				
fresh-raw	3 oz	1	90	10%
TUNA HELPER (See also SEAFOOD ENTREE/DINNER)				
(Betty Crocker) prepared				
Cheesy Noodles	⅕ pkg	8	240	32%
Creamy Noodles	⅕ pkg	14	300	42%
Fettuccine Alfredo	⅕ pkg	13	300	41%
Pot Pie	⅙ pkg	27	420	58%
Romanoff	⅕ pkg	9	290	28%
Tetrazzini	⅕ pkg	8	240	30%
(Bumble Bee) Tuna Mix-Ins				
As Packaged				
Lemon Herb	2 oz	–	25	–
Zesty Tomato	2 oz	–	25	–
TUNA PATTY/homemade	3 oz	3	80	34%
TUNA SALAD				
commercial				
(Carnation)				
The Spreadables	1.875 oz	6	90	60%
homemade-includes salad dressing,				
tuna canned in oil, & no egg	1 cup	19	375	46%
TURBINADO SUGAR				
(Hain)	1 Tbs	–	50	–

Food and Description	Amount	Fat Grams	Total Calories	% Fat Calories
TURBOT/raw	3 oz	2.5	81	28%
TURKEY				
(NOTE: All turkey meat is roasted, unless otherwise stated.)				
all classes/meat, skin, giblets, and neck-roasted-1 whole turkey	~ 9 lb	379.97	8245	42%
dark meat w/skin	~ 2 lb	93	1789	47%
dark meat w/o skin	~ 5 oz	10	262	34%
giblets /simmered	~ 5 oz	7	243	26%
gizzard/simmered	~ 5 oz	5.6	236	21%
heart/simmered	~ 5 oz	8	257	28%
light meat w/skin	2¼ lb	87	206	38%
light meat w/o skin	~ 5 oz	4.5	219	19%
liver/simmered	~ 5 oz	8	237	30%
meat & skin-dark & light-no giblets or neck	~ 4 lb	180.6	3857	42%
(Butterball) deep basted	3.5 oz	9-10	190-200	42%-45%
meat only (dark & light)	~ 5 oz	6.95	238	26%
(Armour Star)				
Broth basted w/sugar	4 oz	10	180	50%
w/o sugar	4 oz	10	180	50%
Butter basted	4 oz	10	190	47%
(Butterball)				
boneless-light & dark-meat only-cooked	3.5 oz	7	140	45%
Deep Basted-dark meat w/o skin	3.5 oz	10	195	46%
light meat w/o skin	3.5 oz	4	160	23%
Li'L Butterball/frozen				
light & dark-meat only-cooked	3.5 oz	7	175	36%
Stuffed/frozen-light-meat only-cooked	3.5 oz	3.5	140	23%
dark meat only-cooked	3.5 oz	7	175	36%
(Butterball) cooked parts w/o skin				
Breast Fillet	3.5 oz	3.5	140	23%
Breast Half	3.5 oz	7	175	36%
Breast Slices	3.5 oz	3.5	140	23%
Drumsticks	3.5 oz	7	175	36%
Thighs	3.5 oz	14	245	51%
Wing Drumettes	3.5 oz	10	280	32%
Wings	3.5 oz	10.5	210	45%
Canned (Tyson) Wholesale Club Item	3.5 oz	3	120	23%
(Hormel) Turkey By George				
Hickory Barbecue	5 oz	5	190	24%
Italian Style Parmesan	5 oz	5	170	26%

Food and Description	Amount	Fat Grams	Total Calories	% Fat Calories
Lemon Pepper	5 oz	4	160	23%
Mustard Tarragon	5 oz	6	180	30%
(Land O'Lakes) Fresh				
Breast	3 oz	1	100	9%
Drumsticks	3 oz	5	120	38%
Thighs	3 oz	10	150	60%
Wings	3 oz	5	120	38%
Butter-basted young turkey	3 oz	8	140	51%
Plain young turkey	3 oz	7	130	49%
Self-basting (broth) young	3 oz	5	120	38%
Turkey Hindquarters Roast	3 oz	8	140	51%
(Louis Rich)				
Fresh Turkey Cuts				
Turkey Breast-cooked	1 oz	2	45	40%
Turkey Breast Roast-cooked	1 oz	1	40	23%
Turkey Breast Slices-cooked	1 oz	1	40	23%
Turkey Breast Steaks-cooked	1 oz	1	40	23%
Turkey Breast Tenderloins-cooked	1 oz	.5	40	11%
Turkey Drumsticks	1 oz	3	55	49%
Turkey Thighs	1 oz	4	65	55%
Turkey Wings	1 oz	3	55	49%
Turkey Wing Drumettes	1 oz	2	50	36%
Turkey Wing Portions	1 oz	3	55	49%
Whole-Fresh	1 oz	3	55	49%
(Perdue) Perdue Done It!/ Cooked as packaged				
Breast Nuggets	1 oz	4.1	69	53%
Turkey Back/meat only-simmered	~ 5 oz	11	274	36%
Turkey Breast/meat & skin				
(½ breast)	~ 2 lb	64	1637	35%
Turkey Breast (Armour)				
Turkey Selects-boneless				
Breast Roast	3 oz	5	120	38%
Breast slices	3 oz	1	90	10%
Breast Tenderloins	3 oz	1	90	10%
Turkey Strips	3 oz	4	100	36%
Turkey Breast/meat only				
Frozen-Cooked				
(Butterball)	3.5 oz	7	175	36%
(Tyson) Wholesale Club Item	3.5 oz	3	160	17%
Turkey Breast of/boneless meat only				
(Butterball) cooked	3.5 oz	3.5	140	23%
Turkey Drumsticks				
(Butterball) Fresh'N Easy Drumettes				
cooked	1 oz	3	80	34%

Food and Description	Amount	Fat Grams	Total Calories	% Fat Calories
Turkey Drumsticks (Butterball)-Fresh'N Easy-cooked	1 oz	2	50	36%
Turkey/flesh only				
dark meat	1 cup	9	223	36%
light meat	1 cup	4	194	19%
Turkey/ground-packaged	2 oz	7	122	52%
(Armour) Golden Star-raw	1 oz	4	50	72%
(Armour) Turkey Selects	3 oz	6	120	45%
Turkey Leg/meat & skin	~ 1 lb	55	1133	41%
Turkey Wing/meat & skin	~ 6.5 oz	23	426	49%
(Butterball) Fresh'N Easy-cooked	1 oz	2	60	30%
(Louis Rich)				
85% lean	1 oz	4	60	60%
90% lean	1 oz	3	50	54%
(Swift Premium) cooked	1 oz	5	70	64%
(Swift Premium) dark meat w/skin-cooked	3.5 oz	14	245	51%
TURKEY ENTREE/DINNER (See also FROZEN ENTREE/DINNER)				
Turkey & Gravy/frozen	5 oz	3.7	95	35%
(Banquet)	8 oz	8	150	48%
(Banquet)-Cook'n Bags	5 oz	6	100	54%
Turkey Dijon/frozen				
(Lean Cuisine)	9.5 oz	5	230	20%
Turkey Loaf/homemade	5 oz	15	280	48%
Turkey (Louis Rich)-breaded-frozen				
Turkey Nuggets-prepared	~ 1 oz	4	65	55%
Turkey Patties-prepared	~ 3 oz	13	220	53%
Turkey Sticks	1 oz	5	80	56%
Turkey Pot Pies				
frozen				
(Banquet)				
Original	7 oz	31	510	55%
Supreme Microwave	7 oz	26	423	55%
(Morton)	7 oz	28	420	60%
(Stouffer's)	10 oz	33	530	56%
(Swanson)				
Hungry Man	16 oz	36	650	50%
Original	7 oz	21	380	50%
(Tyson) Premium	9 oz	18	370	44%
homemade (9"dia)	⅓ serving/			
	~ 8 oz	31	550	51%
Turkey Roast/frozen-light & dark	~ 7 oz	11	304	33%
	3 oz	5	130	35%
Turkey, Scalloped/homemade	~ 7 oz	5.6	253	20%

Food and Description	Amount	Fat Grams	Total Calories	% Fat Calories
Turkey (Schwan's)-frozen-partially or fully cooked unless otherwise stated				
Roll	3.5 oz	7	140	45%
Breast w/Gravy	3.5 oz	5	110	41%
Turkey Breast (unbreaded)	3 oz	< 1	70	6%
Turkey, Sticks/homemade-breaded/battered and fried	5 oz	24	397	54%
Turkey, Stuffed Breast/frozen (Weight Watchers)	8.5 oz	8	270	27%
Turkey (Tyson) Premium Dinners				
Frozen w/Dressing	11.5 oz	11	380	26%
Turkey Tetrazzini/frozen	~ 7 oz	16.6	282	53%
TURKEY PRODUCTS (*See also* LUNCHEON MEAT)				
Turkey Bacon				
(Armour) Turkey Selects	1 strip	2	35	51%
Turkey Bologna	2 slices/2 oz	8.6	113	69%
Turkey Breakfast Strips (Armour)-Golden				
Star-raw	1 strip	4	50	72%
(Armour) Turkey Selects	1 strip	4	50	72%
(Armour)				
barbequed-packaged	1 oz	1	39	23%
(Butterball) Deli-no salt added	1 oz	–	45	–
Fresh Half-cooked	1 oz	2	50	36%
Fresh'N Easy slices-cooked	1 oz	1	40	23%
Oven Prepared Deli w/caramel-skinless	1 oz	–	25	–
Slice'N Serve Hickory Smoked-Breast of turkey	1 oz	1	35	26%
Slice'N Serve BBQ Seasoned-Breast of Turkey	1 oz	2	40	45%
Slice'N Serve oven-prepared w/broth	1 oz	1	30	30%
Slice'N Serve oven-prepared smoked	1 oz	1	30	30%
Slice'N Serve oven-prepared skinless young w/broth	1 oz	1	30	30%
Slice'N Serve oven-roasted				
Breast of turkey	1 oz	1	35	26%
Turkey Breast	1 oz	2	40	45%
(Louis Rich) fully cooked				
Barbecued	1 oz	1	35	26%
Hickory Smoked	1 oz	1	35	26%
Hickory Smoked Dark Roast of Turkey	1 oz	.5	35	13%
Honey Roasted	1 oz	1	35	26%
Oven Roasted	1 oz	1	30	30%

Food and Description	Amount	Fat Grams	Total Calories	% Fat Calories
Roast of Turkey-Breast & Dark (Oscar Meyer) Oven roasted	1 oz	.5	30	15%
97% fat-free	1 slice	.5	20	23%
Smoked-98% fat-free	1 slice	.5	20	23%
Turkey, canned/boned w/broth	2.5 oz	4.87	116	38%
(Hormel) Chunk	6¾ oz	10	230	39%
(Swanson) Premium Chunk White	2.5 oz	2	90	20%
(Swanson) Premium Chunk White & Dark	2.5 oz	3	90	30%
Turkey Frankfurter-Generic	2.5 oz	8	102	71%
Turkey Ham	2 slices/2 oz	2.88	73	36%
(Butterball) Slice'N Serve	1 oz	2	35	51%
Slice'N Serve-Honey cured	1 oz	2	40	45%
(Louis Rich)	1 oz	1	35	26%
w/water added	1 oz	1	35	26%
Turkey Loaf	2 slices/2 oz	.67	47	13%
Turkey Pastrami	2 oz	3.5	80	39%
(Butterball) Slice'N Serve	1 oz	1	35	26%
Turkey Patties/breaded-battered-fried	1(2¼ oz)	11.5	181	57%
Turkey Roll/light	1 oz	2	42	43%
light & dark	2 slices/2 oz	1.98	42	42%
Turkey Salami	2 slices/2 oz	7.8	111	63%
(Butterball) Slice'N Serve	1 oz	4	50	72%
Turkey Sausage-smoked-packaged (Armour) Golden Star-raw				
links or patties	1 oz	4	60	60%
(Armour) Turkey Selects-Heat'N Serve	1 oz	6	80	68%
(Louis Rich) Turkey-Ground Breakfast	1 oz	4	55	66%
TURKEY SOUP (*See* SOUP)				
TURMERIC/ground	1 tsp	–	4	–
TURNIP				
fresh-boiled	½ cup	–	14	–
frozen	½ cup	–	26	–
raw	½ cup	–	18	–
TURNIP GREENS				
fresh-boiled	½ cup	–	15	–
canned				
generic	½ cup	–	17	–
(Luck's) w/diced turnips				
seasoned w/pork	7.5 oz	6	90	60%
frozen				
generic	½ cup	–	24	–
(Pictsweet) w/diced turnips	3.3 oz	–	20	–
raw	½ cup	–	7	–

Food and Description	Amount	Fat Grams	Total Calories	% Fat Calories
TURTLE/Green				
canned	3 oz	.6	91	6%
raw	3 oz	< 1	76	6%

V

Food and Description	Amount	Fat Grams	Total Calories	% Fat Calories
VEAL CUTS				
Breast/lean & fat-braised	3 oz	18	258	63%
Chop				
Lean & fat-fried				
w/ bone-raw	6.5 oz	18.6	282	59%
Lean only w/bone-raw	6.5 oz	6.6	177	34%
Chuck/lean & fat-cooked	3 oz	10.9	200	49%
Cutlet, Steak				
Lean & fat				
Boneless-broiled/				
braised	3 oz	9.4	182	47%
Lean only				
Boneless-broiled/				
braised	3 oz	3.5	140	23%
Ground or patty broiled				
(4 oz raw)	2.4 oz	8.9	156	51%
Loin/lean & fat				
Braised or broiled	3 oz	13	199	59%
Rib Roast/lean & fat				
Roasted	3 oz	14	230	55%
Round w/ Rump				
Roasts & leg cutlets				
Braised or broiled	3 oz	9.0	184	17%
■ **VEAL CUTS, ORGANS**				
Calf				
Heart/braised-chopped	1 cup	13	302	39%
Liver/fried	3 oz	11	222	45%
Sweetbreads/braised	3 oz	2.7	143	17%
Tongue/braised-sliced	~ 1 oz	1.7	45	34%

Food and Description	Amount	Fat Grams	Total Calories	% Fat Calories
VEAL DISHES/Frozen & Homemade (*See also* FROZEN ENTREE/DINNER)				
(NOTE: The data listed in this table may vary slightly, depending on the fat content of the veal cuts used in preparation.)				
Veal Parmigiana				
Frozen				
(Banquet)				
Breaded	5 oz	11	230	43%
w/Sauce & Cheese	~ 6.5 oz	18	282	57%
(Swanson's)	~ 12 oz	22	450	44%
Standard Home Recipe (USDA)	~ 6.5 oz	20	351	51%
Veal Patty Parmigiana				
Frozen (Weight Watchers)	8.44 oz	10	220	41%
Veal Scallopini w/sauce				
Standard Home Recipe (USDA)	~ 3.5 oz	19	255	67%
VEAL STEAKS				
Frozen (Hormel)				
Breaded	4 oz	13	240	49%
Unbreaded	4 oz	4	130	28%
VEGETABLE DISHES (*See also* individual listings of vegetable dishes)				
Broccoli, carrots, & pasta w/lightly seasoned sauce				
frozen (Birds Eye)	⅔ cup	4	87	41%
Broccoli, Cauliflower, Carrots w/cheese sauce				
frozen				
(Birds Eye)	5 oz	5	100	45%
(Green Giant)	½ cup	2	60	30%
	1 pkg/5 oz	2	80	23%
(Stokely) Singles	4 oz	3	70	39%
Broccoli, Cauliflower in Creamy Itailian Cheese Sauce				
frozen (Birds Eye)	½ cup	6	90	60%
Corn, green beans, & pasta curls w/light cream sauce				
frozen (Birds Eye)	½ cup	4.9	108	41%
Garden Salad				
canned (Joan of Arc)	½ cup	–	70	–
Micro Quick				
frozen (Freshlike)				
Broccoli, Pasta, Carrots in Cheese Sauce	4.5 oz	3	100	27%
Corn, Italian Green Beans, Red Peppers in Butter Sauce	5 oz	2	90	20%
Peas, Carrots, Onions-Cheese Sauce	5 oz	3	90	30%

Food and Description	Amount	Fat Grams	Total Calories	% Fat Calories
Peas, Cauliflower, Red Peppers in Butter Sauce	5 oz	2	90	20%
Mixed vegetables in butter sauce frozen (Green Giant)	½ cup	2	60	30%
Mixed vegetables in onion sauce frozen (Birds Eye)	2.6 oz	5	100	45%
Pizza-cheese & vegetable homemade/thin crust	1 slice/ ~ 2 oz	6	163	33%
Stew Vegetables frozen (Ore Ida)	3 oz	–	50	–
Sweet Corn, Pinto Beans, Red Bell Pepper in savory sauce microwave Vegetable Classics (Del Monte)	3⅓ oz	4	110	33%
Vegetable Lasagna (Impromtu Lite) box mix-microwave	10.6 oz	11	290	34%
Vegetable Medley breaded/frozen (Ore Ida)	3 oz	9	160	51%
Vegetables & Pasta in Creamy Stroganoff Sauce frozen (Birds Eye) Custom Cuisine	4.6 oz	5	130	35%
Vegetables in Authentic Oriental Sauce frozen (Birds Eye)Custom Cuisine	3.5 oz	3	70	39%
Vegetables in Creamy Cheese Sauce frozen (Birds Eye)Custom Cuisine	3.5 oz	5	210	21%
Vegetables in Delicate Herb Sauce frozen (Birds Eye) Custom Cuisine	3.5 oz	4	60	60%
Vegetarian Medley frozen (Kibun)	10 oz	2	240	8%
VEGETABLE JUICE COCKTAIL				
(Campbell's) V-8				
No Salt Added	6 oz	–	40	–
Original	6 oz	–	35	–
Spicy Hot	6 oz	–	35	–
Generic	6 oz	–	34	–
Very Veggi/low-cal	8 oz	–	40	–
VEGETABLE SOUP (See SOUP)				
VEGETABLES, MIXED (See also CUCCOTASH)				
Canned				
Beets w/onions	½ cup	–	80	–
Chop Suey Vegetables (La Choy)	½ cup	–	10	–
Fancy Chinese Vegetables (La Choy)	½ cup	–	12	–
Hot & Spicy Garden Mix (Vlasic)	1 oz	–	4	–

Food and Description	Amount	Fat Grams	Total Calories	% Fat Calories
Mixed Vegetables (Del Monte)	½ cup	–	40	–
Mixed Vegetables-Old Fashioned Harvest				
Time (S&W)	½ cup	–	35	–
Peas & carrots	½ cup	–	48	–
(Libby)	½ cup	–	50	–
Peas & onions	½ cup	–	30	–
Succotash (lima beans & corn)				
(Libby)	½ cup	1	80	11%
Country style (S & W)	½ cup	1	80	11%
w/Cream-Style Corn	½ cup	.7	102	6%
w/Whole Kernel Corn	½ cup	.6	81	7%
Veg-All-Homestyle (Larsen's)				
Lite	½ cup	–	35	–
Regular	½ cup	–	35	–
Dehydrated Flakes (French's)	1 Tbs	–	12	–
(Del Monte) Salad Bar Canned				
Marinated Medley	2 oz	–	50	–
3-Bean Salad	2 oz	–	45	–
Frozen (Birds Eye)				
Baby carrots, peas, & pearl onions	~ ½ cup	–	50	–
Broccoli, baby carrots, &				
water chestnuts	~ ½ cup	–	35	–
Broccoli, carrots, & pasta twists	~ ½ cup	4	9	40%
Broccoli, carrots, & water chestnuts	¾ cup	–	45	–
Broccoli, cauliflower, & carrots	~ ½ cup	–	25	–
Broccoli, corn, & red peppers	~ ½ cup	–	50	–
Broccoli, green beans, pearl onions,				
& red peppers	~ ½ cup	–	25	–
Broccoli, red peppers, bamboo shoots,				
& straw mushrooms	~ ½ cup	–	25	–
Brussels sprouts, cauliflower, & carrots	~ ½ cup	–	30	–
Carrots & pasta	~ ½ cup	4	90	40%
Carrots, peas, & pearl onions	~ ½ cup	–	48	–
Cauliflower & carrots	~ ½ cup	2.9	60	44%
Cauliflower, baby carrots, & snow peas	~ ½ cup	–	30	–
Chinese Style - International Recipe	~ ½ cup	3.9	68	52%
Chinese Style - Stir Fry	~ ½ cup	–	36	–
Chow Mein Style - International Recipe	~ ½ cup	4	90	40%
Corn, green beans, & pasta curls	~ ½ cup	5	110	41%
Custom Cuisine-Creamy Mushroom	~ ½ cup	6	107	51%
Vegetables w/herb sauce	~ ½ cup	6	107	51%
Green beans, French, toasted almond	~ ½ cup	2	50	36%
Green peas & pearl onions	~ ½ cup	–	70	–
Italian Style - International Recipe	~ ½ cup	5.5	102	49%

Food and Description	Amount	Fat Grams	Total Calories	% Fat Calories
Japanese Style - International Recipe	~ ½ cup	6	100	54%
Japanese Style - Stir Fry	~ ½ cup	–	30	–
Mandarin Style - International Recipe	~ ½ cup	4	90	40%
Mixed vegetables-regular	~ ½ cup	–	60	–
New England Style - International Recipe	~ ½ cup	6	125	43%
Pasta Primavera Style -International Recipe	~ ½ cup	5	120	38%
Peas & carrots	~ ½ cup	–	38	–
Peas & onions	~ ½ cup	–	40	–
Rice, green peas, & mushrooms	~ ½ cup	–	110	–
San Francisco Style - International Recipe	~ ½ cup	5	100	45%
(Freshlike)				
California Blend	3.3 oz	–	30	–
Chuckwagon Blend	3.3 oz	–	70	–
Italian Blend	3.3 oz	–	30	–
Midwestern Blend	3.3 oz	–	40	–
Mixed Vegetables	3.3 oz	–	70	–
Oriental Blend	3.3 oz	–	25	–
Winter Blend	3.3 oz	–	95	–
Wisconsin Blend	3.3 oz	–	50	–
Scandinavian Blend	3.3 oz	–	45	–
Vegetables For Soup	3.3 oz	–	50	–
Vegetables for Stew	3.3 oz	–	50	–
(Green Giant)				
Microwaveable/Pantry Express				
Corn, Green Beans, Carrots, & Pasta	½ cup	2	80	23%
Green Beans, Potatoes, & Mushrooms	½ cup	2	50	36%
Mixed Vegetables	½ cup	1	35	26%
Mixed Vegetables	4 oz	–	50	–
One Serving Vegetables				
Broccoli, Cauliflower, & Carrots	4 oz	–	30	–
Cauliflower in Cheese-Flavored Sauce	5.5 oz	2	80	23%
(Harvest Fresh) Mixed Vegetables	4 oz	–	45	–
(Ore Ida) Stew Vegetables	4 oz	–	60	–
(Pictsweet)				
Express-microwave				
Broccoli, carrots, & cauliflower	2.5 oz	–	20	–

Food and Description	Amount	Fat Grams	Total Calories	% Fat Calories
Broccoli, carrots, & water chestnuts	2.5 oz	–	25	–
Broccoli & cauliflower	2.5 oz	–	20	–
Broccoli, corn, & red peppers	2.5 oz	–	25	–
Broccoli, French Beans, Onions, & Red Peppers	2.5 oz	–	20	–
Peas, Pearl Onions, & Mushrooms	2.5 oz	–	45	–
Squash, onion, & peppers	2.5 oz	–	18	–
Mixed Vegetables	3.2 oz	–	60	–
Succotash	3.3 oz	1	100	9%
Vegetables Belgian	3.2 oz	–	30	–
Vegetables California	3.2 oz	–	25	–
Vegetables Cantonese	3.2 oz	–	35	–
Vegetables Del Sol	3.2 oz	–	30	–
Vegetables for Stir Fry	3.5 oz	–	35	–
prepared as directed	3.5 oz	4	75	48%
Vegetables Grande	3.2 oz	–	45	–
Vegetables Italian	3.2 oz	–	20	–
Vegetables Japanese	3.2 oz	–	25	–
Vegetables Milano	3.2 oz	–	40	–
Vegetables New England	3.2 oz	–	40	–
Vegetables Oriental	3.2 oz	–	25	–
Vegetables Parisian	3.2 oz	–	30	–
Vegetables Romano	3.2 oz	–	50	–
Vegetables Swiss	3.2 oz	–	25	–
Vegetables Western	3.2 oz	–	50	–
(Stokely)				
Singles Broccoli, carrots, & Water Chestnuts	3 oz	1	30	30%
Singles Broccoli & cauliflower	3 oz	1	20	45%
Singles Broccoli, Cauliflower, & Carrots	3 oz	1	25	36%
Valley Combinations (Pillsbury/Green Giant)				
Broccoli Cauliflower Supreme	½ cup	–	40	–
Broccoli Carrot Fanfare	½ cup	–	20	–
Corn Broccoli Bounty	½ cup	1	45	20%
Sweet Pea Cauliflower Medley	½ cup	–	30	–
Cauliflower Green Bean Festival	½ cup	–	16	–
Valley Combinations (Pillsbury/Green Giant)-Dual Pouch				
American Style				
w/sauce	½ cup	2	70	26%
w/o sauce	½ cup	–	50	–

Food and Description	Amount	Fat Grams	Total Calories	% Fat Calories
Broccoli Cauliflower Medley				
w/sauce	½ cup	2	60	30%
w/o sauce	½ cup	–	30	–
Broccoli Fanfare				
w/sauce	½ cup	2	80	23%
w/o sauce	½ cup	–	50	–
Le Sueur Style				
w/sauce	½ cup	2	70	26%
w/o sauce	½ cup	–	50	–
VEGETARIAN FOOD				
(Amy's) Frozen				
Country Dinner	11.35 oz	20	482	37%
Lasagna (Organic Vegetable)	10 oz	7	310	20%
Macaroni & Cheese	1 serving	10.8	226	43%
Macaroni & Soy Cheese	1 serving	8.45	228	33%
Mexican Tamale Pie (Organic)	8 oz	3	170	16%
Pot Pie				
Broccoli	1 pie	21.26	390	49%
Vegetable Tofu	1 pie	18.5	348	48%
(La Loma)				
Canned & Dry Packed - Meatless				
Big Franks	1.8 oz	6	110	49%
Chicken Supreme Mix (dry)	¼ cup	–	50	–
Dinner Cuts	3.5 oz	1	110	49%
no salt	3.5 oz	1	110	49%
Fried Chicken w/Gravy	3 oz	10	140	64%
Linketts	2.5 oz	8	140	51%
Little Links	1.6 oz	5	90	50%
Nuteena-luncheon loaf	2.3 oz	12	160	68%
Ocean Platter Mix (dry)	¼ cup	–	50	–
Patty Mix (dry)	¼ cup	–	50	–
Proteena-nut loaf	2.5 oz	7	150	42%
Redi-Burger	2.4 oz	6	130	42%
Sandwich Spread	1.7 oz	4	70	51%
Savory Dinner Loaf				
mix unprepared	¼ cup	–	50	–
Sizzle Franks	2.4 oz	13	170	69%
Stew Pack	2 oz	3	90	30%
Swiss Steak w/Gravy	3.3 oz	10	170	53%
Tastee Cuts	2.2 oz	1	60	15%
Tender Bits	2 oz	3	80	34%
Tender Rounds w/gravy	2.6 oz	4	120	30%
Vege-burger mix	½ cup	2	110	16%
no salt	½ cup	2	110	16%

Food and Description	Amount	Fat Grams	Total Calories	% Fat Calories
Vitaburger Chunks	¼ cup	–	70	–
Vitaburger Granules	¾ oz	–	70	–
Frozen Products - Meatless				
Chik Nuggets	5 pieces	20	270	67%
Corn Dogs	2.5 oz	8	190	38%
Fried Chicken	2 oz	14	180	70%
Griddle Steaks	2 oz	7	140	45%
Savoy Meatballs	2.5 oz	8	190	38%
Sizzle Burger	2.5 oz	12	220	49%
(Worthington)				
Canned & Dry Packed - Meatless				
Chik				
Diced-drained	¼ cup	8	90	80%
Sliced-drained	2 slices	8	90	80%
Chili	⅔ cup	10	190	47%
Choplets	2 slices	2	100	18%
Country Stew	9.5 oz	10	220	47%
Fri Chik	2 pieces	13	180	65%
Granburger	6 Tbs	1	110	8%
Harvest Bake				
Lentil Rice Loaf	4 oz	11	200	50%
Vegetarian Cutlets	3.25 oz	2	100	18%
Natural Touch Mix				
Dry-Loaf	4 oz	7	180	35%
Vegetarian	⅔ cup	12	230	41%
Stroganoff	4 oz	3	90	30%
Taco	2 Tbs	2	90	20%
Non Meat Balls	3	6	100	54%
Numete	½" slice	11	150	66%
Prime Stakes	1 piece	10	160	56%
Protose	½" slice	8	180	40%
Saucettes	2 links	11	150	66%
Savory Slices	2 slices	6	100	54%
Super Links	1 link	7	100	63%
Turkee Slices	2 slices	9	130	62%
Vegetable Skallops	½ cup	2	90	20%
no salt	½ cup	1	80	11%
Vegetable Steaks	2½ pieces	2	110	16%
Vegetarian Burger	½ cup	4	150	24%
no salt added	½ cup	6	160	34%
Veja-Links	2 links	10	140	64%
Frozen Products - Meatless				
Beef Pie-Vegetarian	8 oz	16	360	40%
Bolono	2 slices	2	60	30%

Food and Description	Amount	Fat Grams	Total Calories	% Fat Calories
Chic-ketts roll	½ cup	7	160	39%
Chicken				
Diced	½ cup	13	190	62%
Roll	~ 2.5 oz	10	150	60%
Slices	2 slices	9	130	62%
Chicken Pie-Vegetarian	8 oz	20	380	47%
Chik Stiks	1 piece/			
	1.6 oz	7	110	57%
Corned Beef				
Roll	2.5 oz	7	150	42%
Slices	4 slices	6	120	45%
Crispy Chik				
Nuggets	3 oz	19	280	61%
Patties	1 pattie	15	220	61%
Dinner Roast	2 oz	8	120	60%
Egg Rolls-Vegetarian	1	6	160	34%
Fillets-Vegetarian	2 fillets	9	180	45%
Fripats	1 piece	12	180	60%
Golden Croquettes	5 pieces	14	280	45%
Harvest Bake Lentil Rice				
Loaf	2½ slices	9	190	43%
Leanies	1 link	6	100	54%
Multigrain Cutlets	2 slices	2	90	205
Natural Touch Dinner Entree	1 pattie	13	210	56%
Natural Touch Garden Pattie	1 pattie	4	120	30%
Okara Patties	1 pattie	10	160	56%
Pepp-Roni	1 oz	8	100	72%
Prosage				
Links	2 links	9	130	62%
Patties	2 patties	14	210	60%
Roll	~ 2.5 oz	12	180	60%
Salami				
Roll	2 slices	5	90	50%
Slices	2 slices	4	70	51%
Smoked Beef	3 slices	6	120	45%
Smoked Turkey				
Roll	4 slices	12	180	60%
Slices	4 slices	12	180	60%
Stakelets	1 piece	8	150	48%
Stripples	4 strips	9	120	00%
Tuno-roll	2 oz	7	100	63%
Wham				
Roll	3 slices	7	120	53%
Slices	3 slices	7	120	53%

Food and Description	Amount	Fat Grams	Total Calories	% Fat Calories
(Morningstar Farms) Frozen Products - Meatless				
Breakfast Links	3 links	14	190	66%
Breakfast Patties	2 patties	12	190	57%
Breakfast Strips	3 strips	6	80	68%
Country Breakfast				
Cinnamon Swirl French Toast & Patties	6.5 oz	15	380	36%
Scramblers, Links, & Hash Browns	7 oz	23	360	58%
Scramblers, Links, & Pancakes	6.8 oz	19	380	45%
Country Crisp Patties	1 pattie	15	220	61%
Grillers	1 pattie	12	180	60%
Homestyle Country Crisps	3 oz	16	250	58%
Scramblers	¼ cup	3	60	45%
Zesty Country Crisps	3 oz	19	280	61%
VENISON				
Cured-boneless	3 oz	5	151	30%
Raw-boneless steaks	3 oz	5	153	29%
Raw-lean meat	3 oz	3	107	25%
Stewed-boneless	3 oz	5	153	29%
VICHYSSOISE (See SOUP)				
VINEGAR				
Cider	1 oz	–	–	–
	½ cup	–	15	–
Distilled	1 Tbs	–	2	–
	1 cup	–	29	–
(Hain)				
Cider	1 Tbs	–	2	–
Raw Unpasteurized Apple Cider	1 Tbs		2	–
(Progresso)				
Garlic	1 Tbs	–	2	–
Red Wine	1 Tbs	–	2	–
Red Wine Flavored	1 Tbs	–	2	–
(Regina) Wine				
Red	1 oz	–	4	–
Red/Garlic	1 oz	–	4	–
White	1 oz	–	4	–
VITA JUICE-including Beta Carotene	8 oz	–	90	–
VODKA (See LIQUOR, DISTILLED)				

W

Food and Description	Amount	Fat Grams	Total Calories	% Fat Calories
WAFFLE				
Box-Mix (*See also* PANCAKE/WAFFLE MIX)				
(Aunt Jemima)				
Buckwheat	¼ cup	1	107	8%
Buttermilk	⅓ cup	1	75	12%
Original	¼ cup	1	108	8%
Whole wheat	⅓ cup	1	142	6%
(Classique Fare)				
Belgian Waffle Dry Mix	1.66 oz	1.2	172	6%
Frozen				
(Aunt Jemima)				
Apple & Cinnamon	2.5 oz	5.6	176	29%
Blueberry	2.5 oz	5.2	175	27%
Buttermilk	2.5 oz	5.8	179	29%
Lite	1 waffle	1	70	13%
Original	2.5 oz	5.6	173	29%
Whole Grain	2.5 oz	3	150	18%
(Belgian Chef)				
Original	1	2	90	10%
w/oat bran	1	6	140	39%
(Downyflake)				
Blueberry	2	4	180	20%
Buttermilk Jumbo	2	5	190	24%
Crisp & Healthy				
Apple & Cinnamon	1	1	80	11%
Original	1	1	80	11%
Hot-N-Buttery	2	6	180	30%
Multi-grain	2	14	250	50%
Oat Bran	2	13	260	45%
Plain/jumbo	2	4	170	21%
Plain/regular	2	3	120	23%
(Eggo)				
Apple Cinnamon	1	5	130	35%
Blueberry	1	5	130	35%
Buttermilk	1	5	120	38%

Food and Description	Amount	Fat Grams	Total Calories	% Fat Calories
Fruit Top				
Apple	1	6	190	28%
Blueberry	1	6	190	28%
Peach	1	6	190	28%
Strawberry	1	6	190	28%
Homestyle	1	5	120	38%
Mini's	4	3	90	30%
Nut & honey	1	6	130	42%
Oat Bran	1	4	110	33%
Special K-fat free	1	–	80	–
(Eggo/Nutri-Grain)				
Plain	1	5	120	38%
Strawberry	1	5	120	38%
(Roman Meal) plain	2	14	280	45%
(Swanson) Great Starts				
Belgian				
Strawberries in Sausage	3½ oz	8	210	34%
w/Sausage	2⅞ oz	19	280	61%
(Weight Watchers)				
Belgian	1.50 oz	4	120	30%
Multi-grain Belgian	1.50 oz	4	120	30%
Shake 'N Pour Mix (Bisquick)				
Original	2	6	280	19%
Standard Home Recipe (USDA)				
7" round	~2½ oz	7	209	30%
9" square	11 oz	19.6	558	32%
WAFFLE SYRUP (*See* PANCAKE/WAFFLE SYRUP)				
WALNUT				
Black				
Dried	1 oz	16	172	84%
Dried-Chopped	1 cup	70.7	759	84%
(Planters)	1 oz	17	180	85%
English or Persian				
(Azar) Pieces	1 oz	19	190	90%
(Diamond) Pieces	1 oz	19	190	90%
Dried	1 oz	17.57	182	87%
Dried-Pieces	1 cup	74	770	87%
(Planters)	1 oz	20	190	95%
WATER				
Mineral Water (Perrier)				
With-A-Twist Lemon	12 oz	–	–	–
With-A-Twist Lime	12 oz	–	–	–
Plain/all types	UNLIMITED	–	–	–
Quinine Water	12 oz	–	142	–

Food and Description	Amount	Fat Grams	Total Calories	% Fat Calories
Seltzer Water	12 oz	–	–	–
(Crystal Geyser) Light				
Black Cherry Cider	6 oz	–	60	–
Cranberry-Raspberry	6 oz	–	60	–
Kiwi Lemonade	6 oz	–	60	–
Natural Peach	6 oz	–	60	–
Vanilla Creme	6 oz	–	60	–
Generic				
Lemon Flavored	12 oz	–	–	–
Lime Flavored	12 oz	–	–	–
Orange Flavored	12 oz	–	–	–
Strawberry Flavored	12 oz	–	–	–
(Schweppes)				
Black Cherry	6 oz	–	–	–
Lemon	6 oz	–	–	–
Lemon-Lime	6 oz	–	–	–
Lime	6 oz	–	–	–
Orange	6 oz	–	–	–
Peaches'N Cream	6 oz	–	–	–
Plain	6 oz	–	–	–
Wild Raspberry	6 oz	–	–	–
Sparkling				
(Coor's) Rocky Mountain Sparkling Water				
Cherry	8 fl oz	–	–	–
Lemon Lime	8 fl oz	–	–	–
Original	8 fl oz	–	–	–
(Perrier) all flavors	8 fl oz	–	–	–
(Schweppes)				
Black Cherry	6 oz	–	–	–
Lemon	6 oz	–	–	–
Lemon-Lime	6 oz	–	–	–
Lime	6 oz	–	–	–
Orange	6 oz	–	–	–
Peaches'N Cream	6 oz	–	–	–
Plain	6 oz	–	–	–
Wild Raspberry	6 oz	–	–	–
Tonic Water	6 oz	–	125	–
Low Cal	6 oz	–	2	–
(Canada Dry)	6 oz	–	135	–
Diet	6 oz	–	4	–
(Schweppes)	6 oz	–	70	–
Diet	6 oz	–	–	–
Vichy Water				
(Schweppes)	6 oz	–	–	–

Food and Description	Amount	Fat Grams	Total Calories	% Fat Calories
WATER CHESTNUT, CHINESE				
Canned				
Generic				
Sliced	½ cup	–	35	–
(Chun King)				
Sliced	8 oz	.5	179	3%
Whole	8.5 oz	.5	190	2%
Raw-Sliced	½ cup	–	66	–
WATERCRESS				
chopped	½ cup	–	2	–
raw	1 sprig	–	–	–
WATERCRESS SOUP (*See* SOUP)				
WATERMELON				
Fresh				
10" diameter	¹⁄₁₆ wedge	2	152	12%
	1 cup	.68	50	12%
Kernels-dried	1 oz	13	158	74%
	1 cup	51	602	76%
WAX BEAN				
Canned	½ cup	–	25	–
(Del Monte)				
Cut	½ cup	–	20	–
French style	½ cup	–	20	–
(Festal)	½ cup	–	20	–
(Joan of Arc)	½ cup	< 1	25	18%
(S&W) Premium Golden cut	½ cup	–	20	–
WAX GOURD				
fresh-boiled	1 cup	–	23	–
raw	1 cup	–	17	–
WEAKFISH				
broiled w/butter or margarine	3 oz	9.6	177	49%
WHALE/raw	3 oz	6	130	42%
WHEAT (*See* BULGUR)				
WHEAT GERM				
(Kretschmer)				
Honey crunch	¼ cup	3	110	25%
Plain	¼ cup	3	100	27%
(Krusteaz)	1 oz	2	103	18%
WHELK (*See* SNAIL)				
WHEY				
dried	1 cup	–	193	–
acid	1 Tbs	–	10	–
sweet	1 cup	2	512	–
	1 Tbs	–	26	–

Food and Description	Amount	Fat Grams	Total Calories	% Fat Calories
fluid				
acid	1 cup	< 1	60	8%
sweet	1 cup	.7	65	10%
WHIPPED TOPPING (*See also* CREAM, ICE CREAM TOPPING)				
frozen	1 Tbs	1	15	60%
frozen-non dairy	1 Tbs	.8	11	66%
powdered-w/ whole milk	1 Tbs	–	10	–
	1 cup	10	150	60%
powdered-low-calorie	1 Tbs	1	8	100%
pressurized-cream	1 Tbs	1	8	100%
	½ cup	7	75	84%
non dairy	1 Tbs	1	10	81%
	1 cup	16	185	78%
WHISKEY (*See* LIQUOR, DISTILLED)				
WHITE BEANS				
boiled	½ cup	–	125	–
small	½ cup	.58	127	4%
canned	½ cup	–	153	–
WHITE PERCH/raw	3 oz	3	100	27%
WHITE SAUCE (*See* SAUCE)				
WHITEFISH				
Mixed				
(Mother's)				
jellied	1 fishball	1	46	20%
jellied in broth	1 fishball	1	70	13%
Raw		3 oz	4.98	114
Smoked	3 oz	.79	92	8%
WHITEFISH & PIKE				
jar (Manischewitz)	3.5 oz	3.57	99	33%
sweet	3.5 oz	4	129	28%
jellied (Rokeach)	1 fishball	1	60	15%
jellied in broth (Mother's)	1 fishball	1	60	15%
WHITING (*See also* SEAFOOD ENTREE/DINNER)				
breaded & fried	3 oz	9.7	171	51%
cooked-dry heat	3 oz	1	98	9%
raw	3 oz	1	77	12%
WIENER (*See* FRANKFURTER)				
WINE				
(NOTE: Percent refers to alcohol content.)				
Alcohol Removed, white				
(Carl Jung)	3 fl oz	–	20	–
Barbera, white	4 fl oz	–	91	–
Beaujolais-12%	4 fl oz	–	96	–
Bordaux-red-12%	4 fl oz	–	96	–

Food and Description	Amount	Fat Grams	Total Calories	% Fat Calories
Burgundy				
Cooking	¼ cup	–	2	–
Red-12%	4 fl oz	–	96	–
Sparkling-12%	4 fl oz	–	116	–
White-12%	4 fl oz	–	90	–
Cabernet Sauvignon	4 fl oz	–	88	–
Chablis	4 fl oz	–	84	–
Emerald	4 fl oz	–	102	
Gold	4 fl oz	–	97	–
Pink	4 fl oz	–	98	–
Ruby	4 fl oz	–	104	–
Champagne				
Brut	4 fl oz	–	100	–
Domestic	4 fl oz	–	84	–
Extra Dry	4 fl oz	–	105	–
Pink	4 fl oz	–	98	–
Chardonnay	4 fl oz	–	88	–
Chenin Blanc	4 fl oz	–	86	–
Chianti	4 fl oz	–	100	–
Cold Duck	4 fl oz	–	108	–
Desert	4 fl oz	–	180	–
Dubonnet	4 fl oz	–	160	–
French Colombard	4 fl oz	–	88	–
Liebfraumilch-10%	4 fl oz	–	84	–
Madeira-19%	4 fl oz	–	160	–
Muscatelle (Muscatel)	3.5 fl oz	–	158	–
Port				
Ruby-20%	4 fl oz	–	184	–
Tawny-20%	4 fl oz	–	184	–
White	4 fl oz	–	172	–
Reising-12%	4 fl oz	–	90	–
Rhine-11%	4 fl oz	–	96	–
Rhone-12%	4 fl oz	–	96	–
Rose'	4 fl oz	–	90	–
Saki/Sake	1.5 fl oz	–	36	–
Sauterne				
Cooking	¼ cup	–	2	–
12%	4 fl oz	–	116	–
12% dry	4 fl oz	–	108	–
Sauvignon Blanc	4 fl oz	–	80	–
Sherry				
Cooking	¼ cup	–	20	–
Cream-19.5%	4 fl oz	–	200	–
Dry-19%	4 fl oz	–	162	–

Food and Description	Amount	Fat Grams	Total Calories	% Fat Calories
Sweet Wines	4 fl oz	–	165	–
Sylvaner-12%	4 fl oz	–	90	–
Table				
Red	3.5 fl oz	–	74	–
Rose	3.5 fl oz	–	73	–
White	3.5 fl oz	–	70	–
Tokay	4 fl oz	–	164	–
Vermouth				
Dry-17%	4 fl oz	–	136	–
Sweet-17%	4 fl oz	–	180	–
Wine Cooler	7 fl oz	–	101	–
	12 fl oz	–	192	–
(Bartles & Jaymes)				
Light	6 oz	–	67	–
Light Berry	6 oz	–	75	–
Wine Spritzer	5 fl oz	–	61	–
Zinfandel	4 fl oz	–	92	–
White	4 fl oz	–	82	–
WINGED BEAN/boiled	½ cup	5	126	36%
WOLF FISH/raw	3 oz	2	80	23%
WON TON SOUP (*See* SOUP)				
WORCESTERSHIRE SAUCE (*See also* SAUCE)				
Regular	1 Tbs	–	10	–
Smokey	1 Tbs	–	10	–

Y

Food and Description	Amount	Fat Grams	Total Calories	% Fat Calories
YAM				
Canned-candied (S&W)	½ cup	–	180	–
Heavy syrup	½ cup	–	120	–
Light syrup	½ cup	–	110	–
Mashed	½ cup	–	90	–
w/Pineapple orange sauce	½ cup	–	190	–
Canned-whole Southern in extra heavy				
Syrup (S&W)	½ cup	1	139	7%

Food and Description	Amount	Fat Grams	Total Calories	% Fat Calories
Fresh-boiled or baked	1 cup	–	158	–
Mountain Yam-Hawaii				
Cooked-cubed	½ cup	–	59	–
Raw-cubed	½ cup	–	46	–
Raw	1 cup	–	177	–
YAM BEAN-TUBER				
Boiled	4 oz	–	52	–
Raw w/skin	½ lb	< 1	85	5%
w/o skin	4 oz	< 1	47	10%
YARDLONG BEAN				
Boiled	½ cup	–	102	–
YEAST				
Active dry				
Baker's	1 pkg	–	20	–
	1 oz	.5	80	6%
Brewer's	1 Tbs	–	25	–
	1 oz	–	80	–
Compressed-baker's	1 oz	1	24	38%
Torula	1 oz	–	79	–
(Fleischmann's)				
Active Dry & Rapid Rise				
Jar	¼ oz	–	20	–
Package	¼ oz	–	20	–
Fresh Active	.6 oz	–	15	–
Household	.5 oz	–	15	–
(Louis Laboratories) Brewer's	2 Tbs	1	114	8%
YELLOW BEAN				
Baked-canned	½ cup	3	180	15%
Boiled	½ cup	.95	126	7%
Snap				
Cooked	½ cup	–	22	–
Canned	½ cup	–	13	–
Frozen	½ cup	–	18	–
YELLOWEYE BEAN				
Canned-Seasoned w/Pork (Luck's)	7.5 oz	6	220	25%
YELLOWTAIL/raw	3 oz	4.5	124	33%
YOGURT, DAIRY				
Bon Lait (Fromage Frais)				
Peach	6 oz	5	200	23%
Raspberry	6 oz	5	200	23%
Strawberry	6 oz	5	200	23%
(Breyers)				
Black Cherry	8 oz	5	270	17%
Blueberry	8 oz	6	260	21%

Food and Description	Amount	Fat Grams	Total Calories	% Fat Calories
Mixed Berry	8 oz	5	270	17%
Mixed Berry-low fat	8 oz	2	250	7%
Peach	8 oz	5	270	17%
Peach-low fat	8 oz	2	250	7%
Pineapple	8 oz	5	270	17%
Plain	8 oz	8	190	38%
Red Raspberry	8 oz	6	260	21%
Strawberry	8 oz	5	270	17%
Strawberry Banana	8 oz	6	280	19%
Strawberry Banana-low fat	8 oz	2	250	7%
Vanilla Bean	8 oz	7	230	27%
(Columbo) Lite				
Blueberry	8 oz	< 1	190	2%
Cherry	8 oz	< 1	190	2%
Coffee	8 oz	< 1	190	2%
Peach	8 oz	< 1	190	2%
Plain	8 oz	< 1	110	4%
Raspberry	8 oz	< 1	190	2%
Strawberry	8 oz	< 1	190	2%
Strawberry Banana	8 oz	< 1	190	2%
Vanilla	8 oz	< 1	110	4%
(Dannon)				
Blended				
Blueberry	6 oz	–	150	–
French Vanilla	6 oz	–	153	–
Lemon Chiffon	6 oz	–	150	–
Peach	6 oz	–	150	–
Raspberry	6 oz	–	150	–
Strawberry	6 oz	–	150	–
Strawberry Banana	6 oz	–	150	–
Extra Smooth				
Mini-Pack Raspberry/Strawberry/ Banana	4.4 oz	2	130	14%
Mini-Pack Strawberry/ Peach	4.4 oz	2	130	14%
Fruit on the Bottom				
Banana	8 oz	3	240	11%
Blueberry	8 oz	3	240	11%
Blueberry-Fresh Flavors	8 oz	4	200	18%
Boysenberry	8 oz	3	240	11%
Cherry	8 oz	3	240	11%
Coffee-Fresh Flavors	8 oz	3	200	14%
Dutch Apple	8 oz	3	240	11%
Exotic Fruit-Fresh Flavors	8 oz	3	240	11%

Food and Description	Amount	Fat Grams	Total Calories	% Fat Calories
Lemon-Fresh Flavors	8 oz	4	210	17%
Mixed Berry	8 oz	3	240	11%
Nonfat	8 oz	–	110	–
Peach	8 oz	3	240	11%
Pina colada	8 oz	3	240	11%
Plain	8 oz	4	140	26%
Raspberry-Fresh Flavors	8 oz	4	200	18%
Strawberry	8 oz	3	240	11%
Strawberry-Fresh Flavors	8 oz	4	200	18%
Strawberry-Banana	8 oz	3	240	11%
Vanilla-Fresh Flavors	8 oz	3	200	14%
Light				
Blueberry	8 oz	–	100	–
Cherry Vanilla	8 oz	–	100	–
Mini Strawberry/Blueberry	4.4 oz	–	60	–
Mini Strawberry/Peach	4.4 oz	–	60	–
Peach	8 oz	–	100	–
Raspberry	8 oz	–	100	–
Strawberry	8 oz	–	100	–
Strawberry Fruit Cup	8 oz	–	100	–
Strawberry-Banana	8 oz	–	100	–
Vanilla	8 oz	–	100	–
(Del Monte) Yogurt Cup 1½% milkfat				
Awesome Peach	4¾ oz	2	140	13%
Cool Blueberry	4¾ oz	2	140	13%
Rad Raspberry	4¾ oz	2	140	13%
Totally Strawberry	4¾ oz	2	140	13%
(Johnston's) Premium				
Black Cherry	6 oz	5	260	17%
Boysenberry	6 oz	5	260	17%
Lemon Chiffon	6 oz	5	225	20%
Peach	6 oz	5	260	17%
Raspberry Trifle	6 oz	5	225	20%
Strawberry	6 oz	5	260	17%
Vanilla	6 oz	7	200	32%
(Kemps)				
Classic Yogurt Strawberry	6 oz	2	150	12%
Vanilla & Fruit, Strawberry	6 oz	2	160	11%
Yogurt Jr.'s, Strawberry	4 oz	1	130	7%
(Kissle) Creamy Blend (No yogurt culture)				
Blackberry	6 oz	3	180	15%
Blueberry	6 oz	3	180	15%
Cherry	6 oz	3	180	15%
Chocolate	6 oz	4	200	18%

Food and Description	Amount	Fat Grams	Total Calories	% Fat Calories
French Vanilla	6 oz	3	180	15%
Lemon	6 oz	3	180	15%
Milk chocolate	6 oz	4	200	18%
Mixed berry	6 oz	3	180	15%
Peach	6 oz	3	180	15%
Raspberry	6 oz	3	180	15%
Strawberry	6 oz	3	180	15%
Strawberry-Banana	6 oz	3	180	15%
(La Carona) Low fat				
All fruit flavors	8 oz	4	230	16%
Plain	8 oz	5	160	28%
Nonfat/plain	8 oz	< 1	120	4%
(La Yogurt) All fruit flavors	6 oz	4	190	19%
Plain	6 oz	6	140	39%
(La Yogurt-25) All flavors	8 oz	–	200	–
(Light N'Lively)				
Free				
Blueberry	4.4 oz	–	50	–
Red Raspberry	4.4 oz	–	50	–
Strawberry	4.4 oz	–	50	–
Strawberry fruit cup	4.4 oz	–	50	–
99% fat free				
Blueberry	5 oz	1	150	6%
Peach	5 oz	2	150	12%
Pineapple	5 oz	1	150	6%
Red Raspberry	5 oz	2	140	13%
Strawberry	5 oz	2	150	12%
Strawberry Banana	5 oz	1	160	6%
Strawberry Fruit Cup	5 oz	2	150	12%
100-No Sugar Added				
Black Cherry	8 oz	–	100	–
Blueberry	8 oz	–	100	–
Lemon	8 oz	–	100	–
Peach	8 oz	–	100	–
Red Raspberry	8 oz	–	90	–
Strawberry	8 oz	–	90	–
Strawberry Fruit Cup	8 oz	–	90	–
Original				
Black Cherry	8 oz	2	230	8%
Blueberry	8 oz	2	240	8%
	4.4 oz	1	130	7%
Grape	4.4 oz	1	130	7%
Peach	8 oz	2	240	8%
	4.4 oz	1	130	7%

Food and Description	Amount	Fat Grams	Total Calories	% Fat Calories
Pineapple	8 oz	2	230	8%
	4.4 oz	1	130	7%
Red Raspberry	8 oz	2	230	8%
	4.4 oz	1	130	7%
Strawberry	8 oz	2	240	8%
	4.4 oz	1	130	7%
Strawberry Banana	8 oz	2	260	7%
	4.4 oz	1	140	7%
Strawberry Fruit Cup	8 oz	2	240	8%
	4.4 oz	1	130	7%
(Lite-Line) Lowfat Swiss Style-plain				
1½% milkfat	8 oz	2	140	13%
Natural Cherry Vanilla-1% milkfat	8 oz	2	240	8%
Natural Peach -1% milkfat	8 oz	2	230	8%
Natural Strawberry-1% milkfat	8 oz	2	240	8%
Lowfat				
Coffee, Vanilla-lowfat	4 oz	1	97	9%
Fruit-lowfat	4 oz	1	115	8%
Plain-lowfat	4 oz	1.8	72	23%
Part skim (non-fat)	4 oz	–	63	–
Whole milk	4 oz	3.7	70	48%
(Lucerne) Nonfat				
Blueberry	8 oz	–	180	–
Cherry	8 oz	–	180	–
Peach	8 oz	–	180	–
Plain	8 oz	–	130	–
Strawberry	8 oz	–	180	–
(Meadow Gold) Lowfat-Plain				
2% milkfat	8 oz	5	160	28%
Sundae Style-Raspberry				
1.5% milkfat	8 oz	4	250	14%
(Mountain High)				
Black Cherry	8 oz	6	220	25%
Blueberry	8 oz	6	220	25%
Honey Vanilla	8 oz	6	220	25%
Honey Vanilla Blend	8 oz	8	210	34%
Plain	8 oz	9	200	41%
Plain/Acidophilus	8 oz	9	200	41%
Raspberry	8 oz	6	220	25%
Strawberry	8 oz	8	210	34%
(Mountain High) Honey Light				
All flavors	8 oz	< 1	190	2%
(New Country)				
Blueberry Supreme	6 oz	2	150	12%

Food and Description	Amount	Fat Grams	Total Calories	% Fat Calories
Cherry Supreme	6 oz	2	150	12%
Fresh Vanilla	6 oz	2	150	12%
Mixed Berries	6 oz	2	150	12%
Orange Supreme	6 oz	2	150	12%
Peaches'n Cream	6 oz	2	150	12%
Raspberry Supreme	6 oz	2	150	12%
Strawberry Banana Supreme	6 oz	2	150	12%
Strawberry Supreme	6 oz	2	150	12%
(Quality Chekd-Kemps)				
All fruit flavors	8 oz	3	300	9%
Plain	8 oz	3	160	17%
(Scandia) All flavors	6 oz	2	160	11%
(Ultimate 90) All fruit flavors	8 oz	–	90	–
(Weight Watchers)				
Fruit/all flavors	8 oz	1	150	6%
Plain nonfat	8 oz	1	150	6%
(Whitney's)				
Light				
Cherry	6 oz	–	130	–
Peach	6 oz	–	130	–
Strawberry	6 oz	–	130	–
Original				
Apples & Raisins	6 oz	5	200	23%
Blueberry	6 oz	5	200	23%
Boysenberry	6 oz	5	200	23%
Cherry	6 oz	5	200	23%
Coffee	6 oz	6	200	27%
Lemon	6 oz	6	200	27%
Peach	6 oz	5	200	23%
Pina Colada	6 oz	7	210	30%
Plain	6 oz	7	150	42%
Raspberry	6 oz	5	200	23%
Strawberry	6 oz	5	200	23%
Strawberry Banana	6 oz	5	200	23%
Tropical Fruits	6 oz	6	200	27%
Vanilla	6 oz	6	200	27%
Wild Berries	6 oz	5	200	23%
(Yoplait)				
Custard style				
Banana	6 oz	4	190	19%
Cherry	6 oz	4	180	20%
Strawberry	6 oz	4	190	19%
Vanilla	6 oz	4	180	20%
Light/all flavors	6 oz	.5	90	5%

Food and Description	Amount	Fat Grams	Total Calories	% Fat Calories
Light/Nonfat				
Blueberry	6 oz	–	80	–
Cherry	6 oz	–	80	–
Peach	6 oz	–	80	–
Raspberry	6 oz	–	80	–
Strawberry	6 oz	–	80	–
Strawberry Banana	6 oz	–	80	–
Strawberry Peach	6 oz	–	80	–
Low Fat				
Blueberry	6 oz	4	230	16%
Cherry	6 oz	3	210	13%
Strawberry	6 oz	3	210	13%
Strawberry-Banana	6 oz	4	240	15%
Lowfat Breakfast				
Apple Cinnamon	6 oz	4	220	16%
Berries	6 oz	3	220	12%
Cherry w/Almonds	6 oz	3	210	13%
Sunrise Peach	6 oz	3	230	12%
Strawberry Banana	6 oz	3	230	12%
Strawberry w/Almonds	6 oz	3	210	13%
Tropical Fruits	6 oz	4	230	16%
New Light/Nonfat				
Blueberry	4 oz	–	60	–
Raspberry	4 oz	–	60	–
Strawberry	4 oz	–	60	–
Strawberry-Banana	4 oz	–	60	–
Nonfat				
Plain	8 oz	–	120	–
Vanilla	8 oz	–	180	–
Original				
Apple	6 oz	4	190	19%
Blueberry	6 oz	4	190	19%
Boysenberry	6 oz	4	190	19%
Cherry	6 oz	4	190	19%
Lemon	6 oz	4	190	19%
Mixed berry	6 oz	4	190	19%
Orange	6 oz	4	190	19%
Peach	6 oz	4	190	19%
Pina colada	6 oz	4	190	19%
Plain	6 oz	5	130	35%
Raspberry	6 oz	4	190	19%
Strawberry	6 oz	4	190	19%
Strawberry-Banana	6 oz	4	190	19%
Vanilla	6 oz	3	180	15%

Food and Description	Amount	Fat Grams	Total Calories	% Fat Calories
(Yoplait 150) All flavors	6 oz	–	150	–
YOGURT BARS				
(Baskin Robbins)				
Dutch Chocolate Chip	1 bar	14	260	48%
Praline Vanilla	1 bar	14	250	50%
(Kemps)				
Yogurt Dipped On A Stick				
Vanilla	1 bar	7	120	53%
Yogurt On A Stick				
Raspberry	1 bar	1	60	15%
Strawberry	1 bar	1	60	15%
(The Country's Best Yogurt - TCBY)				
Yog-a-bar				
Low-fat vanilla	1 bar	11	170	58%
Sugar-free vanilla	1 bar	9	120	68%
Vanilla w/heath	1 bar	14	220	57%
Toasted almonds	1 bar	17	240	64%
YOGURT DESSERT (Sara Lee)				
Frozen strawberry-light	1 slice	< 1	120	4%
YOGURT DRINKS				
(Dannon) All flavors	8 oz	4	190	19%
(Glen Oaks)				
Banana	8 oz	4	212	17%
Raspberry	8 oz	4	212	17%
Strawberry	8 oz	4	212	17%
Tropical fruit	8 oz	4	212	17%
(Weight Watchers)/Frozen				
Chocolate	7.5 oz	1	220	4%
YOGURT, FROZEN				
(REMINDER—try to stick with the fruit toppings, as other toppings are high in fat.)				
(Baskin Robbins)				
Low fat	½ cup	1	120	8%
Non fat	½ cup	–	110	–
Truly Free	½ cup	–	70	–
(Brice)				
Cappuccino	3 oz	3	90	30%
Chocolate	3 oz	3	100	27%
Strawberry	3 oz	3	100	27%
Vanilla	3 oz	3	90	00%
(Carnation)				
Chocolate	3 oz	1	90	10%
Peach	3 oz	1	90	10%
Raspberry	3 oz	1	90	10%
Vanilla	3 oz	1	80	11%

Food and Description	Amount	Fat Grams	Total Calories	% Fat Calories
(Dannon) On A Stick-All flavors	1.75 oz	1	50	18%
(Danny) Yogurt Bars				
Boysenberry-carob coated	1 bar	8	140	51%
Chocolate	1 bar	1	60	15%
Chocolate-chocolate coated	1 bar	8	130	55%
Pina colada	1 bar	1	70	13%
Raspberry-chocolate coated	1 bar	7	130	49%
Strawberry-chocolate coated	1 bar	7	130	49%
Vanilla	1 bar	1	60	15%
Vanilla-chocolate coated	1 bar	8	130	55%
(Dreyer's) Inspirations				
Low-fat				
Chocolate	3 oz	1	80	11%
Citrus height	3 oz	1	80	11%
Marble fudge	3 oz	3	100	27%
Mocha fudge	3 oz	3	100	27%
Perfectly peach	3 oz	1	80	11%
Raspberry	3 oz	1	80	11%
Raspberry vanilla	3 oz	1	80	11%
Strawberry	3 oz	1	80	11%
Strawberry-banana	3 oz	1	80	11%
Vanilla	3 oz	1	80	11%
Non-fat				
Cherry	3 oz	–	70	–
Chocolate	3 oz	–	80	–
Mocha	3 oz	–	80	–
Strawberry	3 oz	–	70	–
Vanilla	3 oz	–	80	–
(Haagen-Dazs)				
Chocolate	4 oz	4	170	21%
Peach	4 oz	4	160	23%
Strawberry	4 oz	4	170	23%
Vanilla	4 oz	4	170	21%
Vanilla almond crunch	4 oz	6	190	28%
(Honey Hill)				
Chocolate Thunder	3 oz	3	110	25%
Cookie Jar	3 oz	5	130	35%
Peach	3 oz	3	110	25%
Vanilla Velvet	3 oz	4	110	33%
White Almond Chocolate	3 oz	5	120	38%
(Kemps)				
Low-Fat Strawberry	4 oz	1	107	8%
Non-Fat				
Free Vanilla	4 oz	–	40	–

Food and Description	Amount	Fat Grams	Total Calories	% Fat Calories
Strawberry	4 oz	–	93	–
Soft-Serve Vanilla				
Original	1 oz	1	30	30%
Non-Fat	1 oz	–	25	–
(Knudsen) Push Ups/all flavors	3 oz	1	90	10%
(La Corona)				
Blueberry	3 oz	1	80	11%
Chocolate	3 oz	2	90	20%
Strawberry	3 oz	1	80	11%
Strawberry-banana	3 oz	1	90	10%
(La Carona) Frozen Yogurt On A Stick				
All flavors	1	1	50	18%
(Lite Time)				
French vanilla	3 oz	3	90	30%
Strawberry	3 oz	3	90	30%
(Natural Nectar's)				
Fi-Bar Yogurt Lite				
Chocolate	1 sandwich	6	190	28%
Strawberry	1 sandwich	7	210	30%
Vanilla	1 sandwich	7	200	32%
(Rhapsody Farms)				
Mocha almond	4 oz	2	89	20%
Red raspberry	4 oz	2	89	20%
Vanilla	4 oz	2	89	20%
Non Fat				
Chocolate peanut butter	3 oz	–	85	–
Dutch chocolate	3 oz	–	85	–
Mocha Madness	3 oz	–	85	–
Peach	3 oz	–	85	–
Strawberry Extravaganza	3 oz	–	85	–
(Sealtest)				
Black cherry	1/4 pint	2	120	15%
Red raspberry	1/4 pint	1	100	9%
Strawberry	1/4 pint	2	110	16%
Tres Bein (Shamrock)				
French vanilla	3 oz	3	90	30%
Honey nut	3 oz	3	100	27%
Peach	3 oz	2	90	20%
Raspberry	3 oz	2	90	20%
Strawberry	3 oz	2	90	20%
(Yoplait)				
Chocolate	4 oz	3	130	21%
Strawberry	4 oz	3	120	23%
Vanilla	4 oz	3	120	23%

Z

Food and Description	Amount	Fat Grams	Total Calories	% Fat Calories

ZABAGLIONE (*See* CUSTARD)
ZUCCHINI (*See* SQUASH, SUMMER)

Fast food

Food and Description	Amount	Fat Grams	Total Calories	% Fat Calories
GENERIC LISTING (USDA Averages Derived From Several Restaurant Chains)				
■ **BREAKFAST**				
Biscuit-plain	1	13	276	42%
Croissant w/egg & cheese	1	24.7	369	60%
Croissant w/egg, cheese, & bacon	1	28	413	61%
Croissant w/egg, cheese, & ham	1	33.58	475	64%
Croissant w/egg, cheese, & sausage	1	38	524	65%
Danish-cheese	1	24.6	353	63%
Danish-cinnamon	1	16.7	349	43%
Danish-fruit	1	15.9	335	43%
Egg-scrambled	2 eggs	15	200	68%
English Muffin				
w/butter	1	5.76	189	27%
w/cheese & sausage	1	24	394	55%
w/egg, cheese, & Canadian bacon	1	19.76	383	46%
w/egg, cheese, & sausage	1	30.85	487	57%
French Toast w/butter	2 slices	18.76	356	47%
French Toast Sticks	5 sticks	29	479	55%
Omelet-ham & cheese	2 egg	17.7	255	62%
Pancakes w/syrup & butter	3 cakes	13.99	519	24%
Potatoes, hash brown	½ cup	9	151	54%
Sausage	1 patty	8	100	72%
■ **CHICKEN, CHILI, SEAFOOD, PIZZA**				
Chicken/breaded/fried/dark meat	2 pieces	26.7	430	56%
Chicken/breaded/fried/wing & breast	2 pieces	29.5	494	54%
Chicken nuggets				
plain	1 piece	2.95	48	55%
	6 pieces	17.7	290	55%
w/bar-b-q sauce	6 pieces	17.90	330	49%
w/honey	6 pieces	17.5	329	48%
w/mustard sauce	6 pieces	18.9	323	53%
w/sweet & sour sauce	6 pieces	17.95	346	47%
Chili Con Carne	1 cup	8	254	28%
Clams/breaded/fried	¾ cup	26	451	52%
Crab/baked	1 cake	1	88	10%

Food and Description	Amount	Fat Grams	Total Calories	% Fat Calories
Crab-soft shell/fried	1	17.86	334	48%
Crab/fried	1 cake	18.8	290	58%
Fish Fillet battered or breaded fried	1	11	211	47%
Oysters/battered or breaded/fried	6	17.9	368	44%
Pizza-cheese	⅛ of			
	12" pizza	2.5	109	21%
	12" pizza	20	873	21%
Pizza-meat & vegetable	⅛ of			
	12" pizza	4	152	24%
	12" pizza	35	1213	26%
Pizza-pepperoni	⅛ of			
	12" pizza	5	135	33%
	12" pizza	41.55	1081	35%
Pizza-supreme (thin & crispy)	½ of			
	10" pizza	21	510	37%
(thick & chewy)	½ of			
	10" pizza	22	640	31%
Scallops/breaded/fried	6 pieces	19	386	44%
Shrimp/breaded/fried	6-8 pieces	24.9	454	49%
■ CONDIMENTS				
Butter	1 pkt-½ oz	11	100	100%
Catsup	1 pkt-¼ oz	–	3	–
Half & Half	1 pkt-½ oz	1.6	18	80%
Honey	1 pkt-½ oz	–	43	–
Jelly	1 pkt-¾ oz	–	58	–
Lemon	1 pkt-½ oz	–	3	–
Lettuce	2 leaves	–	2	–
Mayonnaise	1 pkt-⅖ oz	9	81	100%
Mustard	1 pkt-⅕ oz	–	4	–
Nondairy Creamer	1 pkt-⅖ oz	3.5	55	57%
Onion	2 slices	–	7	–
Pickle	2 slices	–	2	–
Salad Dressings				
Bleu Cheese	1 pkt-2½ oz	34	342	90%
French	1 pkt-2 oz	20.6	228	81%
Italian	1 pkt-2 oz	34	326	94%
Low Calorie	1 pkt-2 oz	2	50	36%
Oriental	1 pkt-2 oz	1	102	9%
Thousand Island	1 pkt-2½ oz	39	396	89%
Wine Vinegar	1 Tbs	–	2	–
Sugar	1 pkt	–	25	–
Sugar Substitute	1 pkt	–	4	–
Syrup	1 pkt-1½ oz	–	122	–

Food and Description	Amount	Fat Grams	Total Calories	% Fat Calories
Tartar Sauce	1 pkt-½ oz	8	74	97%
Tomato	1 slice	–	5	–
■ DESSERTS				
Brownie	1	10	243	37%
Fried Pies	1	14	266	47%
Ice Cream Cone	Small	3	110	25%
	Medium	7	230	27%
	Large	10	340	27%
Ice Cream Cone dipped in chocolate	Small	7	150	42%
	Medium	13	300	39%
	Large	20	450	40%
Ice Cream Sandwich	1	4	140	26%
Ice Milk (soft serve w/cone)	1 oz	6	164	33%
Sundae				
carmel	1	9	303	27%
hot fudge	1	8.6	284	27%
strawberry	1	7.85	269	26%
■ MEXICAN FOODS				
Burritos				
bean	2	13.5	448	27%
bean & cheese	2	11.7	377	28%
bean & chili peppers	2	14.67	413	32%
bean & meat	2	17.8	508	32%
bean, cheese, & beef	2	13	331	35%
beef	2	20.8	523	36%
beef & chili peppers	2	16.5	426	35%
beef, cheese, & chili peppers	2	24.79	634	35%
Chimichanga				
beef	1	19.67	425	42%
beef & cheese	1	23.45	443	48%
beef & red chili peppers	1	19	424	40%
beef, cheese, & red chili peppers	1	17.55	364	43%
Enchilada				
cheese & beef	1	17.64	324	49%
cheese, beef, & beans	1	16	344	42%
cheese & sour cream	1	18.85	320	53%
Frijoles-cheese	1 cup	7.78	226	31%
Nachos				
cheese	6-8 pieces	18.95	345	49%
cheese & jalapeno pepper	6-8 pieces	34	607	50%
cheese, ground beef, beans & jalapeno pepper	6-8 pieces	30.69	568	49%
cinnamon & sugar	6-8 pieces	35.98	592	55%

Food and Description	Amount	Fat Grams	Total Calories	% Fat Calories
Taco	1 small	20.55	370	50%
	1 large	31.6	569	50%
Taco Salad-lettuce, tomato, chili sauce, ground beef, cheese, & taco shell	1½ cup	14.77	279	47%
Taco Salad w/chili con carne	1½ cup	13	288	41%
Tostada				
bean & cheese	1	9.86	223	40%
bean, beef, & cheese	1	16.9	334	46%
beef & cheese	1	16	315	46%
beef, cheese, & guacomole	2	23	360	58%
■ SALADS & SALAD BAR MISC.				
Alfalfa Sprouts	1 oz	–	10	–
Bacon Bits	2 Tbs	3	54	50%
Broccoli	~ 2 oz	–	6	–
Carrots	~ 2 oz	–	12	–
Cauliflower	~ 2 oz	–	14	–
Cheese				
cheddar-shredded	3 Tbs	7	84	75%
cottage	½ cup	5	117	39%
parmesan	3 Tbs	4.5	70	58%
Cole Slaw	½ cup	8	90	80%
Croutons	18 pieces	1	35	26%
Cucumber-sliced	3 slices	–	2	–
Eggs-hard-cooked/ chopped	2 Tbs	2	30	60%
Garbanzo Beans	1 Tbs	–	11	–
Green Peas	½ cup	–	60	–
Lettuce	½ cup	–	5	–
Mozzarella Cheese	1 oz	7	90	70%
Mushrooms-pieces	¼ cup	–	6	–
Onions	2 Tbs	–	4	–
Peppers, Green	2 Tbs	–	4	–
Salad Dressings (See CONDIMENTS in this category; OILS) REMEMBER: 2 oz = 4 LEVEL TBS!				
Salad-Chef-w/cheese, turkey, ham & egg	1½ cup	16	267	54%
Salad-tossed/no dressing w/lettuce, tomato, radishes, carrots, cabbage, cucumber & green pepper	1½ cup	–	32	–
Salad-tossed				
w/cheese & egg	1½ cup	5.79	102	51%
w/chicken	1½ cup	2	105	17%
w/pasta & seafood	1½ cup	20.85	380	49%
w/shrimp	1½ cup	2	107	17%

Food and Description	Amount	Fat Grams	Total Calories	% Fat Calories
Tomatoes	1 oz	–	6	–

■ SANDWICHES

(NOTE: Meat patty sizes: Regular, single meat patty = 2 oz patty;
Regular, double meat patty = two 2 oz patties; Large, single meat
patty = 4 oz (¼ pound) patty. All sizes of meat patties are served
on appropriate size buns.)

*Does not include condiments or garnishes such as pickle, catsup,
lettuce, onions, tomato, mustard, or mayonnaise/mayonnaise-type
dressing.

Food and Description	Amount	Fat Grams	Total Calories	% Fat Calories
Cheeseburger*	Regular/Single	15	320	42%
Cheeseburger	Regular/Double	28	457	55%
Cheeseburger*-double bun	Regular/Double	21.6	461	42%
Cheeseburger*	Large/Single	32.99	608	49%
Cheeseburger w/bacon	Large/Single	36.76	609	60%
	Large/Double	43.65	706	56%
Cheeseburger*	Large/Triple	50.97	796	57%
Chicken Fillet*	1	29	515	51%
Chicken Fillet w/cheese*	1	38.76	632	55%
Egg & Cheese on bun*	1	19	340	50%
Fish Fillet*	1	22.77	431	48%
Fish Fillet w/tartar sauce/cheese*	1	28.6	524	49%
Hamburger*	Regular/Single	11.8	275	39%
	Regular/Double	27.9	544	46%
Hamburger	Regular/Single	13	279	42%
	Regular/Double	32	576	50%
Hamburger*	Large/Single	22.9	400	52%
Hamburger	Large/Single	27	511	48%
	Large/Triple	41	693	53%
Ham & Cheese on Bun*	1	15	353	38%
Ham, Egg, & Cheese on Bun*	1	16	348	41%
Hot Dog*	1	14.5	242	54%

Food and Description	Amount	Fat Grams	Total Calories	% Fat Calories
Hot Dog w/chili*	1	17.5	324	49%
Hot Dog (i.e., corn dog)*	1	18.9	460	37%
Roast Beef on Bun*	1	13.77	346	36%
Roast Beef w/cheese*	1	18	402	40%
Roast Beef*	1 Super	28	620	41%
Sandwiches on sliced whole wheat bread w/average portions				
Bacon, Lettuce, & Tomato	1	16	290	50%
Bologna/plain	1	16	305	47%
Chicken Salad	1	20	255	71%
Chicken-sliced w/lettuce	1	15	310	44%
Club-Chicken, bacon, & tomato	1	26	570	41%
Corned Beef/plain	1	10	296	30%
Cream Cheese & Jelly	1	16	370	39%
Egg Salad	1	13	285	41%
Ham/plain	1	16	285	51%
Ham & Cheese (Swiss)	1	24	390	55%
Ham Salad	1	17	321	48%
Liverwurst/plain	1	12	260	42%
Peanut Butter	1	20	350	51%
Peanut Butter & Jelly	1	15	385	35%
Roast Beef (hot w/gravy)	1	25	421	53%
Roast Pork (hot w/gravy)	1	31	503	56%
Steak/sirloin (lean & fat-3 oz)	1	12	325	33%
Tunafish Salad	1	14	275	46%
Turkey/plain	1	19	400	43%
■ SIDE ORDERS				
Chili	1 cup	9	268	30%
Coleslaw	¾ cup	10.97	147	67%
Corn on cob w/butter	1 ear	3	155	17%
Corn on cob w/o butter	1 ear	1	125	7%
Hush Puppies	5	11.59	256	41%
Macaroni Salad w/mayonnaise	½ cup	6	168	32%
Onion Rings	8-9	15.5	175	80%
Potato-baked				
w/cheese	1	28.7	475	54%
w/cheese & bacon	1	25.89	451	52%
w/cheese sauce & broccoli	1	21	402	47%
w/cheese sauce & chili	1	21.86	481	41%
w/sour cream & chives	1	22	394	50%
Potatoes-French Fried				
w/beef tallow	Regular	12	237	46%
	Large	18.5	358	47%
w/beef tallow & vegetable oil	Regular	12	237	46%
	Large	18.5	358	47%

Food and Description	Amount	Fat Grams	Total Calories	% Fat Calories
w/vegetable oil	Regular	12	235	46%
	Large	18.5	355	47%
Potatoes-mashed w/whole milk & margarine	⅓ cup	.97	66	13%
Potato Chips	10 chips	7	105	60%
	1 oz	10	148	61%
Potato Salad	⅓ cup	5.7	108	48%
Waldorf Salad	½ cup	5	90	50%

■ SUBS

[NOTE: Following subs are from 6 to 8 inches long (8 to 12 ounces).]

Food and Description	Amount	Fat Grams	Total Calories	% Fat Calories
Sub w/salami, ham, cheese, lettuce, tomato, onion, & roll	1	18.6	456	37%
Sub w/roast beef, lettuce, tomato, & mayonnaise	1	12.96	411	28%
Sub-tuna salad	1	27.99	584	43%

FAST FOOD CHAINS BY NAME
ARBY'S
■ BREAKFAST ITEMS

Food and Description	Amount	Fat Grams	Total Calories	% Fat Calories
Bacon Platter	1	32	860	33%
Biscuit				
Bacon	1	17.9	318	51%
Ham	1	16.6	323	46%
Plain	1	14.9	280	48%
Sausage	1	31.9	460	62%
Blueberry Muffin	1	5.6	200	25%
Cinnamon Nut Danish	1 piece	9.5	340	25%
Croissant				
Bacon/Egg	1	26.2	389	61%
Ham/Cheese	1	20.7	345	54%
Mushroom/Cheese	1	37.7	493	69%
Plain	1	15.6	260	54%
Sausage/Egg	1	39.2	519	68%
Egg Platter	1	24	460	47%
Ham Platter	1	26.2	518	46%
Maple Syrup	1.5 oz	–	43	–
Sausage Platter	1	41	640	58%
Toastix	1 serving	25	420	54%

■ CONDIMENTS

Food and Description	Amount	Fat Grams	Total Calories	% Fat Calories
Arby's Sauce	½ oz	< 1	15	12%
Au Jus	4 oz	–	7	–
Horsey Sauce	½ oz	5	55	82%
Ketchup	½ oz	–	16	–
Mayonnaise	½ oz	10	90	100%
Mustard	½ oz	< 1	11	41%
Sugar Substitute	1 pkt	–	4	–

Food and Description	Amount	Fat Grams	Total Calories	% Fat Calories
■ DESSERTS				
Cheese Cake	3 oz	22.8	306	67%
Chocolate Chip Cookie	1 oz	4	130	28%
Polar Swirl				
Butterfinger	11.6 oz	18.1	457	36%
Heath	11.6 oz	21.8	543	36%
Oreo	11.6 oz	19.7	482	37%
Peanut Butter Cup	11.6 oz	24	517	42%
Snickers	11.6 oz	18.8	511	33%
Turnovers				
Apple	1	18.3	303	54%
Blueberry	1	19	320	53%
Cherry	1	17.8	280	57%
■ DRINKS				
Coca Cola Classic	12 oz	–	141	–
Coffee	8 oz	–	3	–
Diet Coke	12 oz	–	1	–
Diet Seven Up	12 oz	–	4	–
Hot Chocolate	8 oz	1.2	110	10%
Milk (2%)	8 oz	4.4	121	33%
Nehi Orange	12 oz	–	190	–
Orange Juice	6 oz	–	82	–
Pepsi Cola	12 oz	–	159	–
R.C. Cola	12 oz	–	173	–
R.C. Diet Rite	12 oz	–	1	–
R.C. Root Beer	12 oz	–	173	–
Seven Up	12 oz	–	144	–
Upper Ten	12 oz	–	169	–
■ POTATOES				
Baked				
Broccoli & Cheddar	1	17.9	417	39%
Deluxe	1	36.4	621	53%
Mushroom'N Cheese	1	26.7	515	47%
Plain	1	1.9	240	7%
w/Butter/Margarine & Sour Cream	1	25.2	463	49%
Cheddar Fries	5 oz	21.9	399	49%
Curly Fries	3.5 oz	17.7	337	47%
French Fries	2.5 oz	13.2	246	48%
Potato Cakes	3 oz	12	204	53%
■ SALADS (PREPACKAGED)				
Cashew Chicken	1	37	590	56%
Chef	1	11	210	47%
Light	1	9.5	205	42%
Croutons	½ oz	2.2	59	34%

Food and Description	Amount	Fat Grams	Total Calories	% Fat Calories
Dressings				
Blue Cheese	2 oz	31.2	295	95%
Buttermilk Ranch	2 oz	38.5	349	99%
Honey French	2 oz	26.9	322	75%
Light Italian	2 oz	1	23	39%
Thousand Island (Weight Watchers)	2 oz	29.2	298	88%
Creamy French	1 oz	3	48	56%
Creamy Italian	1 oz	3	29	93%
Garden Salad-Light	1 serving	5.2	109	46%
Roast Chicken Salad-Light	1 serving	7	184	34%
Side Salad	1 serving	–	25	–
■ **SANDWICHES**				
Chicken				
Chicken Breast	1	25.8	489	47%
Chicken Cordon Bleu	1	36.7	658	50%
Chicken Fajita Pita	1	9.3	272	31%
Grilled Chicken Barbeque	1	14.4	378	34%
Grilled Chicken Deluxe	1	21.1	426	45%
Roast Chicken Club	1	28.8	513	51%
Roast Chicken Deluxe	1	19.5	373	47%
Other Sandwiches				
Fish Fillet	1	29.1	537	49%
Ham'N Cheese	1	14.7	330	40%
Light				
Chicken Deluxe	1	6	263	21%
Ham Deluxe	1	5.5	255	19%
Roast Beef Deluxe	1	10	294	31%
Roast Turkey Deluxe	1	5	260	17%
Sub Deluxe	1	26	482	49%
Turkey Deluxe	1	20.2	399	46%
Roast Beef				
Bac'N Cheddar Deluxe	1	32.8	532	55%
Beef'N Cheddar	1	19.9	451	40%
French Dip	1	12.2	345	32%
French Dip'N Swiss	1	18.2	425	39%
Giant Roast Beef	1	27.2	530	46%
Junior Roast Beef	1	10.6	218	44%
Philly Beef'N Swiss	1	25.9	408	47%
Regular Roast Beef	1	14.8	353	38%
Super Roast Beef	1	28.2	529	48%
■ **SHAKES**				
Chocolate	12 oz	11.6	451	23%
Jamocha	11.5 oz	10.5	368	26%
Vanilla	11 oz	11.5	330	31%

Food and Description	Amount	Fat Grams	Total Calories	% Fat Calories
■ SOUPS				
Beef w/Vegetables & Barley	8 oz	2.8	96	26%
Boston Clam Chowder	8 oz	10.6	207	46%
Cream of Broccoli	8 oz	8	180	40%
French Onion	8 oz	3.1	67	42%
Lumberjack Mixed Vegetable	8 oz	3.6	89	36%
Old Fashioned Chicken Noodle	8 oz	1.8	99	16%
Pilgrim's Corn Chowder	8 oz	10.6	193	49%
Split Pea w/Ham	8 oz	9.6	200	43%
Tomato Florentine	8 oz	1.5	84	16%
Wisconsin Cheese	8 oz	18.7	287	59%
ARTHUR TREACHER'S				
Chicken Patties	2	21.6	369	53%
Chicken Sandwich	1	19.2	413	42%
Chips	4 oz	13.2	276	43%
Cod Tail Shape, Bake'N Broil	5 oz	14.2	245	52%
Coleslaw	3 oz	8.2	123	60%
Fish	2 pieces	19.8	355	50%
Fish Sandwich	1	24	440	49%
Krunch Pup	1-2 oz	14.8	203	66%
Lemon Luv	1-3 oz	13.9	276	45%
Shrimp	7 pieces	24.4	381	58%
BURGER KING				
■ BEVERAGES				
Coffee	1	–	2	–
Milk				
2%	1	5	121	37%
whole	1	9	157	52%
Orange Juice	1	–	82	–
Shakes				
chocolate	Regular	10	326	34%
chocolate syrup added	Regular	11	409	24%
vanilla syrup added	Regular	10	334	27%
Soft Drinks				
Diet Coke	Medium	–	1	–
Coca Cola Classic	Medium	–	264	–
Sprite	Medium	–	264	–
Tropicana Twister				
Orange Strawberry Banana	6 oz	–	50	–
Orange Cranberry	6 oz	–	50	–
■ BREAKFAST				
Bagel				
Plain	1	6	92	59%
w/Cream Cheese	1	16	370	39%

Food and Description	Amount	Fat Grams	Total Calories	% Fat Calories
Bagel Sandwich				
bacon, egg, & cheese	1	20	453	40%
ham, egg, & cheese	1	17	438	35%
plain w/ egg & cheese	1	16	407	42%
sausage, egg, & cheese	1	36	626	52%
Breakfast Buddy w/Sausage, Egg, & Cheese	1	16	255	56%
Croissan'wich				
bacon, egg, & cheese	1	23	353	59%
ham, egg, & cheese	1	22	351	56%
plain w/ egg & cheese	1	20	315	57%
sausage, egg, & cheese	1	40	534	68%
Danish	1	36	500	65%
French Toast Sticks	1 order	32	538	54%
Hash Browns	1 order	12	213	51%
Mini Muffins, Blueberry	1 order	14	292	43%
Scrambled Egg Platter				
plain	1	34	539	57%
w/bacon	1	39	610	58%
w/sausage	1	53	768	62%
■ BURGERS				
Bacon Double Cheeseburger	1	31	515	54%
Bacon Double Cheeseburger Deluxe	1	38	584	59%
Barbecue Bacon Double Cheeseburger	1	31	536	52%
Burger Buddies	1 pair	17	349	44%
Cheeseburger	1	15	318	42%
Cheeseburger Deluxe	1	23	390	53%
Double Cheeseburger	1	27	483	50%
Double Whopper	1	53	844	57%
Double Whopper w/Cheese	1	61	935	59%
Hamburger	1	11	272	36%
Hamburger Deluxe	1	19	344	50%
Mushroom Swiss Double Cheeseburger	1	27	473	51%
Whopper Sandwich	1	36	614	53%
w/cheese	1	44	706	56%
■ CONDIMENTS				
BK Broiler Sauce	1 Tbs	10	90	100%
Bacon Bits	1 serving	1	16	56%
Bull's Eye Barbecue	1 Tbs	–	22	–
Cream Cheese	1 oz	10	98	92%
Croutons	1 serving	1	31	29%
Dipping Sauces (1 oz servings)				
Barbecue	1 serving	–	45	–
Burger King A.M. Express Dip	1 serving	–	84	–

Food and Description	Amount	Fat Grams	Total Calories	% Fat Calories
Honey	1 serving	–	91	–
Ranch	1 serving	18	171	95%
Sweet & Sour	1 serving	–	45	–
Tartar	1 serving	18	174	93%
Ketchup	1 Tbs	–	17	–
Lettuce	1 piece	–	3	–
Mayonnaise	2 Tbs	21	194	97%
Mushroom Topping	¾ oz	1	13	69%
Mustard	1 serving	–	2	–
Pickle	½ oz	–	1	–
Processed American Cheese	¾ oz	7	92	68%
Processed Swiss Cheese	¾ oz	6	82	66%
Salad Dressing (Newman's Own)				
Bleu Cheese	1 serving	32	300	96%
French	1 serving	22	290	68%
Italian-Light	1 serving	1	30	30%
Ranch	1 serving	37	350	95%
Olive Oil & Vinegar	1 serving	33	310	96%
Thousand Island	1 serving	26	290	81%
(Weight Watchers)				
Caesar Salad	1 serving	< 1	6	45%
Creamy Ranch	1 serving	< 1	35	8%
Tartar Sauce	2 Tbs	14	134	94%
Tomato	1 oz	–	6	–
■ DESSERTS				
Apple Pie	1 piece	14	311	41%
Cherry Pie	1 piece	13	360	33%
Chocolate Brownie (Weight Watchers)	1 piece	3	100	27%
Lemon Pie	1 piece	8	290	25%
Mocha Pie (Weight Watchers)	1 piece	5	160	28%
Snickers Ice Cream Bar	1	14	220	57%
Yogurt, Frozen (Breyers)				
Chocolate	1 serving	3	132	20%
Vanilla	1 serving	3	120	23%
■ SANDWICHES & SIDE ORDERS				
Angel Hair Pasta w/Cheese (Weight Watchers)	1 serving	5	210	21%
Angel Hair Pasta w/o Cheese (Weight Watchers)	1 serving	2	160	11%
BK Broiler Chicken Sandwich	1	8	267	27%
Broiled Chicken Sandwich (no dressing)	1 serving	4	140	26%
Chef Salad (no dressing)	1 serving	9	178	46%
Chicken Sandwich	1	40	685	53%

Food and Description	Amount	Fat Grams	Total Calories	% Fat Calories
Chicken Tenders	1 order	13	236	50%
Chunky Chicken Salad (no dressing)	1 serving	4	142	25%
Fettucini Broiled Chicken (Weight Watchers)	1 serving	11	298	33%
Fish Tenders	1 order	16	267	54%
French Fries	Medium	20	372	48%
Garden Salad (no dressing)	1 serving	5	95	47%
Ocean Catch Fish Fillet Sandwich	1	33	479	62%
Onion Rings	1 order	19	339	50%
Side Salad (no dressing)	1 serving	–	25	–
Veggie Sticks	1 order	1	60	15%

CARL'S JR.
■ BAKERY PRODUCTS

Food and Description	Amount	Fat Grams	Total Calories	% Fat Calories
Blueberry Muffin	1	7	256	25%
Bran Muffin	1	6	220	25%
Chocolate Cake	1	20	380	47%
Chocolate Chip Cookies	1 order	13	330	36%
Danish-variety	1	9	300	27%

■ BEVERAGES

Food and Description	Amount	Fat Grams	Total Calories	% Fat Calories
Carbonated	Regular	–	243	–
Diet Carbonated	Regular	–	2	–
Iced Tea	Regular	–	2	–
Milk-2% low-fat	10 oz	6	175	31%
Orange Juice	Small	1	94	10%
Shakes	Regular	7	353	18%

■ BREAKFAST

Food and Description	Amount	Fat Grams	Total Calories	% Fat Calories
Bacon	2 strips	4	50	72%
English Muffin w/margarine	1	6	180	30%
French Toast Dips	1 order	25	480	47%
Hashed Brown Nuggets	1 order	9	170	48%
Hot Cakes w/margarine	1 order	12	360	30%
Sausage	1 Patty	17	190	81%
Scrambled Eggs	1 order	9	120	68%
Sunrise Sandwich				
w/bacon	1	19	370	46%
w/sausage	1	32	500	58%

■ POTATOES

Food and Description	Amount	Fat Grams	Total Calories	% Fat Calories
Bacon & Cheese	1	34	650	47%
Broccoli & Cheese	1	17	470	33%
Cheese	1	22	550	36%
Fiesta	1	23	550	38%
Lite	1	3	250	11%
Sour Cream & Chive	1	13	350	33%

■ SALAD DRESSINGS

Food and Description	Amount	Fat Grams	Total Calories	% Fat Calories
Bleu Cheese	2 oz	14	150	84%

Food and Description	Amount	Fat Grams	Total Calories	% Fat Calories
House	2 oz	17	186	82%
Italian Reduced-Calorie	2 oz	10	90	100%
Thousand Island	2 oz	23	231	90%
■ SANDWICHES				
American Cheese	1	5	63	71%
California Roast Beef'n Swiss	1	8	360	20%
Charbroiler BBQ Chicken	1	5	320	14%
Charbroiler Chicken Club	1	22	510	39%
Country Fried Steak	1	33	610	49%
Double Western Bacon Cheeseburger	1	53	890	54%
Famous Star Hamburger	1	36	590	55%
Filet of Fish	1	26	550	43%
Happy Star Hamburger	1	8	220	33%
Old Time Star Hamburger	1	17	400	38%
Swiss Cheese	1	4	57	63%
Super Star Hamburger	1	50	770	58%
Western Bacon Cheeseburger	1	33	630	47%
■ SIDE ORDERS				
French Fries	Regular	17	360	43%
Onion Rings	1 order	15	310	44%
Zucchini	1 order	16	300	48%
■ SOUPS				
Boston Clam Chowder	1 order	8	140	51%
Cream of Broccoli	1 order	6	140	39%
Lumber Jack Mix Vegetable	1 order	3	70	39%
Old Fashioned Chicken Noodle	1 order	1	80	11%

CHICK-FIL-A
■ DESSERTS/BEVERAGES

Food and Description	Amount	Fat Grams	Total Calories	% Fat Calories
Fudge Brownie w/nuts	1	19	369	46%
Ice cream	1	4.9	134	33%
Lemon Pie	1 slice	5	329	14%
Lemonade	Regular	–	124	–
Iced Tea	Regular	–	3	–
■ SANDWICHES/NUGGETS				
Chicken Salad Sandwich w/wheat bread	1	26.5	449	53%
Chick-fil-A Chargrilled Chicken Sandwich	1	4.8	258	17%
Chick-fil-A Chargrilled Chicken Deluxe Sandwich w/lettuce & tomato	1	4.9	266	17%
Chick-fil-A Chicken/no bun	1	6.8	219	28%
Chick-fil-A Chicken Sandwich w/bun	1	8.8	426	19%
Chick-fil-A Chicken Deluxe Sandwich	1	8.9	435	18%
Chick-fil-A Nuggets	8 pack	15	287	47%
	12 pack	22.6	430	47%

Food and Description	Amount	Fat Grams	Total Calories	% Fat Calories
■ SALADS/SIDE ORDERS				
Chargrilled Chicken Garden Salad	1	2	126	14%
Chicken Salad-Cup	1	28	309	82%
Chicken Salad-Plate	1	43.5	475	82%
Cole Slaw-cup	1	14	175	72%
Carrot & Raisin Salad-Cup	1	4.8	116	37%
Hearty Breast of Chicken Soup				
small	1	2.7	152	16%
Potato Salad-Cup	1	15	198	68%
Tossed Salad				
plain	1	–	21	–
w/Honey French	1	24	246	88%
w/Lite Italian	1	2	66	27%
w/Ranch dressing	1	16	177	81%
w/Thousand Island	1	21.9	231	85%
Waffle Potato Fries	Regular	13.5	270	45%
CHURCH'S FRIED CHICKEN				
Breast	1	17	287	64%
Breast w/wing	1	20	303	59%
Leg	1	9	147	55%
Thigh	1	22	306	65%
■ SIDE DISHES				
Corn w/butter spread	1	9	237	34%
French Fries	Regular	6	138	39%
DAIRY QUEEN				
■ BEVERAGES				
Malt				
Chocolate	Small	13	520	23%
	Regular	18	760	21%
	Large	25	1060	21%
Vanilla	Regular	14	610	21%
Shake				
Chocolate	Small	13	490	24%
	Regular	14	540	23%
	Large	26	990	24%
Vanilla	Regular	14	520	24%
	Large	16	600	24%
■ MISCELLANEOUS SPECIALTIES				
Banana Split	1	11	510	19%
Blizzard				
Heath	Small	23	560	37%
	Regular	36	820	40%
Strawberry	Small	12	500	22%
	Regular	16	740	19%

Food and Description	Amount	Fat Grams	Total Calories	% Fat Calories
Breeze				
Heath	Small	12	450	24%
	Regular	21	680	28%
Strawberry	Small	< 1	400	1%
	Regular	1	590	2%
Buster Bar	1	29	450	58%
Chocolate Dipped Cone	Small	9	190	43%
	Regular	16	330	44%
	Large	24	570	38%
Chocolate Sundae	Small	4	190	19%
	Regular	7	300	21%
	Large	10	440	21%
Cone				
Chocolate	Regular	7	230	27%
	Large	11	350	28%
Vanilla	Small	4	140	26%
	Regular	7	230	27%
	Large	10	340	27%
DQ Frozen Cake Slice (undecorated)	1 slice	18	380	43%
DQ Sandwich	1	4	140	26%
Dilly Bar	1	13	210	56%
Hot Fudge Brownie Delight Sundae	1	29	710	37%
Mr. Misty	Small	–	190	–
	Regular	–	250	–
	Large	–	340	–
Mr. Misty Float	1	7	390	16%
Mr. Misty Freeze	1	12	500	22%
Nutty Double Fudge	1	22	580	34%
Peanut Buster Parfait	1	32	710	41%
Queen's Choice Big Scoop				
Chocolate	1	14	310	41%
Vanilla	1	14	300	42%
Strawberry Waffle Cone Sundae	1	12	350	31%
Yogurt				
Cone	Regular	< 1	180	3%
	Large	< 1	260	2%
Cup	Regular	< 1	170	3%
	Large	< 1	230	2%
Strawberry Sundae	Regular	< 1	200	2%
■ SANDWICHES				
BBQ	1	4	225	16%
Chicken				
Breaded Fillet				
Plain	1	20	430	42%
w/Cheese	1	25	480	47%

Food and Description	Amount	Fat Grams	Total Calories	% Fat Calories
Grilled Fillet	1	8	300	24%
Fish Fillet				
Plain	1	16	370	39%
w/Cheese	1	21	420	45%
Hamburger				
DQ Homestyle Ultimate Burger	1	47	700	60%
Double				
Plain	1	25	460	49%
w/Cheese	1	34	570	54%
Single				
Plain	1	13	310	38%
w/Cheese	1	18	365	44%
Hot Dog				
Plain	1	16	280	51%
w/Cheese	1	21	330	57%
w/Chili	1	19	320	53%
Super Hot Dog-¼ lb	1	38	590	58%
■ SIDE ORDERS				
French Fries	Small	10	210	43%
	Regular	14	300	42%
	Large	18	390	42%
Garden Salad (no dressing)	1 serving	13	200	59%
Lettuce	1 piece	–	2	–
Onion Rings	1 order	12	240	45%
Salad Dressing				
French Reduced Calorie	1 serving	5	90	50%
Thousand Island	1 serving	21	225	84%
Side Salad (no dressing)	1 serving	–	25	–
Tomato	1 slice	–	3	–
DOMINO'S				
■ CHEESE PIZZA				
12" - serves 4	2 slices	6	340	16%
16" - serves 6	2 slices	8	400	18%
Deluxe	2 slices	20	498	36%
■ PEPPERONI				
12" - serves 4	2 slices	12	380	28%
16" - serves 6	2 slices	14	440	29%
Double Cheese	2 slices	25	545	41%
DRUTHER'S				
■ BREAKFAST				
Bacon & Egg Plate (fried)	1 serving	41.9	721	52%
Bacon & Egg Plate (scrambled)	1 serving	43	742	52%
Bacon & Egg w/Biscuit	1 serving	16.3	258	57%
Biscuits & Gravy	1 serving	14.7	331	40%

Food and Description	Amount	Fat Grams	Total Calories	% Fat Calories
Ham & Egg Plate				
(fried)	1 serving	35.3	681	47%
(scrambled)	1 serving	44.6	762	53%
Ham & Egg w/Biscuit	1 serving	11.2	217	46%
Sausage & Egg Platter				
(fried)	1 serving	43.4	741	53%
(scrambled)	1 serving	44.6	762	53%
Sausage & Egg w/Biscuit	1 serving	15	246	55%
Sausage (1), Biscuit (1)	1 serving	11.1	179	56%
Sausages (2), Biscuits (2)	1 serving	22.3	358	56%
■ CHICKEN & FISH				
Chicken				
8 pieces	1 order	114	3664	28%
12 pieces	1 order	171	5496	28%
Dinner or Snack				
2-piece breast & wing				
w/potatoes & cole slaw	1 order	49.9	970	46%
2-piece breast & wing	1 order	30.7	595	46%
2-piece leg & thigh	1 order	29.8	549	49%
w/potatoes & cole slaw	1 order	49	925	48%
3-piece breast, thigh, & leg	1 order	66.9	1281	47%
3-piece breast, thigh, & wing	1 order	70.3	1309	48%
Fish				
Fish & Chips	1 order	29.8	729	37%
Fish Dinner	1 order	31.3	770	37%
■ SANDWICHES				
Cheeseburger				
Deluxe Quarter	1	37.6	660	51%
Double	1	26.1	500	47%
Regular	1	17.8	380	42%
Fish Sandwich	1	14.4	349	37%
Hamburger	1	13.4	327	37%

GODFATHER'S PIZZA
■ ORIGINAL PIZZA

Food and Description	Amount	Fat Grams	Total Calories	% Fat Calories
Cheese				
Mini	¼ pizza	4	138	26%
Small	⅙ pizza	7	239	26%
Medium	⅛ pizza	8	242	30%
Large	⅒ pizza	8	271	27%
Combo				
Mini	¼ pizza	5	164	27%
Small	⅙ pizza	11	299	33%
Medium	⅛ pizza	12	318	34%
Large	⅒ pizza	12	332	33%

Food and Description	Amount	Fat Grams	Total Calories	% Fat Calories
■ **GOLDEN CRUST**				
Cheese				
Small	⅙ pizza	8	213	34%
Medium	⅛ pizza	9	229	35%
Large	⅒ pizza	11	261	38%
Combo				
Small	⅙ pizza	12	273	40%
Medium	⅛ pizza	13	283	41%
Large	⅒ pizza	15	322	42%
HARDEE'S				
■ **BREAKFAST**				
Bacon Biscuit	1	21	360	53%
Bacon & Egg Biscuit	1	24	410	53%
Bacon, Egg, & Cheese Biscuit	1	28	460	55%
Big Country Breakfast				
w/bacon	1	40	660	55%
w/country ham	1	38	670	51%
w/ham	1	33	620	48%
w/sausage	1	57	850	60%
Biscuit'N'Gravy	1 order	24	440	49%
Canadian Rise'N'Shine Biscuit	1	27	470	52%
Chicken Biscuit	1	22	430	46%
Cinnamon'N'Raisin	1	17	320	48%
Country Ham Biscuit	1	18	350	46%
Country Ham & Egg Biscuit	1	22	400	50%
Ham Biscuit	1	16	320	45%
Ham & Egg Biscuit	1	19	370	46%
Ham, Egg, & Cheese Biscuit	1	23	420	49%
Hash Rounds	1 order	14	230	55%
Margarine/Butter Blend	1	4	35	100%
Rise'N'Shine Biscuit	1	18	320	51%
Sausage Biscuit	1	28	440	57%
Sausage & Egg Biscuit	1	31	490	57%
Steak Biscuit	1	29	500	52%
Steak & Egg Biscuit	1	32	550	52%
Syrup	1	–	120	–
Three Pancakes	1 order	2	280	6%
w/2 bacon strips	1 order	9	350	23%
w/1 sausage pattie	1 order	16	430	34%
■ **HAMBURGERS & SANDWICHES**				
All Beef Hotdog	1	17	300	51%
Bacon Cheeseburger	1	39	610	58%
Big Deluxe Burger	1	30	500	54%
Big Roast Beef	1	11	300	33%

Food and Description	Amount	Fat Grams	Total Calories	% Fat Calories
Big Twin	1	25	450	50%
Cheeseburger	1	14	320	39%
Chicken Fillet	1	13	370	32%
Fisherman's Fillet	1	24	500	43%
Grilled Chicken Breast Sandwich	1	9	310	26%
Hamburger	1	10	270	33%
Hot Ham'N'Cheese	1	12	330	33%
Mushroom'N'Swiss Burger	1	27	490	50%
Quarter Pound Cheeseburger	1	29	500	52%
Regular Roast Beef	1	9	260	31%
The Lean 1	1	18	420	39%
Turkey Club	1	16	390	37%
■ SALADS & SPECIAL ITEMS				
Big Fry	1	23	500	41%
Chef Salad	1	15	240	56%
Chicken'N Pasta Salad	1	3	230	12%
Chicken Stix	6 pieces	9	210	39%
	9 pieces	14	310	41%
Crispy Curls	1 order	16	300	48%
Garden Salad	1	14	210	60%
Large French Fries	1	17	360	43%
Regular French Fries	1	11	230	43%
Side Salad	1	–	20	–
■ SHAKES & DESSERTS				
Apple Turnover	1	12	270	40%
Big Cookie	1	13	250	47%
Cool Twist Cone				
chocolate	1	6	200	27%
vanilla	1	6	190	28%
vanilla/chocolate	1	6	190	28%
Cool Twist Sundae				
caramel	1	10	330	27%
hot fudge	1	12	320	34%
strawberry	1	8	260	28%
Shake				
chocolate	1	8	460	16%
strawberry	1	8	440	16%
vanilla	1	9	400	20%

JACK-IN-THE-BOX
■ BEVERAGES

Coca-Cola Classic	small	–	192	–
Coffee	small	–	2	–
Diet Coke	small	–	1	–
Dr. Pepper	small	–	192	–

Food and Description	Amount	Fat Grams	Total Calories	% Fat Calories
Iced Tea	small	–	4	–
Milk-lowfat (2%)	8.5 oz	5	122	37%
Milk Shake				
Chocolate	11 oz	7	330	19%
Strawberry	11.5 oz	7	320	20%
Vanilla	11 oz	6	320	17%
Orange Juice	6.5 oz	–	80	–
Ramblin' Root Beer	small	–	235	–
Sprite	small	–	192	–
■ BREAKFAST				
Breakfast Jack	1	13	307	38%
Country Crock Spread	1 serving	3	25	100%
Grape Jelly	1 pkt	–	38	–
Hash Browns	1 order	11	156	54%
Pancake Platter	1	22	612	32%
Pancake Syrup	1 pkt	–	121	–
Sausage Crescent	1	43	584	66%
Scrambled Egg Platter	1	32	559	54%
Scrambled Egg Pocket	1	21	431	44%
Sourdough Breakfast Sandwich	1	20	381	47%
Supreme Crescent	1	40	547	66%
■ DESSERTS				
Cheesecake	1	18	309	52%
Double Fudge Cake	1 piece	9	288	28%
Hot Apple Turnover	1	19	354	48%
■ FINGER FOODS				
BBQ Sauce	1 oz	–	44	–
Buttermilk House Dressing	2.5 oz	36	362	90%
Chicken Strips	4 pieces	13	285	41%
	6 pieces	20	451	40%
Chicken Wings	6 pieces	44	846	47%
	9 pieces	66	1270	47%
Egg Rolls	3 pieces	24	437	49%
	5 pieces	41	753	49%
Hot Sauce	1 pkt	–	4	–
Italian Sauce	1.5 oz	–	28	–
Mini Chimichangas	4 pieces	28	571	44%
	6 pieces	42	856	44%
Sweet & Sour Sauce	1 pkt	–	40	–
Toasted Raviolis	7 pieces	28	537	47%
	10 pieces	40	768	77%
■ HAMBURGERS				
Bacon Bacon Cheeseburger	1	45	705	57%
Cheeseburger	1	14	315	40%
Double Cheeseburger	1	27	467	52%

Food and Description	Amount	Fat Grams	Total Calories	% Fat Calories
Grilled Sourdough Burger	1	50	712	63%
Hamburger	1	11	267	37%
Jumbo Jack	1	34	584	52%
w/cheese	1	40	677	53%
Ultimate Cheeseburger	1	69	942	66%
■ MEXICAN FOOD				
Guacamole	1 pkt	3	30	90%
Salsa	1 pkt	–	8	–
Super Taco	1	17	281	54%
Taco	1	11	187	53%
■ SALADS				
Chef Salad	1	18	325	50%
Dressing				
Bleu Cheese Dressing	1 pkt	22	262	76%
Buttermilk House Dressing	1 pkt	36	362	90%
Italian-low calorie	1 pkt	2	25	72%
Thousand Island Dressing	1 pkt	30	312	87%
Side Salad	1	3	51	53%
Taco Salad	1	31	503	56%
■ SANDWICHES				
Chicken & Mushroom Sandwich	1	18	438	38%
Chicken Fajita Pita	1	8	292	25%
Chicken Supreme	1	39	641	56%
Country Fried Steak Sandwich	1	25	450	50%
Fish Supreme	1	27	510	52%
Grilled Chicken Fillet	1	19	431	38%
Mayo-Mustard Sauce	1 pkt	13	124	94%
Mayo-Onion Sauce	1 pkt	15	143	94%
Sirloin Steak Sandwich	1	23	517	40%
■ SIDE ORDERS				
French Fries	Small	11	219	45%
	Regular	17	351	44%
	Jumbo	19	396	43%
Old Fashioned Patty Melt	1	46	713	58%
Onion Rings	1 order	23	380	54%
Seasoned Curly Fries	1 order	20	358	50%
Sesame Breadsticks	1 order	2	70	26%
Tortilla Chips	1 oz	6	139	39%

KENTUCKY FRIED CHICKEN
■ EXTRA TASTY CRISPY CHICKEN

Food and Description	Amount	Fat Grams	Total Calories	% Fat Calories
Center Breast	1 piece	21	344	55%
Drumstick	1 piece	14	205	61%
Side Breast	1 piece	27	379	64%
Thigh	1 piece	31	414	67%
Wing	1 piece	17	231	66%

Food and Description	Amount	Fat Grams	Total Calories	% Fat Calories
■ **HOT & SPICY CHICKEN**				
Center Breast	1 piece	25	382	59%
Drumstick	1 piece	14	207	61%
Side Breast	1 piece	27	398	61%
Thigh	1 piece	30	412	66%
Wing	1 piece	18	244	66%
■ **KFC NUGGETS & SAUCES**				
Nuggets	3.4 oz	18	284	57%
Sauce				
Barbeque	1 oz	< 1	35	13%
Honey	1 oz	–	49	–
Mustard	1 oz	< 1	36	23%
Sweet & Sour	1 oz	< 1	58	9%
■ **KFC SKINFREE CRISPY**				
Center Breast	1 piece	16	296	49%
Drumstick	1 piece	9	166	49%
Side Breast	1 piece	17	293	52%
Thigh	1 piece	17	256	60%
■ **ORIGINAL RECIPE CHICKEN**				
Center Breast	1 piece	14	260	48%
Drumstick	1 piece	9	152	53%
Side Breast	1 piece	15	245	55%
Thigh	1 piece	21	287	66%
Wing	1 piece	11	172	58%
■ **OTHER KFC ITEMS**				
Buttermilk Biscuits	1	12	235	46%
Chicken Littles Sandwich	1	10	169	53%
Cole Slaw	1 order	6	114	47%
Colonel's Chicken Sandwich	1 sandwich	27	482	50%
Corn-on-the-Cob	1	2	90	20%
Crispy Fries	1 order	17	294	52%
French Fries	Regular	12	244	44%
Hot Wings Brand	6 pieces	33	471	63%
Mashed Potatoes & Gravy	1 order	2	71	25%

LITTLE CAESAR'S PIZZA
■ **INDIVIDUAL ORDERS**

Food and Description	Amount	Fat Grams	Total Calories	% Fat Calories
Baby Pan!Pan!	1 pizza	22	525	38%
Crazy Bread	1 piece	1	98	9%
Crazy Sauce	1 serving	–	63	–
Slice!Slice!	1 slice	31	756	37%
■ **PIZZA!PIZZA!**				
Round Cheese				
Small	1 slice	5	138	33%
Medium	1 slice	5	154	29%
Large	1 slice	6	169	32%

Food and Description	Amount	Fat Grams	Total Calories	% Fat Calories
Round Cheese & Pepperoni				
Small	1 slice	6	151	36%
Medium	1 slice	7	168	38%
Large	1 slice	7	185	34%
Square Cheese				
Small	1 slice	6	188	29%
Medium	1 slice	6	185	29%
Large	1 slice	6	188	29%
Square Cheese & Pepperoni				
Small	1 slice	8	204	35%
Medium	1 slice	8	201	36%
Large	1 slice	8	204	35%
■ SALADS & SANDWICHES				
Antipasto Salad (small)	1 serving	5	96	47%
Greek Salad (small)	1 serving	5	85	53%
Ham & Cheese Sandwich	1	27	553	44%
Italian Sandwich	1	35	615	51%
Tossed Salad (small)	1 serving	1	37	24%
Tuna Sandwich	1	31	610	46%
Turkey Sandwich	1	17	450	34%
Veggie Sandwich	1	47	784	54%

LONG JOHN SILVER'S
■ ALA CARTE

Food and Description	Amount	Fat Grams	Total Calories	% Fat Calories
Baked				
Chicken, Light Herb	3.9 oz	4	130	28%
Lemon Crumb 3-Piece Fish	5 oz	1	150	6%
Batter-Dipped Fish	1 piece	12	210	51%
Batter-Dipped Shrimp	1 piece	2	25	72%
Chicken Plank	1 piece	6	130	42%
Cole Slaw (drained on fork)	3.4 oz	6	140	39%
Corn Cobbette (w/spread)	1 piece	8	140	51%
Desserts				
Apple Pie	1 piece	13	320	37%
Cherry Pie	1 piece	13	360	33%
Chocolate Chip Cookie	1 cookie	9	230	35%
Lemon Pie	1 piece	9	340	24%
Oatmeal Raisin Cookie	1 cookie	10	160	56%
Walnut Brownie	1 piece	22	440	45%
Fries	3 oz	6	170	32%
Green Beans	3.5 oz	< 1	20	14%
Homestyle Fish	1 piece	5	110	41%
Hushpuppies	1 piece	2	70	26%
Rice	4 oz	3	160	17%
Roll	1 piece	< 1	110	4%

Food and Description	Amount	Fat Grams	Total Calories	% Fat Calories
Seafood Chowder w/Cod	7 oz	6	140	49%
Seafood Gumbo w/Cod	7 oz	8	120	60%
Small Salad (no dressing)	1.9 oz	–	11	–
■ CONDIMENTS				
Catsup	1 serving	–	12	–
Honey Mustard Sauce	1 serving	< 1	20	23%
Italian, Creamy Dressing	1 oz	3	30	90%
Malt Vinegar	1 serving	–	1	C
Ranch Dressing	1 oz	19	180	95%
Saltine Crackers	1 pkg	1	25	36%
Sea Salad Dressing	1 oz	15	140	96%
Seafood Sauce	1 serving	< 1	14	32%
Sweet & Sour Sauce	1 serving	< 1	20	23%
Tartar Sauce	1 serving	5	50	90%
■ ENTREES (STANDARD)				
Baked				
Chicken	16.8 oz	15	570	24%
Chicken-Light Herb	3.9 oz	4	130	28%
Fish w/Lemon Crumb	3 pieces	12	580	19%
Light Portion Fish w/Lemon Crumb	2 pieces	4	270	13%
Shrimp Scampi	18.1 oz	16	560	26%
Shrimp Scampi Sauce	5.2 oz	5	120	38%
3-Piece Fish Lemon Crumb	5 oz	1	150	6%
Chicken				
Chicken Planks w/Fries	2 pieces	19	440	39%
Chicken Planks w/Fries & Slaw	3 pieces	37	860	39%
Clams w/Fries, Slaw, & 2 Hushpuppies	12.7 oz	44	910	44%
Combinations				
1 Fish, 1 Chicken w/Fries	8.1 oz	25	510	44%
1 Fish, 2 Chicken w/Fries, Slaw, & 2 Hushpuppies	15.2 oz	43	930	42%
2 Fish, 8 Shrimp w/Fries, Slaw, & 2 Hushpuppies	17.2 oz	54	1070	45%
2 Fish, 5 Shrimp, 1 Chicken w/Fries, Slaw, & 2 Hushpuppies	18.1 oz	56	1130	45%
2 Fish, 4 Shrimp, 3 oz Clams w/Fries & Slaw	18.1 oz	61	1200	46%
Fish				
Fish & Fries	2 pieces	30	580	47%
Fish & More w/Fries & Slaw	2 pieces	42	860	44%
Long John's Homestyle Fish w/Fries & Slaw	3 pieces	34	780	39%

Food and Description	Amount	Fat Grams	Total Calories	% Fat Calories
Shrimp w/Fries, Slaw, & 2 Hushpuppies	11.7 oz	34	710	43%
■ FINGER FOODS				
Batter-Dipped Fish	1 piece	12	210	51%
Chicken Planks	2 pieces	13	270	43%
■ KID'S MEALS (Includes 1 Hushpuppy)				
1 Piece Fish & Fries	6.9 oz	21	450	42%
1 Piece Fish, 1 Piece Chicken, & Fries	8.9 oz	27	580	42%
2 Chicken Planks & Fries	7.8 oz	22	510	39%
■ SALADS (w/o salad dressing)				
Ocean Chef	8.2 oz	5	350	13%
Seafood	9.8 oz	31	380	73%
Small	1.9 oz	–	11	–
■ SANDWICHES (w/o sandwich sauce)				
Baked Chicken	6.4 oz	8	310	23%
Batter-Dipped Chicken	2 pieces	17	440	35%
Batter-Dipped Fish	1 piece	16	380	38%

MCDONALD'S
■ BEVERAGES

Food and Description	Amount	Fat Grams	Total Calories	% Fat Calories
Apple Juice	6 oz	–	90	–
Coca-Cola Classic	12 oz	–	140	–
	16 oz	–	190	–
	22 oz	–	260	–
	32 oz	–	380	–
Diet Coke	12 oz	–	1	–
	16 oz	–	1	–
	22 oz	–	2	–
	32 oz	–	3	–
Grapefruit Juice	6 oz	–	80	–
Milk				
1%	8 oz	2	110	16%
Orange Drink	12 oz	–	130	–
	16 oz	–	180	–
	22 oz	–	240	–
	32 oz	–	360	–
Orange Juice	6 oz	–	80	–
Shakes				
chocolate	~ 10.7 oz	10.6	390	24%
lowfat	10.4 oz	1.7	320	5%
strawberry	~ 10.7 oz	10	380	24%
lowfat	10.4 oz	1.3	320	4%
vanilla	~ 10.7 oz	10	350	26%
lowfat	10.4 oz	1.3	320	4%

Food and Description	Amount	Fat Grams	Total Calories	% Fat Calories
Sprite	12 oz	–	140	–
	16 oz	–	190	–
	22 oz	–	260	–
	32 oz	–	380	–
■ BREAKFAST				
Biscuit				
w/bacon, egg, & cheese	1	26	440	53%
w/biscuit spread	1	13	260	45%
w/sausage	1	28	420	60%
w/sausage & egg	1	33	505	59%
Breakfast Burrito	1	17	280	55%
Cheerios	¾ cup	1	80	11%
Danish				
Apple	1	17	390	39%
Cinnamon Raisin	1	21	440	43%
Iced Cheese	1	21	390	48%
Raspberry	1	15	410	33%
Egg McMuffin	1	11	280	35%
English Muffin w/spread	1	4	170	21%
Hashbrown Potatoes	1 Order	7	130	49%
Hotcakes w/margarine & syrup	1 Order	12	440	25%
Pork Sausage	1 Order	15	160	84%
Sausage McMuffin	1	20	345	52%
Sausage McMuffin w/egg	1	25	430	52%
Scrambled Eggs	1 Order	10	140	64%
Wheaties	¾ cup	1	90	10%
■ CHICKEN MCNUGGETS & SAUCES				
Chicken McNuggets	6 pieces	15	270	50%
Sauces				
Barbeque Sauce	1 pkt	.5	50	9%
Honey Sauce	1 pkt	–	45	–
Hot Mustard Sauce	1 pkt	3.6	70	46%
Sweet & Sour Sauce	1 pkt	–	60	–
■ DESSERTS				
Apple Bran Muffin/fat-free	1	–	180	–
Apple Pie	1	15	260	52%
Chocolatey Chip Cookies	~ 2.3 oz	15	330	43%
McDonaldland Cookies	2.3 oz	9	290	28%
Soft Serve Ice Cream	1	4.5	140	29%
Yogurt				
Hot Caramel	6 oz	3	270	10%
Hot Fudge Lowfat Sundae	6 oz	3	240	11%
Strawberry Lowfat Sundae	6 oz	1	210	4%
Vanilla Lowfat Cone	3 oz	1	105	9%

Food and Description	Amount	Fat Grams	Total Calories	% Fat Calories
■ SALADS				
Bacon Bits	1 serving	1	15	60%
Chef	1	9	170	48%
Chicken Salad Chunky	1	4	150	24%
Croutons	1 serving	2	50	36%
Dressings				
Bleu Cheese	1 Tbs	4	50	72%
Lite Vinaigrette	1 Tbs	< 1	12	38%
Ranch	1 Tbs	5	55	82%
Red French low-cal	1 Tbs	2	40	45%
Thousand Island	1 Tbs	3	45	60%
Garden	1	2	50	36%
Side	1	1	30	30%
■ SANDWICHES				
Big Mac	1	26	500	47%
Cheeseburger	1	13	305	38%
Chicken Fajita	1 serving	8	185	39%
Fillet-O-Fish	1	18	370	44%
Hamburger	1	9	255	32%
McLean Deluxe	1	10	320	28%
w/Cheese	1	14	370	34%
McChicken	1	20	415	43%
Quarter Pounder	1	20	410	44%
w/Cheese	1	28	510	49%
■ SIDE ORDERS				
French Fries	Small	12	270	40%
	Medium	17	320	48%
	Large	22	400	50%

PIZZA HUT
■ HAND-TOSSED PIZZA

Food and Description	Amount	Fat Grams	Total Calories	% Fat Calories
Cheese	2 slices/ Medium	20	518	35%
Pepperoni	2 slices/ Medium	23	500	41%
Supreme	2 slices/ Medium	26	540	43%
Super Supreme	2 slices/ Medium	25	556	41%
■ PAN PIZZA				
Cheese	2 slices/ Medium	18	492	33%
Pepperoni	2 slices/ Medium	22	540	37%
Supreme	2 slices/ Medium	30	589	46%

Food and Description	Amount	Fat Grams	Total Calories	% Fat Calories
Super Supreme	2 slices/ Medium	26	563	42%
■ PERSONAL PAN PIZZA				
Pepperoni	Whole Pizza	29	675	39%
Supreme	Whole Pizza	28	647	39%
■ THIN'N CRISPY PIZZA				
Cheese	2 slices/ Medium	17	398	38%
Pepperoni	2 slices/ Medium	20	413	44%
Supreme	2 slices/ Medium	22	459	43%
Super Supreme	2 slices/ Medium	21	463	41%
PONDEROSA				
■ BEVERAGES				
Coffee, Black	6 oz	–	2	–
Milk				
Whole, Chocolate	8 oz	8.5	208	37%
Whole, Plain	8 oz	8.6	159	49%
Tea, Unsweetened	6 oz	–	2	–
■ DESSERTS				
Banana Pudding	1 oz	2.4	52	42%
Ice Milk				
Chocolate	3.5 oz	2.9	152	17%
Vanilla	3.5 oz	2.6	150	16%
Mousse				
Chocolate	1 oz	4.4	78	51%
Strawberry	1 oz	4.6	74	56%
Strawberry Glaze	1 oz	–	37	–
Toppings				
Caramel	1 oz	< 1	100	6%
Chocolate	1 oz	< 1	89	3%
Strawberry	1 oz	< 1	71	3%
Whipped	1 oz	6.4	80	72%
Vanilla Wafer	2 cookies	1	35	26%
■ ENTREES				
Chicken Breast	1 order	2.1	98	19%
Chicken Wings	2 pieces	9	210	39%
Fish, Baked				
Bake'r Broil	1 order	13	230	51%
Baked Scrod	1 order	1	120	8%
Fish, Broiled				
Halibut	1 order	2.4	170	13%
Roughy	1 order	4.8	138	31%

Food and Description	Amount	Fat Grams	Total Calories	% Fat Calories
Salmon	1 order	2.7	192	13%
Swordfish	1 order	9.4	271	31%
Trout	1 order	3.9	228	15%
Fish, Fried	1 order	9	190	43%
Fish Nuggets	1 piece	1.7	31	49%
Hot Dog	1	13	144	81%
Kansas City Strip, precooked	5 oz	5.7	138	37%
New York Strip, precooked	8 oz	10.5	314	30%
	10 oz	14.5	384	34%
Porterhouse, precooked	16 oz	30.9	640	43%
Rib-eye, precooked	6 oz	14.2	282	45%
	5 oz	12.8	219	53%
Shrimp, fried	7 pieces	.5	231	2%
Shrimp, mini	6 pieces	1.7	47	33%
Sirloin, precooked	7 oz	10.8	241	40%
Sirloin Tips, precooked	5 oz	8.2	473	16%
Steak, Chopped, precooked	4 oz	16.2	225	65%
	5.3 oz	21.5	296	65%
Steak Kabobs, meat only, precooked	3 oz	4.8	153	28%
Steak Sandwich	1	11.1	408	24%
Steak Teriyaki, precooked	5 oz	3.1	174	16%
T-Bone, precooked	10 oz	18.4	444	37%
	8 oz	8.5	178	43%
■ SIDE DISHES, SAUCES, AND CONDIMENTS				
BBQ Sauce	1 Tbs	–	25	–
Beans, Baked	4 oz	6	170	32%
Beans, Green	3.5 oz	–	20	–
Carrots	3.5 oz	–	31	–
Cauliflower, Breaded	4 oz	1	115	8%
Cheese, Herb/Garlic Spread	1 Tbs	10	100	90%
Cheese Sauce	4 Tbs	2	52	35%
Corn	3.5 oz	< 1	90	5%
Gravy, Brown	4 Tbs	1	25	36%
Gravy, Turkey	4 Tbs	< 1	25	7%
Macaroni & Cheese	1 oz	< 1	17	26%
Margarine, Liquid	1 Tbs	11	100	100%
Margarine, Whipped	1 Tbs	1.2	34	32%
Okra, Breaded	4 oz	1	124	7%
Onion Rings, Breaded	4 oz	8.8	213	37%
Pasta Shells	2 oz	< 1	78	3%
Peas	3.5 oz	< 1	67	4%
Potatoes				
Baked	1 serving	< 1	145	3%
French Fried	1 serving	4.3	120	32%
Mashed	1 serving	< 1	62	3%

Food and Description	Amount	Fat Grams	Total Calories	% Fat Calories
Wedges	1 serving	6	130	42%
Rice Pilaf	1 serving	4	160	34%
Rolls, Dinner	1	3.4	184	17%
Rolls, Sourdough	1	1	110	8%
Salad Oil	1 Tbs	14	120	100%
Shortening, Liquid	2 Tbs	28.3	249	100%
Sour Cream	1 Tbs	2.5	26	87%
Spaghetti	2 oz	< 1	78	3%
Spaghetti Sauce	4 oz	4	110	33%
Stuffing	4 oz	11	230	43%
Sweet & Sour Sauce	1 oz	< 1	37	12%
Tortilla Chips	1 oz	8	150	48%
Winter Mix	3.5 oz	–	25	–
Zucchini, Breaded	4 oz	< 1	102	6%
■ SALAD BAR SELECTIONS				
Apple, medium	1	1	80	11%
Apple, canned	4 oz	–	90	–
Apple Rings, Spiced	4 oz	–	100	–
Applesauce	4 oz	–	80	–
Banana, medium	1	< 1	87	2%
Banana Chips	2 oz	1.3	25	47%
Beets, Diced	4 oz	< 1	55	7%
Breadsticks				
Italian	1 piece	1	100	9%
Sesame	2 pieces	–	35	–
Broccoli	1 oz	< 1	9	90%
Cabbage, Green	1 oz	–	9	–
Cabbage, Red	1 oz	–	1	–
Cantaloupe	1 wedge	–	13	–
Celery	1 oz	–	4	–
Cheese, Imitation (shredded)	1 oz	7	90	70%
Cheese Spread	1 oz	6.7	98	62%
Cherry Peppers	2 pieces	< 1	7	26%
Chicken Salad	3.5 oz	15.4	213	65%
Chow Mein Noodles	.2 oz	1.2	25	43%
Cocktail Sauce	2 Tbs	1	34	26%
Coconut, Shredded	.2 oz	1.9	25	68%
Cottage Cheese	4 oz	5	120	38%
Crackers, Melba Snacks	2 pieces	–	18	–
Croutons	1 oz	3.7	115	29%
Cucumber	1 oz	–	4	–
Eggs, Diced	2 oz	6.6	94	63%
Fruit Cocktail	4 oz	< 1	97	2%
Garbanzo Beans	1 oz	–	102	–
Gelatin, Plain	4 oz	–	71	–

Food and Description	Amount	Fat Grams	Total Calories	% Fat Calories
Granola	.2 oz	1	24	38%
Grapes	10 pieces	< 1	34	5%
Ham, Diced	2 oz	10	120	75%
Honeydew	1 wedge	< 1	25	7%
Lemon	1 wedge	–	3	–
Lettuce	1 oz	–	5	–
Macaroni Salad	3.5 oz	11.7	335	31%
Mushrooms	1 oz	–	8	–
Olives				
Black	1	< 1	4	90%
Green	1	< 1	3	90%
Onions				
Green	1 piece	–	7	–
Red and Yellow	1 oz	–	11	–
Oranges	1 piece	–	45	–
Pasta Salad, pre-made	3.5 oz	11.7	269	39%
Peaches, Canned	4 oz	–	70	–
Peanuts, granulated	.2 oz	2.3	30	69%
Pears, Canned	4 oz	< 1	98	5%
Pepper, Green	1 oz	–	6	–
Pickles				
Dill Spears	.14 oz	–	< 1	–
Sweet Chips	.14 oz	–	4	–
Pineapple, Fresh	1 wedge	–	11	–
Pineapple, Tidbits	4 oz	< 1	95	2%
Potato Salad	3.5 oz	5.9	126	42%
Radishes	1 oz	–	4	–
Spinach	1 oz	–	7	–
Sprouts				
Alfalfa	1 oz	–	10	–
Bean	1 oz	–	10	–
Strawberries	2 oz	< 1	14	13%
Sunflower Seeds	.2 oz	2.8	32	79%
Tartar Sauce	1 oz	10.5	95	100%
Tomatoes	1 oz	–	6	–
Turkey, Julienne	1 oz	< 1	29	19%
Turkey-Ham Salad	3.5 oz	12.8	186	62%
Watermelon	1 wedge	< 1	111	7%
Yogurt				
Fruit	4 oz	1	115	8%
Vanilla	4 oz	2	110	16%

QUINCY'S
■ MAIN DISHES

Food and Description	Amount	Fat Grams	Total Calories	% Fat Calories
Catfish Fillets	2 pieces	12	309	35%

Food and Description	Amount	Fat Grams	Total Calories	% Fat Calories
Chicken Breast, Grilled	1 piece	< 1	145	2%
Chicken Strips	4 pieces	15	318	42%
Hamburger				
Quarter Pound	1	19	403	42%
Quarter Pound w/Cheese	1	23	451	46%
Shrimp	7 pieces	12	248	44%
Steak				
Chopped	5.8 oz	34	466	66%
Country Style w/Mushroom				
Sauce	6 oz	19	288	59%
Filet	5.6 oz	12	231	47%
Luncheon, Chopped	4 oz	25	350	64%
Rib-eye	7.3 oz	60	665	81%
Sirloin	5.9 oz	54	649	75%
Sirloin, Club	4.8 oz	10	283	32%
Sirloin, Large	7.7 oz	70	852	74%
Sirloin, Petite	4 oz	37	446	75%
Sirloin Tips	4 oz	9	236	34%
T-Bone	7.8 oz	95	1045	82%
■ SIDE DISHES AND CONDIMENTS				
Coleslaw	1 serving	5	60	74%
Cornbread	1 piece	6	178	30%
Green Beans	1 serving	1	40	23%
Margarine	2 Tbs	22	200	100%
Mushroom Sauce	1 serving	< 1	27	17%
Peppers & Onions	1 serving	5	80	56%
Potato, Baked (no butter)	1 serving	< 1	181	2%
Steak Fries	1 serving	21	426	44%
■ SOUPS				
Broccoli, Cream Of	1 serving	14	193	65%
Chili w/Beans	1 serving	16	346	42%
Clam Chowder	1 serving	14	198	64%
Vegetable Beef	1 serving	2	78	23%
RAX				
■ BEVERAGES				
Coke	16 oz	–	205	–
Diet Coke	16 oz	–	1	–
Hot Cocoa Mix				
prepared	6 oz	11	110	90%
■ DESSERTS				
Chocolate Chip Cookies	2 cookies	12	262	41%
Milk Shakes (no whipped topping)				
Chocolate	1	12	445	24%
Strawberry	1	12	445	24%

Food and Description	Amount	Fat Grams	Total Calories	% Fat Calories
Vanilla	1	13	385	30%
Whipped Topping	1 dollop	4	50	72%
■ MEXICAN BAR				
Banana Pepper Rings	1 Tbs	–	2	–
Cheese Sauce	3.5 oz	17	420	36%
Cheese Sauce, Nacho	3.5 oz	22	470	42%
Green Onions	¼ cup	–	10	–
Jalapeno Peppers	1 oz	–	6	–
Olives	3.5 oz	10	110	82%
Refried Beans	3 oz	4	120	30%
Sour Topping	3.5 oz	11	130	76%
Spanish Rice	3.5 oz	< 1	90	5%
Spicy Meat Sauce	3.5 oz	4	80	45%
Taco Sauce	3.5 oz	< 1	30	12%
Tomatoes	1 oz	–	6	–
Tortilla	1 piece	2	110	16%
Tortilla Chips	1 oz	7	140	45%
■ PASTA BAR				
Alfredo Sauce	3.5 oz	3	80	34%
Chicken Noodle Soup	3.5 oz	< 1	40	11%
Cream of Broccoli Soup	3.5 oz	2	50	36%
Parmesan Cheese Substitute	1 oz	4	80	45%
Pasta Shells	3.5 oz	4	170	21%
Pasta Vegetable Blend	3.5 oz	4	100	36%
Rainbow Rotini	3.5 oz	4	180	20%
Spaghetti	3.5 oz	4	140	26%
Spaghetti Sauce	3.5 oz	< 1	80	6%
Spaghetti Sauce w/Meat	3.5 oz	8	150	48%
■ POTATOES				
Baked				
Cheese & Bacon	1 serving	28	780	32%
Cheese & Broccoli	1 serving	26	760	31%
Chili & Cheese	1 serving	23	700	30%
Plain	1 serving	< 1	264	2%
Plain w/Margarine	1 serving	11	364	27%
French Fries (May have unsalted, upon request)				
Large	1 order	20	390	46%
Regular	1 order	14	282	45%
Potato Topping Ingredients				
Bacon Bits	½ oz	2	40	45%
BBQ Meat Sauce	2.5 oz	3	110	25%
Broccoli	1.5 oz	< 1	16	11%
Cheese Sauce	3 oz	15	370	36%
Chili	3 oz	2	80	23%
Liquid Margarine	1 Tbs	11	100	100%

Food and Description	Amount	Fat Grams	Total Calories	% Fat Calories
Onion, Diced	½ oz	–	10	–
Sour Topping	3.5 oz	11	130	76%
■ **SALAD BAR ITEMS**				
Alfalfa Sprouts	1 oz	–	8	–
Applesauce	1 cup	< 1	100	5%
Bacon Bits	½ oz	2	40	45%
Banana Chips	1 oz	< 1	100	5%
Beets	1 cup	< 1	60	5%
Broccoli	½ cup	–	16	–
Cabbage	1 cup	–	16	–
Cantaloupe	2 pieces	< 1	16	17%
Carrots	¼ cup	–	8	–
Cauliflower	½ cup	–	16	–
Celery	½ cup	–	< 1	–
Cheddar Cheese, imitation				
Shredded	1 oz	6	90	60%
Tidbits	1 oz	11	160	62%
Cherry Peppers	1 Tbs	–	6	–
Chow Mein Noodles	1 oz	6	140	39%
Coconut	1 oz	11	160	62%
Cole Slaw	3.5 oz	4	70	51%
Cottage Cheese	1 cup	10	150	60%
Crackers, Plain	2 pieces	< 1	16	17%
Croutons	½ oz	< 1	40	11%
Cucumbers	2 slices	–	2	–
Eggs	1½ oz	5	70	64%
Garbanzo Beans	½ cup	5	360	13%
Gelatin, Lime or Strawberry	½ cup	< 1	90	3%
Grapefruit Sections	1 cup	< 1	80	4%
Grapes	1 cup	< 1	100	5%
Green Pepper	¼ cup	–	8	–
Honeydew Melon	2 pieces	< 1	25	7%
Kale	1 oz	–	16	–
Kidney Beans	1 cup	1	220	4%
Peaches	2 slice	–	16	–
Peas	1 oz	–	25	–
Pickle	1 spear	–	8	–
Pineapple				
Canned	3.5 oz	< 1	100	5%
Fresh	3 oz	< 1	45	10%
Potato Salad	1 cup	17	260	59%
Pudding				
Butterscotch	3.5 oz	6	140	39%
Chocolate	3.5 oz	6	140	39%
Vanilla	3.5 oz	6	140	39%

Food and Description	Amount	Fat Grams	Total Calories	% Fat Calories
Radish	½ oz	–	2	–
Red Cabbage	¼ cup	–	4	–
Salad Dressings				
Blue Cheese	1 Tbs	5	50	90%
Lite	1 Tbs	3	35	77%
French	1 Tbs	4	60	60%
Lite	1 Tbs	2	40	45%
Italian	1 Tbs	4	50	72%
Lite	1 Tbs	3	30	90%
Oil	1 Tbs	14	130	100%
Poppy Seed	1 Tbs	4	60	60%
Ranch	1 Tbs	5	45	100%
Thousand Island	1 Tbs	6	70	77%
Lite	1 Tbs	3	40	68%
Vinegar	1 Tbs	–	2	–
Sesame Sticks	1 oz	10	150	60%
Soynuts	1 oz	7	120	53%
Strawberries	2 oz	–	18	–
Sunflower Seeds w/Raisins	1 oz	10	130	69%
Three-Bean Salad	½ cup	< 1	100	5%
Tomatoes	1 oz	–	6	–
Turkey Bits	2 oz	3	70	39%
Watermelon	2 pieces	–	18	–
■ SALADS (No Dressing)				
Chef Salad	1 serving	14	230	55%
Gourmet Garden	1 serving	6	134	40%
Grilled Chicken Garden	1 serving	9	202	40%
■ SANDWICH ACCOMPANIMENTS				
American Cheese Slice	½ oz	5	60	75%
Bacon	½ oz	7	80	79%
BBC Sauce	¾ oz	16	145	100%
BBQ Meat Topping	3.25 oz	4	140	26%
Bun				
Hoagie, 6"	1	10	280	32%
Kaiser, 4"	1	2	180	10%
Small	1	3	180	15%
Catsup	1 Tbs	< 1	6	75%
Fish	3.5 oz	12	230	47%
Ham	2.5 oz	2	70	26%
Horseradish Sauce	¾ oz	< 1	10	45%
Lettuce, Shredded	¼ cup	–	2	–
Mayonnaise	¾ oz	16	150	96%
Mushroom Sauce	1 oz	–	16	–
Philly Vegetables	2 oz	1	30	30%
Pickle Spear	2.3 oz	< 1	8	23%

Food and Description	Amount	Fat Grams	Total Calories	% Fat Calories
Roast Beef	2.8 oz	9	140	58%
Swiss Cheese Slices	½ oz	2	30	60%
Tartar Sauce	½ oz	5	50	90%
Tomatoes, sliced	½ oz	–	2	–
Turkey	2.5 oz	3	80	34%
■ SANDWICHES				
BBC (Beef, Bacon, & Cheddar)	1	32	523	55%
BBQ	1	14	420	30%
Country Fried Chicken Breast	1	29	618	42%
Fish	1	17	460	33%
Grilled Chicken Breast	1	23	402	51%
Ham & Swiss	1	23	430	48%
Philly Melt	1	16	396	36%
Roast Beef				
Deluxe	1	30	498	54%
Regular	1	10	262	34%
Small (Uncle Al)	1	14	260	48%
Turkey Bacon Club	1	43	670	58%
ROY ROGERS				
■ BEVERAGES				
Coke	12 oz	–	145	–
Diet Coke	12 oz	–	1	–
Hot Chocolate	6 oz	2	123	15%
Milkshake				
chocolate	1	10	358	25%
strawberry	1	10	315	29%
vanilla	1	11	306	32%
■ BREAKFAST				
Crescent Roll	1	18	287	56%
Crescent Sandwich	1	27	401	61%
w/bacon	1	30	431	63%
w/ham	1	29	445	59%
w/sausage	1	29	449	58%
Egg & Biscuit Platter	1	27	394	62%
w/bacon	1	30	435	62%
w/ham	1	29	442	59%
w/sausage	1	29	460	57%
Pancake Platter				
w/syrup & butter	1	15	452	30%
w/bacon	1	18	493	33%
w/ham	1	17	506	30%
w/sausage	1	30	608	44%
■ SANDWICHES				
Bacon Cheeseburger	1	39	581	60%

Food and Description	Amount	Fat Grams	Total Calories	% Fat Calories
Cheeseburger	1	37	563	59%
Hamburger	1	28	456	55%
Roast Beef	Regular	10	317	28%
w/cheese	Regular	19	424	40%
	Large	12	360	30%
w/cheese	Large	19	424	40%
RR Bar Burger	1	39	611	57%
■ CHICKEN				
Breast	1	24	412	52%
Breast & wing combo	1	37	604	55%
Drumstick	1	8	140	51%
Nuggets	6	17	267	57%
Thigh	1	20	296	61%
Thigh & leg combo	1	28	436	58%
Wing	1	13	192	61%
■ DESSERTS				
Brownie	1	11	264	38%
Danish				
apple	1	12	249	43%
cheese	1	12	254	43%
cherry	1	14	271	47%
Strawberry Short Cake	1	19	447	38%
Sundaes				
caramel	1	9	293	28%
hot fudge	1	13	337	35%
strawberry	1	7	216	29%
■ SALAD BAR				
Bacon & Tomato Dressing	2 Tbs	12	136	79%
Bacon Bits	1 Tbs	1	33	27%
Beets-Sliced	¼ cup	–	15	–
Bleu Cheese Dressing	2 Tbs	16	150	96%
Broccoli	½ cup	–	20	–
Carrots-shredded	¼ cup	–	42	–
Cheddar Cheese	¼ cup	9	112	72%
Chinese Noodles	¼ cup	3	55	82%
Croutons	2 Tbs	1	70	13%
Cucumbers	6 slices	–	4	–
Eggs-chopped	2 Tbs	4	55	66%
Green Peas	¼ cup	–	7	–
Lettuce	1 cup	–	10	–
Low-Cal Italian Dressing	2 Tbs	6	70	77%
Macaroni Salad	2 Tbs	4	60	60%
Mushrooms	¼ cup	–	5	–
Potato Salad	2 Tbs	3	50	54%
Ranch Dressing	2 Tbs	14	155	81%

Food and Description	Amount	Fat Grams	Total Calories	% Fat Calories
Sunflower Seeds	1 oz/ ~ 2 Tbs	14	160	79%
Thousand Island Dressing	2 Tbs	16	160	90%
Tomatoes	3 slices	–	20	–
■ SIDE ORDERS				
Biscuit	1	12	231	47%
Cole Slaw	1	7	110	57%
French Fries	Regular	14	268	47%
	Large	18	357	45%
Hot Topped Potato	1	< 1	211	2%
w/bacon & cheese	1	22	397	50%
w/broccoli & cheeese	1	18	376	43%
w/margarine	1	7	274	23%
w/sour cream & chives	1	21	408	46%
w/taco beef & cheese	1	22	463	43%
Macaroni	1	11	186	53%
Potato Salad	1	6	107	51%
7-ELEVEN				
Big Bite				
Regular w/2 oz Beef Wiener	1	18	287	56%
Super w/4 oz Beef Wiener	1	34	460	67%
Burritos				
Bean & Cheese	1 serving	23	616	34%
Beef & Bean				
Green Chili	1 serving	23	617	34%
Plain	1 serving	11.5	308	34%
Red Chili	1 serving	11.5	308	34%
Red Hot				
5 oz	1 serving	11.6	310	34%
10 oz	1 serving	23.2	620	34%
Premium 5.2 oz	1 serving	17	359	43%
Beef, Bean, & Cheese	1 serving	20.5	395	47%
Beef & Potato	1 serving	18.4	394	42%
Chicken & Rice				
Premium	1 serving	5.6	244	21%
Chicken, Breast of	4.8 oz	15.7	405	35%
Chimichanga, Beef	5 oz	14.9	363	37%
Deli-Shoppe Microwave Products				
Bacon Cheeseburger	1 serving	28.7	558	40%
Bagel & Cream Cheese	1 serving	16	338	43%
Char Sandwich, Large	1 serving	47.2	713	60%
Fish Sandwich w/Cheese	1 serving	14.5	433	30%
Sausage, Red Hot, Large	1 serving	59.2	845	63%
Turkey Wedge	1 serving	5.6	193	26%

Food and Description	Amount	Fat Grams	Total Calories	% Fat Calories
Enchilada, Beef & Cheese	6.5 oz	21.7	369	53%
Fajitas	5 oz	11.4	311	33%
Sandito, Ham & Cheese	5 oz	16	347	41%
Sandito, Pizza	5 oz	17	345	44%
Tacos, Soft (Twin)	5.9 oz	19.7	399	44%
SHAKEY'S PIZZA				
Fried Chicken & Potatoes	3 pieces	56	947	53%
	5 pieces	90	1700	48%
Ham & Cheese, Hot	1 order	21	550	34%
Pizza				
Homestyle Pan Crust 12"				
Cheese only	1/10 pizza	13.7	303	41%
Cheese w/Onion, Green Pepper, Black Olives, & Mushrooms	1/10 pizza	14.7	320	41$
Pepperoni	1/10 pizza	15.4	343	40%
Sausage, Mushroom	1/10 pizza	16.9	343	44%
Sausage, Pepperoni	1/10 pizza	19.9	374	48%
Shakey's Special	1/10 pizza	20.7	384	49%
Thick Crust 12"				
Cheese only	1/10 pizza	4.8	170	25%
Cheese w/Green Pepper, Black Olives, & Mushrooms	1/10 pizza	4	162	22%
Pepperoni	1/10 pizza	6.4	185	31%
Sausage, Mushroom	1/10 pizza	5.6	179	28%
Sausage, Pepperoni	1/10 pizza	8	177	41%
Shakey's Special	1/10 pizza	8.3	208	36%
Thin Crust 12"				
Cheese only	1/10 pizza	5.2	133	35%
Cheese w/ Onion, Green Pepper, Black Olives, & Mushrooms	1/10 pizza	4.5	125	32%
Pepperoni	1/10 pizza	6.9	148	42%
Sausage, Mushroom	1/10 pizza	6	141	38%
Sausage, Pepperoni	1/10 pizza	8.4	166	46%
Shakey's Special	1/10 pizza	8.7	171	46%
Potatoes	15 pieces	36	950	34%
Shakey's Super Hot Hero	1 serving	44	810	49%
Spaghetti w/Meat Sauce & Garlic Bread	1 serving	33	940	32%
SHONEY'S				
■ AMERICA'S FAVORITES				
Chicken Tenders	1 serving	20.4	388	47%
Country Fried Steak	1 serving	27.2	449	55%
Lasagna	1 serving	9.8	297	30%
Liver'N Onions	1 serving	22.9	411	50%

Food and Description	Amount	Fat Grams	Total Calories	% Fat Calories
Spaghetti	1 serving	16.3	496	30%
■ BREAKFAST				
Bacon	3 strips	9.4	109	78%
Biscuit	1	8	170	42%
Country Gravy	3 oz	9.8	114	77%
Croissant	1	16	260	55%
Egg, Fried	1 serving	14.7	159	83%
Grits	3 oz serving	3.2	57	51%
Ham, Breakfast	2 slices	2	59	31%
Hashbrowns	3 oz serving	3	90	30%
Home Fries	1 serving	3.7	115	29%
Honey Bun	1	14	265	48%
Muffin, Blueberry	1 order	7	214	29%
Pancake (6")	1 serving	< 1	91	2%
Sausage	1 patty	9.6	103	84%
Sirloin, Charbroiled	6 oz	24.5	357	62%
Syrup, Lo-Cal	2.2 oz	–	98	–
Toast w/Butter	2 slices	5.2	163	29%
■ BURGERS & SANDWICHES				
All-American Burger	1	32.6	501	59%
Bacon Burger	1	40	591	61%
Baked Ham Sandwich	1	10.3	290	32%
Chicken, Charbroiled	1	17	451	34%
Chicken Fillet Sandwich	1	21.2	464	41%
Country Fried Sandwich	1	25.8	588	39%
Fish Sandwich	1	12.7	323	35%
Grilled Bacon & Cheese	1	28.2	440	58%
Grilled Cheese	1	16.9	302	50%
Ham Club on Whole Wheat	1	35.5	642	50%
Mushroom/Swiss Burger	1	41.7	616	61%
Old-Fashioned Burger	1	28.2	470	54%
Patty Melt	1	41.7	640	59%
Philly Steak Sandwich	1	44	673	59%
Reuben Sandwich	1	34.7	596	52%
Slim Jim Sandwich	1	23.9	484	44%
Shoney Burger	1	35.7	498	65%
Turkey Club on Whole Wheat	1	32.7	635	46%
■ DESSERTS				
Apple Pie A La Mode	1 serving	23	492	42%
Carrot Cake	1 serving	26	500	47%
Hot Fudge Cake	1 serving	19.7	522	34%
Hot Fudge Sundae	1 serving	22	451	44%
Strawberry Pie	1 serving	16.7	332	45%
Strawberry Sundae	1 serving	19	380	45%
Walnut Brownie A La Mode	1 serving	33.7	576	53%

Food and Description	Amount	Fat Grams	Total Calories	% Fat Calories
■ **ENTREES**				
Beef Patty, Light	1 serving	22.9	289	71%
Fish, Light Fried	1 serving	14.4	297	44%
Italian Feast	1 serving	19.6	500	35%
Shrimp, Boiled	1 serving	1	93	10%
Shrimp Sampler	1 serving	22.7	412	50%
Steak & Chicken, Charbroiled				
Chicken, Charbroiled	1 serving	7.4	239	28%
Chicken, Hawaiian	1 serving	7.4	262	25%
Half O'Pound	1 serving	34.4	435	71%
Ribeye	8 oz	50.5	605	75%
Sirloin	6 oz	24.5	357	62%
Steak'N Shrimp				
w/Charbroiled Shrimp	1 serving	22.6	361	56%
w/Fried Shrimp	1 serving	32.7	507	58%
■ **SALAD DRESSINGS**				
Biscayne Lo-Cal	2 Tbs	1	62	15%
Blue Cheese	2 Tbs	13	117	100%
French	2 Tbs	12	124	87%
French, Rue	2 Tbs	10	122	74%
Honey Mustard	2 Tbs	17	165	93%
Italian, Creamy	2 Tbs	15	135	100%
Italian, Golden	2 Tbs	15	141	96%
Italian, Weight Watchers	2 Tbs	–	10	–
Ranch	2 Tbs	10	95	95%
Thousand Island	2 Tbs	13	130	90%
■ **SALADS (Prepared)**				
Ambrosia	¼ cup	3.3	75	40%
Apple Grape Surprise	¼ cup	–	19	–
Beet Onion	¼ cup	1.3	25	47%
Broccoli/Cauliflower	¼ cup	8.5	98	78%
Broccoli/Cauliflower/Carrot	¼ cup	4.4	53	75%
Broccoli/Cauliflower/Ranch	¼ cup	6.4	65	89%
Carrot Apple	¼ cup	9	99	82%
Cole Slaw	¼ cup	5	69	65%
Cucumber Lite	¼ cup	–	12	–
Don's Pasta	¼ cup	4.6	82	50%
Fruit Delight	¼ cup	1.6	54	27%
Italian Vegetable	¼ cup	–	11	–
Kidney Bean Salad	¼ cup	2	55	33%
Macaroni	¼ cup	13.9	207	60%
Mixed Fruit	¼ cup	–	37	–
Mixed Squash	¼ cup	4	49	73%
Oriental Salad	¼ cup	2.7	79	31%
Pea Salad	¼ cup	5.5	73	68%

Food and Description	Amount	Fat Grams	Total Calories	% Fat Calories
Rotelli Pasta	¼ cup	4	78	46%
Seigan Salad	¼ cup	3.6	72	45%
Snow Salad	¼ cup	4	72	50%
Spaghetti Salad	¼ cup	4.6	81	51%
Spring Salad	¼ cup	2.9	38	69%
Summer Salad	¼ cup	11.6	114	92%
Three Bean Salad	¼ cup	5	96	47%
Waldorf	¼ cup	5.2	81	58%
■ SAUCES				
BBQ	1 serving	1	41	22%
Cocktail	1 serving	–	36	–
Sweet'N Sour	1 serving	–	58	–
Tartar	1 serving	7.7	84	83%
■ SEAFOOD				
Baked Fish	1 serving	1.4	170	7%
Fish'N Chips w/fries	1 serving	34.8	639	49%
Fish'N Shrimp	1 serving	25.5	487	47%
Seafood Platter	1 serving	28	566	45%
Shrimp, Bite-Size	1 serving	24.7	387	57%
Shrimp, Charbroiled	1 serving	3	138	20%
Shrimper's Feast				
Large	1 serving	33.3	575	52%
Regular	1 serving	22.2	383	52%
■ SIDE DISHES				
Baked Potato	1 serving	< 1	264	1%
French Fries	3 oz serving	7.5	189	36%
	4 oz serving	9.9	252	35%
Grecian Bread	1 serving	2.2	80	25%
Onion Rings	1 piece	3	52	52%
Rice	3.5 oz	3.7	137	24%
Sauteed Mushrooms	3 oz	6.5	75	78%
Sauteed Onions	2.5 oz	2	37	49%
■ SOUPS				
Bean	6 oz	1	63	14%
Beef Cabbage	6 oz	3	86	31%
Broccoli, Cream Of	6 oz	4.6	75	55%
Broccoli/Cauliflower	6 oz	9.2	124	67%
Cheddar Chowder	6 oz	2.3	91	23%
Cheese Florentine Ham	6 oz	7.8	110	64%
Chicken, Cream Of	6 oz	8.9	130	60%
Chicken Gumbo	6 oz	2	60	30%
Chicken Noodle	6 oz	1.4	62	20%
Chicken Rice	6 oz	< 1	72	6%
Chicken Vegetable, Cream	6 oz	1.3	79	15%
Clam Chowder	6 oz	5.4	94	52%

Food and Description	Amount	Fat Grams	Total Calories	% Fat Calories
Corn Chowder	6 oz	4.7	148	29%
Onion	6 oz	2	29	62%
Potato	6 oz	3.4	102	30%
Tomato Florentine	6 oz	1	63	14%
Tomato Vegetable	6 oz	< 1	46	6%
Vegetable Beef	6 oz	1.5	82	16%
STEAK & SHAKE				
Apple Danish	1 danish	23.8	391	55%
Apple Pie	1 piece	17.65	407	39%
Apple Pie A La Mode	1 piece	25.45	549	42%
Baked Beans	1 serving	3.68	173	19%
Baked Ham Sandwich	1	22	451	44%
Brownie	1 piece	11.5	258	40%
Brownie Fudge Sundae	1	35.2	645	49%
Cheese Cake	1 piece	11	368	27%
Cheese Cake w/Strawberries	1 piece	11.35	386	26%
Chef Salad	1 serving	17.6	313	51%
Cherry Pie	1 piece	13.75	334	37%
Cherry Pie A La Mode	1 piece	21.55	476	41%
Chili & Oyster Crackers	1 serving	14	337	37%
Chili Mac & 4 Saltines	1 serving	12.4	311	36%
Chili-3 Ways & 4 Saltines	1 serving	16	402	36%
Chocolate Shake	1	37.8	608	56%
Coca-Cola Float	1	17.2	514	30%
Coffee	6 oz	–	2	–
Cottage Cheese	½ cup	3.63	94	35%
Dr. Pepper	10.5 oz	–	137	–
Egg Sandwich	1	9.9	275	32%
French Fries	1 order	10.2	211	44%
Ham & Egg Sandwich	1	17.2	434	36%
Hot Chocolate	6 oz	18.6	686	24%
Hot Fudge Nut Sundae	1	34.4	530	58%
Hot Tea	7 oz	–	4	–
Iced Tea	7.5 oz	–	6	–
Lemon Drink (small)	1	–	86	–
Lemon Float	1	18.6	555	30%
Lemon Freeze	1	24.9	548	41%
Lettuce & Tomato	1 serving	–	4	–
Lettuce & Tomato Salad w/ 1 oz Thousand Island Dressing	1 serving	15.33	168	82%
Low Calorie Platter	1 serving	13.7	293	42%
Milk	8 oz	7.88	146	49%
Orange Drink (small)	1	–	83	–
Orange Float	1	16.83	502	30%

Food and Description	Amount	Fat Grams	Total Calories	% Fat Calories
Orange Freeze	1	23.8	516	42%
Orange Juice	7 oz	< 1	105	3%
Root Beer	10 oz	–	115	–
Root Beer Float	1	16.7	529	28%
Steakburger	1	7.12	277	23%
w/Cheese	1	13.3	353	34%
Strawberry Shake	1	40	648	56%
Strawberry Sundae	1	21.7	330	59%
Super Steakburger	1	12	375	29%
w/Cheese	1	18.3	451	37%
Toasted Cheese Sandwich	1	13.34	250	48%
Triple Steakburger	1	17	474	32%
w/Cheese	1	29.5	626	42%
Vanilla Ice Cream	1½ scoops	11.7	213	49%
Vanilla Shake	1	38.4	619	56%
TACO BELL				
Bean Burrito	1	14	381	33%
Beef Burito	1	21	431	44%
Burrito Supreme	1	22	440	45%
Chicken Burrito	1	12	334	32%
Chicken Fajita	1	10	226	40%
Chicken Soft Taco	1	10	213	42%
Chilito	1	18	383	42%
Cinnamon Crispas	1 order	15	259	52%
Cinnamon Twists	1 order	8	171	42%
Combination Burrito	1	16	407	35%
Guacamole	1 pkt	2	34	53%
Jalapeno Peppers	1 order	–	20	–
Mexican Pizza	1	37	575	58%
Meximelt				
Beef	1	15	266	51%
Chicken	1	15	257	53%
Nacho Cheese Sauce	1 serving	8	103	70%
Nachos	1 order	18	346	47%
Nachos Bellgrande	1 order	35	649	49%
Nachos Supreme	1 order	27	367	66%
Pico De Gallo	1	–	6	–
Pintos & Cheese	1 order	9	190	43%
Ranch Dressing	1 pkt	25	236	85%
Salsa	1 pkt	–	18	–
Sauce				
Green	1 serving	–	4	–
Red	1 serving	–	10	–
Sour Cream	1 pkt	4	46	78%

Food and Description	Amount	Fat Grams	Total Calories	% Fat Calories
Taco	1	11	183	54%
Taco Salad w/salsa	1 order	61	905	61%
Taco Salad w/salsa w/o shell	1 order	31	484	58%
Taco Sauce	1 pkt	–	2	–
Taco Sauce-hot	1 pkt	–	3	–
Taco-soft	1	12	225	48%
Taco Supreme	1	15	230	59%
Taco Supreme-soft	1	16	272	53%
Tostada	1	11	243	41%
TACO JOHN'S				
Apple Grande	1	8	257	28%
Beans, Refried	1 serving	6	331	16%
Burrito				
Bean	1	6	249	22%
Beef	1	18	355	46%
Combo	1	12	302	36%
Smothered w/Green Chili	1	24	405	53%
Smothered w/Texas Chili	1	24	518	42%
Super	1	11	434	23%
Chili, Texas	1 serving	22	430	46%
Chimi	1	19	487	35%
Churro	1	7	122	52%
Enchilada	1	18	379	43%
Nachos	1 serving	19	407	42%
Nachos, Super	1 serving	34	657	47%
Potato Ole Large	1	6	414	13%
Taco				
Bravo, Super	1	20	485	37%
Burger	1	14	332	38%
Regular	1	13	228	51%
Soft Shell	1	13	276	42%
Taco Salad, Super	1	18	450	36%
Tostada	1	13	228	51%
WENDY'S				
■ BEVERAGES				
Coffee	6 oz	–	2	–
Cola	16 oz	–	100	–
Diet Cola	16 oz	–	1	–
Hot Chocolate	6 oz	1	100	9%
Lemonade	8 oz	–	90	–
Lemon-Lime	16 oz	–	100	–
Milk				
Chocolate	8 oz	5	160	28%
Regular (2%)	8 oz	4	110	33%

Food and Description	Amount	Fat Grams	Total Calories	% Fat Calories
Tea (Hot or Iced)	6 oz	–	1	–
■ **CHICKEN NUGGETS**				
Crispy Chicken Nuggets	6 pieces	20	280	64%
Nuggets Sauce				
Barbecue	1 pkg	–	50	–
Honey	1 pkg	–	45	–
Sweet & Sour	1 pkg	–	45	–
Sweet Mustard	1 pkg	1	50	18%
■ **CHILI, CHEESE, CRACKERS**				
Cheddar Cheese (shredded)	2 Tbs	6	70	77%
Chili				
Small	8 oz	6	190	28%
Large	12 oz	9	290	28%
Crackers	2 pieces	1	25	36%
■ **DESSERTS**				
Chocolate Chip Cookie	1	13	280	42%
Danish-Apple	1	14	360	35%
Cinnamon Raisin	1	18	410	40%
Frosty-Dairy	12 oz	10	340	26%
	16 oz	13	460	25%
	20 oz	17	570	27%
Pudding				
Butterscotch	¼ cup	4	90	40%
Chocolate	¼ cup	4	90	40%
■ **GARDEN SPOT SALAD BAR**				
Alfafa Sprouts	½ cup	–	4	–
Applesauce, Chunky	2 Tbs	–	30	–
Bacon Bits	2 Tbs	2	45	40%
Breadsticks	1	–	14	–
Broccoli	½ cup	–	14	–
California Cole Slaw	2 Tbs	3	45	60%
Cantaloupe	2 pieces	–	20	–
Carrots	¼ cup	–	12	–
Cauliflower	½ cup	–	14	–
Cheddar Chips	2 Tbs	5	70	64%
Cheese (shredded)	2 Tbs	4	50	72%
Chicken Salad	2 Tbs	5	70	64%
Chives	1 Tbs	–	4	–
Chow Mein Noodles	¼ cup	2	35	51%
Cottage Cheese	2 Tbs	1	30	30%
Croutons	2 Tbs	1	30	30%
Crushed Red Peppers	1 oz	4	120	30%
Cucumbers	¼ cup	–	4	–
Dressings				
Blue Cheese	2 Tbs	19	180	95%

Food and Description	Amount	Fat Grams	Total Calories	% Fat Calories
Celery Seed	2 Tbs	11	130	76%
French	2 Tbs	10	120	75%
French Sweet Red	2 Tbs	10	130	69%
(Hidden Valley) Ranch	2 Tbs	10	100	90%
Italian Caesar	2 Tbs	16	150	96%
Reduced Calorie Bacon & Tomato	2 Tbs	4	50	72%
Salad Oil	2 Tbs	14	240	53%
Thousand Island	2 Tbs	13	130	90%
Wine Vinegar	1 Tbs	–	2	–
Eggs	2 Tbs	3	40	68%
Garbanzo Beans	2 Tbs	1	45	20%
Green Peas	½ cup	–	60	–
Green Peppers	2 pieces	–	2	–
Honeydew Melon	1 piece	–	18	–
Jalapeno Peppers	1 Tbs	–	2	–
Lettuce-Iceberg	1 cup	–	8	–
Lettuce-Romaine	1 cup	–	9	–
Mushrooms	¼ cup	–	4	–
Olives, Black	2 Tbs	1	16	56%
Oranges	2 oz	–	26	–
Parmesan Cheese				
Imitation	1 oz	3	80	34%
Natural	1 oz	9	130	62%
Pasta Salad	2 Tbs	4	80	45%
Peaches	2 oz	–	17	–
Pepperoni-sliced	6 pieces	3	30	90%
Pineapple Chunks	½ cup	–	60	–
Potato Salad	2 Tbs	5	70	64%
Pudding				
Chocolate	¼ cup	3	80	34%
Vanilla	¼ cup	3	80	34%
Red Onions	1 Tbs	–	4	–
Saltine Crackers	4 pieces	2	45	40%
Seafood Salad	¼ cup	4	70	51%
Strawberry Banana Dessert	⅕ cup	–	110	–
Strawberries	1 piece	–	8	–
Sunflower Seeds & Raisins	2 Tbs	6	80	68%
Three Bean Salad	2 Tbs	–	30	–
Tomatoes	1 oz	–	8	–
Tuna Salad	2 Tbs	6	100	54%
Turkey Ham	2 Tbs	1	30	30%
Watermelon	1 piece	–	20	–
■ POTATOES				
Baked				
Bacon & Cheese	1	17	510	30%

Food and Description	Amount	Fat Grams	Total Calories	% Fat Calories
Broccoli & Cheese	1	14	450	28%
Cheese	1	24	550	39%
Chili & Cheese	1	25	600	38%
Plain	1	< 1	300	2%
Sour Cream	1 pkt	6	60	90%
Sour Cream & Chives	1	6	370	15%
French Fries	Small	12	240	45%
	Medium	17	360	43%
	Biggie	22	450	44%
■ SALADS				
Fresh-To-Go				
Breadstick	1 piece	3	130	21%
Caesar Side	1	6	160	34%
Deluxe Garden	1	5	110	41%
Grilled Chicken	1	8	200	36%
Side	1	3	60	45%
Taco	1	30	640	42%
■ SANDWICH COMPONENTS				
American Cheese	1 slice	6	70	77%
American Cheese, Jr.	1 slice	4	45	80%
Bacon	1 piece	2	30	90%
Breaded Chicken Fillet	1 piece	10	220	41%
Country Fried Steak	1 piece	16	230	63%
Fish Fillet	1 piece	9	170	48%
Grilled Chicken Fillet	1 piece	3	70	39%
Hamburger ¼ Lb Patty	1 patty	12	190	57%
Honey Mustard-Low Calorie	1 tsp	2	25	72%
Jr. Hamburger Patty	1 patty	6	90	60%
Kaiser Bun	1 bun	3	200	14%
Ketchup	1 serving	–	8	–
Mayonnaise	1 serving	7	70	90%
Mustard	1 serving	–	4	–
Onion	1 serving	–	4	–
Pickles	1 serving	–	2	–
Sandwich Bun	1 bun	3	160	17%
Tartar Sauce	1 serving	14	126	100%
Tomatoes	1 slice	–	4	–
■ SANDWICHES				
Bacon Cheeseburger, Jr.	1	25	440	51%
Big Classic on Kaiser Bun	1	23	480	43%
Breaded Chicken Sandwich	1	20	450	40%
Cheeseburger, Jr.	1	13	320	37%
Cheeseburger Deluxe, Jr.	1	20	390	46%
Cheeseburger 2 oz/Kid's Meal	1	13	310	38%
Chicken Club Sandwich	1	25	520	43%

Food and Description	Amount	Fat Grams	Total Calories	% Fat Calories
Chicken Sandwich	1	19	440	39%
Country Fried Steak Sandwich	1	26	460	51%
Fish Fillet Sandwich	1	25	460	49%
Grilled Chicken Fillet	1	3	70	39%
Grilled Chicken Sandwich	1	7	290	22%
Hamburger, Jr.	1	9	270	30%
Hamburger, Kid's Meal	1	9	270	30%
Plain Single	1	15	350	39%
Single w/Everything	1	23	440	47%
Swiss Deluxe, Jr.	1	18	360	45%
■ MEXICAN FIESTA				
Cheese Sauce	¼ cup	2	40	45%
Picante Sauce	2 Tbs	–	10	–
Refried Beans	¼ cup	2	70	26%
Rice, Spanish	¼ cup	1	60	15%
Sour Topping, Imitation	2 Tbs	4	45	80%
Taco Chips	8 pieces	6	160	34%
Taco Meat	2 Tbs	4	80	45%
Taco Sauce	2 Tbs	–	12	–
Taco Shells	1	3	50	54%
Tortilla, Flour	1	3	100	27%
■ SUPER BAR—PASTA				
Alfredo Sauce	¼ cup	1	30	30%
Fettucini	½ cup	4	120	30%
Garlic Toast	1 piece	3	70	39%
Macaroni & Cheese	½ cup	6	130	42%
Pasta Medley	½ cup	2	60	30%
Red Peppers, Crushed	1 Tbs	1	20	45%
Romano/Parmesan Blend grated	2 Tbs	3	70	39%
Rotini	½ cup	2	90	20%
Spaghetti Sauce	¼ cup	< 1	30	15%
Spaghetti Meat Sauce	¼ cup	1	45	20%

WHATABURGER
■ BEVERAGES

Food and Description	Amount	Fat Grams	Total Calories	% Fat Calories
Orange Juice	6 oz	–	85	–
Vanilla Shake	Small	9	322	25%
■ BREAKFAST				
Breakfast on a bun	1	34	520	59%
Egg Omelette Sandwich	1	15	312	43%
Hash Browns	1 order	9	150	54%
Pancakes	1 order	2.9	199	13%
Pancakes w/sausage	1 order	21.9	407	48%
Pecan Danish	1	15.6	270	52%

Food and Description	Amount	Fat Grams	Total Calories	% Fat Calories
Sausage	1 order	9	150	54%
■ SANDWICHES				
Whataburger	1	24	580	37%
Whataburger/cheese	1	32.6	669	44%
Whataburger, Jr.	1	13.5	304	40%
Whataburger, Jr./cheese	1	18	351	46%
Justaburger	1	11.5	265	39%
Justaburger/cheese	1	15.5	312	45%
Whatacatch	1	27	475	51%
Whatacatch/cheese	1	31	522	53%
Chatachick'n	1	31.7	671	43%
■ SIDE ORDERS				
Apple Pie	1	11.8	236	45%
Fajita Taco	1	11	301	33%
French Fries	Small	12	221	49%
	Regular	18	332	49%
Onion Rings	1 order	13	226	52%
■ TAQUITOS				
Plain	1	18.5	310	54%
w/ Cheese	1	22.5	357	57%
Potato & Egg	1	14	311	41%
Potato & Egg w/cheese	1	18.8	358	47%
WHITE CASTLE				
Cheeseburger	1	11	200	50%
Chicken Sandwich	1	7.5	186	36%
Fish Sandwich-no tartar sauce	1	5	155	29%
French Fries	Regular	15	301	45%
Hamburger	1	8	161	45%
Onion Chips	3.3 oz	17	329	47%
Onion Rings	Regular	13	245	48%
Sausage & Egg Sandwich	1	22	322	62%
Sausage Sandwich	1	12	196	55%
Tartar Sauce	1 Tbs	8	72	100%
White Bun Only	1	< 1	74	6%